AF510214

A Case-Based Approach to Cancer Therapy

A Case-Based Approach to Cancer Therapy

Editor: Gretchen Flammer

AMERICAN
MEDICAL PUBLISHERS
www.americanmedicalpublishers.com

AMERICAN
MEDICAL PUBLISHERS
www.americanmedicalpublishers.com

Cataloging-in-Publication Data

A case-based approach to cancer therapy / edited by Gretchen Flammer.
p. cm.
Includes bibliographical references and index.
ISBN 978-1-63927-618-9
1. Cancer--Treatment. 2. Tumor--Treatment. 3. Cancer--Treatment--Case studies.
4. Tumor--Treatment--Case studies. I. Flammer, Gretchen.
RC270.8 .C37 2023
616.994 06--dc23

© American Medical Publishers, 2023

American Medical Publishers,
41 Flatbush Avenue,
1st Floor, New York,
NY 11217, USA

ISBN 978-1-63927-618-9 (Hardback)

This book contains information obtained from authentic and highly regarded sources. Copyright for all individual chapters remain with the respective authors as indicated. All chapters are published with permission under the Creative Commons Attribution License or equivalent. A wide variety of references are listed. Permission and sources are indicated; for detailed attributions, please refer to the permissions page and list of contributors. Reasonable efforts have been made to publish reliable data and information, but the authors, editors and publisher cannot assume any responsibility for the validity of all materials or the consequences of their use.

Trademark Notice: Registered trademark of products or corporate names are used only for explanation and identification without intent to infringe.

Contents

Preface....VII

Chapter 1 **Serum PD-1/PD-L1 Levels, Tumor Expression and PD-L1 Somatic Mutations in HER2-Positive and Triple Negative Normal-Like Feline Mammary Carcinoma Subtypes**....1
Catarina Nascimento, Ana Catarina Urbano, Andreia Gameiro, João Ferreira, Jorge Correia and Fernando Ferreira

Chapter 2 **The Cellular Prion Protein: A Promising Therapeutic Target for Cancer**....17
Gyeongyun Go and Sang Hun Lee

Chapter 3 **Hypoxia and Macrophages Act in Concert Towards a Beneficial Outcome in Colon Cancer**....31
Flávia Martins, Rosa Oliveira, Bruno Cavadas, Filipe Pinto, Ana Patrícia Cardoso, Flávia Castro, Bárbara Sousa, Marta Laranjeiro Pinto, Ana João Silva, Diogo Adão, José Pedro Loureiro, Nicole Pedro, Rui Manuel Reis, Luísa Pereira, Maria José Oliveira and Angela Margarida Costa

Chapter 4 **Talkin' Toxins: From Coley's to Modern Cancer Immunotherapy**....54
Robert D. Carlson, John C. Flickinger, Jr. and Adam E. Snook

Chapter 5 **Understanding the Effects of Radiotherapy on the Tumour Immune Microenvironment to Identify Potential Prognostic and Predictive Biomarkers of Radiotherapy Response**....77
Shuhui Cheng, Eleanor J. Cheadle and Timothy M. Illidge

Chapter 6 **Botulinum Neurotoxins and Cancer**....97
Shivam O. Mittal and Bahman Jabbari

Chapter 7 **Pro-Inflammatory Cytokines in the Formation of the Pre-Metastatic Niche**....111
Ru Li, Annie Wen and Jun Lin

Chapter 8 **Cnf1 Variants Endowed with the Ability to Cross the Blood–Brain Barrier: A New Potential Therapeutic Strategy for Glioblastoma**....127
Andrea Colarusso, Zaira Maroccia, Ermenegilda Parrilli, Elena Angela Pia Germinario, Andrea Fortuna, Stefano Loizzo, Laura Ricceri, Maria Luisa Tutino, Carla Fiorentini and Alessia Fabbri

Chapter 9 **Investigating Radiotherapy Response in a Novel Syngeneic Model of Prostate Cancer**....141
Charles M. Haughey, Debayan Mukherjee, Rebecca E. Steele, Amy Popple, Lara Dura-Perez, Adam Pickard, Mehjabin Patel, Suneil Jain, Paul B. Mullan, Rich Williams, Pedro Oliveira, Niamh E. Buckley, Jamie Honeychurch, Simon S. McDade, Timothy Illidge, Ian G. Mills and Sharon L. Eddie

Chapter 10 **Inclusion of a Furin Cleavage Site Enhances Antitumor Efficacy against Colorectal Cancer Cells of Ribotoxin α-Sarcin- or RNase T1-Based Immunotoxins** **160**
Javier Ruiz-de-la-Herrán, Jaime Tomé-Amat, Rodrigo Lázaro-Gorines, José G. Gavilanes and Javier Lacadena

Chapter 11 **Cancer Acidity and Hypertonicity Contribute to Dysfunction of Tumor-Associated Dendritic Cells: Potential Impact on Antigen Cross-Presentation Machinery** **180**
Sven Burgdorf, Stefan Porubsky, Alexander Marx and Zoran V. Popovic

Chapter 12 **Tumor Microenvironment as a Regulator of Radiation Therapy: New Insights into Stromal-Mediated Radioresistance** **193**
Varintra E. Krisnawan, Jennifer A. Stanley, Julie K. Schwarz and David G. DeNardo

Chapter 13 **Histone Demethylase KDM5B as a Therapeutic Target for Cancer Therapy** **218**
Anmi Jose, Gautham G. Shenoy, Gabriel Sunil Rodrigues, Naveena A. N. Kumar, Murali Munisamy, Levin Thomas, Jill Kolesar, Ganesha Rai, Praveen P. N. Rao and Mahadev Rao

Permissions

List of Contributors

Index

Preface

Cancer refers to a type of disease where cells of the body divide more quickly than usual. These aberrant cells combine to form a tumor or lump. There are five types of cancer, namely, sarcoma, leukemia, carcinoma, lymphoma and melanoma. There are numerous approaches used to treat cancer, which depend on the type of cancer, its stage, types of treatment that are accessible and the intended outcomes of the treatment. Cancer therapy emphasizes on the management of cancer in patients, which is frequently accomplished through radiotherapy, surgery and chemotherapy. In certain cases of cancer, benefit can be achieved from targeted therapies. A cancer patient may undergo a variety of therapies, including the ones intended to alleviate cancer symptoms. The treatment of cancer encompasses bone marrow transplant, hormone therapy, radiofrequency ablation, immunotherapy and cryoablation. This book unravels the recent studies on cancer therapy. It attempts to understand the various interventions used for the management of this diseases. Different approaches, evaluations, and advanced studies on this topic have been included in this book.

The researches compiled throughout the book are authentic and of high quality, combining several disciplines and from very diverse regions from around the world. Drawing on the contributions of many researchers from diverse countries, the book's objective is to provide the readers with the latest achievements in the area of research. This book will surely be a source of knowledge to all interested and researching the field.

In the end, I would like to express my deep sense of gratitude to all the authors for meeting the set deadlines in completing and submitting their research chapters. I would also like to thank the publisher for the support offered to us throughout the course of the book. Finally, I extend my sincere thanks to my family for being a constant source of inspiration and encouragement.

Editor

Serum PD-1/PD-L1 Levels, Tumor Expression and PD-L1 Somatic Mutations in HER2-Positive and Triple Negative Normal-Like Feline Mammary Carcinoma Subtypes

Catarina Nascimento [1], Ana Catarina Urbano [1], Andreia Gameiro [1], João Ferreira [2], Jorge Correia [1] and Fernando Ferreira [1,*]

1 CIISA—Centro de Investigação Interdisciplinar em Sanidade Animal, Faculdade de Medicina Veterinária, Universidade de Lisboa, Avenida da Universidade Técnica, Lisboa 1300-477, Portugal; catnasc@fmv.ulisboa.pt (C.N.); curbano.ms@gmail.com (A.C.U.); agameiro@fmv.ulisboa.pt (A.G.); jcorreia@fmv.ulisboa.pt (J.C.)

2 Instituto de Medicina Molecular, Faculdade de Medicina, Universidade de Lisboa, Lisboa 1649-028, Portugal; hjoao@medicina.ulisboa.pt

* Correspondence: fernandof@fmv.ulisboa.pt

Abstract: Tumor microenvironment has gained great relevance due to its ability to regulate distinct checkpoints mediators, orchestrating tumor progression. Serum programmed cell death protein-1 (PD-1) and programmed death ligand-1 (PD-L1) levels were compared with healthy controls and with serum cytotoxic T-lymphocyte-associated antigen 4 (CTLA-4) and tumor necrosis factor-alpha (TNF-α) levels in order to understand the role of PD-1/PD-L1 axis in cats with mammary carcinoma. PD-1 and PD-L1 expression was evaluated in tumor-infiltrating lymphocytes (TILs) and cancer cells, as the presence of somatic mutations. Results showed that serum PD-1 and PD-L1 levels were significantly higher in cats with HER2-positive ($p = 0.017$; $p = 0.032$) and triple negative (TN) normal-like mammary carcinomas ($p = 0.004$; $p = 0.015$), showing a strong positive correlation between serum CTLA-4 and TNF-α levels. In tumors, PD-L1 expression in cancer cells was significantly higher in HER2-positive samples than in TN normal-like tumors ($p = 0.010$), as the percentage of PD-L1-positive TILs ($p = 0.037$). *PD-L1* gene sequencing identified two heterozygous mutations in exon 4 (A245T; V252M) and one in exon 5 (T267S). In summary, results support the use of spontaneous feline mammary carcinoma as a model for human breast cancer and suggest that the development of monoclonal antibodies may be a therapeutic strategy.

Keywords: feline mammary carcinoma; PD-1; PD-L1; CTLA-4; TNF-α; biomarkers; immunotherapy

---

1. Introduction

Breast cancer is the most diagnosed tumor among women [1] and feline mammary carcinoma (FMC) is the third most common tumor in the cat. At the molecular level, there are distinct subtypes of breast cancer: Luminal A, Luminal B, HER2-positive and triple-negative (normal-like and basal-like) [2]. The HER2-positive subtype is characterized by a HER2 overexpression and a lack of hormone receptors (estrogen receptor (ER) and/or progesterone receptor (PR)), while the triple negative tumors are defined by the absence of ER, PR and HER2 expression, each representing 15–20% of all breast cancer cases [1,3]. As in human breast cancer [4], FMC presents an aggressive and infiltrative behavior [5,6], with both HER2-positive and triple negative (TN) subtypes showing worse prognosis than luminal A and B subtypes. Furthermore, a surgical approach is often necessary for the treatment of FMC, as the adjuvant chemotherapy (cyclophosphamide, vincristine, doxorubicin) is not useful in some cases [7]. Thus, the identification of novel diagnostic biomarkers and therapeutic targets is needed, not only to improve the clinical outcome of cats with mammary carcinoma but also because FMC shares clinicopathological, histopathological and epidemiological features, as well as the molecular classification with human breast cancer [4,8–10]. Moreover, the use of animal models has been increasing, allowing researchers to understand the mechanisms underlying tumorigenesis; mouse species are the most used due to their small size and short gestation period. Nevertheless, laboratory rodents have several limitations, such as a lack of genetic heterogeneity and discrepancies to the human tumor development [11], while pets that spontaneously develop malignant tumors provide natural models, making them excellent for the study of human breast cancer [12].

In humans, the role of the PD-1/PD-L1 axis is being investigated in different tumor types, with the programmed death ligand-1 (PD-L1) expressed by tumor cells regulating T cell activity, promoting immune suppression and tumor escape [13–15]. This immune checkpoint molecule can be expressed by cancer cells and immune cells, as T and B lymphocytes, macrophages and dendritic cells, being its expression on tumor-infiltrating lymphocytes (TILs) correlated with clinical response to anti-PD-L1-targeted immunotherapy (atezolizumab) [16]. Accordingly, a monoclonal antibody that blocks PD-L1 binding to the programmed cell death protein-1 (PD-1) receptor on T cells was recently approved by the Food and Drug Administration (FDA) to treat different tumor types and also PD-L1 positive unresectable locally advanced and metastatic TN breast cancer [17,18], since, several studies showed that PD-1 and PD-L1 are overexpressed in the most aggressive cancer subtypes (HER2-positive and triple negative) [19–22].

The less studied serum PD-1 (sPD-1) and PD-L1 (sPD-L1) levels may also play an important role in anti-tumor immune responses. Studies in patients with breast cancer, lung cancer, metastatic melanoma and renal cell carcinoma reported higher sPD-1 or sPD-L1 levels than in healthy controls, suggesting that elevated serum PD-1 and PD-L1 levels may promote immunosuppression and are therefore to be considered adverse prognostic factors [23–25]. Furthermore, cytotoxic T-lymphocyte-associated antigen 4 (CTLA-4) is another immune mediator that inhibits T-cell immune function, being also targeted in breast cancer. Accordingly, serum CTLA-4 levels are increased in cats with mammary carcinoma, as well as in human malignant tumors [10]. Some trials are evaluating the combination of anti-PD-1/PD-L1 antibodies with CTLA-4 inhibitors [17,26]. In humans, CTLA-4 regulates T-cell proliferation at the initial stage of immune responses, primarily in lymph nodes, whereas PD-1 suppresses T cells in later stages, typically in peripheral tissues. Additionally, it has been described that certain pro-inflammatory cytokines, such as tumor necrosis factor-alpha (TNF-α), can up-regulate PD-L1 expression in cancer cells, contributing to create an immunosuppressive tumor microenvironment [27,28]. Furthermore, TNF-α is described to be elevated in cats with mammary carcinoma, being positively correlated with serum CTLA-4 levels, as in humans [10].

The *PD-L1* gene encodes for a transmembrane glycoprotein with 290 amino acid residues [29], presenting two extracellular immunoglobulin domains, a cytoplasmic domain and shows a sequence homology of 74.5% with feline *PD-L1* gene (UniProt, accession numbers: *Felis catus*—M3WAP8, *Homo sapiens*—Q9NZQ7).

Considering the above evidences and the lack of knowledge on the role of the PD-1/PD-L1 signaling pathway in tumor progression in the cat, this study aimed to: (i) quantify and compare the sPD-1 and sPD-L1 levels in animals with different mammary carcinoma subtypes and healthy controls; (ii) evaluate the PD-1 and PD-L1 expression in tumor-infiltrating lymphocytes (TILs) and cancer cells; (iii) test for statistical associations between serum PD-1, PD-L1, CTLA-4 and TNF-α levels; (iv) identify genomic mutations in the *PD-L1* gene to validate future checkpoint-blocking therapies.

2. Results

2.1. Cats with HER2-Positive or TN Normal-Like Mammary Carcinoma Showed Higher Serum PD-1 and PD-L1 Levels

Serum PD-1 and PD-L1 levels were measured in cats with mammary carcinoma, grouped according to their tumor subtype and compared with serum levels detected in the healthy control group (Tables 1 and 2).

Table 1. Serum programmed cell death protein-1 (PD-1) levels in healthy cats and queens grouped according to their mammary carcinoma molecular subtype.

Group	n	sPD-1 (pg/mL) Median ± SD	sPD-1 (pg/mL) Mean ± SEM
Control	12	534.0 ± 253.2	459.0 ± 73.1
Luminal A	7	708.8 ± 2165.2	1826.5 ± 818.8
Luminal B	15	590.3 ± 1776.8	1386.3 ± 458.8
HER2-positive	11	1148.9 ± 3386.0	3129.6 ± 1020.9
TN Normal-Like	7	3655.1 ± 31,478.1	21,637.3 ± 11,897.6
TN Basal-Like	6	513.3 ± 145.0	519.3 ± 59.2

Table 2. Serum programmed death ligand-1 (PD-L1) levels detected in healthy cats and queens stratified by their mammary carcinoma molecular subtype.

Group	n	sPD-L1 (pg/mL) Median ± SD	sPD-L1 (pg/mL) Mean ± SEM
Control	13	1835.5 ± 545.6	1762.5 ± 151.3
Luminal A	7	1789.6 ± 941.6	2121.5 ± 355.9
Luminal B	15	1628.0 ± 773.4	1877.6 ± 199.7
HER2-positive	9	5490.4 ± 3789.6	5672.6 ± 1263.2
TN Normal-Like	7	4377.5 ± 8819.4	8313.0 ± 3333.4
TN Basal-Like	6	1436.3 ± 425.6	1534.2 ± 173.8

Results from the Kruskal–Wallis test found significant differences between the mean ranks of at least one pair of groups ($p = 0.044$ for PD-1; $p = 0.006$ for PD-L1). Indeed, cats showing HER2-positive or TN normal-like mammary carcinoma displayed higher serum PD-1 levels than healthy group (1148.9 pg/mL vs. 534.0 pg/mL, $p = 0.017$; 3655.1 pg/mL vs. 534.0 pg/mL, $p = 0.004$, Figure 1A), as well as serum PD-L1 levels (5490.4 pg/mL vs. 1835.5 pg/mL, $p = 0.032$; 3641.4 pg/mL vs. 1835.5 pg/mL, $p = 0.015$, Figure 1B). Furthermore, the optimal cut-off value of serum PD-1 levels was 801.6 pg/mL in cats with HER2-positive mammary carcinoma (AUC = 0.765 ± 0.104, 95% CI: 0.562–0.968, $p = 0.031$; sensitivity = 54.5%; specificity = 91.7%; Figure 1C) and 801.6 pg/mL in cats with TN normal-like mammary carcinoma (AUC = 0.857 ± 0.092, 95% CI: 0.676–1.000, $p = 0.011$; sensitivity = 57.1%; specificity = 91.7%; Figure 1D). Regarding the serum PD-L1 levels, the optimal cut-off value in cats with HER2-positive mammary carcinoma was 2545.0 pg/mL (AUC = 0.778 ± 0.117, 95% CI: 0.548–1.000, $p = 0.030$; sensitivity = 66.7%; specificity = 92.3%; Figure 1E) and 2519.0 pg/mL in cats with TN normal-like tumor subtype (AUC = 0.857 ± 0.123, 95% CI: 0.617–1.000, $p = 0.010$; sensitivity = 85.7%; specificity = 92.3%; Figure 1F). No significant differences were found in serum PD-1 and PD-L1 levels between cats with mammary carcinoma of other molecular subtypes and the control group.

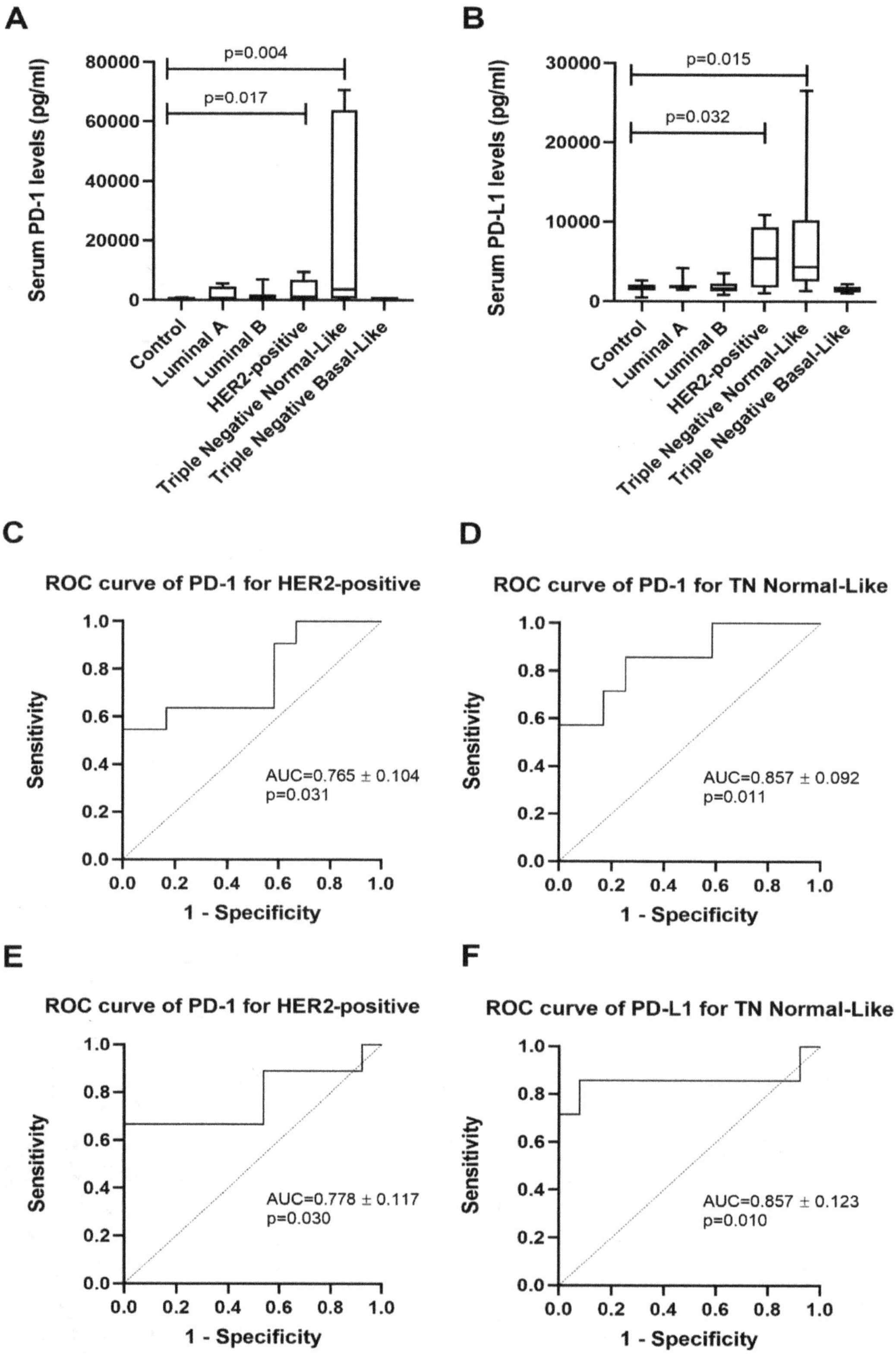

Figure 1. Serum programmed cell death protein-1 (PD-1) and programmed death ligand-1 (PD-L1) levels in cats with HER2-positive and triple negative (TN) normal-like mammary carcinoma. (**A**) Box plot analysis showing the range of serum PD-1 and (**B**) PD-L1 levels in control group and cats with mammary carcinoma stratified according to their molecular subtype. (**C**) Receiver Operating Characteristic (ROC) curve analysis for the identification of the optimal cut-off value of sPD-1 levels for cats with HER2-positive mammary carcinoma and (**D**) for cats with TN normal-like mammary carcinoma. (E) ROC curve analysis of PD-L1 for cats showing HER2-positive mammary carcinoma and (**F**) TN normal-like carcinoma.

The data obtained also revealed a positive correlation between serum PD-1 and PD-L1 levels in cats with mammary carcinoma ($r = 0.780$, $p < 0.0001$, Figure 2A), particularly in those exhibiting HER2-positive ($r = 0.786$, $p = 0.03$, Figure 2B) or TN normal-like tumor subtypes ($r = 0.857$, $p = 0.03$, Figure 2C).

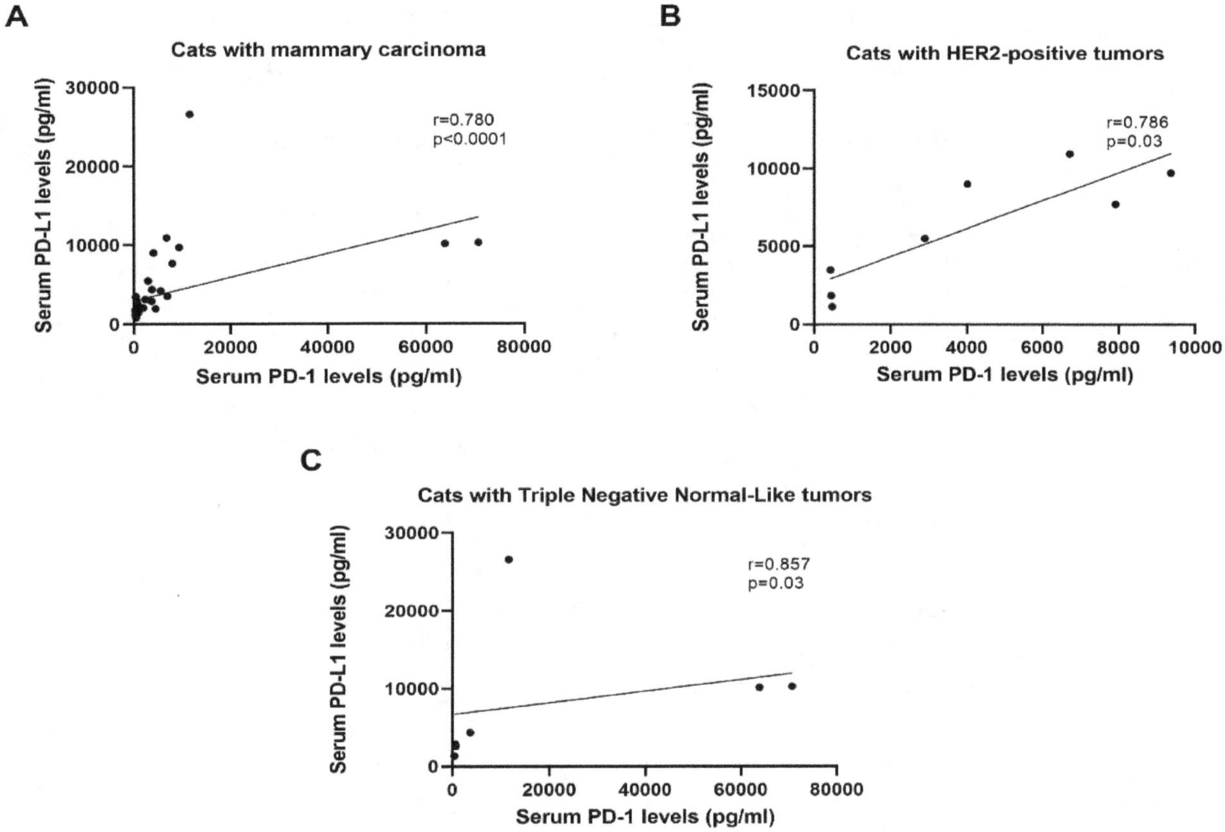

Figure 2. Serum programmed cell death protein-1 (PD-1) and programmed death ligand-1 (PD-L1) levels are strongly correlated in cats with HER2-positive and TN normal-like mammary carcinoma. (**A**) Correlation between sPD-1 and sPD-L1 levels in cats with mammary carcinoma (**B**) and in cats with HER2-positive and (**C**) triple negative (TN) normal-like carcinoma subtypes.

2.2. Serum CTLA-4 and TNF-α Levels are Positively Correlated with Serum PD-1/PD-L1 Levels in Cats with HER2-Positive and TN Normal-Like Tumors

A strong positive correlation was found in cats with HER2-positive mammary carcinomas between the serum PD-1 levels and serum PD-L1 ($r = 0.923$), CTLA-4 ($r = 0.975$) and TNF-α ($r = 0.968$) levels (Table 3). The queens with TN normal-like carcinomas also showed a strong positive correlation between serum PD-1 levels and serum PD-L1 ($r = 0.857$), CTLA-4 ($r = 0.927$) and TNF-α ($r = 0.893$) levels (Table 3).

2.3. TN normal-like Mammary Carcinomas Showed Lower PD-L1 Expression than HER2-Positive Tumors

Considering the high serum PD-L1 levels presented by cats with HER2-positive or TN normal-like mammary carcinomas, we further evaluated the percentage and staining intensity of PD-L1 expression in tumor-infiltrating lymphocytes (TILs) and in cancer cells, by immunostaining of tumor samples. Results showed a higher score of PD-L1-positive TILs in HER2-positive tumors than in TN normal-like ones ($p = 0.037$, Figures 3A and 4A,B,E,F). Besides, the PD-L1 score on cancer cells was significantly higher in HER2-positive tumors than in TN normal-like mammary carcinomas ($p = 0.010$, Figures 3B and 4C–F).

Table 3. Spearman's correlation between serum programmed cell death protein-1 (PD-1), programmed death ligand-1 (PD-L1), cytotoxic T-lymphocyte-associated antigen 4 (CTLA-4) and tumor necrosis factor-alpha (TNF-α) levels in cats with HER2-positive and triple negative (TN) normal-like mammary carcinomas.

HER2-Positive	**PD-1**	**PD-L1**	**CTLA-4**	**TNF-α**
PD-1	–	0.923**	0.975 **	0.968 **
PD-L1	0.923**	–	0.947 **	0.922 **
CTLA-4	0.975**	0.947**	–	0.947 **
TNF-α	0.968**	0.922**	0.947**	–
TN Normal-Like	**PD-1**	**PD-L1**	**CTLA-4**	**TNF-α**
PD-1	–	0.857*	0.927**	0.893**
PD-L1	0.857*	–	0.815*	0.857*
CTLA-4	0.927**	0.815*	–	0.927**
TNF-α	0.893**	0.857*	0.927**	–

* indicates $p < 0.05$, ** indicates $p < 0.01$.

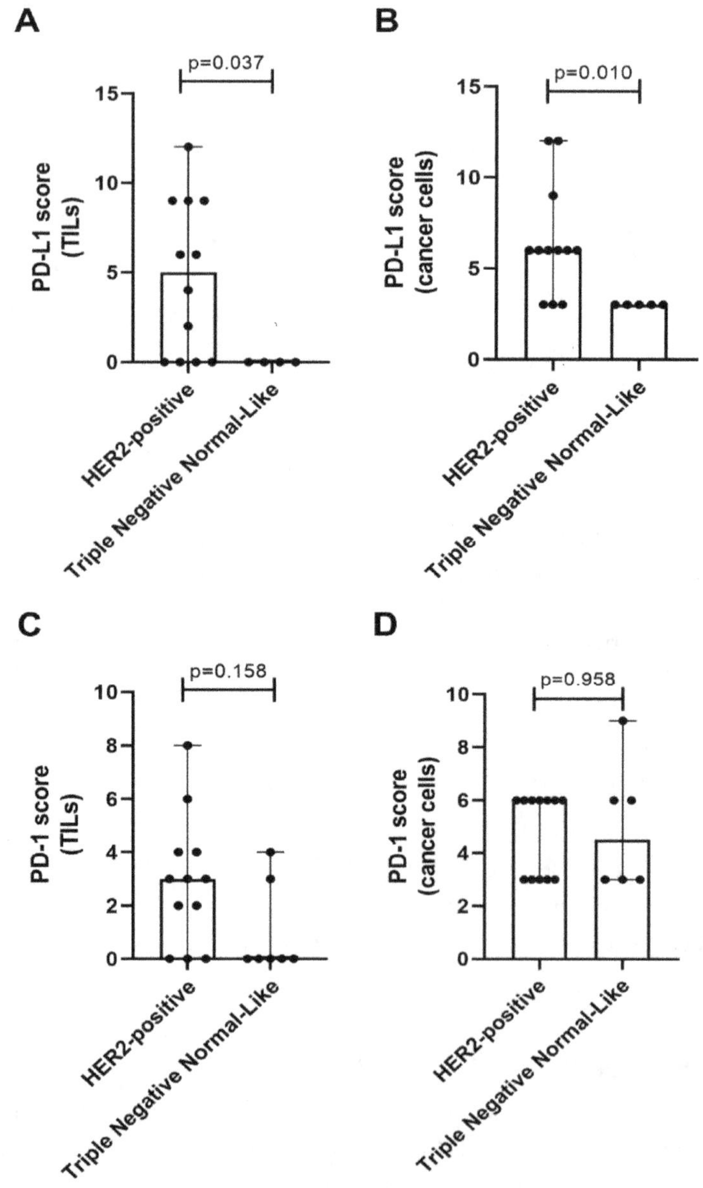

Figure 3. Programmed death ligand-1 (PD-L1) and programmed cell death protein-1 (PD-1) staining analysis of tumor-infiltrating lymphocytes (TILs) and cancer cells in HER2-positive and triple negative (TN) normal-like tumor samples (range values). (**A**) The score of PD-L1-positive TILs (**B**) and cancer cells

in HER2-positive mammary carcinomas in comparison to TN normal-like tumors. (**C**) The score of PD-1-positive TILs between HER2-positive tumors and TN normal-like mammary carcinomas and (**D**) cancer cells.

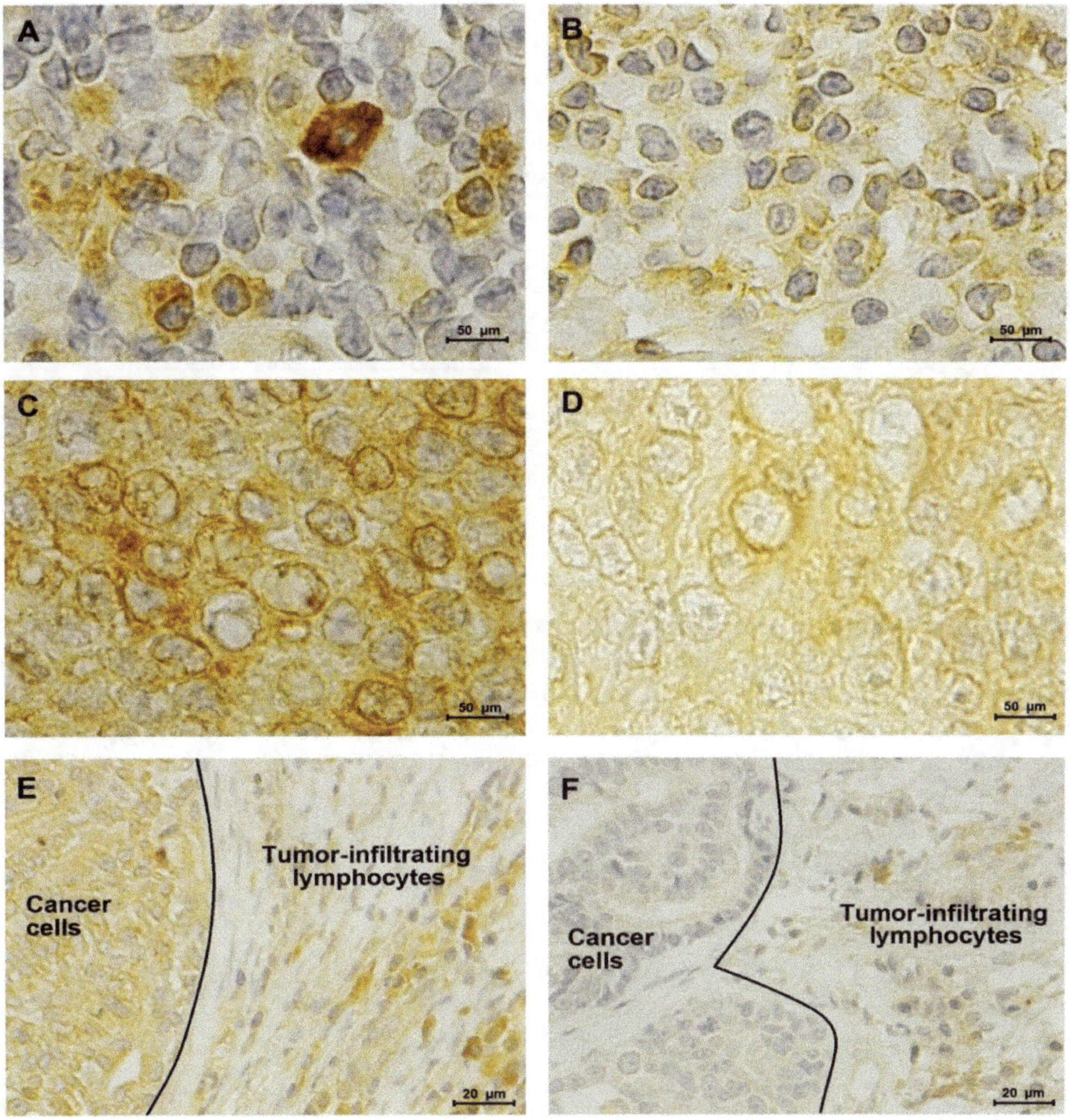

Figure 4. Programmed death ligand-1 (PD-L1) expression in tumor-infiltrating lymphocytes (TILs) and cancer cells of HER2-positive mammary carcinomas and triple negative (TN) normal-like tumors. (**A**) Representative PD-L1 immunostaining of tumor infiltrating lymphocytes in a HER2-positive (**B**) and in a TN normal-like mammary carcinoma (100× objective). (**C**) PD-L1 score intensity 4+ in HER2-positive cancer cells (**D**) and score 1+ in TN normal-like cancer cells (100× objective). Furthermore, in TILs, PD-L1 is localized to the cell membrane and cytoplasm, while in cancer cells it is mainly distributed to cytoplasmic and nuclear membranes. (**E**) Immunohistochemical staining of PD-L1 in a HER2-positive solid carcinoma (**F**) and in a TN normal-like tubulopapillary carcinoma (40× objective).

Regarding PD-1 expression in TILs and cancer cells, no significant differences were found between HER2-positive tumors and TN normal-like mammary carcinomas ($p = 0.158$, Figure 3C; $p = 0.958$, Figure 3D).

2.4. Elevated Serum PD-1/PD-L1 Levels Showed A Higher Concordance with IHC for PD-1 and PD-L1 in Cancer Cells than in TILs

Our results revealed that elevated serum PD-1 levels, PD-1-positive TILs and PD-1-positive cancer cells were found in 61.5%, 41.7% and 100% of cats with HER2-positive mammary carcinoma and in 57.1%, 33.3% and 100% of cats with triple-negative normal-like mammary tumors. In parallel, elevated serum PD-L1 levels, PD-L1-positive TILs and PD-L1-positive cancer cells were detected in 76.9%, 66.7% and 100% of cats with HER2-positive tumors and in 85.7%, 20% and 100% of cats with a triple-negative normal-like tumor subtype (Table 4). Thus, these results demonstrated that serum analysis could provide differential information when compared with the expression of the two immune checkpoint molecules in TILs and cancer cells.

Table 4. Concordance between the animals with elevated serum PD-1/PD-L1 levels (sPD-1, sPD-L1), PD-1/PD-L1–positive TILs infiltration and PD-1/PD-L1-positive cancer cells.

Tumor subtype	sPD-1	TILs	Concordance	sPD-1	Cancer cells	Concordance
HER2-positive	61.5%	41.7%	58.3%	61.5%	100%	66.7%
Triple Negative Normal-Like	57.1%	33.3%	0%	57.1%	100%	66.7%
Tumor subtype	**sPD-L1**	**TILs**	**Concordance**	**sPD-L1**	**Cancer cells**	**Concordance**
HER2-positive	76.9%	66.7%	41.7%	76.9%	100%	75%
Triple Negative Normal-Like	85.7%	20%	20%	85.7%	100%	100%

2.5. Three Non-Redundant Mutations Were Detected in Feline PD-L1 gene

Results from DNA sequencing allowed us to identify three heterozygous mutations in the feline *PD-L1* gene (Figure 5). Two were found in exon 4 (c.16.756G > A; c.16.777G >A), one changing a neutral nonpolar amino acid (alanine-245) to a neutral polar residue (threonine) in 3.8% of the studied population (1/26). The second mutation converted a methionine to a valine (p.V252M), both neutral nonpolar amino acids, in 42.3% of the animals evaluated (11/26). A third mutation was identified in exon 5 (c.18.526A > C), replacing a neutral polar threonine by a neutral polar serine at residue number 267, in 3.8% of the DNA samples (1/26).

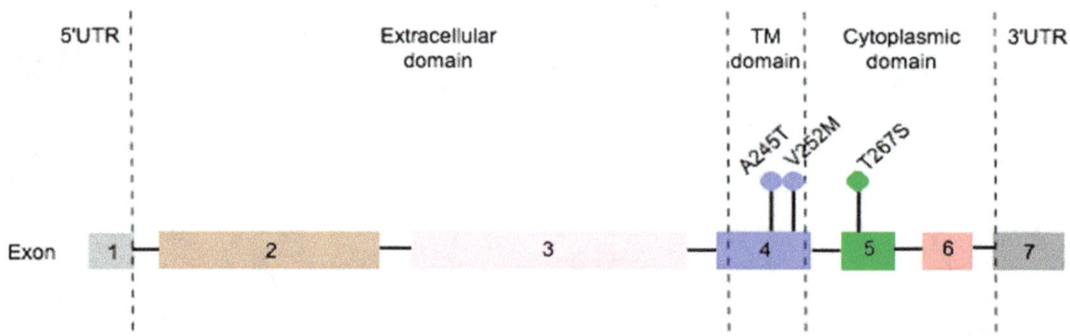

Figure 5. Three heterozygous and non-redundant somatic mutations were found in feline *programmed death ligand-1 (PD-L1)* gene.

3. Discussion

In order to escape the immune system, cancer cells can develop mechanisms to downregulate immune responses. For example, by overexpression of distinct immune checkpoint molecules such as PD-L1. In humans, the interaction between PD-L1 and its receptor has been revealed as an important step in the maintenance of an immunosuppressive tumor microenvironment [30]. Thus, a better understanding of the PD-1/PD-L1 pathway may also contribute to the development of new diagnostic tools and molecular therapies targeting PD-L1 in pets.

The results obtained showed that cats presenting mammary carcinoma subtypes associated with more aggressive features and poor prognosis [31] (HER2-positive and TN normal-like) displayed significantly increased serum PD-1 and PD-L1 levels, as reported in humans with HER2-positive metastatic breast cancer [32], TN breast cancer [23], renal cell carcinoma [25], esophageal cancer [33], gastric cancer [24], advanced pancreatic cancer [34], lung cancer [35] and metastatic melanoma [36] correlated to shorter overall survival and tumor-free survival times [23,25,32,33,35], suggesting a conserved role of the PD-1/PD-L1 axis in both species. Moreover, as reported in humans, our findings uncovered a positive correlation between serum PD-1 and PD-L1 levels, suggesting that both molecules are co-regulated [23,34]. Furthermore, cats with HER2-positive or TN normal-like tumors showed a strong positive correlation between serum PD-1, PD-L1, CTLA-4 and TNF-α levels, which are immune-inhibitory molecules that downregulate T-cell immune responses, suggesting that these animals were immunosuppressed. CTLA-4 is another immune molecule located on the surface of T cells and expressed by regulatory T cells (Tregs), which triggers an inhibitory signal to immune cells [37], also being targeted in breast cancer treatment [26]. Additionally, the higher serum levels of the pro-inflammatory cytokine TNF-α may contribute to the increased tumor cell survival and PD-L1 stabilization on breast tumor cells, playing a critical role for tumor escape from immune surveillance [28]. Accordingly, a previous study also reported elevated serum CTLA-4 levels in cats with mammary carcinoma, being associated with HER2-positive status and TNF-α levels, in accordance with our findings.

Results from the immunostaining analysis revealed that PD-L1 expression in TILs and cancer cells was higher in HER2-positive mammary carcinoma, as reported in humans [2,3,16,20,22], contrasting with TN mammary carcinoma tumor samples. In spite of our findings, previous studies in human breast cancer showed that PD-1 and PD-L1 positive TILs and cancer cells overexpressing PD-L1 were frequently found in triple negative breast cancer subtype [16,23,38–41]. These controversial results may be due to the fact that serum PD-1 levels were higher in cats with TN normal-like carcinomas compared with animals presenting HER2-positive carcinomas, indicating that sPD-1 can bind to PD-L1 attached to the cell membrane of dendritic cells, inhibiting T cell function and proliferation, as previously described [42]. Additionally, recent studies described the presence of tumor-derived exosomes that carry PD-L1, suggesting an effective paracrine mechanism that cancer cells use to communicate and reprogram immune cells and consequently suppress T-cell activation [43–45]. These findings support that HER2-positive cancer cells lead to a local immunosuppressive microenvironment, strengthening the systemic immunosuppression found in cats with this tumor subtype. Moreover, our results revealed PD-L1 expression in cell membrane and cytoplasm of TILs, while in cancer cells the immunostaining was distributed to cytoplasmic and nuclear membranes. Accordingly, in human breast cancer different approaches were used to evaluate the PD-L1 expression, with some studies described only membranous staining and others, in agreement with our findings, registered both membranous and cytoplasmic staining [46,47]. In addition, Ghebeh et al. showed a predominant staining in the cytoplasm near to the nuclear membrane, probably the endoplasmic reticulum, and an expression of PD-L1 in the nucleus, as we described [48]. Additionally, our results showed that elevated serum PD-1/PD-L1 levels were detected more frequently than PD-1/PD-L1 overexpression in TILs of HER2-positive and triple-negative normal-like feline mammary carcinomas. Notably, a high concordance rate was found between elevated serum PD-1/PD-L1 levels and PD-1/PD-L1 overexpression in cancer cells of the same FMC subtypes, suggesting that the serum analysis can be a non-invasive tool for the real-time assessment of these immune checkpoints molecules in feline mammary carcinoma, as reported for breast cancer [49].

Lastly, three non-redundant heterozygous mutations were found in the feline *PD-L1* gene, with none of them located at the PD-L1 extracellular domain, which is recognized by the recent and promising monoclonal antibody approved for the treatment of human metastatic TN breast cancer [29]. This shall not compromise the future development of checkpoint-blocking therapies targeting PD-L1 for FMC treatment. According to the Catalogue of Somatic Mutations in Cancer (COSMIC), six mutations were reported with very low frequency in human breast cancer patients (148/47,194; 0.3%), all different from the ones that we detected.

4. Material and Methods

4.1. Animal Population

Tumor and serum samples were collected from 53 queens with mammary carcinoma that underwent mastectomy and 15 healthy queens presenting for elective ovariohysterectomy at the Small Animal Hospital of the Veterinary Medicine Faculty, University of Lisbon. All mammary lesions were embedded in paraffin after fixation in 10% buffered formalin (pH 7.2) during 24–48 h. Serum was separated from clotted blood by centrifugation (1500× g, 10 min, 4 °C) and stored at −80 °C until further use. All samples that showed hemolysis were discarded, as recommended for humans [50].

For each animal enrolled in the study, the following clinicopathological characteristics were recorded: age, breed, reproductive status, contraceptive administration, treatment performed (none, surgery or surgery plus chemotherapy), number, location and size of tumor lesions, histopathological classification, malignancy grade, presence of tumor necrosis, lymphatic invasion, lymphocytic infiltration, cutaneous ulceration, regional lymph node involvement, stage of the disease (TNM system), disease free-survival (DFS) and overall survival (OS) [31]. Table 5 summarizes the collected clinical data. Briefly, the mean age at diagnosis was 11.8 years (range 6.5–18 years), while the mean size of the primary lesions was 2.6 cm (range 0.3–7 cm). The DFS was 9.2 ± 7.8 months (n = 49; 95% CI: 7.3–11.7 months) and the OS was 15.0 ± 9.8 months (n = 51; 95% CI: 12.2–17.7 months).

Table 5. Clinicopathological features of the 53 female cats with mammary carcinoma enrolled in this study.

Clinicopathological Feature	Number of Animals (%)	Clinicopathological Feature	Number of Animals (%)
Age		Tumor size	
<8 years old	3 (5.7%)	<2 cm	19 (35.8%)
≥ 8 years old	50 (94.3%)	≥ 2 cm	34 (64.2%)
Breed		HP classification	
Not determined	39 (73.6%)	Tubulopapillary carcinoma	21 (39.6%)
Siamese	5 (9.4%)	Solid carcinoma	6 (11.3%)
Persian	6 (11.3%)	Cribriform carcinoma	5 (9.4%)
Norwegian Forest Cat	2 (3.8%)	Papillary-cystic carcinoma	1 (1.9%)
Blue Russian	1 (1.9%)	Tubular carcinoma	12 (22.6%)
Spayed		Mucinous carcinoma	8 (15.2%)
No	28 (52.8%)	Tumor malignancy grade	
Yes	24 (45.3%)	I	3 (5.7%)
Unknown	1 (1.9%)	II	7 (13.2%)
Contraceptive administration		III	43 (81.1%)
No	19 (35.9%)	Tumor necrosis	
Yes	28 (52.8%)	No	13 (24.5%)
Unknown	6 (11.3%)	Yes	40 (75.5%)
Treatment		Tumor lymphatic invasion	
None	1 (1.9%)	No	48 (90.5%)
Mastectomy	48 (90.6%)	Yes	5 (9.5%)
Mastectomy + Chemo	4 (7.5%)	Lymphocytic infiltration	
Multiple tumors		No	17 (32.0%)
No	19 (35.8%)	Yes	34 (64.2%)
Yes	34 (64.2%)	Unknown	2 (3.8%)
Lymph node status		Tumor ulceration	
Negative	32 (60.4%)	No	46 (86.8%)
Positive	17 (32.1%)	Yes	7 (13.2%)
Unknown	4 (7.5%)	Ki-67 index	
TNM classification		Low (<14%)	36 (67.9%)
I	13 (24.5%)	High (>14%)	17 (32.1%)
II	6 (11.3%)	Progesterone status	
III	29 (54.7%)	Negative	28 (52.8%)
IV	5 (9.5%)	Positive	25 (47.2%)
Tumor localization		Estrogen status	
M1	8 (15.1%)	Negative	37 (69.8%)

Table 5. *Cont.*

Clinicopathological Feature	Number of Animals (%)	Clinicopathological Feature	Number of Animals (%)
M2	10 (18.9%)	Positive	16 (30.2%)
M3	20 (37.7%)	HER2 status	
M4	15 (28.3%)	Negative	41 (77.4%)
		Positive	12 (22.6%)

TNM—Tumor, Node, Metastasis; HP—Histopathological.

4.2. Quantification of Serum PD-1, PD-L1, CTLA-4 and TNF-α Levels

Serum PD-1, PD-L1, CTLA-4 and TNF-α levels were quantified by using the commercially available immunoassay kits from R&D systems (Minneapolis, MN, USA) and following the manufacturer's recommendations. PD-1 levels were measured with the PD-1 DuoSet ELISA kit (DY1086,); PD-L1 levels with the PD-L1/B7-H1 DuoSet ELISA kit (DY156); CTLA-4 levels with the CTLA-4 DuoSet ELISA kit (DY476); and the TNF-α levels with the TNF-α DuoSet ELISA kit (DY2586), all based on a solid-phase sandwich enzyme-linked immunosorbent assay (ELISA) technique. The concentration levels of the above molecules were calculated using appropriate standard curves, by making serial dilutions from a stock solution of recombinant PD-1, PD-L1, CTLA-4 and TNF-α (9, 18, 36, 78, 156, 312.5, 625, 1250, 2500, 5000 and 10,000 pg/mL). Serum PD-1 and PD-L1 levels (pg/mL) were calculated using a quadratic regression ($y = ax^2 + bx + c$, $r^2 = 0.99$ for PD-1 and $r^2 = 0.96$ for PD-L1) and serum CTLA-4 and TNF-α concentrations were determined using a curve-fitting equation ($y = mx + c$, $r^2 > 0.99$) [10].

Briefly, quantification of the abovementioned molecules was performed in 96-well microplates incubated overnight with the corresponding capture antibodies (100 μL/well), at room temperature RT). On the next day, plates were washed three times with 400 μL/well of PBS-Tween 0.05% and incubated with 300 μL/well of PBS/BSA blocking agent (1%, *w/v*), at RT for 60 min. Then, plates were washed three times with 400 μL/well PBS-Tween 0.05% and incubated with 100 μL/well of each dilution, in duplicate. For determination of serum PD-1, PD-L1, CTLA-4 and TNF-α levels, serum samples were diluted 20 times in PBS/BSA 1% and 100 μL of each sample was added to the wells. The plates were thereafter sealed and incubated for 2 hours at RT. After another washing step (3 × 400 μL/well PBS-Tween 0.05%), 100 μL/well of detection antibodies was added and incubated for 2 hours at RT. Later and after three washes with 400 μL/well of PBS-Tween 0.05%, 100 μL/well of streptavidin-HRP was added and incubated for 20 min at RT, avoiding placing the microplate in direct light. Afterwards a further washing step (3 × 400 μL/well PBS-Tween 0.05%), 100 μL/well of substrate solution (1:1 mixture of H2O2 and tetramethylbenzidine) was added and incubated for 20 min at RT in the dark. Finally, the reaction was stopped by adding 50 μL/well of 2 N H2SO4 and gently shaking the plate. The absorbance was measured by a spectrophotometer (Fluostar Optima Microplate Reader, BMG, Ortenberg, Germany), following the manufacturer's recommendations.

4.3. Immunohistochemical Staining and Analysis

To analyze PD-1 and PD-L1 expression, two sections of formalin-fixed paraffin-embedded tissues of FMC with 3 μm thickness (Microtome Leica RM2135, Newcastle, UK) were prepared, mounted on adhesive glass slides (SuperFrost Plus, Thermo Fisher Scientific, MA, USA) and placed at 64 °C for 60 min and then at 37 °C overnight. Then deparaffinization, rehydration and epitope retrieval were performed using a PT-Link module (Dako, Agilent, Santa Clara, CA, USA), by immersing glass slides in Antigen Target Retrieval Solution pH 9 from Dako during 40 min at 95 °C. Thereafter, slides were cooled for 30 min at RT and rinsed twice for 5 min in distilled water. The endogenous peroxidase activity was blocked by an incubation period of 20 min with Peroxidase Block Novocastra Solution (Novacastra, Leica Biosystems, Newcastle, UK), and after two washing steps with PBS the nonspecific binding of immunoglobulins was prevented by incubating the tissue slices with the Protein Block Novocastra Solution (Leica Biosystems) for 60 min. Then, before two PBS washes (2 × 5 min), tissue slides were incubated with an anti-PD-1 monoclonal antibody (1:25 dilution, clone J116, Abcam, Cambridge, UK) or with an anti-PD-L1 monoclonal antibody (1:100 dilution, clone 28-8, Abcam), at 4 °C overnight. After two washes with PBS for 5 min, each tissue section was incubated at RT with the Novolink Polymer (Leica Biosystems) for 30 min. Subsequently and after an additional wash in PBS, the staining was performed using the DAB Chromogen Solution (Leica Biosystems) diluted in Novolink DAB Substrate Buffer (Leica Biosystems, 1:20, 5 min). Finally, tissue sections were counterstained with hematoxylin (Leica Biosystems) for 1 min, dehydrated in a graded ethanol series and mounted.

The analyses of PD-1 and PD-L1 immunostaining was scored following the recommendations of the International TILs Working Group 2014, established for breast cancer [52]. Briefly, the area occupied by positive lymphocytes in the stromal compartment was evaluated in whole tumor sections, excluding the TILs outside of the tumor border or in tumor zones with artifacts or necrosis, with 200–400× magnification. In addition, to identify the TILs the pathologists observed their characteristic morphology, as a scarce cytoplasm, a round and small nucleus and the presence of a dense chromatin. The scores of percentages of positive cells were recorded as: 0 (<1%), 1 (1–5%), 2 (6–30%) or 3 (>30%) [10]. The intensity scores were as follows: 0 (negative), 1+ (weak), 2+ (moderate), 3+ (strong) and 4+ (very strong). The percentage of positive cells and intensity scores were then multiplied to obtain a final IHC score. To explore the concordance between the serum PD-1/PD-L1 levels and the PD-1/PD-L1 overexpression in TILs and cancer cells, the cut-off values used were ≥5% and ≥1% for TILs overexpressing PD-1 [41,53] and PD-L1 [18], and ≥1% for cancer cells overexpressing PD-1 or PD-L1 [54,55]. Human placenta and feline lymph node tissues were used as positive controls, whereas sections of healthy mammary tissues were used as negative controls and feline lymph nodes as internal controls. All slides were independently subjected to blind scoring by two independent pathologists.

4.4. DNA Extraction, Amplification and Sequence Analysis of Feline PD-L1 Gene

Genomic DNA extraction was performed in 26 primary mammary tumors using a QIAamp FFPE kit (Qiagen, Dusseldorf, Germany) following the manufacturer's recommendations. Initially, tumor samples were homogenized with Tissue Lyser II (Qiagen) and digested with protease K in a concentration of 20 mg/mL (Qiagen). After several washing steps, the genomic DNA was eluted from the extraction columns and its quantity and quality were measured by NanoDrop ND-100 Spectrophotometer (Thermo Fischer Scientific). Then, the exons of interest in *PD-L1* gene were amplified by using specific primers (Table 6) with a PCR thermal cycler (VWR Thermocycler, Leicestershire, England). PCR procedures were performed with a standard reaction mixture (4 μL/sample of Phusion GC Buffer (Thermo Fischer Scientific), 0.4 μL/sample of dNTPs (Grisp, Porto, Portugal), 0.1 μL/sample of each forward and reverse primers and 0.2 μL/sample of DNA Polymerase (Thermo Fischer Scientific)). In all samples, PCR-grade water and DNA were added to maintain a concentration of 4 ng/mL. For amplification of exons 3 and 6, PCR reactions were performed as follows: denaturation at 98 °C for 30 s, followed by 35 cycles at 98 °C for 10 s, 56 °C for 30 s, 72 °C for 10 s, plus one extension step of 72 °C for 10 min. For exons 2, 4 and 5, the melting temperature was 60 °C. After confirmation of the expected size for each amplified fragment in an agarose gel (2.5%, Sigma-Aldrich, Darmstadt, Germany), DNA fragments were purified and sequenced by Sanger technique (StabVida, Almada, Portugal).

Table 6. Sequence of the primers used for PCR amplification of exons of feline *programmed death ligand-1* (*PD-L1*) gene.

Exons	Forward 5′–3′	Reverse 5′–3′
2	TTTGGGGACAGCAGCTTGTT	TGAACAGACTGACACCGTGG
3	TCTGAGAACCAGCCAGAATTGA	ACTGGAACATAGGGCGTGTT
4	GTCGAAGGCATCTCGCTGT	AGAGCCACTGTGACAACAACA
5	AATTGACCTCAGGGGTTGGAA	GAGGTAAGGAGGAGCCCGTT
6	TACTGCAGAGGTAACTGGACA	GGCCTCTCACATCCGACATC

The identification of PD-L1 exons was performed using BLAST software (Basic Local Alignment Search Tool, NCBI) by comparing the sequence of feline *PD-L1* gene (NC_018735.3) with its transcript

(Ensembl, ENSFCAT00000078517.1). Sequenced fragments were aligned using the ClustalW tool (Bioedit software), while protein mutations and SNP loci were identified by using the Expert Protein Analysis System's (ExPASY) translate tool (XM_006939039).

4.5. Statistical Analysis

The Kruskal–Wallis test and Dunn's multiple comparisons post-test were applied to compare the serum PD-1 and PD-L1 levels between cats with different mammary carcinoma subtypes and healthy controls. Animals that had serum PD-1 or PD-L1 levels that fell more than three standard deviations from the mean were considered outliers and removed from further analysis. The optimal cut-off values were determined using the Youden index and the area under the receiver operating characteristic (ROC) curve values were calculated. Significant differences on the PD-1 and PD-L1 staining of tumor infiltrating lymphocytes and on the staining intensity of cancer cells were evaluated by using the Mann–Whitney test. Spearman's coefficient was used to assess the correlations between serum PD-1, PD-L1, CTLA-4 and TNF-α levels.

Statistical analysis was conducted in SPSS software version 25.0 (IBM, Armonk, NY, USA) and the two-sided p-value < 0.05 was considered statistically significant. Results were presented as median values. GraphPad Prism version 8.1.2 (GraphPad Software, CA, USA) and Microsoft Excel for MacOS (version 16.30, Microsoft Corporation, Redmond, WA, USA) were used to plot the graphs.

5. Conclusions

In conclusion, our data demonstrated that serum PD-1 and PD-L1 levels were elevated in cats with HER2-positive and TN normal-like mammary carcinomas. The strong positive correlations detected between serum PD-1, PD-L1, CTLA-4 and TNF-α levels also suggest a systemic immunosuppression in cats presenting these tumor subtypes. Additionally, the microenvironment of HER2-positive tumors was revealed to be locally immunosuppressed by overexpressing PD-L1, contrasting with the human breast cancer studies that showed a higher PD-1 and PD-L1 expression in triple negative molecular subtype. Altogether, our results indicate that cats presenting HER2-positive or TN normal-like tumors could benefit from immunostimulatory therapies (e.g., anti-PD-L1, anti-CTLA-4) and provide support to the use of spontaneous feline mammary carcinoma as a model for human breast cancer.

Author Contributions: Conceptualization, C.N. and F.F.; Methodology, C.N. and F.F.; Formal analysis, C.N. and A.C.U. and F.F.; Investigation, C.N., A.C.U., A.G., J.F., J.C. and F.F.; Supervision, F.F.; Funding acquisition, F.F.; Project administration, F.F.; Writing—original draft preparation, C.N. and F.F.; Writing—review and editing, C.N., A.C.U., A.G., J.F., J.C., and F.F. All authors have read and agreed to the published version of the manuscript.

Acknowledgments: The authors would like to thank Dra. Maria Soares for the clinical samples and database.

References

1. Soare, G.R.; Soare, C.A. Immunotherapy for Breast Cancer: First FDA Approved Regimen. *Discoveries* **2019**, *7*, 4–6. [CrossRef]
2. Solinas, C.; Carbognin, L.; De Silva, P.; Criscitiello, C.; Lambertini, M. Tumor-infiltrating lymphocytes in breast cancer according to tumor subtype: Current state of the art. *Breast* **2017**, *35*, 142–150. [CrossRef] [PubMed]
3. Padmanabhan, R.; Kheraldine, H.S.; Meskin, N.; Vranic, S.; Al Moustafa, A.E. Crosstalk between HER2 and PD-1/PD-L1 in Breast Cancer: From Clinical Applications to Mathematical Models. *Cancers* **2020**, *12*, 636. [CrossRef] [PubMed]
4. Cannon, C. Cats, Cancer and Comparative Oncology. *Vet. Sci.* **2015**, *2*, 111–126. [CrossRef]
5. Adega, F.; Borges, A.; Chaves, R. Cat Mammary Tumors: Genetic Models for the Human Counterpart. *Vet. Sci.* **2016**, *3*, 17. [CrossRef]
6. Hassan, B.B.; Elshafae, S.M.; Supsavhad, W.; Simmons, J.K.; Dirksen, W.P.; Sokkar, S.M.; Rosol, T.J. Feline Mammary Cancer: Novel Nude Mouse Model and Molecular Characterization of Invasion and Metastasis Genes. *Vet. Pathol.* **2017**, *54*, 32–43. [CrossRef] [PubMed]

7. Michishita, M.; Ohtsuka, A.; Nakahira, R.; Tajima, T.; Nakagawa, T.; Sasaki, N.; Arai, T.; Takahashi, K. Anti-tumor effect of bevacizumab on a xenograft model of feline mammary carcinoma. *J. Vet. Med. Sci.* **2016**, *78*, 685–689. [CrossRef] [PubMed]
8. Soares, M.; Ribeiro, R.; Najmudin, S.; Gameiro, A.; Rodrigues, R.; Cardoso, F.; Ferreira, F. Serum HER2 levels are increased in cats with mammary carcinomas and predict tissue HER2 status. *Oncotarget* **2016**, *7*. [CrossRef] [PubMed]
9. Ferreira, D.; Soares, M.; Correia, J.; Adega, F.; Ferreira, F.; Chaves, R. Assessment of ERBB2 and TOP2α gene status and expression profile in f eline mammary tumors: Findings and guidelines. *Aging* **2019**, *11*. [CrossRef]
10. Urbano, A.C.; Nascimento, C.; Soares, M.; Correia, J.; Ferreira, F. Clinical Relevance of the serum CTLA-4 in Cats with Mammary Carcinoma. *Sci. Rep.* **2020**, *10*, 3822. [CrossRef]
11. Bürtin, F.; Mullins, C.S.; Linnebacher, M. Mouse models of colorectal cancer: Past, present and future perspectives. *World J. Gastroenterol.* **2020**, *26*, 1394–1426. [CrossRef] [PubMed]
12. Soares, M.; Correia, J.; Adega, F.; Ferreira, D. Gene expression association study in feline mammary carcinomas. *PLoS ONE* **2019**, *14*. [CrossRef]
13. Gatalica, Z.; Snyder, C.; Maney, T.; Ghazalpour, A.; Holterman, D.A.; Xiao, N.; Overberg, P.; Rose, I.; Basu, G.D.; Vranic, S.; et al. Programmed cell death 1 (PD-1) and its ligand (PD-L1) in common cancers and their correlation with molecular cancer type. *Cancer Epidemiol. Biomark. Prev.* **2014**, *23*, 2965–2970. [CrossRef]
14. Kim, A.; Lee, S.J.; Kim, Y.K.; Park, W.Y.; Park, D.Y.; Kim, J.Y.; Lee, C.H.; Gong, G.; Huh, G.Y.; Choi, K.U. Programmed death-ligand 1 (PD-L1) expression in tumour cell and tumour infiltrating lymphocytes of HER2-positive breast cancer and its prognostic value. *Sci. Rep.* **2017**, *7*, 11671. [CrossRef] [PubMed]
15. Baptista, M.Z.; Sarian, L.O.; Derchain, S.F.M.; Pinto, G.A.; Vassallo, J. Prognostic significance of PD-L1 and PD-L2 in breast cancer. *Hum. Pathol.* **2016**, *47*, 78–84. [CrossRef]
16. Cimino-Mathews, A.; Thompson, E.; Taube, J.M.; Ye, X.; Lu, Y.; Meeker, A.; Xu, H.; Sharma, R.; Lecksell, K.; Cornish, T.C.; et al. PD-L1 (B7-H1) expression and the immune tumor microenvironment in primary and metastatic breast carcinomas. *Hum. Pathol.* **2016**, *47*, 52–63. [CrossRef]
17. Gu, D.; Ao, X.; Yang, Y.; Chen, Z.; Xu, X. Soluble immune checkpoints in cancer: Production, function and biological significance. *J. Immunother. Cancer* **2018**, *6*, 1–14. [CrossRef]
18. U.S.Food & Drug FDA Approves Atezolizumab for PD-L1 Positive Unresectable Locally Advanced or Metastatic Triple-Negative Breast Cancer. Available online: https://www.fda.gov/drugs/drug-approvals-and-databases/fda-approves-atezolizumab-pd-l1-positive-unresectable-locally-advanced-or-metastatic-triple-negative (accessed on 15 April 2019).
19. Wimberly, H.; Brown, J.R.; Schalper, K.; Haack, H.; Silver, M.R.; Nixon, C.; Bossuyt, V.; Pusztai, L.; Lannin, D.R.; Rimm, D.L. PD-L1 expression correlates with tumor-infiltrating lymphocytes and response to neoadjuvant chemotherapy in breast cancer. *Cancer Immunol. Res.* **2015**, *3*, 326–332. [CrossRef]
20. Solinas, C.; Garaud, S.; De Silva, P.; Boisson, A.; Van den Eynden, G.; de Wind, A.; Risso, P.; Vitória, J.R.; Richard, F.; Migliori, E.; et al. Immune checkpoint molecules on tumor-infiltrating lymphocytes and their association with tertiary lymphoid structures in human breast cancer. *Front. Immunol.* **2017**, *8*, 1412. [CrossRef]
21. Noske, A.; Möbus, V.; Weber, K.; Schmatloch, S.; Weichert, W.; Köhne, C.H.; Solbach, C.; Ingold Heppner, B.; Steiger, K.; Müller, V.; et al. Relevance of tumour-infiltrating lymphocytes, PD-1 and PD-L1 in patients with high-risk, nodal-metastasised breast cancer of the German Adjuvant Intergroup Node–positive study. *Eur. J. Cancer* **2019**, *114*, 76–88. [CrossRef]
22. Vranic, S.; Cyprian, F.S.; Gatalica, Z.; Palazzo, J. PD-L1 status in breast cancer: Current view and perspectives. *Semin. Cancer Biol.* **2019**. [CrossRef] [PubMed]
23. Li, Y.; Cui, X.; Yang, Y.J.; Chen, Q.Q.; Zhong, L.; Zhang, T.; Cai, R.L.; Miao, J.Y.; Yu, S.C.; Zhang, F. Serum sPD-1 and sPD-L1 as biomarkers for evaluating the efficacy of neo-adjuvant chemotherapy in triple-negative breast cancer patients. *Clin. Breast Cancer* **2019**, 326–332. [CrossRef]
24. Zheng, Z.; Bu, Z.; Liu, X.; Zhang, L.; Li, Z.; Wu, A.; Wu, X.; Cheng, X.; Xing, X.; Du, H.; et al. Level of circulating PD-L1 expression in patients with advanced gastric cancer and its clinical implications. *Chin. J. Cancer Res.* **2014**, *26*, 104–111. [CrossRef]

25. Frigola, X.; Inman, B.A.; Lohse, C.M.; Krco, C.J.; Cheville, J.C.; Thompson, R.H.; Leibovich, B.; Blute, M.L.; Dong, H.; Kwon, E.D. Identification of a soluble form of B7-H1 that retains immunosuppressive activity and is associated with aggressive renal cell carcinoma. *Clin. Cancer Res.* **2011**, *17*, 1915–1923. [CrossRef] [PubMed]
26. Makhoul, I.; Atiq, M.; Alwbari, A.; Kieber-Emmons, T. Breast Cancer Immunotherapy: An Update. *Breast Cancer Basic Clin. Res.* **2018**, *12*. [CrossRef] [PubMed]
27. Wang, X.; Yang, L.; Huang, F.; Zhang, Q.; Liu, S.; Ma, L.; You, Z. Inflammatory cytokines IL-17 and TNF-α up-regulated PD-L1 expression in human prostate and colon cancer cells. *Physiol. Behav.* **2016**, *176*, 139–148. [CrossRef]
28. Lim, S.O.; Li, C.W.; Xia, W.; Cha, J.H.; Chan, L.C.; Wu, Y.; Chang, S.S.; Lin, W.C.; Hsu, J.M.; Hsu, Y.H.; et al. Deubiquitination and Stabilization of PD-L1 by CSN5. *Cancer Cell* **2016**, *30*, 925–939. [CrossRef]
29. Lawson, N.L.; Dix, C.I.; Scorer, P.W.; Stubbs, C.J.; Wong, E.; Hutchinson, L.; McCall, E.J.; Schimpl, M.; DeVries, E.; Walker, J.; et al. Mapping the binding sites of antibodies utilized in programmed cell death ligand-1 predictive immunohistochemical assays for use with immuno-oncology therapies. *Mod. Pathol.* **2019**. [CrossRef]
30. Li, S.; Chen, L.; Jiang, J. Role of programmed cell death ligand-1 expression on prognostic and overall survival of breast cancer: A systematic review and meta-analysis. *Medicine* **2019**, *98*. [CrossRef]
31. Soares, M.; Madeira, S.; Correia, J.; Peleteiro, M.; Cardoso, F.; Ferreira, F. Molecular based subtyping of feline mammary carcinomas and clinicopathological characterization. *Breast* **2016**, *27*, 44–51. [CrossRef]
32. Leitzel, K.; Ali, S.M.; Shepherd, L.E.; Parulekar, W.R.; Zhu, L.; Virk, S.; Nomikos, D.; Aparicio, S.; Gelmon, K.A.; Drabick, J.J.; et al. Serum PD-L1 and outcomes in CCTG MA.31 phase 3 trial of anti-HER2 therapy in first-line HER2+ metastatic breast cancer patients (trastuzumab arm only). *J. Clin. Oncol.* **2018**, *36*, 1031. [CrossRef]
33. Ito, M.; Yajima, S.; Suzuki, T.; Oshima, Y.; Nanami, T.; Sumazaki, M.; Shiratori, F.; Funahashi, K.; Tochigi, N.; Shimada, H. High serum PD-L1 level is a poor prognostic biomarker in surgically treated esophageal cancer. *Cancer Med.* **2019**, 1321–1327. [CrossRef] [PubMed]
34. Kruger, S.; Legenstein, M.L.; Rösgen, V.; Haas, M.; Modest, D.P.; Westphalen, C.B.; Ormanns, S.; Kirchner, T.; Heinemann, V.; Holdenrieder, S.; et al. Serum levels of soluble programmed death protein 1 (sPD-1) and soluble programmed death ligand 1 (sPD-L1) in advanced pancreatic cancer. *Oncoimmunology* **2017**, *6*, e1310358. [CrossRef]
35. Abu Hejleh, T.; Furqan, M.; Ballas, Z.; Clamon, G. The clinical significance of soluble PD-1 and PD-L1 in lung cancer. *Crit. Rev. Oncol. Hematol.* **2019**, *143*, 148–152. [CrossRef]
36. Ugurel, S.; Schadendorf, D.; Horny, K.; Sucker, A.; Schramm, S.; Utikal, J.; Pföhler, C.; Herbst, R.; Schilling, B.; Blank, C.; et al. Elevated baseline serum PD-1 or PD-L1 predicts poor outcome of PD-1 inhibition therapy in metastatic melanoma. *Ann. Oncol. Off. J. Eur. Soc. Med. Oncol.* **2020**, *31*, 144–152. [CrossRef] [PubMed]
37. Ward, F.J.; Dahal, L.N.; Wijesekera, S.K.; Abdul-Jawad, S.K.; Kaewarpai, T.; Xu, H.; Vickers, M.A.; Barker, R.N. The soluble isoform of CTLA-4 as a regulator of T-cell responses. *Eur. J. Immunol.* **2013**, *43*, 1274–1285. [CrossRef]
38. Buisseret, L.; Garaud, S.; De Wind, A.; Van Den Eynden, G.; Boisson, A.; Solinas, C. Tumor-infiltrating lymphocyte composition, organization and PD-1 / PD-L1 expression are linked in breast cancer. *Oncoimmunology* **2017**, *6*. [CrossRef]
39. Mittendorf, E.A.; Philips, A.V.; Meric-Bernstam, F.; Qiao, N.; Wu, Y.; Harrington, S.; Su, X.; Wang, Y.; Gonzalez-Angulo, A.M.; Akcakanat, A.; et al. PD-L1 expression in triple-negative breast cancer. *Cancer Immunol. Res.* **2014**, *2*, 361–370. [CrossRef]
40. Polónia, A.; Pinto, R.; Cameselle-Teijeiro, J.F.; Schmitt, F.C.; Paredes, J. Prognostic value of stromal tumour infiltrating lymphocytes and programmed cell death-ligand 1 expression in breast cancer. *J. Clin. Pathol.* **2017**, *70*, 860–867. [CrossRef]
41. Bottai, G.; Raschioni, C.; Losurdo, A.; Di Tommaso, L.; Tinterri, C.; Torrisi, R.; Reis-Filho, J.S.; Roncalli, M.; Sotiriou, C.; Santoro, A.; et al. An immune stratification reveals a subset of PD-1/LAG-3 double-positive triple-negative breast cancers. *Breast Cancer Res.* **2016**, *18*, 121. [CrossRef]
42. Kuipers, H.; Muskens, F.; Willart, M.; Hijdra, D.; van Assema, F.B.J.; Coyle, A.J.; Hoogsteden, H.C.; Lambrecht, B.N. Contribution of the PD-1 ligands/PD-1 signaling pathway to dendritic cell-mediated CD4+ cell activation. *Eur. J. Immunol.* **2006**, *36*, 2472–2482. [CrossRef]

43. Theodoraki, M.N.; Whiteside, T.L.; Gooding, W.E.; Yerneni, S.S.; Hoffmann, T.K. Clinical Significance of PD-L1 + Exosomes in Plasma of Head and Neck Cancer Patients. *Clin. Cancer Res.* **2017**, *24*, 896–905. [CrossRef] [PubMed]
44. Ludwig, S.; Floros, T.; Theodoraki, M.N.; Hong, C.S.; Jackson, E.K.; Lang, S.; Whiteside, T.L. Suppression of lymphocyte functions by plasma exosomes correlates with disease activity in patients with head and neck cancer. *Clin. Cancer Res.* **2017**, *23*, 4843–4854. [CrossRef] [PubMed]
45. Chen, G.; Huang, A.C.; Zhang, W.; Zhang, G.; Wu, M.; Xu, W.; Yu, Z.; Yang, J.; Wang, B.; Sun, H.; et al. Exosomal PD-L1 contributes to immunosuppression and is associated with anti-PD-1 response. *Nature* **2018**, *560*, 382–386. [CrossRef] [PubMed]
46. Stovgaard, E.S.; Dyhl-Polk, A.; Roslind, A.; Balslev, E.; Nielsen, D. PD-L1 expression in breast cancer: Expression in subtypes and prognostic significance: A systematic review. *Breast Cancer Res. Treat.* **2019**, *174*, 571–584. [CrossRef]
47. Beckers, R.K.; Selinger, C.I.; Vilain, R.; Madore, J.; Wilmott, J.S.; Harvey, K.; Holliday, A.; Cooper, C.L.; Robbins, E.; Gillett, D.; et al. Programmed death ligand 1 expression in triple-negative breast cancer is associated with tumour-infiltrating lymphocytes and improved outcome. *Histopathology* **2016**, *69*, 25–34. [CrossRef]
48. Ghebeh, H.; Lehe, C.; Barhoush, E.; Al-Romaih, K.; Tulbah, A.; Al-Alwan, M.; Hendrayani, S.F.; Manogaran, P.; Alaiya, A.; Al-Tweigeri, T.; et al. Doxorubicin downregulates cell surface B7-H1 expression and upregulates its nuclear expression in breast cancer cells: Role of B7-H1 as an anti-apoptotic molecule. *Breast Cancer Res.* **2010**, *12*. [CrossRef]
49. Papadaki, M.A.; Koutsopoulos, A.V.; Tsoulfas, P.G.; Lagoudaki, E.; Aggouraki, D.; Monastirioti, A.; Koutoulaki, C.; Apostolopoulou, C.A.; Merodoulaki, A.C.; Papadaki, C.; et al. Clinical relevance of immune checkpoints on circulating tumor cells in breast cancer. *Cancers* **2020**, *12*, 376. [CrossRef]
50. Lippi, G.; Avanzini, P.; Zobbi, V.; Ippolito, L. Influence of mechanical hemolysis of blood on two D-dimer immunoassays. *Blood Coagul. Fibrinolysis* **2012**, *23*, 461–463. [CrossRef]
51. Soares, M.; Correia, J.; Peleteiro, M.C.; Ferreira, F. St Gallen molecular subtypes in feline mammary carcinoma and paired metastases—Disease progression and clinical implications from a 3-year follow-up study. *Tumor Biol.* **2016**, *37*, 4053–4064. [CrossRef]
52. Salgado, R.; Denkert, C.; Demaria, S.; Sirtaine, N.; Klauschen, F.; Pruneri, G.; Wienert, S.; Van den Eynden, G.; Baehner, F.L.; Penault-Llorca, F.; et al. The evaluation of tumor-infiltrating lymphocytes (TILS) in breast cancer: Recommendations by an International TILS Working Group 2014. *Ann. Oncol.* **2015**, *26*, 259–271. [CrossRef] [PubMed]
53. Wang, Y.; Dong, T.; Xuan, Q.; Zhao, H.; Qin, L.; Zhang, Q. Lymphocyte-Activation Gene-3 Expression and Prognostic Value in Neoadjuvant-Treated Triple-Negative Breast Cancer. *J. Breast Cancer* **2018**, *21*, 124. [CrossRef] [PubMed]
54. Sun, W.Y.; Lee, Y.K.; Koo, J.S. Expression of PD-L1 in triple-negative breast cancer based on different immunohistochemical antibodies. *J. Transl. Med.* **2016**, *14*, 173. [CrossRef] [PubMed]
55. Ács, B.; Madaras, L.; Tőkés, A.M.; Kovács, A.K.; Kovács, E.; Ozsvári-Vidákovich, M.; Karászi, Á.; Birtalan, E.; Dank, M.; Szász, A.M.; et al. PD-1, PD-L1 and CTLA-4 in pregnancy-related and in early-onset breast cancer: A comparative study. *Breast* **2017**, *35*, 69–77. [CrossRef] [PubMed]

2

The Cellular Prion Protein: A Promising Therapeutic Target for Cancer

Gyeongyun Go [1] and Sang Hun Lee [1,2,*]

[1] Department of Biochemistry, Soonchunhyang University College of Medicine, Cheonan 31151, Korea; ggy0227@naver.com

[2] Medical Science Research Institute, Soonchunhyang University Seoul Hospital, Seoul 04401, Korea

* Correspondence: ykckss1114@nate.com

Abstract: Studies on the cellular prion protein (PrP^C) have been actively conducted because misfolded PrP^C is known to cause transmissible spongiform encephalopathies or prion disease. PrP^C is a glycophosphatidylinositol-anchored cell surface glycoprotein that has been reported to affect several cellular functions such as stress protection, cellular differentiation, mitochondrial homeostasis, circadian rhythm, myelin homeostasis, and immune modulation. Recently, it has also been reported that PrP^C mediates tumor progression by enhancing the proliferation, metastasis, and drug resistance of cancer cells. In addition, PrP^C regulates cancer stem cell properties by interacting with cancer stem cell marker proteins. In this review, we summarize how PrP^C promotes tumor progression in terms of proliferation, metastasis, drug resistance, and cancer stem cell properties. In addition, we discuss strategies to treat tumors by modulating the function and expression of PrP^C via the regulation of HSPA1L/HIF-1α expression and using an anti-prion antibody.

Keywords: cellular prion protein; PrP^C; *PRNP*; cancer; cancer stem cell; targeted cancer therapy

---

1. Introduction

The cellular prion protein (PrP^C) is a cell surface glycophosphatidylinositol (GPI)-anchored protein consisting of 208 amino acids, and it is encoded by the *PRNP* gene located on chromosome 20. PrP^C has been intensively studied since it was proposed that misfolding of PrP^C plays a key role in the pathogenesis of neurodegenerative diseases called transmissible spongiform encephalopathies [1–3]. Studies have shown that PrP^C is not simply a cause of neurodegenerative diseases, but it is an important protein involved in many cellular functions such as stress protection, cellular differentiation, mitochondrial homeostasis, circadian rhythm, myelin homeostasis, and immune modulation [4–10]. Furthermore, several studies have shown that PrP^C expression is associated with tumor progression [11–15]. Before addressing the role of PrP^C in tumor progression, we briefly introduce herein some biochemical aspects of PrP^C.

PrP^C is first synthesized as a precursor protein (pre-pro-PrP) comprising 253 amino acids with a signal peptide at the N-terminus and a GPI anchor peptide signaling sequence (GPI-PSS) at the C-terminus. The signal peptide directs pre-pro-PrP into the endoplasmic reticulum (ER), wherein it is cleaved to generate pro-PrP. The pro-PrP is then translocated from the ER to the Golgi complex [16,17] to be further processed by the addition of N-linked glycans, removal of the GPI-PSS, and addition of the pre-assembled GPI anchor [18,19]. Finally, the mature PrP^C of 208 amino acids is translocated to the outer membrane leaflet of cells. However, not all PrP^Cs are present on the cell surface. They are constantly internalized through the recycling endosome and trafficked back repeatedly [20–22]. Through this recycling process, PrP^Cs are also found in the Golgi [22,23], in addition to the nucleus [24,25] and mitochondria [26,27].

The relationship between PrP^C and cancer progression was first discovered when *PRNP* was identified as one of the most-expressed genes in pancreatic cancer cells [28]. Around the same time, other researchers found that PrP^C was overexpressed in a drug-resistant cancer cell line compared to the parental cell line [29]. Based on several studies, it is now well established that PrP^C is involved in the main aspects of cancer biology: proliferation, metastasis, and drug resistance. Moreover, the relationship between PrP^C and cancer stem cell phenotypes has also been uncovered [30,31]. In this review, we summarize the role of PrP^C in tumor progression in terms of proliferation, metastasis, drug resistance, and cancer stem cell properties. Finally, we discuss strategies to control tumor growth by regulating the function and expression of PrP^C.

2. Overview of Physiological Functions of PrP^C

PrP^C is known to regulate several functions of cells, such as stress protection, cellular differentiation, mitochondrial homeostasis, circadian rhythm, myelin homeostasis, and immune modulation. In this review, we briefly summarize the effects of PrP^C on stress protection, cellular differentiation, and mitochondrial homeostasis.

Several studies have shown that PrP^C can directly inhibit apoptosis. PrP^C expression inhibited mitochondria-dependent apoptosis in Bax-overexpressing human primary neurons and MCF-7 breast cancer cells [32,33]. In addition, downregulation of PrP^C reduced the viability of MDA-MB-435 breast cancer cells after serum deprivation [34]. In primary hippocampal neurons, PrP^C protected the cells against staurosporine-induced cell death by interacting with stress-induced phosphoprotein 1 (STI1) [35–37]. PrP^C is also known to protect cells from oxidative stress. For example, the basal levels of ROS and lipid peroxidation were lower in PrP^C-transfected neuroblastoma and epithelial cell lines than in untransfected controls [38,39]. In addition, the expression of PrP^C by primary neurons and astrocytes has been associated with lower levels of damage caused by the addition of various oxidative toxins such as xanthine oxidase, kainic acid, and hydrogen peroxide [40,41]. PrP^C has also been found to be involved in the ER-stress response. When breast carcinoma cells were treated with the ER-stress inducing compounds such as brefeldin A, tunicamycin, and thapsigargin, the expression of PrP^C was induced. Downregulation of PrP^C in several cancer cell lines resulted in an increase in cell death in response to these toxins [13].

Neurite outgrowth is one of the characteristics of neuronal differentiation. Several studies have indicated that PrP^C promotes neurite outgrowth through interactions with other proteins such as neural cell adhesion molecule 1, epidermal growth factor receptor, integrins, laminin, and STI1 [35,42–45]. The downstream signaling of these interactions may include RhoA-Rho kinase-LIMK-cofilin pathway [44]. Activation of various signal pathways, including extracellular signal-regulated kinases 1 and 2 (ERK1/2), phosphatidylinositol-3-kinase (PI3K)/Akt, and mitogen-activated protein kinases (MAPKs), may also induce PrP^C-dependent neurite outgrowth [35,43,46]. It has been reported that PrP^C is also involved in the differentiation of embryonic stem cells. In human embryonic stem cells, downregulation of PrP^C delays spontaneous differentiation into the three germ layers [47]. Similarly, PrP^C expression promotes the differentiation of cultured human embryonic stem cells and multipotent neural precursors to mature neurons, astroglia, and oligodendroglia [47,48].

PrP^C expression also affects mitochondrial homeostasis. Transcriptomic and proteomic analyses of brain tissues and neurons of PrP^C-null and wild-type mice have identified differently expressed proteins. These proteins include cytochrome c oxidase subunits 1 and 2, which are involved in oxidative phosphorylation [49,50]. Furthermore, the absence of PrP^C reduces the number of total mitochondria and increases the number of mitochondria with unusual morphology [49].

3. PrP^C and Cancer Proliferation

PrP^C expression has been reported to promote cancer proliferation in several types of cancer cells, including gastric [51], pancreatic [52], and colon [53–55], as well as in glioblastoma (GBM) [56,57] and schwannanoma [58].

In gastric cancer, PrP^C promotes cell proliferation and metastasis of cancer cells and promotes tumor growth in xenograft mouse models [51]. PrP^C increases the expression of cyclin D1 and thereby promotes their transition from the G0/G1 phase to the S-phase. PrP^C expression also affects Akt signaling. Overexpression of PrP^C increases p-Akt levels, whereas PrP^C knockdown inhibits p-Akt expression [59]. Interestingly, it is known that certain regions of PrP^C influence cell proliferation. Specifically, deletion of amino acids 24–50 of PrP^C significantly reduced cell proliferation. Conversely, deletion of amino acids 51–91 did not affect apoptosis, metastasis cell proliferation, and multidrug resistance in gastric cancer [60].

In pancreatic ductal adenocarcinoma (PDAC), expression of PrP^C increases the proliferation and migration of the cells. In PDAC cell lines, PrP^C exists as a pro-PrP as it retains its GPI-PSS, which has a filamin A (FLNA) binding motif. It was found that the interaction between pro-PrP and FLNA, a cytoplasmic protein involved in actin organization, promotes cell migration [61]. In addition, other studies have shown that PrP^C promote pancreatic cell proliferation by activating the Notch signaling pathway [62].

PrP^C is known to interact with other membrane proteins or extracellular molecules to perform various cellular functions. In human GBM, PrP^C and heat shock 90/70 organizing protein (HOP) are upregulated, and their expression levels correlate with higher proliferation rates and poorer clinical outcomes [56]. Additionally, it has been demonstrated that the binding of HOP to PrP^C promotes proliferation of GBM cell lines and that disruption of PrP^C–HOP interaction inhibits tumor growth and improves the survival of mice [56].

In DLS-1 and SW480 colorectal cancer cells, knockdown of PrP^C significantly reduces the proliferation of cancer cells. It is known that the binding between HIF-2α and the GLUT1 promoter region decreases when PrP^C expression is suppressed, resulting in a decrease in the expression of GLUT1. This may reduce glucose uptake and glycolysis and inhibit cell proliferation [54].

4. PrP^C and Metastasis

It has been demonstrated that PrP^C promotes the invasion and migration of several types of cancer cells, such as gastric [63], pancreatic [62], colon [64], and melanoma [65] cells.

PrP^C expression is higher in metastatic gastric cancer than in non-metastatic gastric cancer. PrP^C increases the invasion and in vivo metastatic ability of gastric cancer cell lines SGC7901 and MKN45, and knockdown of PrP^C significantly reduces cancer cell invasion [63]. PrP^C seems to induce cancer cell invasion by activating the p-ERK1/2 signal and inducing the expression of MMP11. Interestingly, the N-terminal fragment (amino acids 24–90) of PrP^C has been proposed as the region for its invasion-promoting function.

PrP^C levels were found to increase in invasive melanoma, whereas in normal melanocytes, PrP^C was not detected [65]. In melanoma, PrP^C is known to exist as pro-PrP, retaining its GPI-PSS with an FLNA binding motif. As in PDAC earlier, PrP^C promoted migration by binding with FLNA and regulating cytoskeleton organization. PrP^C knockdown significantly reduced the migration of melanoma cells in a wound healing assay [65,66].

In colon cancer, PrP^C is known to promote migration by binding to HOP, also known as stress-induced phosphoprotein 1 (STI1) [64]. It was found that among the colon primary tumor cells, only PrP^C-positive cells were able to promote liver metastasis after injection into immunocompromised mice [67]. Metastasis is highly correlated with epithelial-mesenchymal transition (EMT), a process in which cells lose epithelial markers and interaction between the cell and the extracellular matrix change the cytoskeleton organization and differentiate into mesenchymal phenotype [68]. It is well known that transcription factors such as SNAI1, SNAI2, TWIST1, TWIST2, ZEB1, and ZEB2 induce EMT. *PRNP* expression is highly associated with the EMT signature in colon cancer patients, and PrP^C is known to control the expression of ZEB1 in colon cancer cells [53].

5. PrP^C and Drug Resistance

PrP^C levels were found to be higher in tumor necrosis factor α (TNF-α)-resistant breast cancer cells than in TNF-α-sensitive breast cancer cells [33]. After treatment of TNF-α, the resistant cells did not exhibit cytochrome c release or nuclear condensation. Moreover, PrP^C expression inhibited the Bax translocation to mitochondria and Bax-mediated cytochrome c release. In addition to TNF-α, PrP^C is also involved in the resistance to adriamycin (ADR) and TRAIL-mediated cell death in breast cancer cells as down-regulation of PrP^C increased the sensitivity to these molecules. [69]. Inhibition of PrP^C expression did not inhibit formation of death-inducing signaling complex (DISC); however, it inhibited Bcl-2 expression and promoted Bid cleavage, resulting in cell death [69]. In addition, it has been confirmed that PrP^C co-localization and coexpression with p-glycoprotein (P-gp) occur in ADR-resistant MCF-7 cells. When the expression of PrC^C was inhibited in these cells, the capability of paclitaxel, a P-gp substrate, to induce in vitro invasion of the cells decreased [52]. More importantly, tissue microarray analysis of 756 breast cancer tumors demonstrated that PrP^C was associated with ER-negative breast cancer subsets, and compared with ER-negative/PrP^C-positive cells, ER-negative/PrP^C-negative cells are more sensitive to adjuvant chemotherapy [70].

PrP^C is also involved in drug resistance in colon cancer. Hypoxia-induced PrP^C expression in colorectal cancer cells inhibits TRAIL-induced apoptosis [71]. PrP^C inhibited apoptosis of colon cancer cells by activating the PI3K-Akt pathway [72]. Conversely, deletion of PrP^C resulted in reduced Akt activation and enhanced caspase-3 activation [73]. Our group has demonstrated that PrP^C levels significantly increase in 5-FU-and oxaliplatin-resistant colorectal cancer [74–77]. In addition, knocking down PrP^C expression significantly reduces the drug resistance of colorectal cancer cells. Furthermore, we have shown that PrP^C suppresses the drug-induced activation of stress-associated proteins, such as p38, JNK, and p53. We have also demonstrated that PrP^C inhibits caspase-3 activation by drugs and PARP1 cleavage. These results suggest that the level of PrP^C plays an important role in the development of drug resistance in colorectal cancer cells.

6. PrP^C and Cancer Stem Cells

Cancer stem cells (CSCs) are a subpopulation of cells that are capable of self-renewal, differentiation into various cell types in a determined tumor, and tumor propagation when xenotransplanted into mice [78,79]. CSCs are resistant to conventional medical therapies and have been implicated in cancer recurrence, which has made these cells a key target for therapy [80–82].

Recently, studies on the correlation between PrP^C and CSCs have been conducted. PrP^C activation of Fyn-SP1 pathway in colon cancer cells promoted EMT and resulted in a more aggressive phenotype [83]. EMT is closely connected with CSC properties as EMT enhances metastasis and drug resistance of cancer and cancer microenvironment promotes activation of EMT program [84]. Du et al. demonstrated that PrP^C-positive primary colon cancer cells expressed high levels of the EMT-associated markers, TWIST and N-cadherin, and low levels of the epithelial marker, E-cadherin, as well as exhibiting CSC properties such as the expression of the CSC marker, CD44, and tumor-initiating capacity [67].

In line with this finding, PrP^C has been shown to interact with CD44 in multidrug-resistant breast cancer cells [85]. Furthermore, in primary GBM cells, PrP^C silencing reduces the expression of the CSC markers, Sox2 and Nanog, as well as the self-renewal and tumorigenic potential of CSCs [57]. Similar findings were demonstrated by Iglesia et al., who worked on GBM cell lines grown as neurospheres [86].

CSCs are one of the most-studied recent topics in cancer biology. They have emerged as pivotal components that can initiate and maintain tumors [79]. PrP^C is known to interact with CD44, and its expression correlates with resistance to chemotherapy in breast cancer cell lines [85]. Moreover, the CD44-positive and PrP^C-positive subpopulations of colorectal tumor cells have CSC properties, including tumorigenic and metastatic capacities [67], indicating that PrP^C contributes to tumor maintenance by modulating CSC behaviors.

Our group confirmed the correlation between PrP^C and CSC by demonstrating that the levels of PrP^C and CSC marker proteins such as Oct4, Nanog, Sox2, and ALDH1A1 significantly increased in human colorectal cancer tissues and colorectal cancer cells [31]. In addition, knockdown of PrP^C reduced the expression of CSC markers in the CSCs. More specifically, PrP^C inhibited the anticancer drug-induced degradation of Oct4, but did not inhibit the degradation of other stem cell markers such as Nanog, Sox2, and ALDH1A1. Oct4 is a master regulator involved in the self-renewal and pluripotency of CSCs. It has been reported that tumor sphere formation ability is activated in breast cancer cells overexpressing Oct4 [87,88]. Cancer cells overexpressing Oct4 also overexpress other CSC markers such as CD133, CD34, and ALDH1. Oct4 is also involved in the survival, self-renewal, metastasis, and drug resistance of CSCs [89–92]. These results indicate that PrP^C directly regulates Oct4 expression, whereas it indirectly regulates Nanog, Sox2, and ALDH1A to promote the self-renewal and survival of CSCs [31].

In summary, Figure 1 shows the proteins and signaling pathways that seem to be affected by PrP^C expression. The information on these interactions was retrieved from several studies that have been already mentioned in this review. Although PrP^C appear to interact and activate several interaction partners and signaling pathways to promote tumor progression, it is difficult to say that this applies to all cancer cells. The role of PrP^C in cancer needs to be interpreted differently depending on the cell type and interaction partner.

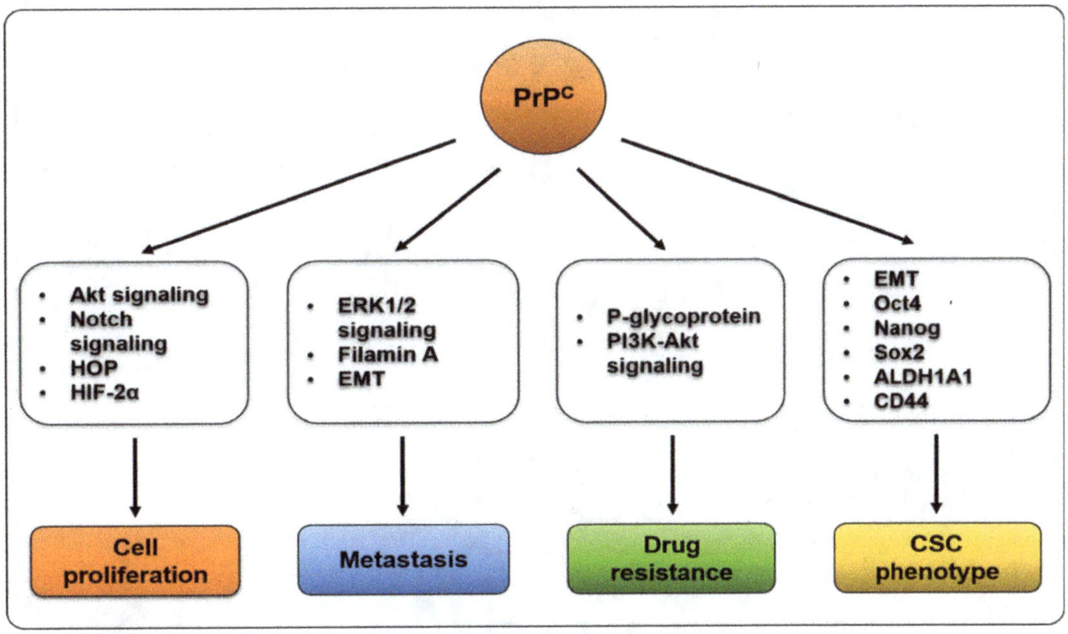

Figure 1. Proteins and signaling pathways that seem to be affected by PrP^C expression. Various proteins and signaling pathways reportedly interact with or are modulated by PrP^C. Some of the proteins shown are known to be regulated indirectly through other proteins rather than direct interaction with PrP^C. PrP^C: prion protein, ECM: extracellular matrix, CSC: cancer stem cell.

7. Cancer Treatment by Targeting PrP^C

Cancer growth can be inhibited by inhibiting the interaction between PrP^C and other proteins. Lopes et al. used a peptide named HOP/STI1230–245 corresponding to the prion binding site of HOP to inhibit the interaction between PrP^C and HOP [56]. Treatment with only the peptide did not inhibit cell proliferation, but co-treatment with HOP inhibited the interaction between HOP and PrP^C and HOP-induced cell proliferation. In addition, HOP/STI1230–245 treatment of orthotopic xenografts inhibited tumor growth and improved animal survival while maintaining cognitive performance [56]. It should be noted that the blockage of PrP^C and HOP may be deleterious, because long-term [93] but not short-term [94] intracranial infusion of antibodies against PrP^C, particularly those against its globular domain, can be neurotoxic [93].

Recently, our group identified that HSP family A (Hsp 70) member 1-like, HSPA1L, regulates the expression of PrP^C [77]. It was confirmed that the expression of HSPA1L increased in colon cancer cells and cancer tissues. We also demonstrated that HSPA1L increases the stability of HIF-1α by binding with HIF-1α and promotes the accumulation of PrP^C. When HSPA1L expression was knocked down, HIF-1α stability and PrP^C expression decreased [77]. In addition, we also showed that HSPA1L binds to GP78 and inhibits its ubiquitination activity, thereby reducing the ubiquitination of PrP^C. Several studies have indicated that deregulation of several E3 ligases affects the growth and metastasis of cancer and the growth of CSCs [95–98]. GP78 is an ER membrane-anchored E3 ligase that regulates the progression of cancer cells through ubiquitin ligase activity. For example, downregulation of GP78-mediated ubiquitination is known to inhibit metastasis in breast cancer cells [99]. We hypothesized that HIF-1α and HSPA1L are major therapeutic targets for colorectal cancer. Indeed, knockdown of HIF-1α and HSPA1L using siRNAs inhibited cancer sphere formation in HT-29 and S707 cells. In an in vivo xenograft model, knockdown of HIF-1α or HSPA1L inhibited tumor growth and liver metastasis (Figure 2). In addition, when both genes were knocked down simultaneously, cancer growth and liver metastasis were further suppressed [77]. These results indicated that PrP^C is important in tumor progression, and the suppression of PrP^C expression by targeting HIF-1α and HSPA1L could be a promising therapeutic strategy to treat cancer.

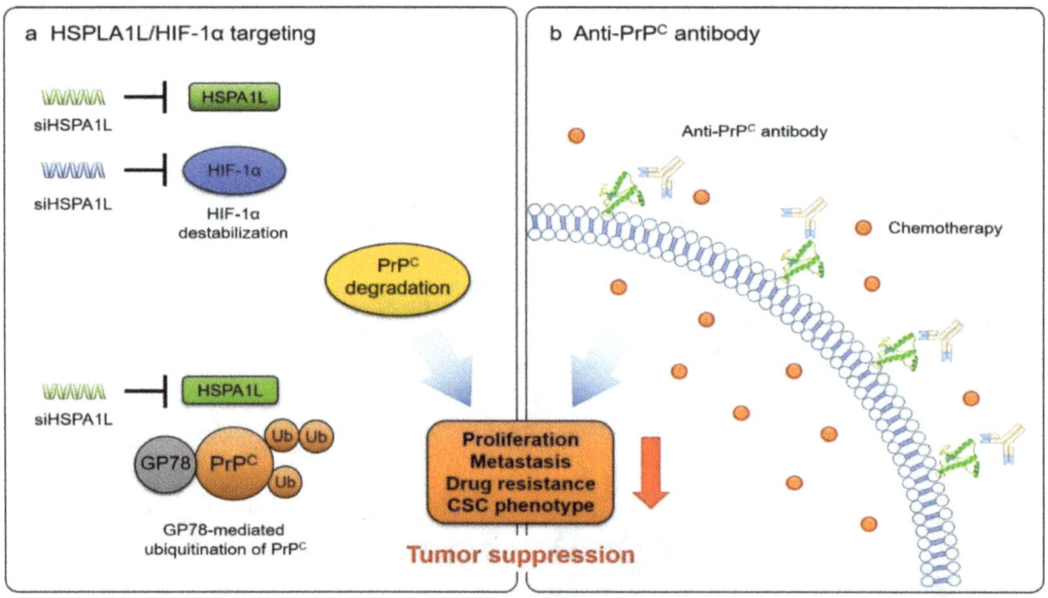

Figure 2. Strategies to suppress the tumor progression by regulating the expression and function of PrP^C. (**a**) In tumor niche, the expression of HSPA1L is increased. HSPA1L binds and stabilizes HIF-1α. HSPA1L directly binds to GP78 and inhibits its ubiquitination activity. Overall, PrP^C expression is increased in tumor cells. Therefore, knocking down HSPA1L and HIF-1α expression induces degradation of PrP^C and tumor suppression. (**b**) Direct targeting of PrP^C using anti-PrP^C antibodies has been demonstrated as a potent cancer therapy. Anti-PrP^C antibody also can be used as a combination therapy with conventional anticancer drugs.

Anti-prion antibodies can be utilized for the treatment of cancer. Antibody therapeutics have been used in the treatment of cancer, unlike existing anticancer drugs, as they have fewer side effects and exhibit high efficacy. For the development of effective antibody therapeutics, the discovery of specific molecular biomarkers in a wide range of solid malignancies is a key process [100]. The functions of PrP^C in the growth, metastasis, drug resistance, and CSC properties of various types of cancer suggest that it is a promising therapeutic target for cancer treatment. We confirmed that an anti-prion antibody showed anticancer effects in a xenograft model and that superior therapeutic effects appeared when the conventional anticancer drugs and anti-prion antibody were applied in combination (unpublished data) (Figure 2). Furthermore, compared to cetuximab, an EGFR-targeting antibody, the anti-prion antibody showed similar anticancer effects with 10 times lower dose in the xenograft mouse model (unpublished data).

Similar to our data, a previous study has revealed the effective epitope of PrP^C for antibody-mediated colon cancer therapy [101]. In colon cancer cell line HCT116 cells, epitope 139–142 and epitope 141–151 targeting anti-PrP antibodies highly inhibited the proliferative capacity of cells, compared with those of epitope 93–109 and epitope 101–112 [101]. Furthermore, epitope 141–151 targeting anti-PrP was approximately 10-fold more active than that of epitope 93–109 targeting anti-PrP [101]. These data indicate that effectiveness of anti-PrP antibodies might be related to the epitope-binding region. Further studies on anti-PrP structure and its targeting epitope site for cancer therapy are needed. One study has shown that N-terminal domain of PrP^C is a direct binding and sequestering site on anti-tumor drug, doxorubicin, in breast cancer [67]. This study suggests that N-terminal-domain-targeting anti-PrP antibodies might be effective antibody therapy when combined with anti-tumor drugs, for cancer treatment.

Although antibody therapy is a promising cancer treatment, resistance may arise due to the characteristics of cancer cells, such as intrinsic phenotypic variation and adaptive phenotypic modifications [100,102–105]. Antibody-drug conjugates (ADCs), which are novel antibody-based therapeutics, are another option for treating tumors. ADC is a technology that focuses on targeting only cancer cells by exploiting the advantages of antibodies: specificity, non-toxicity in circulation, and pharmacokinetics. ADC is known to enter cells through clathrin-mediated endocytosis [106]. The endosome that harbors ADC binds to other vesicles in the cell and forms an endo-lysosome. A protease cleaves the linker of the ADC and activates free drugs to move into the cytoplasm. The drugs bind to the molecular target, causing apoptosis of the tumor cells. A representative example of a successful ADC is Trastuzumab Emtansine (T-DM1) [107–109]. T-DM1 significantly prolonged progression-free and overall survival with less toxicity than lapatinib plus capecitabine in patients with HER2-positive advanced breast cancer who were previously treated with trastuzumab and a taxane. Anti-prion antibodies, such as T-DM1, are expected to be developed as anticancer agents in the form of ADCs.

8. Conclusions

Several studies have suggested that PrP^C promotes tumor progression. It has been demonstrated that PrP^C is overexpressed in various types of cancer cells and tumor tissues, including gastric, pancreatic, breast, and colon cancers, as well as melanoma, GBM, and schwannoma. In addition, it has been shown that PrP^C regulates cell proliferation, metastasis, drug resistance, and cancer stem cell properties through signaling pathways, such as PI3K-Akt and Notch, and interaction with ECM, cell surface molecules, and cancer stem cell markers. It should be noted that the function of PrP^C in cancer should be interpreted depending on the cell type and the molecule that interacts with it. Nevertheless, further research is needed to elucidate the function of PrP^C in tumor progression. However, there seems to be no disagreement that PrP^C is a promising target for cancer treatment.

In addition to PrP^C, the misfolded prion protein (PrP^{Sc}) may be highly expressed in cancer patients compared to the healthy people. Recently, somatic mutations in *PRNP* were analyzed in 10,967 cancer patients using the Cancer Genome atlas (TCGA) database [110]. A total of 48 mutations in *PRNP* gene were identified in cancer patient. Among them, eight somatic mutations— G131V, D167N, V180I, D202N, V203I, R208C, R208H, and E211Q—are known as pathogenic mutations of prion diseases. Interestingly, it has been reported that PrP^{Sc} was also detected in healthy people, who had not been diagnosed with prion diseases [111]. These results may indicate that cancer patients carrying pathogenic somatic mutations of *PRNP* may produce PrP^{Sc} and may not be diagnosed with prion disease.

In this review, we suggest that prion targeting is a promising strategy to treat cancer. Regulating the expression of HSPL1A and HIF-1α, which are involved in the stability and degradation of PrP^C, effectively inhibits cancer growth and metastasis. In addition, an anti-prion antibody has been used to inhibit the growth of cancer. Nevertheless, further studies are needed to verify the anticancer effect and safety of prion targeting in various cancer models. To date, no clinical trials using prion targeting have been conducted; therefore, the effectiveness and safety of cancer treatment strategies using prion targeting should also be verified.

Author Contributions: G.G.: designed and drafted the manuscript; S.H.L.: drafted the manuscript, procured funding, and supervised the study. All authors have read and agreed to the published version of the manuscript.

Acknowledgments: This work was supported by a grant from the National Research Foundation funded by the Korean government (2016R1D1A3B01007727). The funders had no role in the manuscript design, preparation of the manuscript, or decision to publish.

References

1. Prusiner, S.B. Novel proteinaceous infectious particles cause scrapie. *Science* **1982**, *216*, 136–144. [CrossRef] [PubMed]
2. Caughey, B.; Chesebro, B. Prion protein and the transmissible spongiform encephalopathies. *Trends Cell Biol.* **1997**, *7*, 56–62. [CrossRef]
3. Aguzzi, A.; Heppner, F.L. Pathogenesis of prion diseases: A progress report. *Cell Death Differ.* **2000**, *7*, 889–902. [CrossRef] [PubMed]
4. Castle, A.R.; Gill, A.C. Physiological Functions of the Cellular Prion Protein. *Front. Mol. Biosci.* **2017**, *4*, 19. [CrossRef] [PubMed]
5. Dupiereux, I.; Falisse-Poirrier, N.; Zorzi, W.; Watt, N.T.; Thellin, O.; Zorzi, D.; Pierard, O.; Hooper, N.M.; Heinen, E.; Elmoualij, B. Protective effect of prion protein via the N-terminal region in mediating a protective effect on paraquat-induced oxidative injury in neuronal cells. *J. Neurosci. Res.* **2008**, *86*, 653–659. [CrossRef] [PubMed]
6. Graner, E.; Mercadante, A.F.; Zanata, S.M.; Martins, V.R.; Jay, D.G.; Brentani, R.R. Laminin-induced PC-12 cell differentiation is inhibited following laser inactivation of cellular prion protein. *FEBS Lett.* **2000**, *482*, 257–260. [CrossRef]
7. Ramljak, S.; Asif, A.R.; Armstrong, V.W.; Wrede, A.; Groschup, M.H.; Buschmann, A.; Schulz-Schaeffer, W.; Bodemer, W.; Zerr, I. Physiological role of the cellular prion protein (PrPc): Protein profiling study in two cell culture systems. *J. Proteome Res.* **2008**, *7*, 2681–2695. [CrossRef]
8. Tobler, I.; Gaus, S.E.; Deboer, T.; Achermann, P.; Fischer, M.; Rulicke, T.; Moser, M.; Oesch, B.; McBride, P.A.; Manson, J.C. Altered circadian activity rhythms and sleep in mice devoid of prion protein. *Nature* **1996**, *380*, 639–642. [CrossRef]
9. Bremer, J.; Baumann, F.; Tiberi, C.; Wessig, C.; Fischer, H.; Schwarz, P.; Steele, A.D.; Toyka, K.V.; Nave, K.A.; Weis, J.; et al. Axonal prion protein is required for peripheral myelin maintenance. *Nat. Neurosci.* **2010**, *13*, 310–318. [CrossRef]
10. Haddon, D.J.; Hughes, M.R.; Antignano, F.; Westaway, D.; Cashman, N.R.; McNagny, K.M. Prion protein expression and release by mast cells after activation. *J. Infect. Dis* **2009**, *200*, 827–831. [CrossRef]
11. Santos, T.G.; Lopes, M.H.; Martins, V.R. Targeting prion protein interactions in cancer. *Prion* **2015**, *9*, 165–173. [CrossRef] [PubMed]
12. Gao, Z.; Peng, M.; Chen, L.; Yang, X.; Li, H.; Shi, R.; Wu, G.; Cai, L.; Song, Q.; Li, C. Prion Protein Protects Cancer Cells against Endoplasmic Reticulum Stress Induced Apoptosis. *Virol. Sin.* **2019**, *34*, 222–234. [CrossRef] [PubMed]
13. Dery, M.A.; Jodoin, J.; Ursini-Siegel, J.; Aleynikova, O.; Ferrario, C.; Hassan, S.; Basik, M.; LeBlanc, A.C. Endoplasmic reticulum stress induces PRNP prion protein gene expression in breast cancer. *Breast Cancer Res.* **2013**, *15*, R22. [CrossRef]
14. Mehrpour, M.; Codogno, P. Prion protein: From physiology to cancer biology. *Cancer Lett.* **2010**, *290*, 1–23. [CrossRef] [PubMed]

15. Tang, Z.; Ma, J.; Zhang, W.; Gong, C.; He, J.; Wang, Y.; Yu, G.; Yuan, C.; Wang, X.; Sun, Y.; et al. The Role of Prion Protein Expression in Predicting Gastric Cancer Prognosis. *J. Cancer* **2016**, *7*, 984–990. [CrossRef] [PubMed]
16. Tanaka, S.; Maeda, Y.; Tashima, Y.; Kinoshita, T. Inositol deacylation of glycosylphosphatidylinositol-anchored proteins is mediated by mammalian PGAP1 and yeast Bst1p. *J. Biol. Chem.* **2004**, *279*, 14256–14263. [CrossRef] [PubMed]
17. Bonnon, C.; Wendeler, M.W.; Paccaud, J.P.; Hauri, H.P. Selective export of human GPI-anchored proteins from the endoplasmic reticulum. *J. Cell Sci.* **2010**, *123*, 1705–1715. [CrossRef]
18. Sarnataro, D.; Campana, V.; Paladino, S.; Stornaiuolo, M.; Nitsch, L.; Zurzolo, C. PrP(C) association with lipid rafts in the early secretory pathway stabilizes its cellular conformation. *Mol. Biol. Cell* **2004**, *15*, 4031–4042. [CrossRef]
19. Campana, V.; Sarnataro, D.; Zurzolo, C. The highways and byways of prion protein trafficking. *Trends Cell Biol.* **2005**, *15*, 102–111. [CrossRef]
20. Shyng, S.L.; Huber, M.T.; Harris, D.A. A prion protein cycles between the cell surface and an endocytic compartment in cultured neuroblastoma cells. *J. Biol. Chem.* **1993**, *268*, 15922–15928.
21. Sunyach, C.; Jen, A.; Deng, J.; Fitzgerald, K.T.; Frobert, Y.; Grassi, J.; McCaffrey, M.W.; Morris, R. The mechanism of internalization of glycosylphosphatidylinositol-anchored prion protein. *EMBO J.* **2003**, *22*, 3591–3601. [CrossRef] [PubMed]
22. Magalhaes, A.C.; Silva, J.A.; Lee, K.S.; Martins, V.R.; Prado, V.F.; Ferguson, S.S.; Gomez, M.V.; Brentani, R.R.; Prado, M.A. Endocytic intermediates involved with the intracellular trafficking of a fluorescent cellular prion protein. *J. Biol. Chem.* **2002**, *277*, 33311–33318. [CrossRef] [PubMed]
23. Lee, K.S.; Magalhaes, A.C.; Zanata, S.M.; Brentani, R.R.; Martins, V.R.; Prado, M.A. Internalization of mammalian fluorescent cellular prion protein and N-terminal deletion mutants in living cells. *J. Neurochem.* **2001**, *79*, 79–87. [CrossRef] [PubMed]
24. Gu, Y.; Hinnerwisch, J.; Fredricks, R.; Kalepu, S.; Mishra, R.S.; Singh, N. Identification of cryptic nuclear localization signals in the prion protein. *NeuroBiol. Dis.* **2003**, *12*, 133–149. [CrossRef]
25. Morel, E.; Fouquet, S.; Strup-Perrot, C.; Pichol Thievend, C.; Petit, C.; Loew, D.; Faussat, A.M.; Yvernault, L.; Pincon-Raymond, M.; Chambaz, J.; et al. The cellular prion protein PrP(c) is involved in the proliferation of epithelial cells and in the distribution of junction-associated proteins. *PLoS ONE* **2008**, *3*, e3000. [CrossRef]
26. Hachiya, N.S.; Yamada, M.; Watanabe, K.; Jozuka, A.; Ohkubo, T.; Sano, K.; Takeuchi, Y.; Kozuka, Y.; Sakasegawa, Y.; Kaneko, K. Mitochondrial localization of cellular prion protein (PrPC) invokes neuronal apoptosis in aged transgenic mice overexpressing PrPC. *Neurosci. Lett.* **2005**, *374*, 98–103. [CrossRef]
27. Satoh, J.; Onoue, H.; Arima, K.; Yamamura, T. The 14-3-3 protein forms a molecular complex with heat shock protein Hsp60 and cellular prion protein. *J. Neuropathol. Exp. Neurol* **2005**, *64*, 858–868. [CrossRef]
28. Han, H.; Bearss, D.J.; Browne, L.W.; Calaluce, R.; Nagle, R.B.; Von Hoff, D.D. Identification of differentially expressed genes in pancreatic cancer cells using cDNA microarray. *Cancer Res.* **2002**, *62*, 2890–2896.
29. Zhao, Y.; You, H.; Liu, F.; An, H.; Shi, Y.; Yu, Q.; Fan, D. Differentially expressed gene profiles between multidrug resistant gastric adenocarcinoma cells and their parental cells. *Cancer Lett.* **2002**, *185*, 211–218. [CrossRef]
30. Domingues, P.H.; Nanduri, L.S.Y.; Seget, K.; Venkateswaran, S.V.; Agorku, D.; Vigano, C.; von Schubert, C.; Nigg, E.A.; Swanton, C.; Sotillo, R.; et al. Cellular Prion Protein PrP(C) and Ecto-5′-Nucleotidase Are Markers of the Cellular Stress Response to Aneuploidy. *Cancer Res.* **2017**, *77*, 2914–2926. [CrossRef]
31. Lee, J.H.; Yun, C.W.; Han, Y.S.; Kim, S.; Jeong, D.; Kwon, H.Y.; Kim, H.; Baek, M.J.; Lee, S.H. Melatonin and 5-fluorouracil co-suppress colon cancer stem cells by regulating cellular prion protein-Oct4 axis. *J. Pineal. Res.* **2018**, *65*, e12519. [CrossRef] [PubMed]
32. Bounhar, Y.; Zhang, Y.; Goodyer, C.G.; LeBlanc, A. Prion protein protects human neurons against Bax-mediated apoptosis. *J. Biol. Chem.* **2001**, *276*, 39145–39149. [CrossRef] [PubMed]
33. Roucou, X.; Giannopoulos, P.N.; Zhang, Y.; Jodoin, J.; Goodyer, C.G.; LeBlanc, A. Cellular prion protein inhibits proapoptotic Bax conformational change in human neurons and in breast carcinoma MCF-7 cells. *Cell Death Differ.* **2005**, *12*, 783–795. [CrossRef] [PubMed]

34. Yu, G.; Jiang, L.; Xu, Y.; Guo, H.; Liu, H.; Zhang, Y.; Yang, H.; Yuan, C.; Ma, J. Silencing prion protein in MDA-MB-435 breast cancer cells leads to pleiotropic cellular responses to cytotoxic stimuli. *PLoS ONE* **2012**, *7*, e48146. [CrossRef] [PubMed]
35. Lopes, M.H.; Hajj, G.N.; Muras, A.G.; Mancini, G.L.; Castro, R.M.; Ribeiro, K.C.; Brentani, R.R.; Linden, R.; Martins, V.R. Interaction of cellular prion and stress-inducible protein 1 promotes neuritogenesis and neuroprotection by distinct signaling pathways. *J. Neurosci.* **2005**, *25*, 11330–11339. [CrossRef] [PubMed]
36. Beraldo, F.H.; Arantes, C.P.; Santos, T.G.; Queiroz, N.G.; Young, K.; Rylett, R.J.; Markus, R.P.; Prado, M.A.; Martins, V.R. Role of alpha7 nicotinic acetylcholine receptor in calcium signaling induced by prion protein interaction with stress-inducible protein 1. *J. Biol. Chem.* **2010**, *285*, 36542–36550. [CrossRef]
37. Ostapchenko, V.G.; Beraldo, F.H.; Mohammad, A.H.; Xie, Y.F.; Hirata, P.H.; Magalhaes, A.C.; Lamour, G.; Li, H.; Maciejewski, A.; Belrose, J.C.; et al. The prion protein ligand, stress-inducible phosphoprotein 1, regulates amyloid-beta oligomer toxicity. *J. Neurosci.* **2013**, *33*, 16552–16564. [CrossRef]
38. Rachidi, W.; Vilette, D.; Guiraud, P.; Arlotto, M.; Riondel, J.; Laude, H.; Lehmann, S.; Favier, A. Expression of prion protein increases cellular copper binding and antioxidant enzyme activities but not copper delivery. *J. Biol. Chem.* **2003**, *278*, 9064–9072. [CrossRef]
39. Zeng, F.; Watt, N.T.; Walmsley, A.R.; Hooper, N.M. Tethering the N-terminus of the prion protein compromises the cellular response to oxidative stress. *J. Neurochem.* **2003**, *84*, 480–490. [CrossRef]
40. Brown, D.R.; Nicholas, R.S.; Canevari, L. Lack of prion protein expression results in a neuronal phenotype sensitive to stress. *J. Neurosci. Res.* **2002**, *67*, 211–224. [CrossRef]
41. Anantharam, V.; Kanthasamy, A.; Choi, C.J.; Martin, D.P.; Latchoumycandane, C.; Richt, J.A.; Kanthasamy, A.G. Opposing roles of prion protein in oxidative stress- and ER stress-induced apoptotic signaling. *Free Radic. Biol. Med.* **2008**, *45*, 1530–1541. [CrossRef] [PubMed]
42. Santuccione, A.; Sytnyk, V.; Leshchyns'ka, I.; Schachner, M. Prion protein recruits its neuronal receptor NCAM to lipid rafts to activate p59fyn and to enhance neurite outgrowth. *J. Cell Biol.* **2005**, *169*, 341–354. [CrossRef] [PubMed]
43. Llorens, F.; Carulla, P.; Villa, A.; Torres, J.M.; Fortes, P.; Ferrer, I.; del Rio, J.A. PrP(C) regulates epidermal growth factor receptor function and cell shape dynamics in Neuro2a cells. *J. Neurochem.* **2013**, *127*, 124–138. [CrossRef] [PubMed]
44. Loubet, D.; Dakowski, C.; Pietri, M.; Pradines, E.; Bernard, S.; Callebert, J.; Ardila-Osorio, H.; Mouillet-Richard, S.; Launay, J.M.; Kellermann, O.; et al. Neuritogenesis: The prion protein controls beta1 integrin signaling activity. *FASEB J.* **2012**, *26*, 678–690. [CrossRef]
45. Graner, E.; Mercadante, A.F.; Zanata, S.M.; Forlenza, O.V.; Cabral, A.L.; Veiga, S.S.; Juliano, M.A.; Roesler, R.; Walz, R.; Minetti, A.; et al. Cellular prion protein binds laminin and mediates neuritogenesis. *Brain Res. Mol. Brain Res.* **2000**, *76*, 85–92. [CrossRef]
46. Caetano, F.A.; Lopes, M.H.; Hajj, G.N.; Machado, C.F.; Pinto Arantes, C.; Magalhaes, A.C.; Vieira Mde, P.; Americo, T.A.; Massensini, A.R.; Priola, S.A.; et al. Endocytosis of prion protein is required for ERK1/2 signaling induced by stress-inducible protein 1. *J. Neurosci.* **2008**, *28*, 6691–6702. [CrossRef]
47. Lee, Y.J.; Baskakov, I.V. The cellular form of the prion protein guides the differentiation of human embryonic stem cells into neuron-, oligodendrocyte-, and astrocyte-committed lineages. *Prion* **2014**, *8*, 266–275. [CrossRef]
48. Steele, A.D.; Emsley, J.G.; Ozdinler, P.H.; Lindquist, S.; Macklis, J.D. Prion protein (PrPc) positively regulates neural precursor proliferation during developmental and adult mammalian neurogenesis. *Proc. Natl. Acad. Sci. USA* **2006**, *103*, 3416–3421. [CrossRef]
49. Miele, G.; Jeffrey, M.; Turnbull, D.; Manson, J.; Clinton, M. Ablation of cellular prion protein expression affects mitochondrial numbers and morphology. *Biochem. Biophys. Res. Commun.* **2002**, *291*, 372–377. [CrossRef]
50. Stella, R.; Cifani, P.; Peggion, C.; Hansson, K.; Lazzari, C.; Bendz, M.; Levander, F.; Sorgato, M.C.; Bertoli, A.; James, P. Relative quantification of membrane proteins in wild-type and prion protein (PrP)-knockout cerebellar granule neurons. *J. Proteome Res.* **2012**, *11*, 523–536. [CrossRef]
51. Liang, J.; Luo, G.; Ning, X.; Shi, Y.; Zhai, H.; Sun, S.; Jin, H.; Liu, Z.; Zhang, F.; Lu, Y.; et al. Differential expression of calcium-related genes in gastric cancer cells transfected with cellular prion protein. *Biochem. Cell Biol.* **2007**, *85*, 375–383. [CrossRef] [PubMed]

52. Li, Q.Q.; Cao, X.X.; Xu, J.D.; Chen, Q.; Wang, W.J.; Tang, F.; Chen, Z.Q.; Liu, X.P.; Xu, Z.D. The role of P-glycoprotein/cellular prion protein interaction in multidrug-resistant breast cancer cells treated with paclitaxel. *Cell Mol. Life Sci.* **2009**, *66*, 504–515. [CrossRef] [PubMed]
53. Le Corre, D.; Ghazi, A.; Balogoun, R.; Pilati, C.; Aparicio, T.; Martin-Lanneree, S.; Marisa, L.; Djouadi, F.; Poindessous, V.; Crozet, C.; et al. The cellular prion protein controls the mesenchymal-like molecular subtype and predicts disease outcome in colorectal cancer. *EBioMedicine* **2019**, *46*, 94–104. [CrossRef] [PubMed]
54. Li, Q.Q.; Sun, Y.P.; Ruan, C.P.; Xu, X.Y.; Ge, J.H.; He, J.; Xu, Z.D.; Wang, Q.; Gao, W.C. Cellular prion protein promotes glucose uptake through the Fyn-HIF-2alpha-Glut1 pathway to support colorectal cancer cell survival. *Cancer Sci.* **2011**, *102*, 400–406. [CrossRef]
55. Chieng, C.K.; Say, Y.H. Cellular prion protein contributes to LS 174T colon cancer cell carcinogenesis by increasing invasiveness and resistance against doxorubicin-induced apoptosis. *Tumour. Biol.* **2015**, *36*, 8107–8120. [CrossRef]
56. Lopes, M.H.; Santos, T.G.; Rodrigues, B.R.; Queiroz-Hazarbassanov, N.; Cunha, I.W.; Wasilewska-Sampaio, A.P.; Costa-Silva, B.; Marchi, F.A.; Bleggi-Torres, L.F.; Sanematsu, P.I.; et al. Disruption of prion protein-HOP engagement impairs glioblastoma growth and cognitive decline and improves overall survival. *Oncogene* **2015**, *34*, 3305–3314. [CrossRef]
57. Corsaro, A.; Bajetto, A.; Thellung, S.; Begani, G.; Villa, V.; Nizzari, M.; Pattarozzi, A.; Solari, A.; Gatti, M.; Pagano, A.; et al. Cellular prion protein controls stem cell-like properties of human glioblastoma tumor-initiating cells. *Oncotarget* **2016**, *7*, 38638–38657. [CrossRef]
58. Provenzano, L.; Ryan, Y.; Hilton, D.A.; Lyons-Rimmer, J.; Dave, F.; Maze, E.A.; Adams, C.L.; Rigby-Jones, R.; Ammoun, S.; Hanemann, C.O. Cellular prion protein (PrP(C)) in the development of Merlin-deficient tumours. *Oncogene* **2017**, *36*, 6132–6142. [CrossRef]
59. Liang, J.; Ge, F.; Guo, C.; Luo, G.; Wang, X.; Han, G.; Zhang, D.; Wang, J.; Li, K.; Pan, Y.; et al. Inhibition of PI3K/Akt partially leads to the inhibition of PrP(C)-induced drug resistance in gastric cancer cells. *FEBS J.* **2009**, *276*, 685–694. [CrossRef]
60. Liang, J.; Wang, J.; Luo, G.; Pan, Y.; Wang, X.; Guo, C.; Zhang, D.; Yin, F.; Zhang, X.; Liu, J.; et al. Function of PrPC (1-OPRD) in biological activities of gastric cancer cell lines. *J. Cell Mol. Med.* **2009**, *13*, 4453–4464. [CrossRef]
61. Li, C.; Xin, W.; Sy, M.S. Binding of pro-prion to filamin A: By design or an unfortunate blunder. *Oncogene* **2010**, *29*, 5329–5345. [CrossRef] [PubMed]
62. Wang, Y.; Yu, S.; Huang, D.; Cui, M.; Hu, H.; Zhang, L.; Wang, W.; Parameswaran, N.; Jackson, M.; Osborne, B.; et al. Cellular Prion Protein Mediates Pancreatic Cancer Cell Survival and Invasion through Association with and Enhanced Signaling of Notch1. *Am. J. Pathol.* **2016**, *186*, 2945–2956. [CrossRef] [PubMed]
63. Pan, Y.; Zhao, L.; Liang, J.; Liu, J.; Shi, Y.; Liu, N.; Zhang, G.; Jin, H.; Gao, J.; Xie, H.; et al. Cellular prion protein promotes invasion and metastasis of gastric cancer. *FASEB J.* **2006**, *20*, 1886–1888. [CrossRef]
64. De Lacerda, T.C.; Costa-Silva, B.; Giudice, F.S.; Dias, M.V.; de Oliveira, G.P.; Teixeira, B.L.; Dos Santos, T.G.; Martins, V.R. Prion protein binding to HOP modulates the migration and invasion of colorectal cancer cells. *Clin. Exp. Metastasis.* **2016**, *33*, 441–451. [CrossRef] [PubMed]
65. Li, C.; Yu, S.; Nakamura, F.; Pentikainen, O.T.; Singh, N.; Yin, S.; Xin, W.; Sy, M.S. Pro-prion binds filamin A, facilitating its interaction with integrin beta1, and contributes to melanomagenesis. *J. Biol. Chem.* **2010**, *285*, 30328–30339. [CrossRef] [PubMed]
66. Yang, L.; Gao, Z.; Hu, L.; Wu, G.; Yang, X.; Zhang, L.; Zhu, Y.; Wong, B.S.; Xin, W.; Sy, M.S.; et al. Glycosylphosphatidylinositol anchor modification machinery deficiency is responsible for the formation of pro-prion protein (PrP) in BxPC-3 cells and increases cancer cell motility. *J. Biol. Chem.* **2016**, *291*, 6785. [CrossRef] [PubMed]
67. Du, L.; Rao, G.; Wang, H.; Li, B.; Tian, W.; Cui, J.; He, L.; Laffin, B.; Tian, X.; Hao, C.; et al. CD44-positive cancer stem cells expressing cellular prion protein contribute to metastatic capacity in colorectal cancer. *Cancer Res.* **2013**, *73*, 2682–2694. [CrossRef]
68. Lu, W.; Kang, Y. Epithelial-Mesenchymal Plasticity in Cancer Progression and Metastasis. *Dev. Cell* **2019**, *49*, 361–374. [CrossRef]
69. Meslin, F.; Hamai, A.; Gao, P.; Jalil, A.; Cahuzac, N.; Chouaib, S.; Mehrpour, M. Silencing of prion protein sensitizes breast adriamycin-resistant carcinoma cells to TRAIL-mediated cell death. *Cancer Res.* **2007**, *67*, 10910–10919. [CrossRef]

70. Meslin, F.; Conforti, R.; Mazouni, C.; Morel, N.; Tomasic, G.; Drusch, F.; Yacoub, M.; Sabourin, J.C.; Grassi, J.; Delaloge, S.; et al. Efficacy of adjuvant chemotherapy according to Prion protein expression in patients with estrogen receptor-negative breast cancer. *Ann. Oncol.* **2007**, *18*, 1793–1798. [CrossRef]
71. Park, J.Y.; Jeong, J.K.; Lee, J.H.; Moon, J.H.; Kim, S.W.; Lee, Y.J.; Park, S.Y. Induction of cellular prion protein (PrPc) under hypoxia inhibits apoptosis caused by TRAIL treatment. *Oncotarget* **2015**, *6*, 5342–5353. [CrossRef] [PubMed]
72. Vassallo, N.; Herms, J.; Behrens, C.; Krebs, B.; Saeki, K.; Onodera, T.; Windl, O.; Kretzschmar, H.A. Activation of phosphatidylinositol 3-kinase by cellular prion protein and its role in cell survival. *Biochem. Biophys. Res. Commun.* **2005**, *332*, 75–82. [CrossRef] [PubMed]
73. Weise, J.; Sandau, R.; Schwarting, S.; Crome, O.; Wrede, A.; Schulz-Schaeffer, W.; Zerr, I.; Bahr, M. Deletion of cellular prion protein results in reduced Akt activation, enhanced postischemic caspase-3 activation, and exacerbation of ischemic brain injury. *Stroke* **2006**, *37*, 1296–1300. [CrossRef] [PubMed]
74. Lee, J.H.; Yun, C.W.; Lee, S.H. Cellular Prion Protein Enhances Drug Resistance of Colorectal Cancer Cells via Regulation of a Survival Signal Pathway. *Biomol. Ther. (Seoul)* **2018**, *26*, 313–321. [CrossRef] [PubMed]
75. Lee, J.H.; Yoon, Y.M.; Han, Y.S.; Yun, C.W.; Lee, S.H. Melatonin Promotes Apoptosis of Oxaliplatin-resistant Colorectal Cancer Cells Through Inhibition of Cellular Prion Protein. *Anticancer Res.* **2018**, *38*, 1993–2000. [CrossRef] [PubMed]
76. Go, G.; Yun, C.W.; Yoon, Y.M.; Lim, J.H.; Lee, J.H.; Lee, S.H. Role of PrP(C) in Cancer Stem Cell Characteristics and Drug Resistance in Colon Cancer Cells. *Anticancer Res.* **2020**, *40*, 5611–5620. [CrossRef]
77. Lee, J.H.; Han, Y.S.; Yoon, Y.M.; Yun, C.W.; Yun, S.P.; Kim, S.M.; Kwon, H.Y.; Jeong, D.; Baek, M.J.; Lee, H.J.; et al. Role of HSPA1L as a cellular prion protein stabilizer in tumor progression via HIF-1alpha/GP78 axis. *Oncogene* **2017**, *36*, 6555–6567. [CrossRef]
78. Al-Hajj, M.; Clarke, M.F. Self-renewal and solid tumor stem cells. *Oncogene* **2004**, *23*, 7274–7282. [CrossRef]
79. Beck, B.; Blanpain, C. Unravelling cancer stem cell potential. *Nat. Rev. Cancer* **2013**, *13*, 727–738. [CrossRef]
80. Ho, M.M.; Ng, A.V.; Lam, S.; Hung, J.Y. Side population in human lung cancer cell lines and tumors is enriched with stem-like cancer cells. *Cancer Res.* **2007**, *67*, 4827–4833. [CrossRef]
81. Tehranchi, R.; Woll, P.S.; Anderson, K.; Buza-Vidas, N.; Mizukami, T.; Mead, A.J.; Astrand-Grundstrom, I.; Strombeck, B.; Horvat, A.; Ferry, H.; et al. Persistent malignant stem cells in del(5q) myelodysplasia in remission. *N. Engl. J. Med.* **2010**, *363*, 1025–1037. [CrossRef]
82. Dean, M.; Fojo, T.; Bates, S. Tumour stem cells and drug resistance. *Nat. Rev. Cancer* **2005**, *5*, 275–284. [CrossRef] [PubMed]
83. Wang, Q.; Qian, J.; Wang, F.; Ma, Z. Cellular prion protein accelerates colorectal cancer metastasis via the Fyn-SP1-SATB1 axis. *Oncol. Rep.* **2012**, *28*, 2029–2034. [CrossRef] [PubMed]
84. Shibue, T.; Weinberg, R.A. EMT, CSCs, and drug resistance: The mechanistic link and clinical implications. *Nat. Rev. Clin. Oncol.* **2017**, *14*, 611–629. [CrossRef] [PubMed]
85. Cheng, Y.; Tao, L.; Xu, J.; Li, Q.; Yu, J.; Jin, Y.; Chen, Q.; Xu, Z.; Zou, Q.; Liu, X. CD44/cellular prion protein interact in multidrug resistant breast cancer cells and correlate with responses to neoadjuvant chemotherapy in breast cancer patients. *Mol. Carcinog.* **2014**, *53*, 686–697. [CrossRef]
86. Iglesia, R.P.; Prado, M.B.; Cruz, L.; Martins, V.R.; Santos, T.G.; Lopes, M.H. Engagement of cellular prion protein with the co-chaperone Hsp70/90 organizing protein regulates the proliferation of glioblastoma stem-like cells. *Stem Cell Res. Ther.* **2017**, *8*, 76. [CrossRef]
87. Kreso, A.; Dick, J.E. Evolution of the cancer stem cell model. *Cell Stem Cell* **2014**, *14*, 275–291. [CrossRef]
88. Kim, R.J.; Nam, J.S. OCT4 Expression Enhances Features of Cancer Stem Cells in a Mouse Model of Breast Cancer. *Lab. Anim. Res.* **2011**, *27*, 147–152. [CrossRef]
89. Yin, X.; Zhang, B.H.; Zheng, S.S.; Gao, D.M.; Qiu, S.J.; Wu, W.Z.; Ren, Z.G. Coexpression of gene Oct4 and Nanog initiates stem cell characteristics in hepatocellular carcinoma and promotes epithelial-mesenchymal transition through activation of Stat3/Snail signaling. *J. Hematol. Oncol.* **2015**, *8*, 23. [CrossRef]
90. Wang, Y.J.; Herlyn, M. The emerging roles of Oct4 in tumor-initiating cells. *Am. J. Physiol. Cell Physiol.* **2015**, *309*, C709–C718. [CrossRef]
91. Lin, Y.; Yang, Y.; Li, W.; Chen, Q.; Li, J.; Pan, X.; Zhou, L.; Liu, C.; Chen, C.; He, J.; et al. Reciprocal regulation of Akt and Oct4 promotes the self-renewal and survival of embryonal carcinoma cells. *Mol. Cell* **2012**, *48*, 627–640. [CrossRef] [PubMed]

92. Wang, X.Q.; Ongkeko, W.M.; Chen, L.; Yang, Z.F.; Lu, P.; Chen, K.K.; Lopez, J.P.; Poon, R.T.; Fan, S.T. Octamer 4 (Oct4) mediates chemotherapeutic drug resistance in liver cancer cells through a potential Oct4-AKT-ATP-binding cassette G2 pathway. *Hepatology* **2010**, *52*, 528–539. [CrossRef] [PubMed]
93. Sonati, T.; Reimann, R.R.; Falsig, J.; Baral, P.K.; O'Connor, T.; Hornemann, S.; Yaganoglu, S.; Li, B.; Herrmann, U.S.; Wieland, B.; et al. The toxicity of antiprion antibodies is mediated by the flexible tail of the prion protein. *Nature* **2013**, *501*, 102–106. [CrossRef]
94. Coitinho, A.S.; Lopes, M.H.; Hajj, G.N.; Rossato, J.I.; Freitas, A.R.; Castro, C.C.; Cammarota, M.; Brentani, R.R.; Izquierdo, I.; Martins, V.R. Short-term memory formation and long-term memory consolidation are enhanced by cellular prion association to stress-inducible protein 1. *NeuroBiol. Dis.* **2007**, *26*, 282–290. [CrossRef] [PubMed]
95. Jones, M.F.; Hara, T.; Francis, P.; Li, X.L.; Bilke, S.; Zhu, Y.; Pineda, M.; Subramanian, M.; Bodmer, W.F.; Lal, A. The CDX1-microRNA-215 axis regulates colorectal cancer stem cell differentiation. *Proc. Natl. Acad. Sci. USA* **2015**, *112*, E1550–E1558. [CrossRef] [PubMed]
96. Li, N.; Lorenzi, F.; Kalakouti, E.; Normatova, M.; Babaei-Jadidi, R.; Tomlinson, I.; Nateri, A.S. FBXW7-mutated colorectal cancer cells exhibit aberrant expression of phosphorylated-p53 at Serine-15. *Oncotarget* **2015**, *6*, 9240–9256. [CrossRef]
97. Zhang, T.; Kho, D.H.; Wang, Y.; Harazono, Y.; Nakajima, K.; Xie, Y.; Raz, A. Gp78, an E3 ubiquitin ligase acts as a gatekeeper suppressing nonalcoholic steatohepatitis (NASH) and liver cancer. *PLoS ONE* **2015**, *10*, e0118448. [CrossRef]
98. Tsai, Y.C.; Mendoza, A.; Mariano, J.M.; Zhou, M.; Kostova, Z.; Chen, B.; Veenstra, T.; Hewitt, S.M.; Helman, L.J.; Khanna, C.; et al. The ubiquitin ligase gp78 promotes sarcoma metastasis by targeting KAI1 for degradation. *Nat. Med.* **2007**, *13*, 1504–1509. [CrossRef]
99. Chang, Y.W.; Tseng, C.F.; Wang, M.Y.; Chang, W.C.; Lee, C.C.; Chen, L.T.; Hung, M.C.; Su, J.L. Deacetylation of HSPA5 by HDAC6 leads to GP78-mediated HSPA5 ubiquitination at K447 and suppresses metastasis of breast cancer. *Oncogene* **2016**, *35*, 1517–1528. [CrossRef]
100. Cruz, E.; Kayser, V. Monoclonal antibody therapy of solid tumors: Clinical limitations and novel strategies to enhance treatment efficacy. *Biologics* **2019**, *13*, 33–51. [CrossRef]
101. McEwan, J.F.; Windsor, M.L.; Cullis-Hill, S.D. Antibodies to prion protein inhibit human colon cancer cell growth. *Tumour. Biol.* **2009**, *30*, 141–147. [CrossRef] [PubMed]
102. Slamon, D.J.; Leyland-Jones, B.; Shak, S.; Fuchs, H.; Paton, V.; Bajamonde, A.; Fleming, T.; Eiermann, W.; Wolter, J.; Pegram, M.; et al. Use of chemotherapy plus a monoclonal antibody against HER2 for metastatic breast cancer that overexpresses HER2. *N. Engl. J. Med.* **2001**, *344*, 783–792. [CrossRef] [PubMed]
103. Graham, J.; Muhsin, M.; Kirkpatrick, P. Cetuximab. *Nat. Rev. Drug Discov.* **2004**, *3*, 549–550. [CrossRef] [PubMed]
104. Reslan, L.; Dalle, S.; Dumontet, C. Understanding and circumventing resistance to anticancer monoclonal antibodies. *MAbs* **2009**, *1*, 222–229. [CrossRef]
105. Viloria-Petit, A.; Crombet, T.; Jothy, S.; Hicklin, D.; Bohlen, P.; Schlaeppi, J.M.; Rak, J.; Kerbel, R.S. Acquired resistance to the antitumor effect of epidermal growth factor receptor-blocking antibodies in vivo: A role for altered tumor angiogenesis. *Cancer Res.* **2001**, *61*, 5090–5101.
106. Sutherland, M.S.; Sanderson, R.J.; Gordon, K.A.; Andreyka, J.; Cerveny, C.G.; Yu, C.; Lewis, T.S.; Meyer, D.L.; Zabinski, R.F.; Doronina, S.O.; et al. Lysosomal trafficking and cysteine protease metabolism confer target-specific cytotoxicity by peptide-linked anti-CD30-auristatin conjugates. *J. Biol. Chem.* **2006**, *281*, 10540–10547. [CrossRef]
107. Verma, S.; Miles, D.; Gianni, L.; Krop, I.E.; Welslau, M.; Baselga, J.; Pegram, M.; Oh, D.Y.; Dieras, V.; Guardino, E.; et al. Trastuzumab emtansine for HER2-positive advanced breast cancer. *N. Engl. J. Med.* **2012**, *367*, 1783–1791. [CrossRef]
108. Hardy-Werbin, M.; Quiroga, V.; Cirauqui, B.; Romeo, M.; Felip, E.; Teruel, I.; Garcia, J.J.; Erasun, C.; Espana, S.; Cucurull, M.; et al. Real-world data on T-DM1 efficacy - results of a single-center retrospective study of HER2-positive breast cancer patients. *Sci. Rep.* **2019**, *9*, 12760. [CrossRef]
109. Von Minckwitz, G.; Huang, C.S.; Mano, M.S.; Loibl, S.; Mamounas, E.P.; Untch, M.; Wolmark, N.; Rastogi, P.; Schneeweiss, A.; Redondo, A.; et al. Trastuzumab Emtansine for Residual Invasive HER2-Positive Breast Cancer. *N. Engl. J. Med.* **2019**, *380*, 617–628. [CrossRef]

110. Kim, Y.C.; Won, S.Y.; Jeong, B.H. Identification of Prion Disease-Related Somatic Mutations in the Prion Protein Gene (PRNP) in Cancer Patients. *Cells* **2020**, *9*, 1480. [CrossRef]
111. Gill, O.N.; Spencer, Y.; Richard-Loendt, A.; Kelly, C.; Brown, D.; Sinka, K.; Andrews, N.; Dabaghian, R.; Simmons, M.; Edwards, P.; et al. Prevalence in Britain of abnormal prion protein in human appendices before and after exposure to the cattle BSE epizootic. *Acta Neuropathol.* **2020**, *139*, 965–976. [CrossRef] [PubMed]

3

Hypoxia and Macrophages Act in Concert Towards a Beneficial Outcome in Colon Cancer

Flávia Martins [1,2,3,4,†], Rosa Oliveira [1,2,†], Bruno Cavadas [1,3], Filipe Pinto [1,3], Ana Patrícia Cardoso [1,2], Flávia Castro [1,2,5], Bárbara Sousa [1,3], Marta Laranjeiro Pinto [1,2,6], Ana João Silva [1,2], Diogo Adão [1,2], José Pedro Loureiro [1,7], Nicole Pedro [1,3], Rui Manuel Reis [8,9,10], Luísa Pereira [1,3,4], Maria José Oliveira [1,2,4,5] and Angela Margarida Costa [1,2,*]

1 i3S-Institute for Research and Innovation in Health, University of Porto, 4200-135 Porto, Portugal
2 INEB-Institute of Biomedical Engineering, University of Porto, 4200-135 Porto, Portugal
3 IPATIMUP-Institute of Molecular Pathology and Immunology, University of Porto, 4200-135 Porto, Portugal
4 Department of Pathology and Oncology, Faculty of Medicine, University of Porto, 4200-319 Porto, Portugal
5 ICBAS-Institute of Biomedical Sciences Abel Salazar, University of Porto, 4050-313 Porto, Portugal
6 CNC-Center for Neuroscience and Cell Biology, University of Coimbra, 3004-517 Coimbra, Portugal
7 IBMC-Institute of Molecular and Cellular Biology, University of Porto, 4200-135 Porto, Portugal
8 Molecular Oncology Research Center, Barretos Cancer Hospital, 14.784-400 Barretos-SP, Brazil
9 Life and Health Sciences Research Institute (ICVS), School of Medicine, University of Minho, 4710-057 Braga, Portugal
10 ICVS/3B's-PT Government Associate Laboratory, 4710-057 Braga, Portugal
* Correspondence: angela.amorimcosta@ineb.up.pt
† These authors contributed equally to this paper.

Abstract: In colon cancer, the prognostic value of macrophages is controversial, and it is still unknown how hypoxia modulates macrophage–cancer cell crosstalk. To unravel this, co-cultures of human primary macrophages and colon cancer cells were performed at 20% and 1% O_2, followed by characterization of both cellular components. Different colon cancer patient cohorts were analyzed for hypoxia and immune markers, and their association with patient overall survival was established. A positive correlation between *HIF1A* and *CD68* in colon cancer patients was identified but, unexpectedly, in cases with higher macrophage infiltration, *HIF1A* expression was associated with a better prognosis, in contrast to breast, gastric, and lung cancers. Under hypoxia, co-cultures' secretome indicated a shift towards a pro-inflammatory phenotype. These alterations occurred along with increased macrophage phagocytic activity and decreased SIRPα expression. Cancer cells were more invasive and exhibited higher CD47 expression. We hypothesize that the better prognosis associated with $HIF1A^{High}CD68^{High}$ tumors could occur due to macrophagic pro-inflammatory pressure. Indeed, we found that tumors $HIF1A^{High}CD68^{High}$ expressed increased levels of *CD8A*, which is positively correlated with *HIF1A*. In conclusion, we show that in colon cancer, hypoxia drives macrophages into a pro-inflammatory phenotype, concomitant with increased infiltration of anti-tumor immune cells, favoring better disease outcome.

Keywords: hypoxia; macrophages; colon cancer; tumor microenvironment; immune cell infiltration; prognosis

1. Introduction

It is recognized that the non-malignant component of the tumor microenvironment (TM) has a pivotal role in both tumorigenesis and tumor progression. To improve cancer therapy, it is crucial to better understand cancer cell behavior and the associated molecular mechanisms, which cannot be achieved without knowing how the different TM components influence each other's behavior, driving disease outcomes. As an ecosystem, the TM is composed of different entities besides cancer cells, namely, immune cells, fibroblasts, adipocytes, and the extracellular matrix (ECM), which communicate and modulate each other's activities [1].

Macrophages are abundant in the TM, and their high infiltration is associated, in several malignancies, with poor prognosis and therapy resistance [2]. Due to their plasticity, macrophages can polarize into pro-inflammatory and anti-tumor or into anti-inflammatory and pro-tumor [3], being, therefore, interesting therapeutic targets. In fact, it is known that a pro-inflammatory environment is a driving force for the tumorigenic process, driving mutagenesis, while in the context of an established tumor, the pro-inflammatory environment could favor the elimination of already-transformed cells [4].

In colon cancer, the role of macrophages is controversial, with some authors claiming that a high infiltration is associated with better prognosis, while others report that their presence is associated with increased tumor progression-associated activities [5]. Our group has previously evidenced that macrophages induce gastric and colon cancer cell invasion, in a process partially mediated by secreted factors, and that the secretome of macrophages differs from that of macrophages co-cultured with cancer cells [6].

Due to aberrant cancer cell growth and abnormal vascularization, the TM is generally hypoxic. This condition leads to reactive oxygen species accumulation and acidosis, both associated with enhanced invasion, metastasis, and therapy resistance [7], hypoxia being an independent prognostic factor in several types of cancer [8]. Nevertheless, the mechanisms through which hypoxia interferes with the non-malignant components of TM are still a matter of study.

It has been reported that macrophages preferentially accumulate within tumor hypoxic regions, and that hypoxia leads to the genetic reprogramming of both cancer cells and macrophages, mainly through hypoxia inducible factor (HIF) transcription factors. HIF1α, the most important of them, is constitutively expressed and is targeted to degradation at normal oxygen tension, but stabilized under hypoxia [9,10]. The activation of HIF downstream targets leads to cellular adjustments such as metabolic alterations and expression of ECM-remodeling enzymes [11]. It is also known that HIF can affect the immunogenicity of hypoxic breast cancer by inducing the expression of CD47, a cell surface receptor that impairs macrophage pro-phagocytic signaling [12]. Due to its importance, HIF-inhibitors are under consideration as anti-cancer agents [13]. However, the experiments studying the colon cancer cells–macrophages interplay were not performed under hypoxia, nor were the studies about hypoxia focused on this crosstalk, resulting in an incomplete understanding of the role of hypoxia in the colon cancer microenvironment. Giving the controversial role of macrophages in colon cancer, the study of this interplay will provide a deeper understanding of the colon cancer microenvironment complexity.

In the present study, we characterize the effect of low oxygen levels on macrophage behavior and the modulation of macrophages and cancer cells crosstalk. The influence of hypoxia and macrophages is also analyzed in different cohorts of colon cancer patients. The data gathered in this work increases the insight on colon TM specificity and provides information that can result in the development of novel and more efficient therapeutic strategies.

2. Results

2.1. CD68 and HIF1A Are Positively Correlated in Colon Cancer Patients, and the Population $CD68^{High}HIF1A^{High}$ Presents Better Prognosis

To understand the relevance of hypoxia on the modulation of macrophage behavior in colon cancer patients, we took advantage of TCGA and Oncomine databases. Therefore, the expression levels of

CD68, a macrophage lineage marker, and of *HIF1A*, a master hypoxia regulator, in which slight mRNA changes can cause significant alterations in its activity and protein levels, were analyzed [14]. Since TCGA compiles expression data from normal and cancer colon tissues, we focused our analysis in *HIF1A* in *CD68*^{High} and *CD68*^{Low} populations, in both tissues, assuming that *CD68*^{High} population has a higher degree of macrophagic infiltration. As normal colon tissue could have some endogenous degree of inflammation, the threshold used to subdivide the population between *CD68*^{High} and *CD68*^{Low} was defined based on the median *CD68* expression in the normal tissue. Moreover, we found that *HIF1A* expression was significantly higher in tumors from patients with elevated macrophage infiltration (*CD68*^{High}) and that *CD68* expression positively correlated with *HIF1A* expression (Figure 1A). It is described that colon carcinomas exhibit increased nuclear expression of HIF1-α [15]. However, as it may be rapidly targeted to degradation, we evaluated the expression levels of HIF1-α downstream targets that are upregulated under hypoxia conditions, specifically *CA9* and *LOX* (Figure 1B). Using the previous approach, we found a significant increase in *CA9* and *LOX* expression in tumor tissue, which was significantly more pronounced in *CD68*^{High} patients (Figure 1B). Due to the present focus on the role of macrophages on the TM, we particularly evaluated the *CD68*^{High} population. By dividing this population between *HIF1A*^{High} and *HIF1A*^{Low}, we found that *CA9* and *LOX* expression levels are significantly higher in the *HIF1A*^{High} population (Figure 1C). The positive correlation between *CD68* and *HIF1A*, and the increased *CA9* and *LOX* expression in *CD68*^{High}*HIF1A*^{High} patients were validated on the Oncomine database (colon cancer Bittner cohort, with the highest number of patients) (Figure 1D). *CA9* or LOX were not used in further analysis as hypoxic markers due to statistical constraints when the number of patients needed to be sub-divided into *CD68*^{High} and *CD68*^{Low}, and *HIF1A*^{High} and *HIF1A*^{Low}.

A major point of interest was to investigate whether the association between high macrophage infiltration and enhanced expression of hypoxic markers had any impact on patient prognosis. Surprisingly, we found that the *CD68*^{High}*HIF1A*^{High} population presented a significantly better prognosis than the CD68^{High}*HIF1A*^{Low} population (Figure 1E). To check whether this was a common feature in cancers where macrophagic infiltration was associated with prognosis, we used the same TCGA approach to analyze gastric, breast, and lung cancer patients. Despite the low number of patients in some populations, this specific association only occur in colon cancer (Figure 1F). The same analysis was not performed in the Oncomine cohort since survival data is not available.

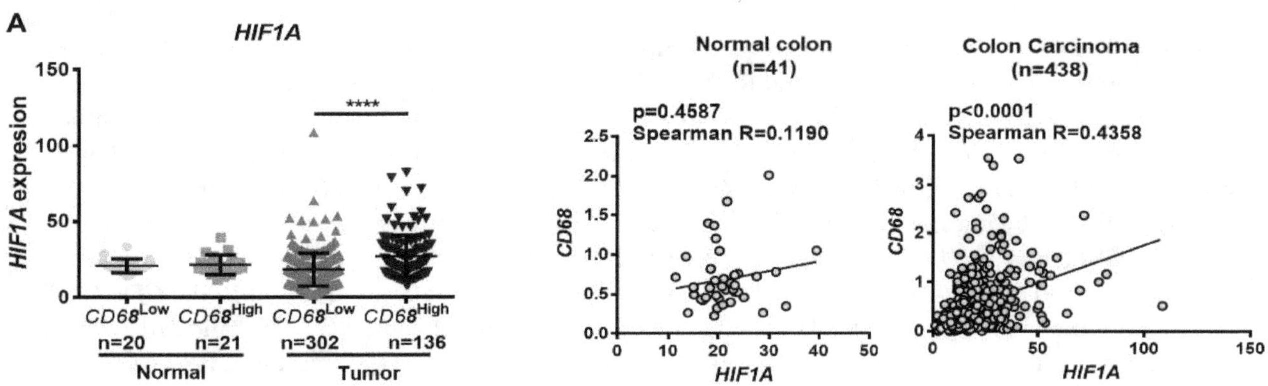

Figure 1. *Cont.*

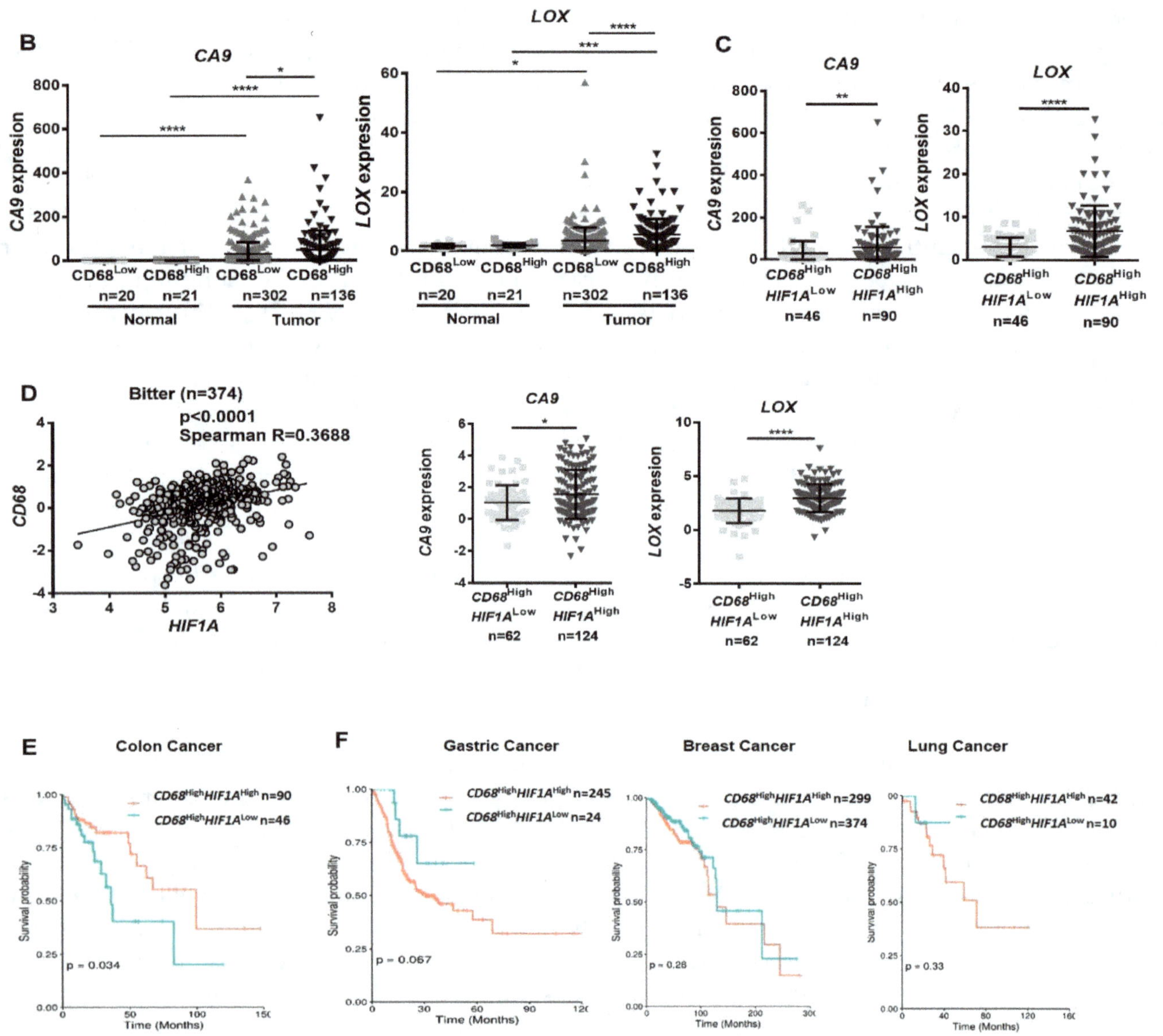

Figure 1. *CD68* and *HIF1A* are positively correlated in colon cancer, and *CD68*^{High}*HIF1A*^{High} tumors present better prognosis. Microarray and RNASeq expression data were downloaded from The Cancer Genome Atlas (TCGA) (**A–C**, **E–F**) and from Oncomine databases (**D**). (**A–C**) Normal and tumor samples were divided into *CD68*^{Low} and *CD68*^{High}, according to the median levels of *CD68* expression in normal samples. In each group, the expression of the hypoxic marker *HIF1A* (**A**), *CA9* and *LOX* (**B**,**C**) genes, known to be regulated by HIF1α in hypoxic conditions, was evaluated. (**A**) The correlation between *CD68* and *HIF1A* was assessed. (**B**,**C**) The expression of *CA9* and *LOX* was evaluated in both normal and tumor samples, in *CD68*^{High} and *CD68*^{Low} populations, and within the *CD68*^{High} population, the expression levels of both genes were compared between *HIF1A*^{Low} and *HIF1A*^{High}, according to the median levels of *HIF1A* expression in normal samples. (**D**) Correlations between *CD68* and *HIF1A*, and *LOX* and *CA9* expression in *CD68*^{High}*HIF1A*^{High} patients were confirmed on Bittner's colon cancer cohort from Oncomine. (**E**,**F**) Kaplan–Meier curves were made with patients' survival data, comparing the populations *CD68*^{High}*HIF1A*^{High} and *CD68*^{High}*HIF1A*^{Low}. The division high/low expression was made according to the median expression of the selected genes in normal tissue (**A–C**; **E–F**), or by the median expression of tumor (**D**). Data from colon (**E**), gastric, breast, and lung (**F**) cancer patients were analyzed. Kruskal–Wallis, Mann–Whitney, or unpaired *t*-test were used to compare gene expression among groups. Spearman's statistical test was used to assess correlation, which was considered moderate positive when Spearman Rs were between 0.2500 and 0.3500, and strong positive when Spearman R > 0.3500. Long-rank (Mantel–Cox) test was performed in the analysis of the survival curves. **** $p < 0.0001$; *** $p < 0.001$; ** $p < 0.01$; * $p < 0.05$.

2.2. *Hypoxia Impacts Macrophage Antigen-Presentation Associated Molecules*

In order to understand the impact of the hypoxic microenvironment on macrophage–colon cancer cell crosstalk, and particularly on macrophage function, indirect co-cultures of macrophages with cancer cells were established at both 20% and 1% O_2 (Figure S1A). The significant increase in cancer cell *CA9* expression at 1% O_2 validates the cellular sensing of the hypoxic stimulus, to which both cells were simultaneously exposed to (Figure S1B), without affecting cellular viability between the conditions (Figure S1C). This indirect co-culture system enables the analysis of differences induced by exchanged secreted factors, but in conditions that allow the full recovery of both cellular populations for further independent studies. The selection of primary macrophages instead of the widely used and modified human monocytic cell line, THP-1, added variability to our equation, being more representative of the existent individual differences. Besides more closely mimicking the TM, human macrophages were preferred in relation to their murine counterparts, given the described interspecies variability regarding polarization markers and activation programs [16].

Macrophages are professional antigen-presenting cells, and immune evasion of cancer cells is a major cancer hallmark. To analyze whether hypoxia can trigger some alterations in the expression of key molecules involved in antigen presentation, macrophage major histocompatibility complexes (MHC) class I (HLA–ABC) and class II (HLA–DR) molecules, and of the co-stimulatory receptor CD86, were investigated by flow cytometry (gating strategy described in Figure S2A). Our results at 1% O_2 evidenced a slight reduction in the percentage of macrophages expressing HLA–ABC ($p < 0.0533$) and CD86 ($p < 0.0938$) (Figure 2A,B,D), with a significant decrease in the percentage of cells expressing HLA–DR (Figure 2A,C) and in the intensity of CD86 expressed by each cell (Figure 2A,D).

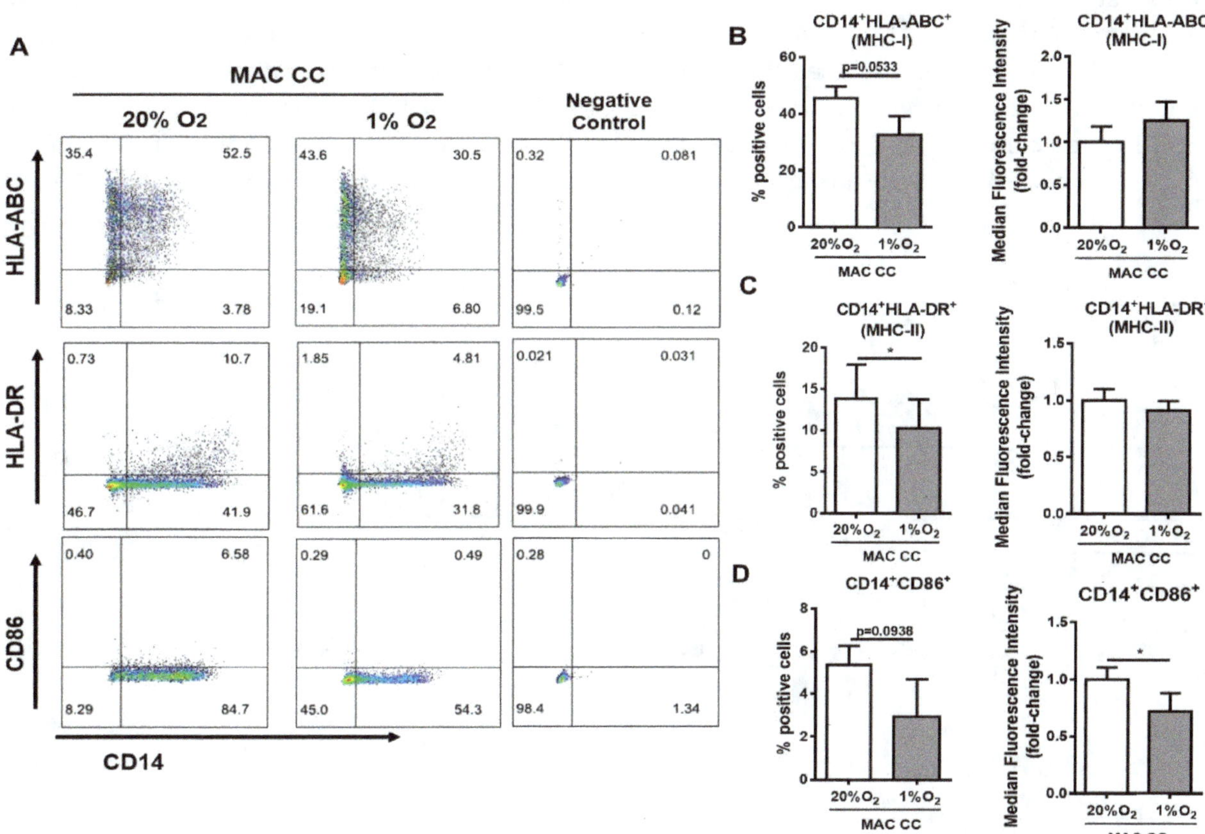

Figure 2. Hypoxia impacts macrophage antigen-presentation associated molecules. Macrophages were indirectly co-cultured with colon cancer cells RKO (MAC CC), at 20% or 1% O_2 for 72 h. Expression of the monocyte/macrophage lineage marker CD14, HLA-ABC (MHC-I), HLA-DR (MHC-II), and CD86 was determined by flow cytometry. (**A**) Pseudo-color plots display the gating strategy for flow cytometry created with FlowJo. (**B–D**) Graphs represent the percentage and median fluorescence

intensity, which is presented as fold-change relatively to 20% O_2 condition of (**B**) CD14+HLA-ABC+, (**C**) CD14+HLA-DR+, or (**D**) CD14+CD86+ cells. Graphs represent the mean values with standard deviations, and are representative of $n = 7$ (HLA-ABC); $n = 10$ (HLA-DR); $n = 6$ (CD86) independent experiments. The statistical tests Wilcox or paired t-test were used; * $p < 0.05$. The p-values between 0.05 and 0.1 were presented and considered a tendency.

2.3. Hypoxia Modulates Macrophage Phagocytic Activity and SIRPα Expression, and CD47 Expression on Cancer Cells

One of the major functions of macrophages is to phagocyte foreign or self-cellular components targeted to degradation. This is particularly important in the context of macrophage defensive functions against pathogens, their role in regeneration, and also in anti-tumor activities. Noteworthy, it is known that cancer cells express "don't eat me" signals, as the CD47 receptor, which will bind to SIRPα in macrophages, and impairs phagocytosis.

In the present study, we exploited whether hypoxia alters macrophage phagocytic activity, in a similar process already described in breast cancer [12], using hypoxic cancer cells as a phagocytic stimulus. Accordingly, macrophages were co-cultured with cancer cells for 72 h at 20% or 1% O_2 (Figure S1A). Then, cancer cells were removed, and macrophages were directly stimulated with CFSE (Carboxyfluorescein Diacetate Succinimidyl Ester)-labeled cancer cells, previously cultured at 1% O_2 for 72 h. Although no differences were observed in the percentage of phagocytic macrophages, the amount of phagocyted CFSE-labeled cancer cells almost doubled on macrophages pre-conditioned by hypoxia and cancer cells (Figure 3A and Figure S2A,B). Afterwards, we explored alterations in SIRPα levels in the phagocytic macrophages, those engulfing CFSE+ cancer cells (CD14+CFSE+). Interestingly, we found a significant decrease in the percentage of phagocytic macrophages expressing SIRPα, when previously maintained at 1% O_2 in comparison to those at 20% O_2 (Figure 3B and Figure S2A,B). Based on these results, we further analyzed the SIRPα expression in macrophages and CD47 in cancer cells from the indirect co-cultures, maintained for 72 h at 20% or 1% O_2, before the direct contact with the CFSE-labeled cancer cells. Notably, we found that the co-cultures were already sufficient to trigger a decrease in macrophage SIRPα (Figure 3C), and an increase in cancer cells CD47 (Figure 3D).

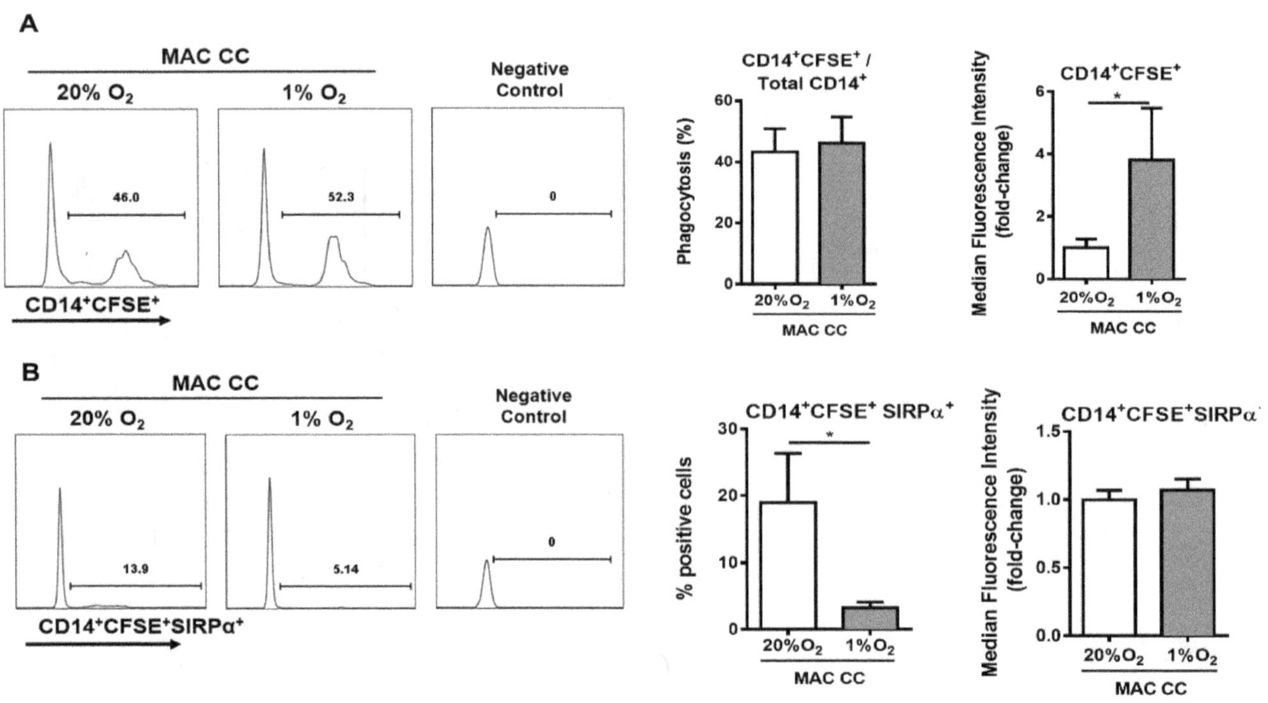

Figure 3. *Cont.*

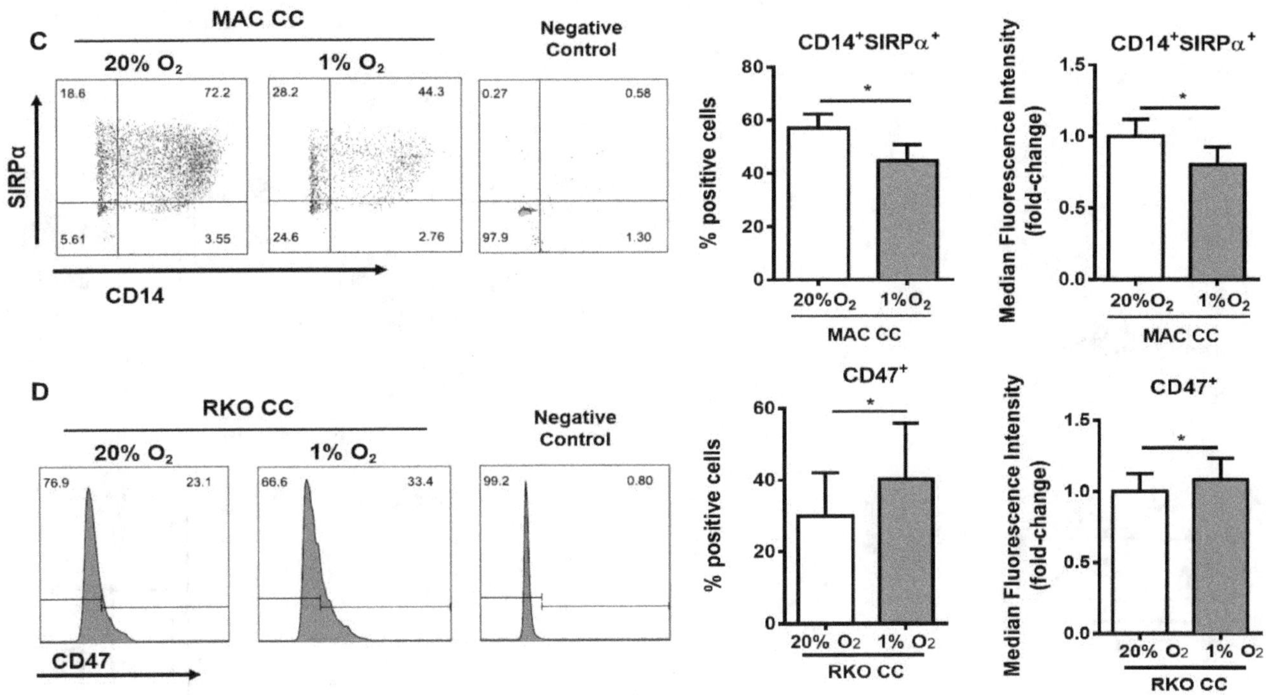

Figure 3. Hypoxia modulates macrophage phagocytic activity and SIRPα expression and CD47 expression on cancer cells. (**A**,**B**) Macrophages that were indirectly co-cultured with RKO (MAC CC) cells, at 20% or 1% O_2 for 72 h, were posteriorly directly stimulated with CFSE-labeled RKO cells for 2 h. Macrophages were analyzed by flow cytometry. Histograms display the gating strategy for flow cytometry created with FlowJo. (**A**) Phagocytic activity was calculated as the ratio of CD14+CFSE+ cells/Total CD14+ cells. (**B**) Graphs represent the percentage of CD14+CFSE+SIRPα+ cells, and the median fluorescence intensity, which is presented as fold-change relatively to 20% O_2 condition. (**C**,**D**) Macrophages were indirectly co-cultured with RKO, at 20% or 1% O_2 for 72 h. Expression of the monocyte/macrophage lineage marker CD14 and SIRPα was evaluated on macrophages (**C**) and of CD47 on cancer cells (**D**) by flow cytometry. Pseudo-color plots (**C**) and histograms (**D**) display the gating strategy for flow cytometry. Graphs represent the percentage and median fluorescence intensity, which is presented as fold-change relatively to 20% O_2 condition of (**C**) CD14+SIRPα+, or (**D**) CD47 cells. Graphs represent the mean values with standard deviations, and are representative of $n = 11$ (phagocytosis); $n = 7$ (CFSE+SIRPα+); $n = 10$ (SIRPα); $n = 11$ (CD47) independent experiments. The statistical tests Wilcox or paired t-test were used; * $p < 0.05$.

2.4. Hypoxia Decreases the Anti-Inflammatory Pressure and Increases IL-1β Secretion

It is described that, depending on the stimulation, macrophages may polarize as pro- or anti-inflammatory, sustaining thereafter anti- or pro-tumor activities, respectively [3]. Therefore, we investigated the impact of hypoxia on the polarization profile of macrophages co-cultured with cancer cells, analyzing the expression of a panel of pro- and anti-inflammatory markers [17] by flow cytometry and ELISA. Despite the fact that hypoxia is usually associated with a worse prognosis and with cellular features related to tumor progression, we found that 1% O_2 treatment resulted in a mixed macrophage phenotype, with alterations in both pro and anti-inflammatory markers. However, the clear decrease in anti-inflammatory markers CD163, TGFβ, CCL18, and IL-10 (Figure 4A,B), along with the increased expression of the pro-inflammatory cytokine IL-1β (Figure 4B), which seems to sustain a hypoxia-induced pro-inflammatory effect, is relevant. Nevertheless, we also observed a significant decrease in pro-inflammatory marker CCR7 (Figure 4A).

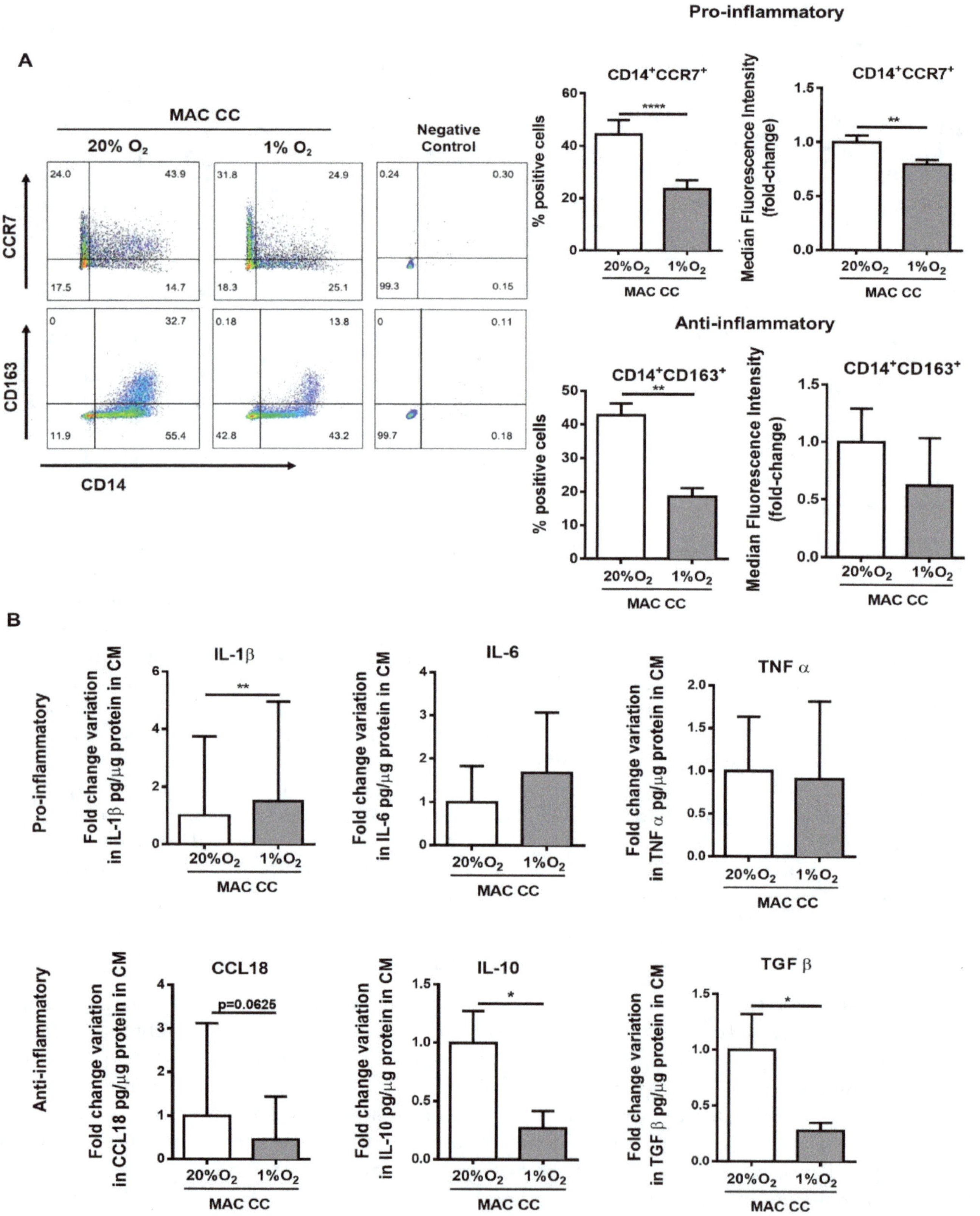

Figure 4. Hypoxia decreases the anti-inflammatory pressure and increases IL-1β secretion. Macrophages were indirectly co-cultured with RKO (MAC CC), at 20% or 1% O_2 for 72 h. (**A**) Expression of CD14 and of the polarization markers CCR7 and CD163 was evaluated on macrophages by flow cytometry. Pseudo-color plots display the gating strategy for flow cytometry. Graphs represent the percentage and median fluorescence intensity, which is presented as fold-change relatively to 20% O_2 condition.

(**B**) Concentration of secreted molecules was measured by ELISA, and normalized to conditioned media (CM) protein levels. Graphs represent cytokine concentration of pro- and anti-inflammatory markers, as a fold change variation to macrophages cultured at 20% O_2. Graphs display the mean values with standard deviations, and are representative of $n = 12$ (CCR7); $n = 5$ (CD163); $n = 10$ (IL-1β); $n = 8$ (IL-6); $n = 5$ (TNF-α); $n = 5$ (CCL18); $n = 5$ (IL-10); $n = 7$ (TGF-β) independent experiments. The statistical tests Wilcox or paired *t*-test were used **** $p < 0.0001$; ** $p < 0.01$; * $p < 0.05$. The *p*-values between 0.05 and 0.1 were presented and considered a tendency.

2.5. Hypoxia Impacts Colon Cancer Cell Behavior, Increasing Invasion and Glucose Consumption

Given the alterations in macrophage behavior induced by the hypoxic environment, as well as differences regarding a patient's overall survival, we decided to assess whether hypoxia and macrophages influence cancer cell behavior.

No differences were observed in both cell proliferation and cell death in cancer cells when co-cultured with macrophages at 20% or 1% O_2 (Figure 5A,B).

As it is well reported that hypoxia can modulate cancer cell metabolism favoring glycolysis, we evaluated the levels of glucose consumption, lactate production, and pH in indirect co-cultures media, established at 20% and 1% O_2. It is important to note that the glucose and lactate levels in co-cultures conditioned media (CM) results from both macrophages and cancer cells, being impossible to discriminate the specific contribution of each cellular population. To obtain additional information, cancer cell expression levels of *SLC2A1*, the gene that codifies the glucose transporter GLUT-1, and of *LDHA*, the gene that codifies an enzyme involved in lactate production were also analyzed. Interestingly, at 1% O_2, we found a significant increase in glucose consumption, which was accompanied by enhanced expression of the glucose-transporter codifying gene (*SLC2A1*) (Figure 5C). Nevertheless, no differences in lactate production were observed, despite the increase in *LDHA* expression, as well as a significant decrease in pH levels (Figure 5C). Noteworthy, all the differences found resulted from the combination of both macrophages and hypoxia.

When we looked into the invasive capacity of cancer cells, we observed that macrophages and hypoxia alone were sufficient to promote cancer cell invasion and, most importantly, this is potentiated when both factors are combined (Figure 5D).

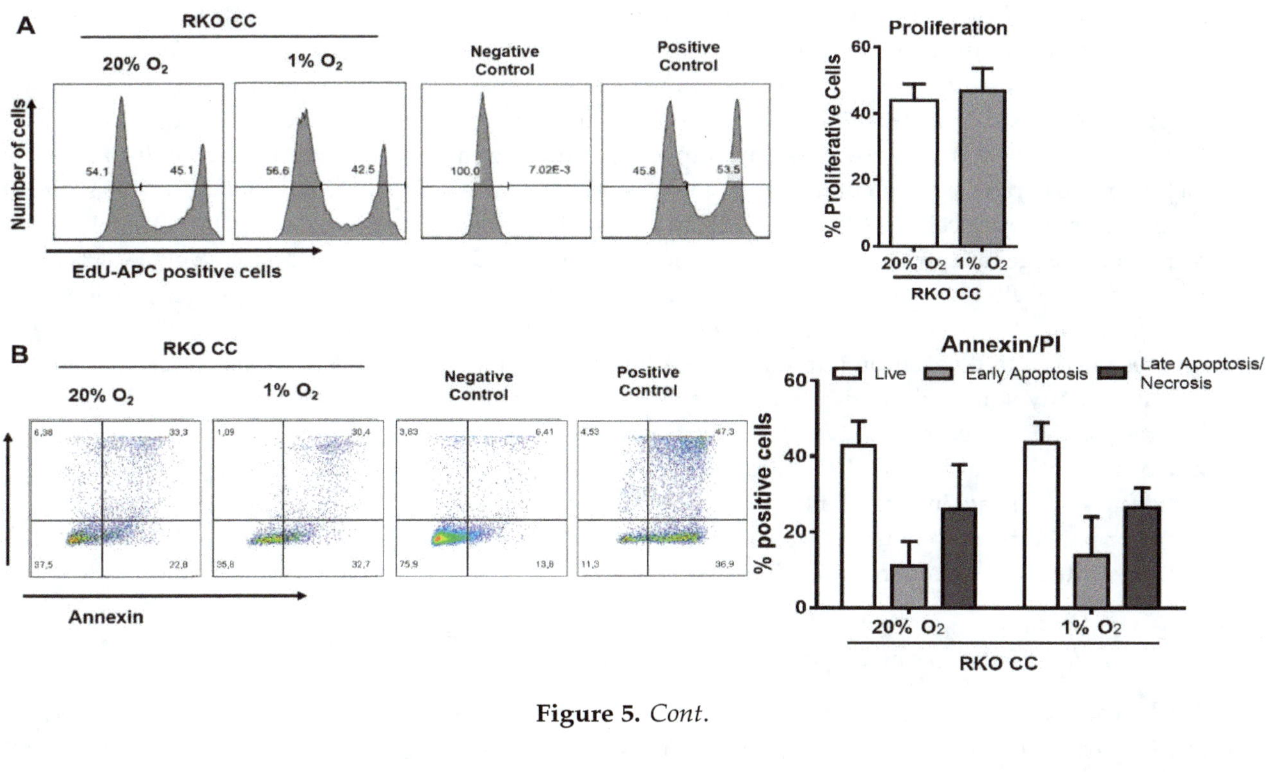

Figure 5. *Cont.*

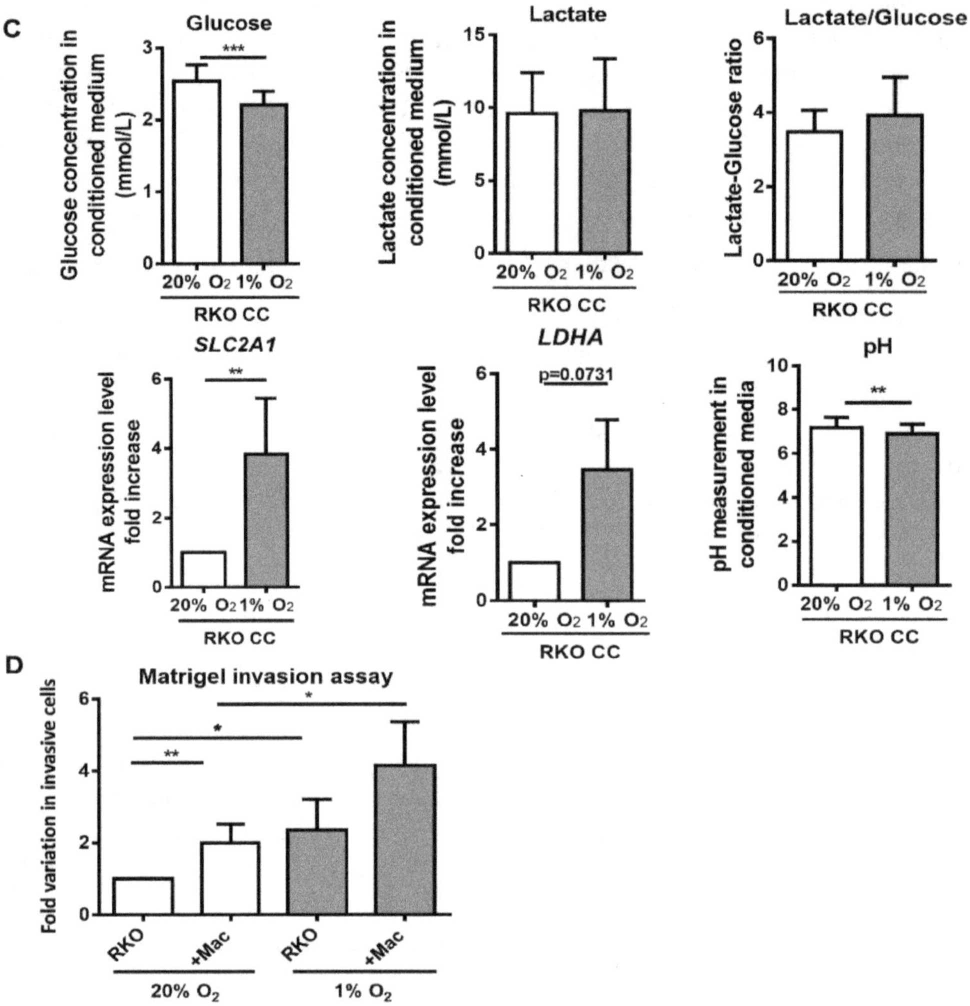

Figure 5. Hypoxia impacts colon cancer cell behavior, increasing invasion and glucose consumption. (**A–C**) Macrophages were indirectly co-cultured with RKO, at 20% or 1% O_2 for 72 h, and (**A**) proliferation of cancer cells was assessed for that period. Data are presented as percentage of proliferative cells. (**B**) AnnexinV/PI assay was used to quantify the percentage of viable (AnnexinV/PI negative), early apoptotic (AnnexinV positive/PI negative), and late apoptotic/necrotic (Annexin V/PI positive) cells. (**C**) Lactate production, glucose consumption, and pH measurements were made on co-cultures CM. Lactate/glucose ratio was calculated with the glucose and lactate concentration values of the same experiments. Cancer cells *SLC2A1* and *LDHA* mRNA levels were measured by qRT–PCR. Relative expression changes are presented as fold variation *SLC2A1/ACTB* and *LDHA/ACTB* relatively to 20% O_2 condition. (**D**) Cells maintained at 20% or 1% O_2, and stimulated or not with macrophages previously maintained at 20% or 1% O_2 were cultured for 24 h on Matrigel coated filters, at 20% or 1% O_2. Data are presented as fold variation in the number of invasive cells relative to RKO cells cultured at 20% O_2 without any stimulation with macrophages. Graphs represent the mean values with standard deviations, and are representative of $n = 5$ (proliferation assay); $n = 6$ (Annexin V/PI assay); $n = 10$ (glucose quantification); $n = 11$ (lactate quantification); $n = 6$ (*SLC2A1*); $n = 5$ (*LDHA*); $n = 9$ (pH); $n = 10$ (invasion assay) independent experiments. The statistical tests Friedman, RM one-way ANOVA, Wilcox or paired *t*-test were used *** $p < 0.001$; ** $p < 0.01$; * $p < 0.05$. The *p*-values between 0.05 and 0.1 were presented and considered a tendency.

2.6. Colon Cancer Patients with CD68^{High}HIF1A^{High} Phenotype Present Increased Expression of Pro-Inflammatory Cytokines and Iincreased Infiltration of Cytotoxic T-Cells

While the in vitro results indicated that hypoxia was associated with features related both with worse prognosis (increased invasion, decreased expression of macrophage antigen-presenting molecules) and good prognosis (increase in phagocytosis and secretion of pro-inflammatory cytokines), the colon cancer patient's survival data evidenced that the *CD68*^{High}*HIF1A*^{High} population correlates with better prognosis. These led us to hypothesize that the in vitro cellular features associated with better prognosis may prevail in vivo, particularly the secretion of pro-inflammatory cytokines, which could lead to the recruitment of other anti-tumor immune cells.

Initially, the expression of the three pro-inflammatory cytokines previously analyzed, IL-1β, IL-6, and TNF-α, were compared between *CD68*^{High}*HIF1A*^{High} and *CD68*^{High}*HIF1A*^{Low} patients, using the TCGA and Oncomine databases. A significantly increased expression of the three cytokines was confirmed in *CD68*^{High}*HIF1A*^{High} tumors (Figure 6A). Moreover, in *CD68*^{High} tumors, a positive correlation between *HIF1A* and the expression of the three pro-inflammatory cytokines was found (Figure 6B). These results corroborate our in vitro findings, in which the analysis of the total lysates of macrophages or cancer cells exposed to 20% or 1% O_2 for 72 h evidenced that the main contributor to the pro-inflammatory IL-1β cytokine, detected in co-cultures CM, is indeed the macrophages and not the cancer cells (Figure 6C and Figure S4). Since it is known that a pro-inflammatory pressure can contribute to the recruitment and activation of anti-tumor immune cells [18–20], we assessed whether *CD68*^{High}*HIF1A*^{High} enriched tumors presented an increased expression of markers of natural killer (NK) cells (*NCAM1*, within the *CD3D*^{Low} population), cytotoxic T-cells (*CD8A*, within the *GZMB*^{High} population), and Th1 cells (*TBX21*, within the *IFNG*^{High} population). Our results confirmed a significant increase in the expression of *NCAM1* and *CD8A*, and an increase, although not statistically significant, of *TBX21* (Figure 6D). Nevertheless, of the two markers that presented significant differences, only CD8A evidenced a positive correlation with *HIF1A* expression on the *CD68*^{High} tumors (Figure 6E).

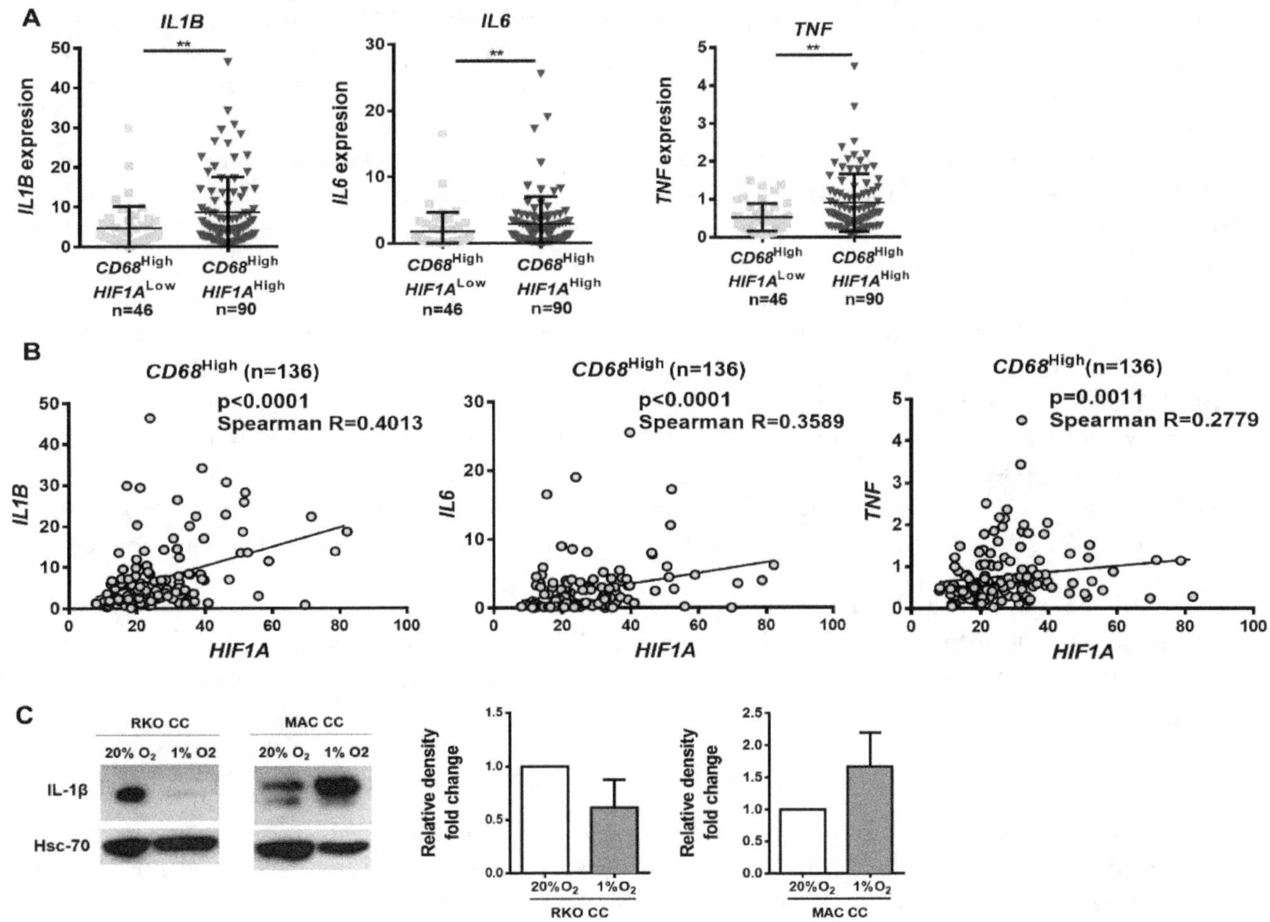

Figure 6. *Cont.*

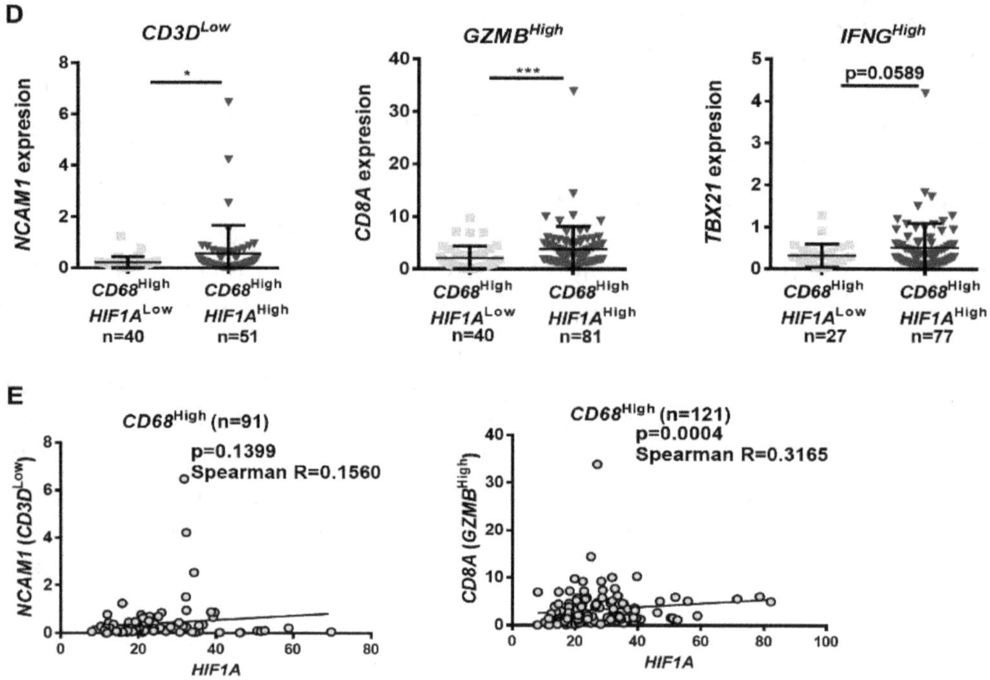

Figure 6. $CD68^{High}HIF1A^{High}$ tumors present increased expression of pro-inflammatory cytokines and increased infiltration of cytotoxic T-cells. RNASeq expression data were downloaded from TCGA. (**A**) The expression of *IL1B, IL6,* and *TNF* was evaluated within the $CD68^{High}$ population, between $HIF1A^{Low}$ and $HIF1A^{High}$, according to the median levels of *CD68* and *HIF1A* expression in normal samples. (**B**) The correlation between *IL1B, IL6, TNF,* and *HIF1A* was assessed within the $CD68^{High}$ population. (**C**) IL-1β protein levels were evaluated in total lysates from co-cultured RKO cells (RKO CC) and macrophages (MAC CC), by Western blot, and band densitometry quantification presented. Hsc70 was used as loading control, and the figure is representative of 3 independent experiments. (**D**) The expressions of *NCAM1, CD8A,* and *TBX21* were evaluated within the $CD68^{High}$ population, between $HIF1A^{Low}$ and $HIF1A^{High}$ subpopulations, according to the median levels of *CD68* and *HIF1A* expression in normal samples. *NCAM1* levels were evaluated within the $CD3D^{Low}$ population, *CD8A* levels were evaluated within the $GZMB^{High}$ population, and *TBX21* levels were evaluated within the $IFNG^{High}$ population. $CD3D^{Low}$, $GZMB^{High}$, and $IFNG^{High}$ populations were established according to the median levels of each marker expression in normal samples. (**E**) Correlations between $NCAM1(CD3D^{Low})$, $CD8A(GZMB^{High})$, and *HIF1A* were assessed within the $CD68^{High}$ population. Mann–Whitney statistical test was used to compare expression between groups. Spearman statistical test was used to assess correlation, which was considered moderate positive when Spearman Rs were between 0.2500 and 0.3500, and strong positive when Spearman R > 0.3500. **** $p < 0.0001$; *** $p < 0.001$; ** $p < 0.01$; * $p < 0.05$. The p-values between 0.05 and 0.1 were presented and considered a tendency.

The results from the TCGA data analysis were confirmed using the Oncomine Bittner colon cancer cohort (Figure S3). Of note, since this cohort does not include data regarding *IFNG* expression, only the levels of *TBX21*, a Th1 cell-specific transcription factor which controls the expression of the hallmark Th1 cytokine IFN-γ was used.

2.7. The Pressure of Hypoxia on Macrophages at the CMS1-MSI-Immune Colon Cancer Type

We anticipated that the observed phenotype might be more relevant in the consensus molecular subtype 1–microsatellite instable (CMS1–MSI)-immune colon cancer subtype [21], due to the increased immune infiltration. To test our hypothesis, we compared the *HIF1A* expression in distal and proximal colon, within the tumors expressing $CD68^{High}$, as the proximal colon is associated with the aforementioned colon cancer subtype. Accordingly, we found that *HIF1A* expression is significantly higher in the proximal than on the distal colon (Figure 7A). In addition, the correlation between *CD68* and *HIF1A* was only observed in proximal tumors (Figure 7B), supporting our hypothesis. Despite no significant differences being found on the survival rates of patients harboring *CD68*^{High}*HIF1A*^{High} and *CD68*^{High}*HIF1A*^{Low} proximal and distal colon tumors, it is possible to observe that the pattern between the two locations is clearly different, suggesting that *CD68*^{High}*HIF1A*^{High} patients might have a better prognosis than *CD68*^{High}*HIF1A*^{Low} patients (Figure 7C). This question should be clarified by increasing the sample size. Since the CMS1–MSI-immune colon cancer subtype is also characterized by high MSI, high levels of *BRAF* mutations, and low levels *KRAS* mutations, we decided to explore whether *CD68*^{High} tumors presented differences in *HIF1A* expression comparing MSI/MSS, and *BRAF* and *KRAS* wild-type versus mutated. Despite the low number of cases available at TCGA with the characterization of the MSI status and *BRAF* and *KRAS* mutations, our analysis showed that, in *CD68*^{High} tumors, the *HIF1A* expression is significantly higher in MSI and *BRAF* mutated cases (Figure 7D). Given these differences, we also looked to *HIF1A* expression in tumors with and without loss of mismatch repair proteins, but no significant difference was found (Figure 7E).

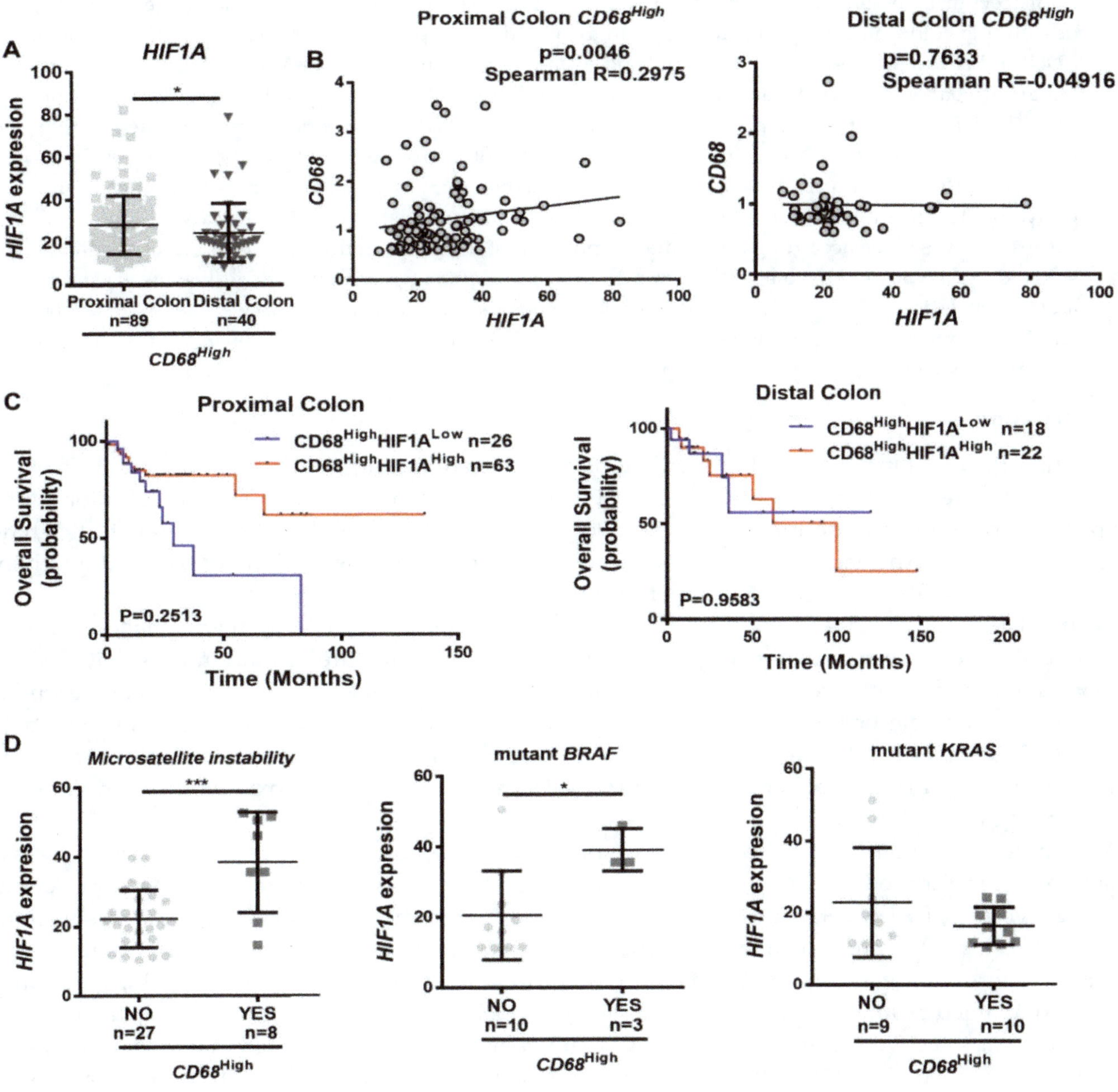

Figure 7. *Cont.*

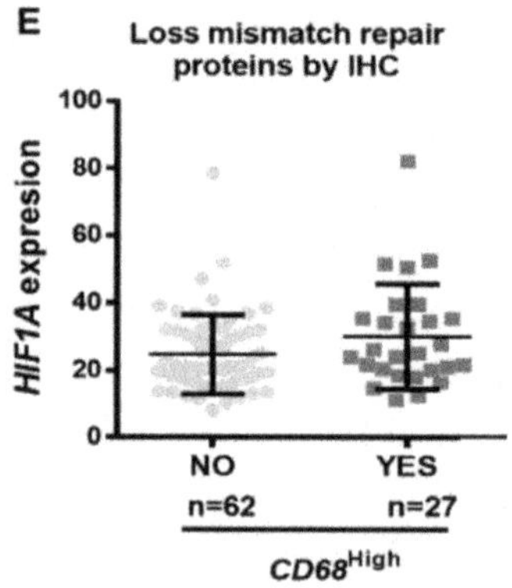

Figure 7. The pressure of hypoxia on macrophages at the consensus molecular subtype 1–microsatellite instable (CMS1–MSI)-immune colon cancer type. Microarray and RNASeq expression data were downloaded from TCGA. (**A**) *HIF1A* expression was evaluated between patients with tumors in proximal colon (cecum, ascending colon, hepatic flexure, and transverse colon) and in distal colon (splenic flexure, descending colon, and sigmoid colon), within the *CD68*^{High} population. (**B**) The correlation between *CD68* and *HIF1A* was assessed in proximal and distal colon population. (**C**) Kaplan–Meier curves were made with patients' survival data, comparing the populations *CD68*^{High}*HIF1A*^{High} with the population *CD68*^{High}*HIF1A*^{Low}, on distal and proximal colon patients. (**D**) *HIF1A* expression was evaluated, within the *CD68*^{High} population, between patients with or without microsatellite instability, BRAF and KRAS mutations. (**E**) *HIF1A* expression was evaluated, within the *CD68*^{High} population, between patients with or without loss of mismatch repair proteins, evaluated by immunohistochemistry. The division high/low expression was made according the median expression of the genes in normal tissue. Mann–Whitney statistical test was used to compare expression between groups. Spearman statistical test was used to assess correlation, which was considered moderate positive when Spearman Rs were between 0.2500 and 0.3500, and strong positive when Spearman R > 0.3500. Long-rank (Mantel–Cox) test to the analysis of the survival curves. ** $p < 0.01$; * $p < 0.05$.

3. Discussion

The full understanding of the interactions established among the distinct TM components is crucial for the development of novel and more efficient anti-tumor therapies. The case of colon cancer is particularly relevant due to the high incidence and mortality, and because several studies have described a very particular behavior of colon cancer cells, in comparison with other tissues, underlying the importance of the colon cancer microenvironment.

In this work, we focused our attention on the crosstalk established between macrophages and colon cancer cells, and on its modulation by hypoxia. Hypoxia is a key feature of solid tumors that has been reported to critically influence cancer cell behavior and is often disregarded. In fact, most of the studies focusing on the role of hypoxia at the tumor microenvironment explored cancer cell metabolic changes [8], while its influence in the non-tumor compartment is still poorly explored. Therefore, the present work brings pioneer information concerning the study of hypoxia on the modulation of macrophage and colon cancer cell interactions.

When exploring tumor databases, we demonstrated that colon tumors exhibit distinct levels of macrophage infiltration, where the most infiltrated tumors are also the most hypoxic ones, presenting higher levels of *HIF1A*, *CA9*, and *LOX* expression. Although the novelty of these findings in colon cancer, these results are not unexpected since it has been previously reported, in other tumors, that hypoxic areas are the ones with enhanced inflammatory infiltration [9]. Notably, this association was accompanied by improved survival rates, clearly evident in *CD68*^{High} tumors, which could reinforce the idea of a protective anti-tumor and pro-inflammatory effect of the recruited macrophages. Indeed, it was previously reported that chemotactic HIF is essential for myeloid cell infiltration and activation through a VEGF-independent mechanism [22]. Here, we assume that *HIF1A* is produced by both tumor and non-tumor cells at the microenvironment, contributing to this immune cell recruitment, but it will be important to determine which population is the main contributor to pursue possible therapeutic applications. It will also be interesting to evaluate the role of HIF2α in this process, as it was reported that HIF1α and HIF2α have opposing roles [23]. In contrast to our results, previous reports in colon cancer described that HIF1α had no association [24], or was associated with worse prognosis [25]. However, none of these studies took the immune component of the microenvironment into consideration.

Importantly, the macrophage infiltration considered in the tumor databases is mainly derived from the tumor core, which is generally the most hypoxic area. It is possible that, depending on localization, macrophage might function in different ways. As our group and others reported, the macrophage inflammatory profile varies according to their location: adjacent tissue, invasive front or intratumor region [2,26]. It will therefore be interesting to assess in patients' samples whether hypoxia influences other macrophage populations besides the ones from the core of the tumor, which is the main region represented in the TCGA patients' samples.

Paradoxically, we found that in vitro hypoxia decreases the expression of macrophage antigen-presenting molecules, namely, HLA-ABC and HLA-DR, and of the co-stimulatory receptor CD86. These results are in line with other reports conducted with macrophage monocultures under hypoxia [27]. Nevertheless, antigen-presentation may still occur at the expense of other immune cells, such as dendritic cells.

This is the first study demonstrating that, although not affecting the percentage of phagocytic macrophages, colon cancer cells and hypoxia enhance macrophage phagocytic capacity. This characteristic might be important in vivo given the increase in necrosis, resulting in enhanced cell debris to collect. In addition, at the molecular level, this finding may suggest the inexistence of a functional anti-phagocytic SIRPα/CD47 system. In line with previous reports in other tumors, we found that hypoxic stimulation leads to an increase of CD47 levels on cancer cells [12,28]. In our system, the enhanced expression of this "don't eat me" signal is counteracted by a decrease in macrophage SIRPα expression. In fact, it seems that less SIRPα expression is associated with increased phagocytosis. In agreement, we found that the percentage of SIRPα+ phagocytic macrophages significantly decreases at 1% O_2, explaining the increased macrophage phagocytic capacity. Accordingly, other authors have described that silencing or blocking of SIRPα in RAW264.7 macrophages promoted the phagocytosis of osteosarcoma cancer cells [29]. Our findings regarding phagocytosis are divergent from previously reported work on breast cancer [12] but are in line with other results showing that macrophagic HIF1α enhances phagocytosis [30], suggesting that this might be a feature dependent on the cancer type. For the first time, we described that, in colon cancer, hypoxia impacts the SIRPα/CD47 axis through the decrease of macrophage SIRPα expression, which may favor their phagocytic capacity. Importantly, the molecular mechanisms associated with this apparent impairment of the SIRPα/CD47 axis need further elucidation.

Regarding the impact of macrophages and hypoxia on cancer cells, we found that despite the increased levels of glucose consumption and *SLC2A1* expression, there was no increase of lactate production, despite the increase in *LDHA* expression and acidosis. Previous reports have stated that lactate polarizes macrophages into an anti-inflammatory phenotype [31]. In our model, where no major alterations on lactate secretion were detected, we also did not find a clear-cut shift on macrophage phenotype. We found that hypoxia potentiated the already described ability of macrophage to induce cancer cell invasion [6]. The maintenance of this pro-tumor feature, despite the secretion of pro-inflammatory cytokines, had already been reported by our group, when macrophage and colon cancer cell co-cultures were treated with ionizing radiation [32].

Some authors have claimed that hypoxia leads to macrophage recruitment and polarization into an anti-inflammatory phenotype [33], while others have reported that hypoxia is not a major driver of macrophage polarization, but instead only triggers fine-tuning of metabolic genes in anti-inflammatory macrophages [34]. Others have described that *HIF1A* depleted macrophages exhibit increased anti-inflammatory markers [35]. In our model, we found alterations in both anti- and pro-inflammatory markers, and, at the secretome level, a shift into a pro-inflammatory phenotype is suggested. For the first time, we demonstrated that macrophages under the influence of colon cancer cells and hypoxia significantly decreased CCR7 expression, in line with other reports of macrophages monocultures [27]. Nevertheless, no impact in the pro-inflammatory markers IL-6 and TNF-α was observed. Interestingly, it has been recently described that HIF and IL-6 expression is increased in colorectal tumors, being both markers positively correlated [36]. In fact, we observed a slight increase in IL-6 secretion levels at 1% O_2, although without statistical significance. In line with our findings, THP-1 macrophages under hypoxia exhibit decreased CD163 mRNA levels [37]; also being reported is that there is a decrease in CCL18 and IL-10 and an increase in IL-1β secretion in macrophages monocultures [27,38]. Accordingly, in our work, the analysis of CM of co-cultures combined with the total lysates of macrophages and cancer cells, evidenced that macrophages are the main producers of secreted IL-1β. While in macrophages, hypoxia is triggering increased IL-1β expression, on cancer cells, the opposite was observed. Overall, our results suggest that hypoxia triggers a decrease in macrophage anti-inflammatory pressure.

Importantly, we found that in $CD68^{High}$ tumors, hypoxia is associated with the expression of pro-inflammatory cytokines, such as *IL1B*, *IL6*, and *TNF*, previously associated with the recruitment of other anti-tumor immune cells [18–20], suggesting the establishment of a pro-inflammatory TM. Interestingly, some authors described that hypoxia-associated anti-inflammatory macrophages repress T-cell activity [9], while others reported that (1) macrophages without HIF had less capacity to stimulate CD8 T-cell proliferation [39]; (2) hypoxia protected activated T-cells from death [40]; (3) CD8 T-cells with constitutive HIF expression delayed T-cell differentiation into effector cells but increased their cytotoxic function, through increased expression of granzyme B [41]. Notably, the $CD68^{High}HIF1A^{High}$ tumors are those presenting higher levels of infiltrated NK and cytotoxic T-cells, which could be related to the improved survival rate observed in these patients. In fact, these findings are in accordance with other reports demonstrating that colon tumors with higher T-cell infiltration are the ones associated with improved survival [42].

We hypothesize that the results described in this work might be particularly important in the CMS1 MSI-immune tumors, those characterized by an immune infiltrate mainly composed of Th1, NK, and cytotoxic T-cells, and with upregulation of proteins involved in immune response pathways [21,43]. Also, it was described that the number of tumors infiltrating macrophages is higher in MSI colon tumors, those associated with better prognosis [44]. Those tumors are generally associated with the proximal colon, and we confirmed that *HIF1A* was significantly upregulated in this region. Interestingly, it was only in those tumors located in the proximal colon that we found a positive correlation between *CD68* and *HIF1A*, and, furthermore, the survival curves associated with these two colon regions were clearly different from each other. It will be important to validate these results in bigger series of colon cancers, comparing distal and proximal tumors. Moreover, it is known that HIF1α represses DNA repair genes [45], which could account for an increased mutation burden and tumor immunogenicity. However, in our analysis, *HIF1A* expression could not be associated with mismatch repair protein expression. Interestingly, it is also known that mutant *BRAF*, a common event on CMS1 tumors, regulates HIF-1α expression in melanoma, affecting cell survival under hypoxic conditions [46]. Indeed, the colon cancer cases with *BRAF* mutation presented a significantly higher expression of *HIF1A*, while no differences were found on *KRAS* mutated cases. It will be interesting to further explore these associations among hypoxia, *BRAF* mutation and MSI status, and macrophage infiltration on colon tumors. In addition, given the documented relevance of the microbiome in cancer progression, the knowledge that there is a particular microbiota organization in proximal colon [47], and that colon bacterial products modulate HIF1-α expression and activation [48,49], it may also be important to explore the impact of the microbiome on macrophage–colon cancer cell crosstalk, within an hypoxic environment.

Despite the well documented influence of hypoxia in triggering different hallmarks of cancer, this work highlights that, depending on the component of the microenvironment, the tumor origin, and even on its localization, hypoxia can play a beneficial role in the combat against the tumor.

4. Materials and Methods

4.1. Bioinformatic Analysis

TCGA

The Cancer Genome Atlas (TCGA; https://cancergenome.nih.gov/) dataset of colon carcinomas was analyzed, and for comparison purposes, gastric, breast ductal, and lung adenocarcinoma datasets were used. Survival plots were performed in R using survival and survminer packages. Median values were calculated in normal tissue and used as threshold to define "high" and "low" expression levels in cancer patients. The expression of genes was quantified as FPKM (fragments per kilobase million), which are provided by TCGA consortium. The number of individuals with information simultaneously on gene expression and survival were 136 for colon, 269 for gastric, 673 for breast ductal, and 52 for lung adenocarcinoma. Clinical and somatic mutation metadata were also provided by the TCGA consortium at https://gdc.cancer.gov/.

4.2. Oncomine

CD68, HIF1A, CA9, LOX, IL1B, IL6, TNF, CD3D, NCAM, GZMB, CD8A, and *TBX21* mRNA expression was assessed in the Bittner colon cancer dataset from Oncomine database (https://www.oncomine.org), encompassing a total of 374 cases. Categorization of patient samples was assigned into low (lowest 50%) and high (highest 50%) subgroups according to the log2 median-centered intensity levels of mRNA expression.

4.3. Ethics Statement

The buffy coats used for monocyte isolation are highly leukocyte-enriched waste-products that results from a whole blood donation of healthy blood donors. The isolation of immune cells from healthy blood donors was approved by the Centro Hospitalar Universitário São João Ethics Committee (protocol 90/19) after collecting each donor's informed consent.

4.4. Human Monocyte Isolation and Macrophage Differentiation

Human monocytes were isolated from buffy coats from healthy blood donors, as previously described (6). Isolated cells were resuspended in RPMI1640 supplemented with 10% fetal bovine serum (FBS, Biowest, Nuaillé, France) and 100 U/mL penicillin and 100 μg/mL streptomycin (PS, Invitrogen, Carlsbad, CA, USA). Then, 1.2×10^6 monocytes were plated per 6-well culture plates and differentiated into macrophages for 10 days. In the first 7 days, macrophages were supplemented with M-CSF (50 ng/mL, ImmunoTools, Friesoythe, Germany). Cells were maintained at 37 °C and 5% CO_2 humidified atmosphere.

4.5. Cancer Cell Culture

RKO colon cancer cell line, from American Type Culture Collection (ATCC), was cultured in RPMI1640 (Invitrogen), supplemented with 10% FBS and 1% PS, and maintained at 37 °C and 5% CO_2 humidified atmosphere.

4.6. Macrophage and Cancer Cell Indirect Co-Cultures

For co-cultures, 1×10^5 RKO cells were seeded into 6-well-plate permeable transwell inserts (PET inserts with 1-μm pore, Corning, Corning, NY, USA) positioned on top of a macrophage culture, 10 days after monocyte isolation. Co-cultures between macrophages and cancer cells were maintained in complete RPMI medium for 72 h at 37 °C, at 20% O_2 or 1% O_2 (94% N_2), 5% CO_2 humidified atmosphere.

4.7. RNA Extraction, cDNA Preparation, and Quantitative Real-Time PCR Analysis

Total RNA was extracted using TRIzol reagent (Invitrogen), according to the manufacturer's instructions. cDNA was synthesized using 1 μg of RNA, using NZY M-MuLV Reverse Transcriptase enzyme (NZYTech, Lisboa, Portugal), according to the manufacturer's instructions. Quantitative real-time PCR (qRT–PCR) was performed with Kapa Probe Fast qPCR Master Mix (Kapa Biosystems, Roche, Basel, Switzerland) using the probes to *ACTB* (Hs01060665), *CA9* (Hs00154208), *LDHA* (Hs.PT.58.22929122), and *SLC2A1* (Hs.PT.58.25872862) (Applied Biosystems, Foster City, CA, USA). Relative mRNA expression of the target genes was normalized to the levels of the housekeeping gene, using the comparative $\Delta\Delta$Ct method. ACTB was used as a housekeeping gene to RKO cells.

4.8. Viability Assay

Macrophage and cancer cell viability was measured by resazurin reduction assay. After 3 days of co-culture, resazurin redox dye (0.01 mg/mL, Sigma-Aldrich, St.Louis, MO, USA) was added (1/10 of the total volume of culture medium) to cell culture, incubated for 4 h at 37 °C and 5% CO_2, and the fluorescence intensity was measured at 530/590 nm in a Synergy Mx fluorometer.

4.9. Flow Cytometry

Macrophages and cancer cells were incubated with accutase (eBioscience, Affymetrix, Santa Clara, CA, USA) at 37 °C for 30 min and harvested by gently scraping. Cells were washed and resuspended in FACS buffer (PBS, 2% FBS (Biowest), 0.01% sodium azide) containing appropriate conjugated antibodies, and stained in the dark for 40 min at 4 °C. Macrophages were immunostained with the following antibodies: anti-human CD14-APC (clone MEM-12), CD14-PE/FITC (clone 18D11), CD14-PerCP/Cy5.5 (clone OFC14D), CD86-FITC (clone BU63), HLA-ABC-PE (clone W6/32), HLA-DR-PE/FITC (clone MEM-12) (Immunotools), CCR7-PerCP/Cy5.5 (G043H7), SIRPα-APC (clone SE5A5) (Biolegend, San Diego, CA, USA), CD163-PE (clone GHI/61) (BD Bioscience, Franklin Lakes, NJ, USA). Cancer cells were stained with anti-human CD47-FITC (clone MEM-122) (Immunotools). Unstained cells and single stained with antibodies or with the respective isotype IgGs were used as control. After additional washing steps, cell fluorescence was acquired on a FACS Canto Flow Cytometer (BD Biosciences) using FACS Diva Software. Data analysis was performed with FlowJo software.

4.10. Phagocytosis Assay

Colon cancer cells were grown for 72 h at 1% O_2, and after this period, suspension of 1×10^7 cells/mL was stained with 2.5 μM CellTrace™ CFSE (Invitrogen), according to the manufacturer's protocol. Macrophages that were previously indirectly co-cultured with cancer cells, for 72 h, were incubated in serum-free medium for 2 h before adding 2.4×10^6 CFSE-labeled cancer cells (1 macrophage:2 cancer cells). After coculture for 2 h at 37 °C, macrophages were harvested and evaluated by flow cytometry, with anti-CD14 and anti-SIRPα antibodies. Phagocytosis was calculated as the percentage of CD14+CFSE+ cells among total CD14+.

4.11. Enzyme-Linked Immunosorbent Assay (ELISA)

Cytokine levels were measured in the CM of mono and co-cultures by ELISA to TGF-β, TNF-α, IL-10, IL-1β, IL-6 (Biolegend), and CCL18 (Abcam, Cambridge, UK) according to the manufacturer's instructions. Concentrations were normalized to the CM total protein concentration, which was measured using the DCProtein assay kit (BioRad, Hercules, CA, USA), following the manufacturer's instructions.

4.12. *Proliferation Assay*

Cell proliferation was determined through the use of the Click-iTTM Plus EdU Flow Cytometry Assay Kit (Invitrogen), according to the manufacturer's instructions. RKO cells cultured in 6-well plates without EdU treatment were used as a negative control, while RKO treated with EdU was used as a positive control.

4.13. *Cell Death Quantification Assay*

Cell death was measured using the FITC Annexin V Apoptosis Detection kit (BD Pharmigen, BD Bioscience, Franklin Lakes, NJ, USA) according to the manufacturer's instructions. Untreated RKO cells cultured in a 6-well plate were used as a negative control, and cells treated with H_2O_2 were used as a positive control.

4.14. *Glucose Quantification Assay*

Glucose levels were measured in the CM of the co-cultures using the enzymatic colorimetric kit, Glucose Assay Kit (Roche), following the manufacturer's instructions. The standard curve for glucose quantification was done using serial dilutions of RPMI, with known glucose concentration.

4.15. *Lactate Quantification Assay*

An enzymatic colorimetric kit (Spinreact, Girona, Spain) was used to determine lactate concentration in co-cultures CM, according to the manufacturer's instructions.

4.16. *pH Measurement*

The CM pH was measured using the Electro Kinetic Analyzer (EKA) (Anton Paar, Graz, Austria).

4.17. *Matrigel Invasion Assay*

Invasion was measured using Matrigel-coated invasion inserts of 8μm pore (Corning), according to the manufacturer's instructions. In the upper compartment, 2.5×10^4 RKO cells were cultured at 20% O_2 or 1% O_2 conditions, either alone or stimulated with macrophages cultured at 20% O_2 or 1% O_2 at the lower compartment. Cells were allowed to invade for 24 h at 37 °C, at 20% O_2 or 1% O_2, respectively. After this period, the inserts were washed with PBS and fixed in 4% PFA for 20 min at RT, and the non-invading cells in the upper compartment of the inserts were removed. The filters were mounted in Vectashield Mounting Medium with DAPI (Vector Laboratories, Burlingame, CA, USA), and the invading cells were visualized and counted with a Leica DM2000 fluorescence microscope (Leica Microsystems, Wetzlar, Germany).

4.18. *Western Blot*

Cell lysates were prepared with Rippa buffer (50 mM Tris HCl pH = 7.5; 1% NonidetP (NP)-40; 150 mM NaCl and 2 mM EDTA) with proteases/phosphatases inhibitors cocktails (Sigma-Aldrich). Protein concentration was determined using the DCProtein assay kit (BioRad) and 20 μg of protein were loaded and run in a 12.5% SDS-polyacrylamide gel. Afterwards, gels were transferred to nitrocellulose membranes (GE Healthcare, Chicago, IL, USA), blocked with 5% non-fat powder milk in PBS + 0.1% Tween-20 (PBS-T 0.1%) for 30 min, and incubated overnight with primary antibodies rabbit anti-IL-1β (GeneTex, Irvine, CA, USA), and mouse anti-Hsc-70 (Santa Cruz, Dallas, TX, USA). HRP-conjugated anti-mouse and anti-rabbit (GE Healthcare, Chicago, IL, USA) were used as secondaries antibodies. Membranes were incubated with Clarity Western ECL Substrate (BioRad) for signal detection. Bands intensity measurements were performed with ImageJ.

4.19. Statistical Analysis

Data were expressed as the mean with standard deviation (SD), and collected from at least three independent experiments with macrophages from different donors. The normality of the distribution was evaluated using the Kolmogorov–Smirnov test. For comparison between two independent groups, *t*-test (paired, Wilcoxon, and Mann–Whitney) was used. For comparison among four independent groups, one-way ANOVA (RM one-way ANOVA, Friedman, and Kruskal–Wallis), with Dunn's multiple comparison was used. Correlations were tested with the Spearman test and considered moderate positive when Spearman Rs were between 0.2500 and 0.3500, and strong positive when Spearman R > 0.3500. Survival curves were analyzed with the log-rank (Mantel–Cox) test. Statistical tests were performed in GraphPad Prism 8. Differences were considered significant at $p < 0.05$.

5. Conclusions

Our results demonstrate the importance of considering hypoxia as a major player on the tumor microenvironment modulation. In particular, we found that in colon tumors with high macrophage infiltration, hypoxia is associated with better prognosis, possibly due to the pro-inflammatory pressure induced by macrophages, which could potentiate the recruitment of other anti-cancer immune cells. This phenomenon appears to be tissue-specific and even dependent on tumor localization within the colon.

Altogether, these data underlie the need to consider the specificities of each tumor microenvironment, since the particular context in which cancer cells are enclosed can have a major impact in disease prognosis and the selection of therapeutic options.

Author Contributions: Conceptualization, A.M.C. and B.S.; Data curation, A.M.C., F.M., R.O., B.C., F.P., F.C., and B.S.; Formal analysis, A.M.C., F.M., R.O., B.C., F.P., A.P.C., F.C., R.M.R., L.P., and M.J.O.; Funding acquisition, M.J.O.; Investigation, A.M.C., F.M., R.O., A.P.C., M.L.P., A.J.S., D.A., and J.P.L.; Methodology, A.M.C., A.P.C., F.C., B.S., M.L.P., A.J.S., D.A., and J.P.L.; Software, B.C., F.P., R.M.R., and L.P.; Supervision, A.M.C.; Validation, A.M.C.; Writing—original draft, A.M.C.; Writing—review and editing, A.M.C., N.P., and M.J.O. All authors have read and agreed to the published version of the manuscript.

Acknowledgments: We acknowledge Sérgia Velho's team for the scientific discussion, Cecília Durães and Tânia Cruz for the help with statistics. We acknowledge all the help from i3S Scientifics Platforms technicians: Catarina Meireles and Emília Cardoso from the Translational Cytometry Unit, Dalila Pedro and Ricardo Vidal from the Biointerfaces and Nanotechnology Unit, Mafalda Rocha and Rob Mensink from the Genomics Unit. The authors would like to thank Serviço de Imunohemoterapia of Centro Hospitalar Universitário de São João (CHUSJ), for kindly donating Buffy Coats.

References

1. Colangelo, T.; Polcaro, G.; Muccillo, L.; D'Agostino, G.; Rosato, V.; Ziccardi, P.; Lupo, A.; Mazzoccoli, G.; Sabatino, L.; Colantuoni, V. Friend or foe? The tumour microenvironment dilemma in colorectal cancer. *Biochim. Biophys. Acta* **2017**, *1867*, 1–18. [CrossRef]
2. Yang, M.; McKay, D.; Pollard, J.W.; Lewis, C.E. Diverse Functions of Macrophages in Different Tumor Microenvironments. *Cancer Res.* **2018**, *78*, 5492–5503. [CrossRef] [PubMed]
3. Mosser, D.M.; Edwards, J.P. Exploring the full spectrum of macrophage activation. Nature reviews. *Immunology* **2008**, *8*, 958–969. [CrossRef] [PubMed]
4. Crusz, S.M.; Balkwill, F.R. Inflammation and cancer: Advances and new agents. *Nat. Rev. Clin. Oncol.* **2015**, *12*, 584–596. [CrossRef] [PubMed]
5. Zhong, X.; Chen, B.; Yang, Z. The Role of Tumor-Associated Macrophages in Colorectal Carcinoma Progression. *Cell. Physiol. Biochem.* **2018**, *45*, 356–365. [CrossRef]
6. Cardoso, A.P.; Pinto, M.L.; Pinto, A.T.; Oliveira, M.I.; Pinto, M.T.; Goncalves, R.; Relvas, J.B.; Figueiredo, C.; Seruca, R.; Mantovani, A.; et al. Macrophages stimulate gastric and colorectal cancer invasion through EGFR Y(1086), c-Src, Erk1/2 and Akt phosphorylation and smallGTPase activity. *Oncogene* **2014**, *33*, 2123–2133. [CrossRef]
7. Semenza, G.L. The hypoxic tumor microenvironment: A driving force for breast cancer progression. *Biochim. Biophys. Acta* **2016**, *1863*, 382–391. [CrossRef]

8. Vaupel, P.; Mayer, A. Hypoxia in cancer: Significance and impact on clinical outcome. *Cancer Metastasis Rev.* **2007**, *26*, 225–239. [CrossRef]
9. Henze, A.T.; Mazzone, M. The impact of hypoxia on tumor-associated macrophages. *J. Clin. Investig.* **2016**, *126*, 3672–3679. [CrossRef]
10. Palazon, A.; Goldrath, A.W.; Nizet, V.; Johnson, R.S. HIF Transcription Factors, Inflammation, and Immunity. *Immunity* **2014**, *41*, 518–528. [CrossRef]
11. Semenza, G.L. Targeting HIF-1 for cancer therapy. *Nat. Rev. Cancer* **2003**, *3*, 721–732. [CrossRef] [PubMed]
12. Zhang, H.; Lu, H.; Xiang, L.; Bullen, J.W.; Zhang, C.; Samanta, D.; Gilkes, D.M.; He, J.; Semenza, G.L. HIF-1 regulates CD47 expression in breast cancer cells to promote evasion of phagocytosis and maintenance of cancer stem cells. *Proc. Natl. Acad. Sci. USA* **2015**, *112*, E6215–E6223. [CrossRef] [PubMed]
13. Onnis, B.; Rapisarda, A.; Melillo, G. Development of HIF-1 inhibitors for cancer therapy. *J. Cell. Mol. Med.* **2009**, *13*, 2780–2786. [CrossRef] [PubMed]
14. Kenneth, N.S.; Mudie, S.; van Uden, P.; Rocha, S. SWI/SNF Regulates the Cellular Response to Hypoxia. *J. Biol. Chem.* **2009**, *284*, 4123–4131. [CrossRef] [PubMed]
15. Simiantonaki, N.; Taxeidis, M.; Jayasinghe, C.; Kurzik-Dumke, U.; Kirkpatrick, C.J. Hypoxia-inducible factor 1 alpha expression increases during colorectal carcinogenesis and tumor progression. *BMC Cancer* **2008**, *8*, 320. [CrossRef]
16. Martinez, F.O.; Helming, L.; Milde, R.; Varin, A.; Melgert, B.N.; Draijer, C.; Thomas, B.; Fabbri, M.; Crawshaw, A.; Ho, L.P.; et al. Genetic programs expressed in resting and IL-4 alternatively activated mouse and human macrophages: Similarities and differences. *Blood* **2013**, *121*, E57–E69. [CrossRef]
17. Dalton, H.J.; Armaiz-Pena, G.N.; Gonzalez-Villasana, V.; Lopez-Berestein, G.; Bar-Eli, M.; Sood, A.K. Monocyte subpopulations in angiogenesis. *Cancer Res.* **2014**, *74*, 1287–1293. [CrossRef]
18. Okada, M.; Kitahara, M.; Kishimoto, S.; Matsuda, T.; Hirano, T.; Kishimoto, T. Il-6 Bsf-2 Functions as a Killer Helper Factor in the Invitro Induction of Cyto-Toxic T-Cells. *J. Immunol.* **1988**, *141*, 1543–1549.
19. Ben-Sasson, S.Z.; Hogg, A.; Hu-Li, J.; Wingfield, P.; Chen, X.; Crank, M.; Caucheteux, S.; Ratner-Hurevich, M.; Berzofsky, J.A.; Nir-Paz, R.; et al. IL-1 enhances expansion, effector function, tissue localization, and memory response of antigen-specific CD8 T cells. *J. Exp. Med.* **2013**, *210*, 491–502. [CrossRef]
20. Turner, M.D.; Nedjai, B.; Hurst, T.; Pennington, D.J. Cytokines and chemokines: At the crossroads of cell signalling and inflammatory disease. *Biochim. Biophys. Acta* **2014**, *1843*, 2563–2582. [CrossRef]
21. Guinney, J.; Dienstmann, R.; Wang, X.; de Reynies, A.; Schlicker, A.; Soneson, C.; Marisa, L.; Roepman, P.; Nyamundanda, G.; Angelino, P.; et al. The consensus molecular subtypes of colorectal cancer. *Nat. Med.* **2015**, *21*, 1350–1356. [CrossRef] [PubMed]
22. Cramer, T.; Yamanishi, Y.; Clausen, B.E.; Forster, I.; Pawlinski, R.; Mackman, N.; Haase, V.H.; Jaenisch, R.; Corr, M.; Nizet, V.; et al. HIF-1alpha is essential for myeloid cell-mediated inflammation. *Cell* **2003**, *112*, 645–657. [CrossRef]
23. Keith, B.; Johnson, R.S.; Simon, M.C. HIF1 alpha and HIF2 alpha: Sibling rivalry in hypoxic tumour growth and progression. *Nat. Rev. Cancer* **2012**, *12*, 9–22. [CrossRef] [PubMed]
24. Jubb, A.M.; Turley, H.; Moeller, H.C.; Steers, G.; Han, C.; Li, J.L.; Leek, R.; Tan, E.Y.; Singh, B.; Mortensen, N.J.; et al. Expression of delta-like ligand 4 (Dll4) and markers of hypoxia in colon cancer. *Br. J. Cancer* **2009**, *101*, 1749–1757. [CrossRef]
25. Baba, Y.; Nosho, K.; Shima, K.; Irahara, N.; Chan, A.T.; Meyerhardt, J.A.; Chung, D.C.; Giovannucci, E.L.; Fuchs, C.S.; Ogino, S. HIF1A overexpression is associated with poor prognosis in a cohort of 731 colorectal cancers. *Am. J. Pathol.* **2010**, *176*, 2292–2301. [CrossRef]
26. Pinto, M.L.; Rios, E.; Doraes, C.; Ribeiro, R.; Machado, J.C.; Mantovani, A.; Barbosa, M.A.; Carneiro, F.; Oliveira, M.J. The Two Faces of Tumor-Associated Macrophages and Their Clinical Significance in Colorectal Cancer. *Front. Immunol.* **2019**, *10*. [CrossRef]
27. Raggi, F.; Pelassa, S.; Pierobon, D.; Penco, F.; Gattorno, M.; Novelli, F.; Eva, A.; Varesio, L.; Giovarelli, M.; Bosco, M.C. Regulation of Human Macrophage M1-M2 Polarization Balance by Hypoxia and the Triggering Receptor Expressed on Myeloid Cells-1. *Front. Immunol.* **2017**, *8*, 1097. [CrossRef]
28. Romano, E.; Rufo, N.; Korf, H.; Mathieu, C.; Garg, A.D.; Agostinis, P. BNIP3 modulates the interface between B16-F10 melanoma cells and immune cells. *Oncotarget* **2018**, *9*, 17631–17644. [CrossRef]
29. Ray, M.; Lee, Y.W.; Hardie, J.; Mout, R.; Yesilbag Tonga, G.; Farkas, M.E.; Rotello, V.M. CRISPRed Macrophages for Cell-Based Cancer Immunotherapy. *Bioconjug. Chem.* **2018**, *29*, 445–450. [CrossRef]

30. Anand, R.J.; Gribar, S.C.; Li, J.; Kohler, J.W.; Branca, M.F.; Dubowski, T.; Sodhi, C.P.; Hackam, D.J. Hypoxia causes an increase in phagocytosis by macrophages in a HIF-1 alpha-dependent manner. *J. Leukoc. Biol.* **2007**, *82*, 1257–1265. [CrossRef]
31. Colegio, O.R.; Chu, N.Q.; Szabo, A.L.; Chu, T.; Rhebergen, A.M.; Jairam, V.; Cyrus, N.; Brokowski, C.E.; Eisenbarth, S.C.; Phillips, G.M.; et al. Functional polarization of tumour-associated macrophages by tumour-derived lactic acid. *Nature* **2014**, *513*, 559–563. [CrossRef]
32. Pinto, A.T.; Pinto, M.L.; Cardoso, A.P.; Monteiro, C.; Pinto, M.T.; Maia, A.F.; Castro, P.; Figueira, R.; Monteiro, A.; Marques, M.; et al. Ionizing radiation modulates human macrophages towards a pro-inflammatory phenotype preserving their pro-invasive and pro-angiogenic capacities. *Sci. Rep.* **2016**, *6*. [CrossRef]
33. Leblond, M.M.; Gerault, A.N.; Corroyer-Dulmont, A.; MacKenzie, E.T.; Petit, E.; Bernaudin, M.; Valable, S. Hypoxia induces macrophage polarization and re-education toward an M2 phenotype in U87 and U251 glioblastoma models. *Oncoimmunology* **2016**, *5*, e1056442. [CrossRef]
34. Laoui, D.; Van Overmeire, E.; Di Conza, G.; Aldeni, C.; Keirsse, J.; Morias, Y.; Movahedi, K.; Houbracken, I.; Schouppe, E.; Elkrim, Y.; et al. Tumor hypoxia does not drive differentiation of tumor-associated macrophages but rather fine-tunes the M2-like macrophage population. *Cancer Res.* **2014**, *74*, 24–30. [CrossRef] [PubMed]
35. Kumar, V.; Gabrilovich, D.I. Hypoxia-inducible factors in regulation of immune responses in tumour microenvironment. *Immunology* **2014**, *143*, 512–519. [CrossRef] [PubMed]
36. Xu, K.; Zhan, Y.; Yuan, Z.; Qiu, Y.; Wang, H.; Fan, G.; Wang, J.; Li, W.; Cao, Y.; Shen, X.; et al. Hypoxia Induces Drug Resistance in Colorectal Cancer through the HIF-1a/miR-338-5p/IL-6 Feedback Loop. *Mol. Ther.* **2019**. [CrossRef] [PubMed]
37. Ye, X.J.; Zhang, J.; Lu, R.; Zhou, G. Signal regulatory protein a associated with the progression of oral leukoplakia and oral squamous cell carcinoma regulates phenotype switch of macrophages. *Oncotarget* **2016**, *7*, 81305–81321. [CrossRef] [PubMed]
38. Song, J.; Cheon, S.Y.; Jung, W.; Lee, W.T.; Lee, J.E. Resveratrol induces the expression of interleukin-10 and brain-derived neurotrophic factor in BV2 microglia under hypoxia. *Int. J. Mol. Sci.* **2014**, *15*, 15512–15529. [CrossRef]
39. Bhandari, T.; Olson, J.; Johnson, R.S.; Nizet, V. HIF-1 alpha influences myeloid cell antigen presentation and response to subcutaneous OVA vaccination. *J. Mol. Med.* **2013**, *91*, 1199–1205. [CrossRef]
40. Makino, Y.; Nakamura, H.; Ikeda, E.; Ohnuma, K.; Yamauchi, K.; Yabe, Y.; Poellinger, L.; Okada, Y.; Morimoto, C.; Tanaka, H. Hypoxia-inducible factor regulates survival of antigen receptor-driven T cells. *J. Immunol.* **2003**, *171*, 6534–6540. [CrossRef]
41. Doedens, A.L.; Phan, A.T.; Stradner, M.H.; Fujimoto, J.K.; Nguyen, J.V.; Yang, E.; Johnson, R.S.; Goldrath, A.W. Hypoxia-inducible factors enhance the effector responses of CD8(+) T cells to persistent antigen. *Nat. Immunol.* **2013**, *14*, 1173–1182. [CrossRef] [PubMed]
42. Galon, J.; Costes, A.; Sanchez-Cabo, F.; Kirilovsky, A.; Mlecnik, B.; Lagorce-Pages, C.; Tosolini, M.; Camus, M.; Berger, A.; Wind, P.; et al. Type, density, and location of immune cells within human colorectal tumors predict clinical outcome. *Science* **2006**, *313*, 1960–1964. [CrossRef]
43. Vasaikar, S.; Huang, C.; Wang, X.; Petyuk, V.A.; Savage, S.R.; Wen, B.; Dou, Y.C.; Zhang, Y.; Shi, Z.A.; Arshad, O.A.; et al. Proteogenomic Analysis of Human Colon Cancer Reveals New Therapeutic Opportunities. *Cell* **2019**, *177*, 1035–1049.e19. [CrossRef]
44. Bauer, K.; Michel, S.; Reuschenbach, M.; Nelius, N.; Doeberitz, M.V.; Kloor, M. Dendritic cell and macrophage infiltration in microsatellite-unstable and microsatellite-stable colorectal cancer. *Fam. Cancer* **2011**, *10*, 557–565. [CrossRef] [PubMed]
45. Yoo, Y.G.; Hayashi, M.; Christensen, J.; Huang, L.E. An Essential Role of the HIF-1 alpha-c-Myc Axis in Malignant Progression. *Ann. N. Y. Acad. Sci.* **2009**, *1177*, 198–204. [CrossRef] [PubMed]
46. Kumar, S.M.; Yu, H.; Edwards, R.; Chen, L.; Kazianis, S.; Brafford, P.; Acs, G.; Herlyn, M.; Xu, X. Mutant V600E BRAF increases hypoxia inducible factor-1alpha expression in melanoma. *Cancer Res.* **2007**, *67*, 3177–3184. [CrossRef]
47. Dejea, C.M.; Wick, E.C.; Hechenbleikner, E.M.; White, J.R.; Welch, J.L.M.; Rossetti, B.J.; Peterson, S.N.; Snesrud, E.C.; Borisy, G.G.; Lazarev, M.; et al. Microbiota organization is a distinct feature of proximal colorectal cancers. *Proc. Natl. Acad. Sci. USA* **2014**, *111*, 18321–18326. [CrossRef]

48. Zgouras, D.; Wachtershauser, A.; Frings, D.; Stein, J. Butyrate impairs intestinal tumor cell-induced angiogenesis by inhibiting HIF-1alpha nuclear translocation. *Biochem. Biophys. Res. Commun.* **2003**, *300*, 832–838. [CrossRef]
49. Koury, J.; Deitch, E.A.; Homma, H.; Abungu, B.; Gangurde, P.; Condon, M.R.; Lu, Q.; Xu, D.Z.; Feinman, R. Persistent HIF-1alpha activation in gut ischemia/reperfusion injury: Potential role of bacteria and lipopolysaccharide. *Shock* **2004**, *22*, 270–277. [CrossRef]

4

Talkin' Toxins: From Coley's to Modern Cancer Immunotherapy

Robert D. Carlson †, John C. Flickinger, Jr. † and Adam E. Snook *

Department of Pharmacology and Experimental Therapeutics, Thomas Jefferson University, 1020 Locust Street, Philadelphia, PA 19107, USA; Robert.Carlson@jefferson.edu (R.D.C.); John.Flickinger@jefferson.edu (J.C.F.J.)
* Correspondence: adam.snook@jefferson.edu
† These authors contributed equally to this work.

Abstract: The ability of the immune system to precisely target and eliminate aberrant or infected cells has long been studied in the field of infectious diseases. Attempts to define and exploit these potent immunological processes in the fight against cancer has been a longstanding effort dating back over 100 years to when Dr. William Coley purposefully infected cancer patients with a cocktail of heat-killed bacteria to stimulate anti-cancer immune processes. Although the field of cancer immunotherapy has been dotted with skepticism at times, the success of immune checkpoint inhibitors and recent FDA approvals of autologous cell therapies have pivoted immunotherapy to center stage as one of the most promising strategies to treat cancer. This review aims to summarize historic milestones throughout the field of cancer immunotherapy as well as highlight current and promising immunotherapies in development.

Keywords: cancer; immunotherapy; vaccine; immune checkpoint inhibitors; adoptive cell therapy; cytokine therapy; Coley's Toxins

Key Contribution: This review summarizes the pivotal milestones in cancer immunotherapy development from Coley's Toxins to modern day.

---

1. Introduction

The understanding of immune system governance in neoplastic growth and development has made significant leaps in recent years [1], but its origins can be traced back well over a century ago. Incidence of tumors spontaneously regressing following infectious or pyretic periods have been described throughout history [2–4]. However, advancements made in histological diagnosis and assessment of tumor malignancies over the past 100 years have given credence to these claims of immune system modulation in cancer.

2. Pivotal Observations in Cancer Immunotherapy

It is possible that cancer has existed ever since the evolution from unicellular organisms into multicellular entities. However, the oldest record of cancer to date is from a 240 million-year-old fossil containing a shell-less stem turtle, *Pappochelys rosinae*, with evidence of osteosarcoma [5]. Until recently, the treatment of cancer has historically focused on tumor excision, cytotoxic chemotherapeutic agents, and radiation therapy. Only after the turn of the 21st century did immunotherapy to treat cancer take stage [Figure 1].

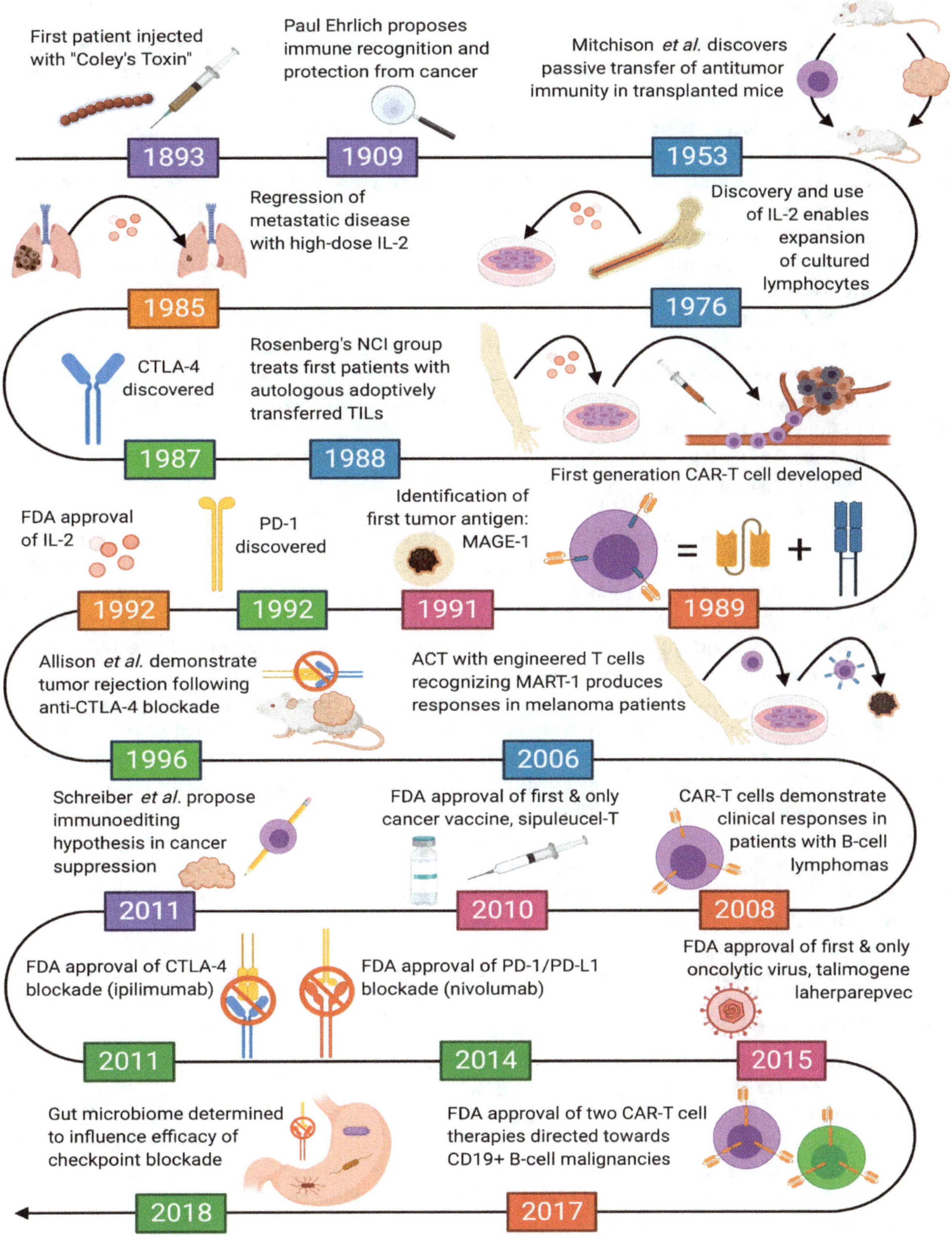

Figure 1. Milestones in the History of Cancer Immunotherapy.

2.1. The Story of Coley's Toxins

William Coley, often regarded as the "Father of Immunotherapy", was a bone surgeon in New York from 1890–1936 who famously developed a cocktail of heat-killed bacteria, called "Coley's Toxins", to treat patients with osteosarcoma. Inspiration for developing this treatment apparently started with one of his first patients, a young woman with osteosarcoma of the hand. Despite his surgical intervention (amputation of the forearm), she succumbed to metastatic disease within months of the operation. This episode had a profound impact on Coley and motivated him to learn more about her disease. He began by reviewing hospital medical records from ninety sarcoma patients, an analysis he later published [6]. While conducting his review, one patient's course of disease was of particular intrigue. Coley came across the description of a patient with an inoperable sarcoma whose tumor completely regressed after developing erysipelas [7], a type of skin infection [8]. Upon reading this account, Coley wondered if it was possible to induce erysipelas in patients as a means to treat cancer. Fortunately for Coley, a German surgeon named Friedrich Fehleisen had only a few years earlier, in 1883, identified *Streptococcus pyogenes* as the bacterium responsible for erysipelas [9]. Thus, Coley was able to test his hypothesis and began injecting sarcoma patients with *Streptococcus pyogenes,* a primitive version of what would later be named Coley's Toxins.

Over the course of Coley's career, from 1888–1933, he tested over a dozen different preparations of his toxin. Developing his infamous toxin required striking a balance between safety and efficacy. Indeed, early preparations were highly variable. Some preparations were impotent and failed to produce any signs of infection while other preparations were highly infectious and led to mortality [10]. Eventually, Coley settled on a combination of heat-killed *Streptococcus pyogenes* and *Serratia marcescens* [11]. Although Coley was not the first person to make a connection between infection and cancer regression, nor the first to inject bacteria into a patient as a means to mediate tumor rejection, Coley's efforts were the most comprehensive and influential. In total, it is estimated that Coley himself injected more than 1000 cancer patients and published over 150 papers related to the topic [11].

Coley reported remarkable success with his toxins and published many reports of his toxins inducing tumor regression [12,13]. However, at the time, his findings were highly controversial and were met with harsh criticism by many of his colleagues. Notable critiques include those in the *Journal of the American Medical Association* in 1894 issuing a statement criticizing the use of his toxins as well as the FDA re-categorizing of "Coley's Toxins" in 1963 as an investigational drug that lacked safety and efficacy data, despite over 70 years of use and numerous publications [11]. This recategorization made it illegal to prescribe Coley's Toxins outside of clinical trial testing. In the end, history would be on the side of William Coley. Years after his death, his toxins were re-evaluated in a controlled trial and were demonstrated to mediate antitumor effects [14]. Moreover, advancements in fundamental understanding of cancer and the immune system have allowed his findings to become more widely accepted and to lay a foundation for future studies of cancer immunotherapy.

2.2. Evidence the Immune System Targets Cancer

Although Coley never fully understood the mechanism by which his toxins functioned, he gathered substantial evidence linking the immune system and cancer. Further clarity and development of this connection would come years later in the form of the immunosurveillance hypothesis. The idea that the immune system possesses a capacity to recognize and eliminate cancer cells was first postulated by Paul Ehrlich in 1909 [15]. While direct experimental evidence during this time period was lacking, Ehrlich reasoned that the incidence of cancer is relatively low but that the formation of aberrant cells is a common phenomenon, suggesting the existence of a host defense system against cancer. Over 50 years later, these ideas were further developed by Burnet and Thomas and formally coined the "immune surveillance" hypothesis [16,17].

Early experimental evidence for the existence of tumor-specific immunity derives from transplantation studies. In 1943, Luwik Gross utilized methylcholanthrene (MCA) to chemically induce sarcoma in a C3H mouse and then transplanted this sarcoma into syngeneic mice. While inoculation with high doses of tumor cells often killed mice, Gross found that inoculation with low doses of tumor cells led to a period of growth followed by gradual tumor regression. In these surviving mice, tumor challenge using high doses of tumor cells invariably led to rejection, suggesting these animals developed immunity to the tumor [18]. Further support for immunosurveillance comes from a seminal study by Prehn and Main in 1953. In these studies, an array of sarcomas from multiple syngeneic mice were generated using MCA. Prehn and Main found that inoculation of a mouse with sarcoma from one source protected that mouse from future challenge using the same sarcoma source but did not protect against challenge using sarcoma derived from a different mouse [19]. Moreover, Prehn and Main demonstrated that transplantation of skin tissue from a donor mouse did not sensitize the recipient mouse to the donor's sarcoma, directly addressing a common critique at the time that rejection was mediated by subtle differences in genetic backgrounds. Collectively, these studies further supported the existence of tumor-specific immunity, adding the nuance that tumor antigens are highly unique to a tumor even in tumors of the same histological type, induced by the same chemical means, and from mice of the same genetic background [19].

While studies in partially immunocompromised mouse models over the following decades failed to support the immunosurveillance hypothesis, definitive demonstration of immunosurveillance came in the early 2000s following a series of studies conducted in novel, specifically immunocompromised, mouse strains. In 2001, Robert Schreiber's group compared the incidence of spontaneous neoplasms between wild-type and *Rag2*$^{-/-}$ mice (*Rag2* encodes a protein necessary for somatic recombination and thus *Rag2*$^{-/-}$ mice lack mature T and B lymphocytes) [20]. In mice over 15 months old, fewer than 20% of wild-type mice contained neoplastic disease while 100% of surveyed *Rag2*$^{-/-}$ mice developed spontaneous neoplastic lesions in various tissues, suggesting functional T and B lymphocytes suppress the development of cancer. Moreover, the same study observed that *Rag2*$^{-/-}$ mice, as well as *Ifngr1*$^{-/-}$ and *Stat1*$^{-/-}$ mice, which are deficient in vital immune signaling pathways, develop higher incidences of sarcoma compared to wild-type mice in MCA-induced tumor models [21]. Similarly, higher incidences of MCA-induced tumors were reported by additional investigators using mice deficient in other vital immune-signaling molecules such as perforin or TNF-related apoptosis-inducing ligand (TRAIL) [22,23]. These experimental studies in mice are mirrored by clinical evidence that humans with compromised immune systems develop higher incidences of cancer. Indeed, individuals born with genetic defects in immune-related genes develop higher incidences of lymphoma [24]. Moreover, people with otherwise normal immune function who acquire AIDS infection or transplant patients who receive immunosuppressive drugs are both at higher risk for developing Non-Hodgkin's lymphoma and virus-induced Kaposi Sarcoma [25,26].

Since the emergence of the immunosurveillance hypothesis, the interplay between the immune system and cancer has been further refined and renamed as the process of "immunoediting" [27]. Immunoediting posits that the immune system and cancer intersect at three stages: elimination, equilibrium, and escape. During the elimination stage, the immune system recognizes and destroys many, but not all aberrant cells. During equilibrium, the immune system and the tumor exert opposing forces, effectively resulting in containment of the tumor. Over time, as the cancer acquires additional mutations and as the immune system exerts a selective pressure eliminating immunogenic cells and leaving behind non-immunogenic cells, the cancer eventually fully escapes immune surveillance. In this final escape stage, the cancer has fully circumvented detection by the immune system and undergoes rapid and uncontrolled growth. Evidence for equilibrium and escape stages is supported by experiments in mice with stagnant tumor sizes who then undergo rapid growth after immune cell depletion [28]. Additionally, tumors arising from immunocompromised mice are more frequently rejected when transplanted into a wild-type host compared to tumors arising from immunocompetent mice [21], partly reflecting immune-induced antigen loss in the presence of an intact immune system [29] (immunoediting). Thus, the fundamental goal of cancer immunotherapy is to overcome the years to decades of immunoediting to generate antitumor immunity that is sufficient to completely eliminate the patient's cancer and cure their disease.

3. Immunomodulatory Agents

Immunomodulators comprise a variety of therapeutic agents and treatment strategies that aid in normalizing, or in the context of cancer, re-engaging or boosting immune cell function to counter uncontrolled cell proliferation. By definition, a tumor that presents in the clinic can be said to have escaped normal immune control, even if tumor-reactive T cells are detected in the blood or have infiltrated the tumor tissue [30]. Although tumor cells themselves possess intrinsic immunosuppressive behaviors, such as cultivating a hypoxic microenvironment [31,32] or generating lactic acid [33], the majority of suppressive influence comes from the normal functions of suppressive immune cells, cytokines, and inhibitory surface molecules [34,35]. Under normal physiological circumstances, these mechanisms suppress T-cell priming and cytotoxic T-cell function to stave off unwarranted autoinflammatory responses [36]. Therefore, many of the immunomodulatory agents described herein aim to directly oppose these immunosuppressive mechanisms and to re-engage the immune system.

3.1. Cytokine Therapy

Prior to understanding their therapeutic immunomodulatory potential in cancer, cytokines were first recognized as systemic soluble factors that could regulate lymphocyte function and inflammatory responses. In 1972, a group from Yale University School of Medicine first characterized a "lymphocyte activating factor" that spurred lymphocyte proliferation in response to soluble agents released by other syngeneic immune cells [37]. These agents were partially purified from antigen-stimulated, lymphocyte-conditioned media and characterized further as "T-cell growth factor" that could support cytotoxic T cells capable of killing autologous leukemic myeloblasts [38]. Shortly thereafter, this key growth factor was definitively purified and described as interleukin-2 (IL-2) [39], which not only allowed T lymphocytes to be cultured in large quantities ex vivo, but also allowed recombinant IL-2 to be administered as a high-dose single-agent [40], or used in tandem with preconditioned and transplanted cancer-specific lymphoid cells [41,42]. A comprehensive report published in 1987 by the NCI's Surgery Branch documented objective responses to high-dose IL-2 and regression of tumors in patients with metastatic melanoma and renal cell cancer [43]. Adjustments made to IL-2 dose scheduling would largely combat acute toxicities, the most prominent being capillary leak syndrome and hypovolemia [44]. These results and safety measures would spur numerous and larger cohort studies utilizing IL-2 in a metastatic setting [45,46], culminating with FDA approval of high-dose intravenous IL-2 for patients with metastatic renal cancer in 1992, and metastatic melanoma several years later. This would be noted as one of the first FDA-approved cancer immunotherapies [47].

Other cytokines that have demonstrated translational applications include interleukin-15 (IL-15), interferon-alpha (IFNα), and granulocyte macrophage colony-stimulating factor (GM-CSF). While both structurally similar and capable of stimulating early T-cell proliferation and NK cell engagement much like IL-2, IL-15 additionally supports memory CD8$^+$ T-cell persistence, a known mediator of long-term antitumor immunity [48]. IL-15 has also proven to be an effective mediator of antitumor protection in murine models of cancer [49–52]. In support of these claims, phase 1 clinical trials utilizing recombinant IL-15 alone, and in conjunction with B-cell-depleting antibodies, are currently underway for treating both solid and liquid tumors, respectively [NCT01021059, NCT03759184].

IFNα, another cytokine originally described in the context of mediating antiviral immune response [53,54], was also identified to inhibit tumor neovasculature, upregulate MHC class I expression, mediate dendritic cell maturation, activate B and T cells, and induce apoptosis—all favorable antitumor attributes [55]. Thanks to the efforts of blood banking that began in the late 1970s [56], adequate quantities of purified IFNα spurred a burst of clinical evaluations in patients with hematological malignancies [57,58] and solid tumors, such as renal cell cancers and malignant melanoma [59,60]. These trials culminated in FDA approval of IFNα as an adjuvant therapy first in rare forms of leukemia, and later in patients with high-risk stage II and stage III melanoma [61].

As the name suggests, GM-CSF was originally identified as a regulator of granulocyte and macrophage differentiation, as well as general hematopoiesis of multi-lineage progenitors [62]. However, in 1993,

Dranoff and colleagues transduced B16 melanoma cells with ten known pro-inflammatory mediators, vaccinated mice with these constructs, and then challenged them with live B16 cells. Of the ten, GM-CSF conferred the largest magnitude of antitumor immunity [63]. These findings prompted strategies to deliver GM-CSF to patients, either by vaccinating patients with irradiated tumor cells engineered to secrete the cytokine [64], or by single-agent dosing [65]. Although the exploration of GM-CSF-expressing tumor vaccines has waned in recent years due to limited clinical efficacy [66], combination strategies employing recombinant GM-CSF with other immunomodulatory agents, such as checkpoint inhibitors [67] and additional cytokines [68] have enhanced overall survival in melanoma patient trials.

3.2. *Immune Checkpoint Inhibitors*

Suppression of immune cell activation, infiltration, and effector functions required for tumor cell clearance can be largely attributed to the immunosuppressive conditions within the tumor microenvironment [69]. In several studies, "dysfunctional" $CD8^+$ T cells were retrieved from patient tumors and nearby draining lymph nodes and said to be lacking the expected differentiation profiles [70], or impaired by the accumulation of repressive $Foxp3^+$ regulatory T cells (Tregs) [71]. A similar phenomenon was originally described in mice infected with a lymphocytic choriomeningitis virus, whereby chronic antigen stimulation induced an "exhausted" T-cell state proceeded by T-cell receptor (TCR) downregulation [72]. The discovery of other requisite activating co-stimulatory signals in addition to canonical antigen stimulation with the TCR [73], which was now known to be insufficient for fully functional T-cell activation [74], gave clues to the complex nature of balancing activation with self-antigen tolerance [75]. Immune homeostasis is dependent upon these co-stimulatory/co-inhibitory receptor-ligand interactions, which in the correct context, safeguard against chronic immune activation and excessive inflammatory responses [76]. Addressing these phenomena directly, immune checkpoint blockade selectively restricts these co-inhibitory signaling mechanisms that have been co-opted by cancer cells, thereby enhancing antitumor T-cell activity.

Although initially identified in 1987 [77], the 1994 discovery of cytotoxic T lymphocyte-associated antigen-4 (CTLA-4) co-inhibitory receptor pairing with the B7 co-stimulatory ligand is perhaps the most substantial [78]. Upregulation of CTLA-4 on both $CD4^+$ and $CD8^+$ T lymphocytes was identified as a negative regulator of T-cell activation and effector functions [79,80], while murine models deficient in CTLA-4 experienced massive lymphoproliferation and tissue infiltration due to over-activation of resident T cells [81,82]. In the late 1990s, Dr. James Allison's group at University of California, administered an inhibitory antibody to block the CTLA-4 co-inhibitory synapse in mice burdened with tumors. Both orthotopic and pre-established tumor cells were rejected following administration of the anti-CTLA-4 antibody, indicating that blockade of inhibitory signals associated with the co-stimulatory pathway can enhance antitumor immunity [83]. These indications prompted the application of CTLA-4 blockade in patients with stage III/IV unresectable melanoma with remarkable success [84], culminating in the 2011 FDA approval of the anti-CTLA-4 monoclonal antibody (mAb), ipilimumab, as an adjuvant therapy for patients with cutaneous melanoma. Retrospective studies have revealed marked increases in survival benefit compared to traditional chemotherapy regimens [85,86], with modest gains observed in other solid tumor types currently in various phases of clinical trials [87].

In an effort to identify genes associated with apoptosis, Dr. Tasuku Honjo's group at Kyoto University discovered programmed cell death protein 1 (PD-1), a lymphoid cell surface protein that the group hypothesized to be a cell-death inducer [88]. Several years later in 1999, the same group generated a PD-1 deficient mouse model that spontaneously developed several autoimmune-like symptoms and systemic graft-versus-host-like disease [89]. Like CTLA-4, PD-1 was identified as a negative regulator of adaptive immune responses. PD-1 ligand 1 (PD-L1) was discovered that same year at the Mayo Clinic and characterized as functionally homologous to the CTLA-4 ligand, B7, but co-stimulated T cells through some additional unknown receptor [90], later identified to be PD-1 [91]. Engagement of PD-1 with its ligand prevented T-cell proliferation and cytokine production when synthetically stimulated, identifying it as an intrinsic inhibitory mechanism of autoreactive lymphocyte activation [91]. PD-L1 surface expression on tumor cells was also discovered to suppress the cytolytic effector functions of $CD8^+$ T cells, with additional speculation that PD-1/PD-L1 blockade could serve as an effective strategy to combat tumor cell escape [92]. Speculation became reality when several groups tested PD-L1 blockade in murine tumor models and concluded that antibodies directed at this co-stimulatory interaction could enhance cancer immunotherapy [93–95]. In one step closer to the clinic, PD-L1 was determined to be a prognostic marker of patient outcome, with higher levels of ligand in resected specimens correlated with poorer patient survival [96]. Within the past 10 years, several high-profile trials employing anti-PD-1/PD-L1 mAbs under various conditions, dosing strategies, and cancer types, have indicated that blockade of this co-inhibitory pathway is both well-tolerated and associated with durable objective responses in patients [97–99]. Consequently, FDA approval was granted first to nivolumab, a humanized PD-1 mAb for metastatic melanoma in 2014, and subsequently for pembrolizumab, a PD-1 mAb alternative. Both therapies elicited greater overall patient survival compared to their anti-CTLA-4 counterpart [100,101]. In 2016, a third antibody was developed, this time directed at the PD-L1 ligand to treat patients with urothelial carcinoma and non-small cell lung cancer with much success [102,103]. This fully humanized anti-PD-L1 mAb, atezolizumab, was granted FDA approval for bladder cancer patients ineligible for traditional cisplatin-based chemotherapies [104]. Recent studies have expanded the number of indications for anti-PD-1/PD-L1 blockade alone [105], and in combination with anti-CTLA-4 [106], both proving to be summarily efficacious.

Although CTLA-4 and PD-1 blockade strategies have demonstrated unprecedented clinical success and accelerated FDA approval, there remains a population of non-responders. These individuals either fail to respond to checkpoint blockade from treatment onset due to innate resistance mechanisms, or acquire secondary resistance resulting in relapse. Retrospective studies of large-cohort clinical trials may expose novel biomarkers capable of predicting resistance to checkpoint therapies [107]. Additional co-inhibitory receptors, each with unique functions, have since been identified to influence negative immune regulation by various mechanisms [108]. Likewise, recent findings have demonstrated that the resident gut microbiome has the ability to influence patient responses to checkpoint blockade, with individuals who had consumed oral antibiotics prior to therapy experiencing poorer anti-PD-1 responses [109,110]. Nonetheless, immune checkpoint inhibitors continue to represent the vast majority of new immunotherapies for the treatment of cancer. These therapies would not be possible without seminal discoveries made in the blockade of negative immune regulatory elements by Drs. James Allison and Tasuku Honjo, for which they were awarded the 2018 Nobel Prize in Physiology or Medicine.

4. Vaccines

While immunomodulatory agents broadly stimulate the immune system, cancer vaccines aim to more precisely steer an immune response towards cancer. At its purest form, a cancer vaccine consists of one or more tumor antigens combined with an adjuvant to enhance the immune response. As will later be described, the type of tumor antigen, delivery method of the antigen, and adjuvant varies greatly. Cancer vaccines can be administered as a therapeutic vaccine in patients with existing malignancies or as a preventive vaccine in healthy or high-risk individuals (primary prevention) or patients in remission (secondary prevention) to protect against future tumor development or recurrence, respectively.

4.1. Tumor Antigens

Initial attempts at vaccination occurred before the identification of specific tumor antigens. These trials utilized cellular-based vaccines consisting of modified or irradiated tumor cells derived from a patient (autologous) or from a cancer cell line (allogeneic) injected with adjuvant [111–113]. With the identification of the first human tumor antigen, MAGE-1, by Thierry Boon's group in 1991, a more refined approach of vaccinating against specific targets was born [114]. Since then, over 75 tumor-associated antigens have been identified [115]. There are two categories of tumor antigens: tumor-associated antigens and tumor-specific antigens. By definition, tumor-associated antigens share expression with some normal tissues while tumor-specific antigens are unique to cancer cells. Notable examples of tumor-associated antigens that have been a focus of multiple immunotherapies include the cancer-testis antigens NY-ESO-1 [116] and MAGE-1 [117], which are expressed by germ cells and ectopically re-expressed in cancers; the oncofetal antigens CEA [118] and alpha-1-fetoprotein [119], which are present during fetal development and re-expressed by cancers; differentiation antigens, such as prostate-specific antigen (PSA) [120] and CD19 [121], which are expressed by cells derived from a specific tissue-type and retained in cancers; and antigens that are over-expressed by cancers relative to normal tissue, including HER2 [122] and telomerase [123]. In contrast to tumor-associated antigens, which share expression with healthy tissue, tumor-specific antigens are exclusively expressed by tumors. Tumor-specific antigens, also known as neoantigens, are mutated peptides created by unique genetic aberrations or may be viral antigens in the case of virus-associated cancers [124].

4.2. Therapeutic Cancer Vaccines

In 1995 and 1996, the first clinical trials testing cancer vaccines against tumor-associated antigens were published. These trials utilized either peptide vaccines [125], or peptide-pulsed dendritic-cell vaccines composed of patient-derived dendritic cells that have been incubated with a peptide prior to re-infusion [126,127]. Other popular methods of cancer vaccination include the use of recombinant viral and bacterial vectors. As microorganisms potently stimulate the immune system, the use of these vectors to deliver tumor antigen in the context of an infection is hypothesized to enhance antitumor immune responses. Common vectors used to deliver tumor antigens include poxvirus [128], adenovirus [129], *Salmonella typhimurium* [130], and *Listeria monocytogenes* [131]. As methods of gene therapy have advanced over the years, the use of DNA and RNA vaccines has become increasingly common [132].

Despite thousands of cancer vaccine clinical trials, only one therapeutic cancer vaccine, Sipuleucel-T, is FDA-approved [133]. Sipuleucel-T is an autologous cell vaccine composed of patient peripheral blood mononuclear cells (PBMCs) pulsed with a chimeric protein consisting of the tumor-associated antigen prostate alkaline phosphatase (PAP) fused to the immunomodulating cytokine GM-CSF. A phase III clinical trial in men with metastatic castration-resistant prostate cancer found that three infusions of Sipuleucel-T led to the induction of PAP-specific immune responses and a 4.1-month improvement in median survival [134].

Limited success in therapeutic settings may be, in part, attributed to poor immunogenicity of the vaccine target and immunosuppressive tumor microenvironments. One approach to overcome poorly immunogenic tumor-associated antigens is the recent trend towards targeting neoantigens. Compared to tumor-associated antigens, neoantigens may be more immunogenic due to a lack of immunological tolerance mechanisms [135]. Until recently, the identification of neoantigens was impractical as the cost and time to sequence patient genomes for unique mutations presented a formidable barrier. However, with advancements in next-generation sequencing, it has become feasible to sequence a patient's normal and tumor genome to identify unique tumor-specific antigens. Personalized therapeutic neoantigen vaccines have shown promise in phase I trials for melanoma [136] and glioblastoma [137]. However, these neoantigen vaccines are in early clinical testing, and thus the efficacy and feasibility of this approach is yet to be determined.

4.3. Preventive Cancer Vaccines

Recently, there has been a trend towards testing cancer vaccines as preventive therapies. Vaccination in preventive settings may be preferable to therapeutic ones as it may allow for the induction of antitumor immunity before the development of immunosuppressive microenvironments [138]. This strategy has shown promise against multiple viral-based cancers. Indeed, vaccination against oncogenic viruses including hepatitis B and human papillomavirus have led to reductions in hepatic [139] and cervical [140] cancers, respectively. However, for non-virally associated cancers, a target antigen and clinical setting to administer preventive vaccines is often less clear. For example, vaccinating a healthy patient against a tumor-associated antigen may carry an unnecessary risk of autoimmunity. Additionally, preventive vaccination against neoantigens, while reducing the risk of autoimmunity, may be impractical as neoantigens are often widely variable between patients. However, preventive vaccination in some settings may be possible. One such example is vaccination against the mucin 1 (MUC1) antigen in patients at high-risk of colorectal cancer. In tumors, MUC1 is hypoglycosylated relative to normal tissues, allowing for the induction of selective antitumor responses [141]. A phase I/II study in patients with a history of colorectal adenoma demonstrated MUC1 immunogenicity and a phase II trial investigating the ability of MUC1 vaccine to prevent adenoma recurrence is currently ongoing [142].

4.4. *Oncolytic Virotherapy*

An emerging immunotherapeutic strategy that is often categorized as a cancer vaccine is the use of oncolytic viruses. Oncolytic viruses preferentially infect and kill tumor cells compared to normal tissue. Selective infection of tumor cells is achieved through a combination of factors including the overexpression of viral receptors on tumor cells which can facilitate viral entry, a proliferative cell cycle that promotes viral replication, and a tumor cell deficiency in type I interferon production leading to limited viral clearance [143]. In addition to mediating tumor regression by direct cell lysis, viral infection activates components of the innate and adaptive immune system, thereby contributing further to tumor cell death. For example, oncolytic viral infection activates NK cells to clear virally-infected tumor cells [144]. Moreover, immunogenic cell death of virally infected tumor cells releases both tumor-associated antigens and neoantigens that can be acquired and presented by antigen-presenting cells, leading to the induction of antitumor $CD8^+$ T cell responses (an approach often described as "in situ vaccination") [145,146].

The potential of oncolytic virotherapy was first noted by George Dock in 1904. Similar to Coley, Dock noticed that a patient with acute leukemia underwent remission after acquiring an influenza infection [147]. Many other case reports followed over the years, eventually leading to hundreds of clinical trials testing oncolytic viruses [148]. In 2015, the first oncolytic viral therapy, talimogene laherparepvec ("T-VEC"), was approved by the FDA for use in metastatic melanoma [143,149]. T-VEC is an attenuated herpes simplex virus harboring various genetic deletions and insertions designed to enhance the antitumor immune response, such as the deletion of an immune-evasive viral gene *ICP47* and the insertion of a human GM-CSF gene [145]. Compared to GM-CSF administration alone, T-VEC led to a 4.4 month increase in median survival in a phase III trial in patients with advanced and metastatic melanoma [143,149].

5. Adoptive Cell Therapy

5.1. *Tumor-Infiltrating Lymphocytes and Engineered T-Cell Receptors*

The antitumor activity of T lymphocytes was first elucidated in the 1950s and 1960s with seminal discoveries made in allograft rejection of sarcomas in experimental rodent models [150,151]. In 1953, Mitchison investigated the passive transfer of tumor immunity via transplantation of lymph nodes from mice inoculated with lymphosarcomas to equivalently challenged, but non-inoculated, mice [152]. A decade later, two groups made similar observations of transferrable tumor immunity by isolating and transplanting the cells of lymphatic tissues, rather than the organs themselves. Cells were collected from the lymphatic ducts and spleens of donor animals previously immunized with sarcoma cells that developed palpable tumors. Administration of those lymphoid cells back into syngeneic and non-syngeneic recipients inoculated with tumors, saw sustained regression indicating that these lymphocytes were "educated" by prior exposure to tumor antigens [153,154].

The means to exploit these T lymphocytes for their antitumor potential was limited by the inherent difficulty of expanding cells ex vivo. In 1976, a group at the NIH first described the co-culture of isolated human bone marrow with conditioned media containing IL-2 that could induce growth and differentiation of bone marrow cells to T lymphocyte precursors [155]. With the advent of commercially synthesized IL-2, T lymphocytes could now be cultured in large quantities, or in the context of an adjuvant, to boost the therapeutic effects of tumor-sensitized and adoptively transferred T lymphocytes [156]. This subset of cytokine-activated lymphocytes was identified to be among those infiltrating the stroma of transplanted tumors. Dr. Steven Rosenberg's group confirmed that tumor-infiltrating lymphocytes (TILs) isolated from resected tumor could recognize syngeneic tumor cells in vitro [157], as well as mediate durable antitumor responses when re-administered back into autologous animal models [158] and cancer patients with metastatic disease [159].

The relatively pure populations of $CD8^+$ and $CD4^+$ T cells cultured from resected tumors appeared to dissipate quickly when returned to patients, meaning that therapeutic responses were often transient. However, in 2002, prior application of a lymphodepleting, nonmyeloablative chemotherapy regimen, originally designed for allogeneic bone marrow transplantation [160], greatly enhanced TIL engraftment and clonal persistence in patients, with some individuals harboring up to 80% $CD8^+$ T cells many months post-infusion [161,162]. Shortly thereafter, another milestone was achieved when the Rosenberg group retrovirally transduced patient-derived peripheral blood lymphocytes with a TCR recognizing the common melanoma antigen, MART-1. Objective cancer regression was observed in 2 out of 15 patients (13%) when engineered T lymphocytes were adoptively transferred back into patients [163], with a subsequent report demonstrating an improved 30% objective response rate [164]. Additional trials employing engineered TCRs targeting NY-ESO-1 in synovial cell sarcoma [165], the GD2 disialoganglioside in neuroblastoma [166], and carcinoembryonic antigen (CEA) in colorectal cancer [167] demonstrated objective clinical responses, thereby broadening the application to additional tumor types. More recently, personalized strategies using whole-exome sequencing of patient tumors has given researchers the ability to target neoantigens with high specificity [168,169]. Classically unmanipulated TIL therapy will continue to serve a patient population with shared and broadly targetable antigens [170], while more nuanced TILs recognizing neoantigens will continue to pace evolving therapies in the age of personalized medicine [171].

5.2. Chimeric Antigen Receptor T Cell (CAR-T Cell) Therapy

Although adoptive transfer of tumor-sensitized and antigen-reactive TILs with prefatory lymphodepletion and IL-2 dosing regimens had proven effective in the clinic, patient responses were often transient: shrinkage in metastatic lesions could occur, without objective response to treatment [172]. Native TCRs are often limited by their ability to recognize post-translationally or aberrantly modified proteins, such as those observed in tumor-associated antigens of malignant cells [173,174]. Likewise, T cells dependent on antigen presentation by MHC molecules are routinely hindered by MHC class I downregulation, a selective mechanism of tumor immune escape [175].

In 1989, an Israeli group at the Weizmann Institute of Science devised the first proof-of-concept strategy using an engineered chimeric antigen receptor (CAR) to circumvent the need for MHC-mediated antigen presentation for T-cell activation. By combining the intracellular T-cell receptor circuitry with the antigen-recognizing variable domains of an antibody raised against 2,4,6-trinitrophenyl (TNP), the researchers were able to elicit a non-MHC-restricted response in transfected T lymphocytes to target cells bearing TNP on their surface [176]. The unprecedented antibody-type specificity, now liberated from MHC presentation and paired to effector T-cell function, could conceivably target post-translationally modified proteins characteristic of tumor cells undergoing selection or escape. Several years later, the same group successfully generated CARs directed towards HER2, a cell surface antigen commonly overexpressed in adenocarcinomas. These CAR-T cells selectively lysed $HER2^+$ cancer cells in vitro, providing evidence that mAbs directed towards common tumor cell antigens, could be reassembled into single chain variable fragments (scFvs) to facilitate immune effector function directly [177]. That same year, a joint venture between Weizmann Institute and the NIH expanded the spectrum of available targets by targeting folate receptors commonly overexpressed in ovarian carcinoma cells and further demonstrating the potential of adoptively transferring these CAR-T cells into cancer patients [178].

In an effort to improve CAR-T cell activation, CD28 costimulatory molecules were added in a single tandem gene product with the intracellular CD3ζ-chain. Tumor cells often lack costimulatory molecules entirely, a barrier to persistent activation in first-generation CAR-T cells. Much like conventional T cells, an "exhausted" phenotype was observed in T cells expressing first-generation constructs encountering tumor cells in excess. In contrast, second-generation CAR-T cells containing additional built-in CD28 costimulatory moieties demonstrated superior signaling functionality, persistence, and cytokine production [179,180], as well as antitumor activity [181]. Over the next decade, second-generation CARs would be the basis for many first-in-human studies: first targeting carbonic anhydrase IX (CAIX), an antigen commonly overexpressed in renal cell carcinoma (RCC), and shortly thereafter, the ovarian cancer–associated antigen α-folate receptor (FR). CAIX-directed CAR-T cells produced grade 2–4 liver toxicity in patients due to CAIX self-antigen present in normal bile duct epithelium, with no overall response in RCC tumors [182]. Likewise, FR-directed CAR-T cells in a parallel phase 1 study, produced no reduction in ovarian tumor burden, albeit with lower grade 1–2 toxicity and no detectable off-tumor or off-target responses [183].

Major clinical breakthroughs were not seen until several years later when CAR-T cell therapy strategy switched from targeting primarily solid tumors, to liquid tumors, such as B-cell lymphomas and leukemias. In 2008, a group at University of Washington pioneered a proof-of-concept clinical trial in which refractory B-cell lymphoma patients received 20 infusions of autologous CD20-directed CAR-T cells. Treatment was well-tolerated in patients, with minimal toxicities and modified T cells persisting up to 9 weeks. Of the seven patients, two were noted as having complete response to treatment [184]. With phase 1 clinical trials rapidly taking shape around B-cell targets, methods for manufacturing and validating clinical-grade autologous CAR-T cells were developed to support increasing demand [185]. Shortly thereafter, the Rosenberg group within the NCI's Surgery Branch, demonstrated in vivo antigen-specific activity of CAR-T cells directed towards the B-cell-specific antigen, CD19, in advanced-stage follicular lymphoma [186]. Paralleling this seminal study, Dr. Carl June's group at the University of Pennsylvania demonstrated specific and effective on-target killing of $CD19^+$ malignant B cells in patients with advanced chronic lymphocytic leukemia (CLL) using CD19-directed CAR-T cells. In that study, two out of three patients experienced complete remission of disease, with a portion of CAR-T cells retaining potent effector function six months after initial infusion, indicating a possible memory CAR-T cell phenotype [187,188]. The CAR employed by the University of Pennsylvania possessed a 4-1BB (CD137) costimulatory domain, rather than CD28, that promoted in vivo persistence and antileukemic function that outperformed conventional CARs with either CD3ζ and CD28 costimulatory molecules or CD3ζ alone [187,189].

Over the next few years, both groups continued to advance the field by targeting various $CD19^+$ hematological malignancies with great success. However, unanticipated and oftentimes severe neurological toxicities in the form of cytokine release syndrome were observed in patients. This toxicity can manifest as fevers, headaches, aphasia, and in some cases, hallucinations, delirium, and seizures [190]. Cytokine blockade strategies to control the abundance of systemically released cytokines, namely administering the IL-6-blocking antibody tocilizumab with and without corticosteroids, were developed to combat acute neural toxicity [191–195]. Although major clinical gains have been achieved with $CD19^+$ hematologic malignancies, the same successes have yet to be fully realized in solid tumors. Despite abundant antigenic heterogeneity, difficulties in trafficking to tumor sites, and an intrinsic immunosuppressive tumor microenvironment [196,197], CAR-T cell therapies against solid tumor malignancies have entered early-phase clinical trials with varying degrees of success [Table 1].

Table 1. Summary of active clinical trials for CAR-T cell therapy in solid tumors.

Antigen Target	Cancer Type	Phase	ClinicalTrials.gov Designation
CD117	Osteoid Sarcoma, Ewing Sarcoma	I/II	NCT03356782
CD133	Liver, Pancreatic, Brain, Breas, Ovarian, Colorectal, Acute Myeloid and Lymphoid Leukemias	I/II	NCT02541370
	Osteoid Sarcoma, Ewing Sarcoma	I/II	NCT03356782
CD171	Neuroblastoma, Ganglioneuroblastoma,	I	NCT02311621
CEA	Colorectal	I/II	NCT02959151
	Lung, Colorectal, Gastric, Breast, Pancreatic	I	NCT02349724
EGFR	Colorectal	I/II	NCT03152435
EGFRvIII	Glioma, Glioblastoma, Gliosarcoma	I/II	NCT01454596
EpCAM	Colon, Esophageal, Pancreatic, Prostate, Gastric, Hepatic	I/II	NCT03013712
EphA2	Glioma	I/II	NCT02575261
ErbB	Head and Neck	I/II	NCT01818323
FRα	Urothelial Bladder	I/II	NCT03185468
GD2	Glioma	I/II	NCT03252171
	Neuroblastoma	I/II	NCT03373097
		I	NCT01822652
		II	NCT02765243
	Cervical	I/II	NCT03356795
	Osteoid Sarcoma, Ewing Sarcoma	I/II	NCT03356782
	Sarcoma, Osteosarcoma, Neuroblastoma, Melanoma	I	NCT02107963
GPC3	Hepatocellular Carcinoma	I/II	NCT02723942
			NCT02959151
			NCT03084380
HER2	Breast	I/II	NCT02547961
	Sarcoma	I	NCT00902044
IL-13Rα2	Glioma, Glioblastoma	I	NCT02208362
Mesothelin	Pancreatic	I/II	NCT02959151
	Cervical	I/II	NCT03356795
	Advanced Solid Tumors	I/II	NCT03615313
	Pancreatic, Ovarian, Mesothelioma	I	NCT02159716
	Malignant Pleural Disease, Mesothelioma, Lung, Breast	I	NCT02414269
MUC1	Cervical	I/II	NCT03356795
	Esophageal	I/II	NCT03706326
	Non-Small Cell Lung	I/II	NCT03525782
	Osteoid Sarcoma, Ewing Sarcoma	I/II	NCT03356782
	Intrahepatic Cholangiocarcinoma	I/II	NCT03633773
MUC-16	Ovarian	I	NCT02498912
PSMA	Urothelial Bladder	I/II	NCT03185468
	Cervical	I/II	NCT03356795
	Prostate	I	NCT01140373

6. Conclusions

The late 19th century observation that tumors could be treated with cocktails of heat-killed bacteria has proven highly influential. Unbeknownst to William Coley and his contemporaries, this would prove to be one of the first documented cases of tumor regression by induced activation of the immune system. Coley's legacy would help spur subsequent hypotheses of immunosurveillance mechanisms capable of mediating steady-state tumor recognition and elimination. Over the next century, exploitation of these mechanisms was to become a major priority as immunotherapies continued to evolve.

Treatment regimens using recombinant cytokines that activate immune cell proliferation and effector functions are efficacious in treating selected patient populations. Likewise, strategies employing immune checkpoint blockade against tumor cells that express co-inhibitory molecules have reached clinical milestones once thought to be unachievable. Vaccines against tumor-associated antigens have demonstrated clinical benefit, with applications turning towards neoantigens as patient-specific tumor sequencing becomes feasible. FDA approval of the oncolytic virotherapy, T-VEC, may also offer another option for locally-acting immune stimulation and antitumor activity when resection, chemotherapy, or radiation are not amenable. Moreover, the success of CAR-T cell therapy in patients with hematological malignancies has established adoptive cell therapy as a viable treatment modality. As the costs associated with patient and tumor genome sequencing continue to decrease, the rapidly evolving "omics"-level of data acquisition and processing may enable precise treatment strategies for these patients. Deconvoluting patient-specific tumor heterogeneity with the assistance of "big data" may enable clinicians and researchers to select the best candidate immunotherapy from the start, while taking proactive approaches to overcome resistance mechanisms in an adaptive tumor microenvironment [198]. The previous ~150 years of immuno-oncology research without significant clinical success has now enabled "hockey stick" growth in exploration of the safety and efficacy of immune-centric therapies in clinical trials. Just as William Coley's fundamental discoveries have shaped modern cancer immunotherapy, so too shall current efforts influence the future of cancer treatment.

Author Contributions: R.D.C., J.C.F.J., and A.E.S. conceived the review, R.D.C. and J.C.F.J. wrote the manuscript, and A.E.S. revised. All authors have read and agreed to the published version of the manuscript.

References

1. Couzin-Frankel, J. Breakthrough of the year 2013. Cancer immunotherapy. *Science* **2013**, *342*, 1432–1433. [CrossRef] [PubMed]
2. Challis, G.B.; Stam, H.J. The spontaneous regression of cancer. A review of cases from 1900 to 1987. *Acta Oncol.* **1990**, *29*, 545–550. [CrossRef] [PubMed]
3. Papac, R.J. Spontaneous regression of cancer. *Cancer Treat. Rev.* **1996**, *22*, 395–423. [CrossRef]
4. Smith, J.L.; Stehlin, J.S. Spontaneous regression of primary malignant melanomas with regional metastases. *Cancer* **1965**, *18*, 1399–1415. [CrossRef]
5. Haridy, Y.; Witzmann, F.; Asbach, P.; Schoch, R.R.; Fröbisch, N.; Rothschild, B.M. Triassic Cancer-Osteosarcoma in a 240-Million-Year-Old Stem-Turtle. *JAMA Oncol.* **2019**, *5*, 425–426. [CrossRef] [PubMed]
6. Coley, W.B., II. contribution to the knowledge of sarcoma. *Ann. Surg.* **1891**, *14*, 199–220. [CrossRef] [PubMed]
7. Coley, W.B. The treatment of malignant tumors by repeated inoculations of erysipelas: With a report of ten original cases. 1. *Am. J. Med. Sci.* **1893**, *105*, 487. [CrossRef]
8. Stevens, D.L.; Bryant, A.E. Impetigo, erysipelas and cellulitis. In *Streptococcus Pyogenes: Basic Biology to Clinical Manifestations*; Ferretti, J.J., Stevens, D.L., Fischetti, V.A., Eds.; University of Oklahoma Health Sciences Center: Oklahoma City, OK, USA, 2016.
9. Fehleisen, F. *Die Aetiologie des Erysipels*; Theodor Fischer: Berlin, Germany, 1883.
10. Cann, S.A.H.; Van Netten, J.P.; Van Netten, C. Dr William Coley and tumour regression: A place in history or in the future. *Postgrad. Med.* **2003**, *79*, 672–680.
11. McCarthy, E.F. The toxins of William B. Coley and the treatment of bone and soft-tissue sarcomas. *Iowa Orthop. J.* **2006**, *26*, 154–158.
12. Coley, W.B. The therapeutic value of the mixed toxins of the streptococcus of erysipelas and bacillus prodigiosus in the treatment of one hundred and sixty cases. *Am. J. Med. Sci.* **1896**, *112*, 251. [CrossRef]

13. Coley, W.B. The Treatment of Inoperable Sarcoma by Bacterial Toxins (the Mixed Toxins of the Streptococcus erysipelas and the Bacillus prodigiosus). *Proc. R. Soc. Med.* **1910**, *3*, 1–48. [CrossRef] [PubMed]
14. Johnston, B.J.; Novales, E.T. Clinical effect of Coley's toxin. II. A seven-year study. *Cancer Chemother. Rep.* **1962**, *21*, 43–68. [PubMed]
15. Ehrlich, P. Über den jetzigen Stand der Karzinomforschung. *Ned Tijdschr Geneeskd.* **1909**, *5*, 273–290.
16. Burnet, F.M. The concept of immunological surveillance. *Immunol. Asp. Neoplasia* **1970**, *13*, 1–27.
17. Thomas, L. On immunosurveillance in human cancer. *Yale J. Biol. Med.* **1982**, *55*, 329–333.
18. Gross, L. Intradermal immunization of C3H mice against a sarcoma that originated in an animal of the same line. *Cancer Res.* **1943**, *3*, 326–333.
19. Prehn, R.T.; Main, J.M. Immunity to methylcholanthrene-induced sarcomas. *J. Natl. Cancer Inst.* **1957**, *18*, 769–778.
20. Shinkai, Y.; Rathbun, G.; Lam, K.P.; Oltz, E.M.; Stewart, V.; Mendelsohn, M.; Charron, J.; Datta, M.; Young, F.; Stall, A.M. RAG-2-deficient mice lack mature lymphocytes owing to inability to initiate V(D)J rearrangement. *Cell* **1992**, *68*, 855–867. [CrossRef]
21. Shankaran, V.; Ikeda, H.; Bruce, A.T.; White, J.M.; Swanson, P.E.; Old, L.J.; Schreiber, R.D. IFNgamma and lymphocytes prevent primary tumour development and shape tumour immunogenicity. *Nature* **2001**, *410*, 1107–1111. [CrossRef]
22. Cretney, E.; Takeda, K.; Yagita, H.; Glaccum, M.; Peschon, J.J.; Smyth, M.J. Increased susceptibility to tumor initiation and metastasis in TNF-related apoptosis-inducing ligand-deficient mice. *J. Immunol.* **2002**, *168*, 1356–1361. [CrossRef]
23. van den Broek, M.E.; Kägi, D.; Ossendorp, F.; Toes, R.; Vamvakas, S.; Lutz, W.K.; Melief, C.J.; Zinkernagel, R.M.; Hengartner, H. Decreased tumor surveillance in perforin-deficient mice. *J. Exp. Med.* **1996**, *184*, 1781–1790. [CrossRef] [PubMed]
24. Mayor, P.C.; Eng, K.H.; Singel, K.L.; Abrams, S.I.; Odunsi, K.; Moysich, K.B.; Fuleihan, R.; Garabedian, E.; Lugar, P.; Ochs, H.D.; et al. Cancer in primary immunodeficiency diseases: Cancer incidence in the United States Immune Deficiency Network Registry. *J. Allergy Clin. Immunol.* **2018**, *141*, 1028–1035. [CrossRef] [PubMed]
25. Engels, E.A.; Pfeiffer, R.M.; Fraumeni, J.F.; Kasiske, B.L.; Israni, A.K.; Snyder, J.J.; Wolfe, R.A.; Goodrich, N.P.; Bayakly, A.R.; Clarke, C.A.; et al. Spectrum of cancer risk among US solid organ transplant recipients. *JAMA* **2011**, *306*, 1891–1901. [CrossRef] [PubMed]
26. Goedert, J.J.; Coté, T.R.; Virgo, P.; Scoppa, S.M.; Kingma, D.W.; Gail, M.H.; Jaffe, E.S.; Biggar, R.J. Spectrum of AIDS-associated malignant disorders. *Lancet* **1998**, *351*, 1833–1839. [CrossRef]
27. Schreiber, R.D.; Old, L.J.; Smyth, M.J. Cancer immunoediting: Integrating immunity's roles in cancer suppression and promotion. *Science* **2011**, *331*, 1565–1570. [CrossRef] [PubMed]
28. Koebel, C.M.; Vermi, W.; Swann, J.B.; Zerafa, N.; Rodig, S.J.; Old, L.J.; Smyth, M.J.; Schreiber, R.D. Adaptive immunity maintains occult cancer in an equilibrium state. *Nature* **2007**, *450*, 903–907. [CrossRef]
29. DuPage, M.; Mazumdar, C.; Schmidt, L.M.; Cheung, A.F.; Jacks, T. Expression of tumour-specific antigens underlies cancer immunoediting. *Nature* **2012**, *482*, 405–409. [CrossRef]
30. Miescher, S.; Whiteside, T.L.; Moretta, L.; von Fliedner, V. Clonal and frequency analyses of tumor-infiltrating T lymphocytes from human solid tumors. *J. Immunol.* **1987**, *138*, 4004–4011.
31. Li, Y.; Patel, S.P.; Roszik, J.; Qin, Y. Hypoxia-Driven Immunosuppressive Metabolites in the Tumor Microenvironment: New Approaches for Combinational Immunotherapy. *Front. Immunol.* **2018**, *9*, 1591. [CrossRef]
32. Barsoum, I.B.; Koti, M.; Siemens, D.R.; Graham, C.H. Mechanisms of hypoxia-mediated immune escape in cancer. *Cancer Res.* **2014**, *74*, 7185–7190. [CrossRef]
33. Fischer, K.; Hoffmann, P.; Voelkl, S.; Meidenbauer, N.; Ammer, J.; Edinger, M.; Gottfried, E.; Schwarz, S.; Rothe, G.; Hoves, S.; et al. Inhibitory effect of tumor cell-derived lactic acid on human T cells. *Blood* **2007**, *109*, 3812–3819. [CrossRef] [PubMed]
34. Togashi, Y.; Shitara, K.; Nishikawa, H. Regulatory T cells in cancer immunosuppression—Implications for anticancer therapy. *Nat. Rev. Clin. Oncol.* **2019**, *16*, 356–371. [CrossRef] [PubMed]
35. Butt, A.Q.; Mills, K.H.G. Immunosuppressive networks and checkpoints controlling antitumor immunity and their blockade in the development of cancer immunotherapeutics and vaccines. *Oncogene* **2014**, *33*, 4623–4631. [CrossRef] [PubMed]

36. Sakaguchi, S.; Yamaguchi, T.; Nomura, T.; Ono, M. Regulatory T cells and immune tolerance. *Cell* **2008**, *133*, 775–787. [CrossRef]
37. Gery, I.; Gershon, R.K.; Waksman, B.H. Potentiation of the T-lymphocyte response to mitogens. I. The responding cell. *J. Exp. Med.* **1972**, *136*, 128–142. [CrossRef]
38. Mier, J.W.; Gallo, R.C. Purification and some characteristics of human T-cell growth factor from phytohemagglutinin-stimulated lymphocyte-conditioned media. *Proc. Natl. Acad. Sci. USA* **1980**, *77*, 6134–6138. [CrossRef]
39. Welte, K.; Wang, C.Y.; Mertelsmann, R.; Venuta, S.; Feldman, S.P.; Moore, M.A. Purification of human interleukin 2 to apparent homogeneity and its molecular heterogeneity. *J. Exp. Med.* **1982**, *156*, 454–464. [CrossRef]
40. Rosenberg, S.A.; Mulé, J.J.; Spiess, P.J.; Reichert, C.M.; Schwarz, S.L. Regression of established pulmonary metastases and subcutaneous tumor mediated by the systemic administration of high-dose recombinant interleukin 2. *J. Exp. Med.* **1985**, *161*, 1169–1188. [CrossRef]
41. Eberlein, T.J.; Rosenstein, M.; Rosenberg, S.A. Regression of a disseminated syngeneic solid tumor by systemic transfer of lymphoid cells expanded in interleukin 2. *J. Exp. Med.* **1982**, *156*, 385–397. [CrossRef]
42. Rosenberg, S.A.; Lotze, M.T.; Muul, L.M.; Leitman, S.; Chang, A.E.; Ettinghausen, S.E.; Matory, Y.L.; Skibber, J.M.; Shiloni, E.; Vetto, J.T. Observations on the systemic administration of autologous lymphokine-activated killer cells and recombinant interleukin-2 to patients with metastatic cancer. *N. Engl. J. Med.* **1985**, *313*, 1485–1492. [CrossRef]
43. Rosenberg, S.A.; Lotze, M.T.; Muul, L.M.; Chang, A.E.; Avis, F.P.; Leitman, S.; Linehan, W.M.; Robertson, C.N.; Lee, R.E.; Rubin, J.T. A progress report on the treatment of 157 patients with advanced cancer using lymphokine-activated killer cells and interleukin-2 or high-dose interleukin-2 alone. *N. Engl. J. Med.* **1987**, *316*, 889–897. [CrossRef] [PubMed]
44. Schwartz, R.N.; Stover, L.; Dutcher, J. Managing toxicities of high-dose interleukin-2. *Oncology* **2002**, *16*, 11–20. [PubMed]
45. Rosenberg, S.A.; Yang, J.C.; Topalian, S.L.; Schwartzentruber, D.J.; Weber, J.S.; Parkinson, D.R.; Seipp, C.A.; Einhorn, J.H.; White, D.E. Treatment of 283 consecutive patients with metastatic melanoma or renal cell cancer using high-dose bolus interleukin 2. *JAMA* **1994**, *271*, 907–913. [CrossRef] [PubMed]
46. Dillman, R.O.; Church, C.; Oldham, R.K.; West, W.H.; Schwartzberg, L.; Birch, R. Inpatient continuous-infusion interleukin-2 in 788 patients with cancer. The National Biotherapy Study Group experience. *Cancer* **1993**, *71*, 2358–2370. [CrossRef]
47. Lee, S.; Margolin, K. Cytokines in cancer immunotherapy. *Cancers* **2011**, *3*, 3856–3893. [CrossRef]
48. Ku, C.C.; Murakami, M.; Sakamoto, A.; Kappler, J.; Marrack, P. Control of homeostasis of CD8+ memory T cells by opposing cytokines. *Science* **2000**, *288*, 675–678. [CrossRef]
49. Evans, R.; Fuller, J.A.; Christianson, G.; Krupke, D.M. IL-15 mediates anti-tumor effects after cyclophosphamide injection of tumor-bearing mice and enhances adoptive immunotherapy: The potential role of NK cell. *Cell. Immunol.* **1997**, *178*, 197. [CrossRef]
50. Kobayashi, H.; Dubois, S.; Sato, N.; Sabzevari, H.; Sakai, Y.; Waldmann, T.A.; Tagaya, Y. Role of trans-cellular IL-15 presentation in the activation of NK cell-mediated killing, which leads to enhanced tumor immunosurveillance. *Blood* **2005**, *105*, 721–727. [CrossRef]
51. Waldmann, T.A. The biology of interleukin-2 and interleukin-15: Implications for cancer therapy and vaccine design. *Nat. Rev. Immunol.* **2006**, *6*, 595–601. [CrossRef]
52. Bessard, A.; Solé, V.; Bouchaud, G.; Quéméner, A. High antitumor activity of RLI, an interleukin-15 (IL-15)–IL-15 receptor α fusion protein, in metastatic melanoma and colorectal cancer. *Mol. Cancer Ther.* **2009**, *8*, 2736–2745. [CrossRef]
53. Howie, J.W. Experiments with interferon in man: A report to the medical research council from the scientific committee on interferon. *Lancet* **1965**, *1*, 505. [PubMed]
54. Müller, U.; Steinhoff, U.; Reis, L.F.; Hemmi, S.; Pavlovic, J.; Zinkernagel, R.M.; Aguet, M. Functional role of type I and type II interferons in antiviral defense. *Science* **1994**, *264*, 1918–1921. [CrossRef]
55. Waldmann, T.A. Cytokines in cancer immunotherapy. *Cold Spring Harb. Perspect. Biol.* **2017**, *10*. [CrossRef] [PubMed]
56. Cantell, K.; Hirvonen, S.; Koistinen, V. [71] Partial purification of human leukocyte interferon on a large scale. In *Methods in Enzymology*; Academic Press: Cambridge, MA, USA, 1981.

57. Merigan, T.C.; Sikora, K.; Breeden, J.H.; Levy, R.; Rosenberg, S.A. Preliminary observations on the effect of human leukocyte interferon in non-Hodgkin's lymphoma. *N. Engl. J. Med.* **1978**, *299*, 1449–1453. [CrossRef] [PubMed]
58. Quesada, J.R.; Hersh, E.M.; Gutterman, J.U. Hairy cell leukemia: Induction of remission with alpha interferon. *Blood* **1983**, *62* (Suppl. 1), 207. [CrossRef] [PubMed]
59. Quesada, J.R.; Swanson, D.A.; Trindade, A.; Gutterman, J.U. Renal cell carcinoma: Antitumor effects of leukocyte interferon. *Cancer Res.* **1983**, *43*, 940–947.
60. Krown, S.E.; Burk, M.W.; Kirkwood, J.M.; Kerr, D. Human leukocyte (alpha) interferon in metastatic malignant melanoma. *Am. Cancer Soc. Phase II Trial* **1984**, *68*, 723–726.
61. Kirkwood, J.M.; Ibrahim, J.G.; Sondak, V.K.; Richards, J.; Flaherty, L.E.; Ernstoff, M.S.; Smith, T.J.; Rao, U.; Steele, M.; Blum, R.H. High-and low-dose interferon alfa-2b in high-risk melanoma: First analysis of intergroup trial E1690/S9111/C9190. *J. Clin. Oncol.* **2000**, *18*, 2444–2458. [CrossRef]
62. Hercus, T.R.; Thomas, D.; Guthridge, M.A.; Ekert, P.G.; King-Scott, J.; Parker, M.W.; Lopez, A.F. The granulocyte-macrophage colony-stimulating factor receptor: Linking its structure to cell signaling and its role in disease. *Blood* **2009**, *114*, 1289–1298. [CrossRef]
63. Dranoff, G.; Jaffee, E.; Lazenby, A.; Golumbek, P.; Levitsky, H.; Brose, K.; Jackson, V.; Hamada, H.; Pardoll, D.; Mulligan, R.C. Vaccination with irradiated tumor cells engineered to secrete murine granulocyte-macrophage colony-stimulating factor stimulates potent, specific, and long-lasting anti-tumor immunity. *Proc. Natl. Acad. Sci. USA* **1993**, *90*, 3539–3543. [CrossRef]
64. Soiffer, R.; Lynch, T.; Mihm, M.; Jung, K.; Rhuda, C.; Schmollinger, J.C.; Hodi, F.S.; Liebster, L.; Lam, P.; Mentzer, S.; et al. Vaccination with irradiated autologous melanoma cells engineered to secrete human granulocyte-macrophage colony-stimulating factor generates potent antitumor immunity in patients with metastatic melanoma. *Proc. Natl. Acad. Sci. USA* **1998**, *95*, 13141–13146. [CrossRef] [PubMed]
65. Small, E.J.; Reese, D.M.; Um, B.; Whisenant, S.; Dixon, S.C.; Figg, W.D. Therapy of advanced prostate cancer with granulocyte macrophage colony-stimulating factor. *Clin. Cancer Res.* **1999**, *5*, 1738–1744. [PubMed]
66. Lawson, D.H.; Lee, S.; Zhao, F.; Tarhini, A.A.; Margolin, K.A.; Ernstoff, M.S.; Atkins, M.B.; Cohen, G.I.; Whiteside, T.L.; Butterfield, L.H.; et al. Randomized, Placebo-Controlled, Phase III Trial of Yeast-Derived Granulocyte-Macrophage Colony-Stimulating Factor (GM-CSF) Versus Peptide Vaccination Versus GM-CSF Plus Peptide Vaccination Versus Placebo in Patients With No Evidence of Disease After Complete Surgical Resection of Locally Advanced and/or Stage IV Melanoma: A Trial of the Eastern Cooperative Oncology Group-American College of Radiology Imaging Network Cancer Research Group (E4697). *J. Clin. Oncol.* **2015**, *33*, 4066–4076. [CrossRef] [PubMed]
67. Hodi, F.S.; Lee, S.; McDermott, D.F.; Rao, U.N.; Butterfield, L.H.; Tarhini, A.A.; Leming, P.; Puzanov, I.; Shin, D.; Kirkwood, J.M. Ipilimumab plus sargramostim vs ipilimumab alone for treatment of metastatic melanoma: A randomized clinical trial. *JAMA* **2014**, *312*, 1744–1753. [CrossRef]
68. O'Day, S.J.; Atkins, M.B.; Boasberg, P. Phase II multicenter trial of maintenance biotherapy after induction concurrent Biochemotherapy for patients with metastatic melanoma. *J. Clin. Oncol.* **2009**, *27*, 6207–6212. [CrossRef]
69. Tang, H.; Qiao, J.; Fu, Y.-X. Immunotherapy and tumor microenvironment. *Cancer Lett.* **2016**, *370*, 85–90. [CrossRef]
70. Mortarini, R.; Piris, A.; Maurichi, A.; Molla, A.; Bersani, I.; Bono, A.; Bartoli, C.; Santinami, M.; Lombardo, C.; Ravagnani, F.; et al. Lack of terminally differentiated tumor-specific CD8+ T cells at tumor site in spite of antitumor immunity to self-antigens in human metastatic melanoma. *Cancer Res.* **2003**, *63*, 2535–2545.
71. Deng, L.; Zhang, H.; Luan, Y.; Zhang, J.; Xing, Q.; Dong, S.; Wu, X.; Liu, M.; Wang, S. Accumulation of foxp3+ T regulatory cells in draining lymph nodes correlates with disease progression and immune suppression in colorectal cancer patients. *Clin. Cancer Res.* **2010**, *16*, 4105–4112. [CrossRef]
72. Gallimore, A.; Glithero, A.; Godkin, A.; Tissot, A.C.; Plückthun, A.; Elliott, T.; Hengartner, H.; Zinkernagel, R. Induction and exhaustion of lymphocytic choriomeningitis virus-specific cytotoxic T lymphocytes visualized using soluble tetrameric major histocompatibility complex class I-peptide complexes. *J. Exp. Med.* **1998**, *187*, 1383–1393. [CrossRef]

73. Joffre, O.; Nolte, M.A.; Spörri, R.; Reis e Sousa, C. Inflammatory signals in dendritic cell activation and the induction of adaptive immunity. *Immunol. Rev.* **2009**, *227*, 234–247. [CrossRef]
74. Shahinian, A.; Pfeffer, K.; Lee, K.P.; Kündig, T.M.; Kishihara, K.; Wakeham, A.; Kawai, K.; Ohashi, P.S.; Thompson, C.B.; Mak, T.W. Differential T cell costimulatory requirements in CD28-deficient mice. *Science* **1993**, *261*, 609–612. [CrossRef] [PubMed]
75. Chen, L.; Flies, D.B. Molecular mechanisms of T cell co-stimulation and co-inhibition. *Nat. Rev. Immunol.* **2013**, *13*, 227–242. [CrossRef] [PubMed]
76. Hargadon, K.M.; Johnson, C.E.; Williams, C.J. Immune checkpoint blockade therapy for cancer: An overview of FDA-approved immune checkpoint inhibitors. *Int. Immunopharmacol.* **2018**, *62*, 29–39. [CrossRef] [PubMed]
77. Brunet, J.F.; Denizot, F.; Luciani, M.F.; Roux-Dosseto, M.; Suzan, M.; Mattei, M.G.; Golstein, P. A new member of the immunoglobulin superfamily—CTLA-4. *Nature* **1987**, *328*, 267–270. [CrossRef]
78. Walunas, T.L.; Lenschow, D.J.; Bakker, C.Y.; Linsley, P.S.; Freeman, G.J.; Green, J.M.; Thompson, C.B.; Bluestone, J.A. CTLA-4 can function as a negative regulator of T cell activation. *Immunity* **1994**, *1*, 405–413. [CrossRef]
79. Qureshi, O.S.; Zheng, Y.; Nakamura, K.; Attridge, K.; Manzotti, C.; Schmidt, E.M.; Baker, J.; Jeffery, L.E.; Kaur, S.; Briggs, Z.; et al. Trans-endocytosis of CD80 and CD86: A molecular basis for the cell-extrinsic function of CTLA-4. *Science* **2011**, *332*, 600–603. [CrossRef]
80. Krummel, M.F.; Allison, J.P. CD28 and CTLA-4 have opposing effects on the response of T cells to stimulation. *J. Exp. Med.* **1995**, *182*, 459–465. [CrossRef]
81. Tivol, E.A.; Borriello, F.; Schweitzer, A.N.; Lynch, W.P.; Bluestone, J.A.; Sharpe, A.H. Loss of CTLA-4 leads to massive lymphoproliferation and fatal multiorgan tissue destruction, revealing a critical negative regulatory role of CTLA-4. *Immunity* **1995**, *3*, 541–547. [CrossRef]
82. Waterhouse, P.; Penninger, J.M.; Timms, E.; Wakeham, A.; Shahinian, A.; Lee, K.P.; Thompson, C.B.; Griesser, H.; Mak, T.W. Lymphoproliferative disorders with early lethality in mice deficient in Ctla-4. *Science* **1995**, *270*, 985–988. [CrossRef]
83. Leach, D.R.; Krummel, M.F.; Allison, J.P. Enhancement of antitumor immunity by CTLA-4 blockade. *Science* **1996**, *271*, 1734–1736. [CrossRef]
84. Hodi, F.S.; O'Day, S.J.; McDermott, D.F.; Weber, R.W.; Sosman, J.A.; Haanen, J.B.; Gonzalez, R.; Robert, C.; Schadendorf, D.; Hassel, J.C.; et al. Improved survival with ipilimumab in patients with metastatic melanoma. *N. Engl. J. Med.* **2010**, *363*, 711–723. [CrossRef] [PubMed]
85. Robert, C.; Thomas, L.; Bondarenko, I.; O'Day, S.; Weber, J.; Garbe, C.; Lebbe, C.; Baurain, J.-F.; Testori, A.; Grob, J.-J.; et al. Ipilimumab plus dacarbazine for previously untreated metastatic melanoma. *N. Engl. J. Med.* **2011**, *364*, 2517–2526. [CrossRef] [PubMed]
86. Schadendorf, D.; Hodi, F.S.; Robert, C.; Weber, J.S.; Margolin, K.; Hamid, O.; Patt, D.; Chen, T.-T.; Berman, D.M.; Wolchok, J.D. Pooled Analysis of Long-Term Survival Data From Phase II and Phase III Trials of Ipilimumab in Unresectable or Metastatic Melanoma. *J. Clin. Oncol.* **2015**, *33*, 1889–1894. [CrossRef] [PubMed]
87. Darvin, P.; Toor, S.M.; Sasidharan Nair, V.; Elkord, E. Immune checkpoint inhibitors: Recent progress and potential biomarkers. *Exp. Mol. Med.* **2018**, *50*, 165. [CrossRef] [PubMed]
88. Ishida, Y.; Agata, Y.; Shibahara, K.; Honjo, T. Induced expression of PD-1, a novel member of the immunoglobulin gene superfamily, upon programmed cell death. *EMBO J.* **1992**, *11*, 3887–3895. [CrossRef] [PubMed]
89. Nishimura, H.; Nose, M.; Hiai, H.; Minato, N.; Honjo, T. Development of lupus-like autoimmune diseases by disruption of the PD-1 gene encoding an ITIM motif-carrying immunoreceptor. *Immunity* **1999**, *11*, 141–151. [CrossRef]
90. Dong, H.; Zhu, G.; Tamada, K.; Chen, L. B7-H1, a third member of the B7 family, co-stimulates T-cell proliferation and interleukin-10 secretion. *Nat. Med.* **1999**, *5*, 1365–1369. [CrossRef]
91. Freeman, G.J.; Long, A.J.; Iwai, Y.; Bourque, K.; Chernova, T.; Nishimura, H.; Fitz, L.J.; Malenkovich, N.; Okazaki, T.; Byrne, M.C.; et al. Engagement of the PD-1 immunoinhibitory receptor by a novel B7 family member leads to negative regulation of lymphocyte activation. *J. Exp. Med.* **2000**, *192*, 1027–1034. [CrossRef]
92. Iwai, Y.; Ishida, M.; Tanaka, Y.; Okazaki, T.; Honjo, T.; Minato, N. Involvement of PD-L1 on tumor cells in the escape from host immune system and tumor immunotherapy by PD-L1 blockade. *Proc. Natl. Acad. Sci. USA* **2002**, *99*, 12293–12297. [CrossRef]

93. Curiel, T.J.; Wei, S.; Dong, H.; Alvarez, X.; Cheng, P.; Mottram, P.; Krzysiek, R.; Knutson, K.L.; Daniel, B.; Zimmermann, M.C.; et al. Blockade of B7-H1 improves myeloid dendritic cell-mediated antitumor immunity. *Nat. Med.* **2003**, *9*, 562–567. [CrossRef]
94. Strome, S.E.; Dong, H.; Tamura, H.; Voss, S.G.; Flies, D.B.; Tamada, K.; Salomao, D.; Cheville, J.; Hirano, F.; Lin, W.; et al. B7-H1 blockade augments adoptive T-cell immunotherapy for squamous cell carcinoma. *Cancer Res.* **2003**, *63*, 6501–6505.
95. Iwai, Y.; Terawaki, S.; Honjo, T. PD-1 blockade inhibits hematogenous spread of poorly immunogenic tumor cells by enhanced recruitment of effector T cells. *Int. Immunol.* **2005**, *17*, 133–144. [CrossRef] [PubMed]
96. Hamanishi, J.; Mandai, M.; Iwasaki, M.; Okazaki, T.; Tanaka, Y.; Yamaguchi, K.; Higuchi, T.; Yagi, H.; Takakura, K.; Minato, N.; et al. Programmed cell death 1 ligand 1 and tumor-infiltrating CD8+ T lymphocytes are prognostic factors of human ovarian cancer. *Proc. Natl. Acad. Sci. USA* **2007**, *104*, 3360–3365. [CrossRef] [PubMed]
97. Brahmer, J.R.; Tykodi, S.S.; Chow, L.Q.M.; Hwu, W.-J.; Topalian, S.L.; Hwu, P.; Drake, C.G.; Camacho, L.H.; Kauh, J.; Odunsi, K.; et al. Safety and activity of anti-PD-L1 antibody in patients with advanced cancer. *N. Engl. J. Med.* **2012**, *366*, 2455–2465. [CrossRef] [PubMed]
98. Topalian, S.L.; Hodi, F.S.; Brahmer, J.R.; Gettinger, S.N.; Smith, D.C.; McDermott, D.F.; Powderly, J.D.; Carvajal, R.D.; Sosman, J.A.; Atkins, M.B.; et al. Safety, activity, and immune correlates of anti-PD-1 antibody in cancer. *N. Engl. J. Med.* **2012**, *366*, 2443–2454. [CrossRef]
99. Garon, E.B.; Rizvi, N.A.; Hui, R.; Leighl, N.; Balmanoukian, A.S.; Eder, J.P.; Patnaik, A.; Aggarwal, C.; Gubens, M.; Horn, L.; et al. KEYNOTE-001 Investigators Pembrolizumab for the treatment of non-small-cell lung cancer. *N. Engl. J. Med.* **2015**, *372*, 2018–2028. [CrossRef]
100. Weber, J.S.; D'Angelo, S.P.; Minor, D.; Hodi, F.S.; Gutzmer, R.; Neyns, B.; Hoeller, C.; Khushalani, N.I.; Miller, W.H.; Lao, C.D.; et al. Nivolumab versus chemotherapy in patients with advanced melanoma who progressed after anti-CTLA-4 treatment (CheckMate 037): A randomised, controlled, open-label, phase 3 trial. *Lancet Oncol.* **2015**, *16*, 375–384. [CrossRef]
101. Schachter, J.; Ribas, A.; Long, G.V.; Arance, A.; Grob, J.-J.; Mortier, L.; Daud, A.; Carlino, M.S.; McNeil, C.; Lotem, M.; et al. Pembrolizumab versus ipilimumab for advanced melanoma: Final overall survival results of a multicentre, randomised, open-label phase 3 study (KEYNOTE-006). *Lancet* **2017**, *390*, 1853–1862. [CrossRef]
102. Powles, T.; Durán, I.; van der Heijden, M.S.; Loriot, Y.; Vogelzang, N.J.; De Giorgi, U.; Oudard, S.; Retz, M.M.; Castellano, D.; Bamias, A.; et al. Atezolizumab versus chemotherapy in patients with platinum-treated locally advanced or metastatic urothelial carcinoma (IMvigor211): A multicentre, open-label, phase 3 randomised controlled trial. *Lancet* **2018**, *391*, 748–757. [CrossRef]
103. Rittmeyer, A.; Barlesi, F.; Waterkamp, D.; Park, K.; Ciardiello, F.; von Pawel, J.; Gadgeel, S.M.; Hida, T.; Kowalski, D.M.; Dols, M.C.; et al. OAK Study Group Atezolizumab versus docetaxel in patients with previously treated non-small-cell lung cancer (OAK): A phase 3, open-label, multicentre randomised controlled trial. *Lancet* **2017**, *389*, 255–265. [CrossRef]
104. Narayan, P.; Wahby, S.; Gao, J.J.; Amiri-Kordestani, L.; Ibrahim, A.; Bloomquist, E.; Tang, S.; Xu, Y.; Liu, J.; Fu, W.; et al. FDA Approval Summary: Atezolizumab plus paclitaxel protein-bound for the treatment of patients with advanced or metastatic TNBC whose tumors express PD-L1. *Clin. Cancer Res.* **2020**. [CrossRef] [PubMed]
105. Kaufman, H.L.; Russell, J.; Hamid, O.; Bhatia, S.; Terheyden, P.; D'Angelo, S.P.; Shih, K.C.; Lebbé, C.; Linette, G.P.; Milella, M.; et al. Avelumab in patients with chemotherapy-refractory metastatic Merkel cell carcinoma: A multicentre, single-group, open-label, phase 2 trial. *Lancet Oncol.* **2016**, *17*, 1374–1385. [CrossRef]
106. Motzer, R.J.; Tannir, N.M.; McDermott, D.F.; Arén Frontera, O.; Melichar, B.; Choueiri, T.K.; Plimack, E.R.; Barthélémy, P.; Porta, C.; George, S.; et al. CheckMate 214 Investigators Nivolumab plus Ipilimumab versus Sunitinib in Advanced Renal-Cell Carcinoma. *N. Engl. J. Med.* **2018**, *378*, 1277–1290. [CrossRef]
107. Jenkins, R.W.; Barbie, D.A.; Flaherty, K.T. Mechanisms of resistance to immune checkpoint inhibitors. *Br. J. Cancer* **2018**, *118*, 9–16. [CrossRef] [PubMed]
108. Anderson, A.C.; Joller, N.; Kuchroo, V.K. Lag-3, Tim-3, and TIGIT: Co-inhibitory Receptors with Specialized Functions in Immune Regulation. *Immunity* **2016**, *44*, 989–1004. [CrossRef] [PubMed]

109. Routy, B.; Le Chatelier, E.; Derosa, L.; Duong, C.P.M.; Alou, M.T.; Daillère, R.; Fluckiger, A.; Messaoudene, M.; Rauber, C.; Roberti, M.P.; et al. Gut microbiome influences efficacy of PD-1-based immunotherapy against epithelial tumors. *Science* **2018**, *359*, 91–97. [CrossRef]
110. Gopalakrishnan, V.; Spencer, C.N.; Nezi, L.; Reuben, A.; Andrews, M.C.; Karpinets, T.V.; Prieto, P.A.; Vicente, D.; Hoffman, K.; Wei, S.C.; et al. Gut microbiome modulates response to anti-PD-1 immunotherapy in melanoma patients. *Science* **2018**, *359*, 97–103. [CrossRef]
111. Hanna, M.G.; Peters, L.C. Specific immunotherapy of established visceral micrometastases by BCG-tumor cell vaccine alone or as an adjunct to surgery. *Cancer* **1978**, *42*, 2613–2625. [CrossRef]
112. Murray, D.R.; Cassel, W.A.; Torbin, A.H.; Olkowski, Z.L.; Moore, M.E. Viral oncolysate in the management of malignant melanoma. II. Clinical studies. *Cancer* **1977**, *40*, 680–686. [CrossRef]
113. McIllmurray, M.B.; Embleton, M.J.; Reeves, W.G.; Langman, M.J.; Deane, M. Controlled trial of active immunotherapy in management of stage IIB malignant melanoma. *Br. Med. J.* **1977**, *1*, 540–542. [CrossRef]
114. van der Bruggen, P.; Traversari, C.; Chomez, P.; Lurquin, C.; De Plaen, E.; Van den Eynde, B.; Knuth, A.; Boon, T. A gene encoding an antigen recognized by cytolytic T lymphocytes on a human melanoma. *Science* **1991**, *254*, 1643–1647. [CrossRef] [PubMed]
115. Cheever, M.A.; Allison, J.P.; Ferris, A.S.; Finn, O.J.; Hastings, B.M.; Hecht, T.T.; Mellman, I.; Prindiville, S.A.; Viner, J.L.; Weiner, L.M.; et al. The prioritization of cancer antigens: A national cancer institute pilot project for the acceleration of translational research. *Clin. Cancer Res.* **2009**, *15*, 5323–5337. [CrossRef] [PubMed]
116. Thomas, R.; Al-Khadairi, G.; Roelands, J.; Hendrickx, W.; Dermime, S.; Bedognetti, D.; Decock, J. NY-ESO-1 Based Immunotherapy of Cancer: Current Perspectives. *Front. Immunol.* **2018**, *9*, 947. [CrossRef] [PubMed]
117. Zajac, P.; Schultz-Thater, E.; Tornillo, L.; Sadowski, C.; Trella, E.; Mengus, C.; Iezzi, G.; Spagnoli, G.C. MAGE-A Antigens and Cancer Immunotherapy. *Front. Med.* **2017**, *4*, 18. [CrossRef] [PubMed]
118. Turriziani, M.; Fantini, M.; Benvenuto, M. Carcinoembryonic antigen (CEA)-based cancer vaccines: Recent patents and antitumor effects from experimental models to clinical trials. *Recent Pat. Anti-Cancer Drug Discov.* **2012**, *7*, 265–296. [CrossRef]
119. Evdokimova, V.N.; Butterfield, L.H. Alpha-fetoprotein and other tumour-associated antigens for immunotherapy of hepatocellular cancer. *Expert Opin. Biol. Ther.* **2008**, *8*, 325–336. [CrossRef] [PubMed]
120. Westdorp, H.; Sköld, A.E.; Snijer, B.A.; Franik, S.; Mulder, S.F.; Major, P.P.; Foley, R.; Gerritsen, W.R.; de Vries, I.J.M. Immunotherapy for prostate cancer: Lessons from responses to tumor-associated antigens. *Front. Immunol.* **2014**, *5*, 191. [CrossRef]
121. Scheuermann, R.H.; Racila, E. CD19 antigen in leukemia and lymphoma diagnosis and immunotherapy. *Leuk. Lymphoma* **1995**, *18*, 385–397. [CrossRef]
122. Ayoub, N.M.; Al-Shami, K.M.; Yaghan, R.J. Immunotherapy for HER2-positive breast cancer: Recent advances and combination therapeutic approaches. *Breast Cancer (Dove Med Press)* **2019**, *11*, 53–69. [CrossRef]
123. Liu, J.-P.; Chen, W.; Schwarer, A.P.; Li, H. Telomerase in cancer immunotherapy. *Biochim. Biophys. Acta* **2010**, *1805*, 35–42. [CrossRef]
124. Jiang, T.; Shi, T.; Zhang, H.; Hu, J.; Song, Y.; Wei, J.; Ren, S.; Zhou, C. Tumor neoantigens: From basic research to clinical applications. *J. Hematol. Oncol.* **2019**, *12*, 93. [CrossRef] [PubMed]
125. Goydos, J.S.; Elder, E.; Whiteside, T.L.; Finn, O.J.; Lotze, M.T. A phase I trial of a synthetic mucin peptide vaccine. Induction of specific immune reactivity in patients with adenocarcinoma. *J. Surg. Res.* **1996**, *63*, 298–304. [CrossRef]
126. Mukherji, B.; Chakraborty, N.G.; Yamasaki, S.; Okino, T.; Yamase, H.; Sporn, J.R.; Kurtzman, S.K.; Ergin, M.T.; Ozols, J.; Meehan, J. Induction of antigen-specific cytolytic T cells in situ in human melanoma by immunization with synthetic peptide-pulsed autologous antigen presenting cells. *Proc. Natl. Acad. Sci. USA* **1995**, *92*, 8078–8082. [CrossRef] [PubMed]
127. Hsu, F.J.; Benike, C.; Fagnoni, F.; Liles, T.M.; Czerwinski, D.; Taidi, B.; Engleman, E.G.; Levy, R. Vaccination of patients with B-cell lymphoma using autologous antigen-pulsed dendritic cells. *Nat. Med.* **1996**, *2*, 52–58. [CrossRef] [PubMed]
128. Kim, J.W.; Gulley, J.L. Poxviral vectors for cancer immunotherapy. *Expert Opin. Biol. Ther.* **2012**, *12*, 463–478. [CrossRef]
129. Gallo, P.; Dharmapuri, S.; Cipriani, B.; Monaci, P. Adenovirus as vehicle for anticancer genetic immunotherapy. *Gene Ther.* **2005**, *12* (Suppl. 1), S84–S91. [CrossRef]

130. Roland, K.L.; Brenneman, K.E. Salmonella as a vaccine delivery vehicle. *Expert Rev. Vaccines* **2013**, *12*, 1033–1045. [CrossRef]
131. Flickinger, J.C.; Rodeck, U.; Snook, A.E. Listeria monocytogenes as a Vector for Cancer Immunotherapy: Current Understanding and Progress. *Vaccines* **2018**, *6*, 48. [CrossRef]
132. Jahanafrooz, Z.; Baradaran, B.; Mosafer, J.; Hashemzaei, M.; Rezaei, T.; Mokhtarzadeh, A.; Hamblin, M.R. Comparison of DNA and mRNA vaccines against cancer. *Drug Discov. Today* **2019**. [CrossRef]
133. Palucka, K.; Banchereau, J. Dendritic-cell-based therapeutic cancer vaccines. *Immunity* **2013**, *39*, 38–48. [CrossRef]
134. Kantoff, P.W.; Higano, C.S.; Shore, N.D.; Berger, E.R.; Small, E.J.; Penson, D.F.; Redfern, C.H.; Ferrari, A.C.; Dreicer, R.; Sims, R.B.; et al. IMPACT Study Investigators Sipuleucel-T immunotherapy for castration-resistant prostate cancer. *N. Engl. J. Med.* **2010**, *363*, 411–422. [CrossRef]
135. Peng, M.; Mo, Y.; Wang, Y.; Wu, P.; Zhang, Y.; Xiong, F.; Guo, C.; Wu, X.; Li, Y.; Li, X.; et al. Neoantigen vaccine: An emerging tumor immunotherapy. *Mol. Cancer* **2019**, *18*, 128. [CrossRef] [PubMed]
136. Ott, P.A.; Hu, Z.; Keskin, D.B.; Shukla, S.A.; Sun, J.; Bozym, D.J.; Zhang, W.; Luoma, A.; Giobbie-Hurder, A.; Peter, L.; et al. An immunogenic personal neoantigen vaccine for patients with melanoma. *Nature* **2017**, *547*, 217–221. [CrossRef] [PubMed]
137. Keskin, D.B.; Anandappa, A.J.; Sun, J.; Tirosh, I.; Mathewson, N.D.; Li, S.; Oliveira, G.; Giobbie-Hurder, A.; Felt, K.; Gjini, E.; et al. Neoantigen vaccine generates intratumoral T cell responses in phase Ib glioblastoma trial. *Nature* **2019**, *565*, 234–239. [CrossRef] [PubMed]
138. Finn, O.J. The dawn of vaccines for cancer prevention. *Nat. Rev. Immunol.* **2018**, *18*, 183–194. [CrossRef]
139. Chang, M.-H. Hepatitis B virus and cancer prevention. *Recent Results Cancer Res.* **2011**, *188*, 75–84. [CrossRef]
140. Guo, F.; Cofie, L.E.; Berenson, A.B. Cervical cancer incidence in young U.S. females after human papillomavirus vaccine introduction. *Am. J. Prev. Med.* **2018**, *55*, 197–204. [CrossRef]
141. Singh, R.; Bandyopadhyay, D. MUC1: A target molecule for cancer therapy. *Cancer Biol. Ther.* **2007**, *6*, 481–486. [CrossRef]
142. Kimura, T.; McKolanis, J.R.; Dzubinski, L.A.; Islam, K.; Potter, D.M.; Salazar, A.M.; Schoen, R.E.; Finn, O.J. MUC1 vaccine for individuals with advanced adenoma of the colon: A cancer immunoprevention feasibility study. *Cancer Prev. Res.* **2013**, *6*, 18–26. [CrossRef]
143. Lawler, S.E.; Speranza, M.-C.; Cho, C.-F.; Chiocca, E.A. Oncolytic viruses in cancer treatment: A review. *JAMA Oncol.* **2017**, *3*, 841–849. [CrossRef]
144. Alvarez, C.A. NK cells impede glioblastoma virotherapy through NKp30 and NKp46 natural cytotoxicity receptors. *Nat. Med.* **2012**, *18*, 1827. [CrossRef]
145. Yung, W.K.A.; Vence, L.M.; Gomez, C. Delta-24-RGD oncolytic adenovirus elicits anti-glioma immunity in an immunocompetent mouse model. *PloS ONE* **2014**, *9*, e97407.
146. Nguyen, T.; Avci, N.G.; Shin, D.H.; Martinez, N. Tune up in situ autovaccination against solid tumors with oncolytic viruses. *Cancers* **2018**, *10*, 171. [CrossRef]
147. Dock, G. The influence of complicating diseases upon leukaemia. *Am. J. Med Sci.* **1904**, *127*, 563. [CrossRef]
148. Larson, C.; Oronsky, B.; Scicinski, J.; Fanger, G.R.; Stirn, M.; Oronsky, A.; Reid, T.R. Going viral: A review of replication-selective oncolytic adenoviruses. *Oncotarget* **2015**, *6*, 19976–19989. [CrossRef] [PubMed]
149. Andtbacka, R.H.I.; Kaufman, H.L.; Collichio, F.; Amatruda, T.; Senzer, N.; Chesney, J.; Delman, K.A.; Spitler, L.E.; Puzanov, I.; Agarwala, S.S.; et al. Talimogene laherparepvec improves durable response rate in patients with advanced melanoma. *J. Clin. Oncol.* **2015**, *33*, 2780–2788. [CrossRef]
150. Rosenberg, S.A.; Restifo, N.P. Adoptive cell transfer as personalized immunotherapy for human cancer. *Science* **2015**, *348*, 62–68. [CrossRef]
151. Cohen, J.E.; Merims, S.; Frank, S.; Engelstein, R.; Peretz, T.; Lotem, M. Adoptive cell therapy: Past, present and future. *Immunotherapy* **2017**, *9*, 183–196. [CrossRef]
152. Mitchison, N.A. Passive transfer of transplantation immunity. *Nature* **1953**, *171*, 267–268. [CrossRef] [PubMed]
153. Delorme, E.J.; Alexander, P. Treatment of primary fibrosarcoma in the rat with immune lymphocytes. *Lancet* **1964**, *2*, 117–120. [CrossRef]
154. Fefer, A. Immunotherapy and chemotherapy of Moloney sarcoma virus-induced tumors in mice. *Cancer Res.* **1969**, *29*, 2177–2183. [PubMed]

155. Morgan, D.A.; Ruscetti, F.W.; Gallo, R. Selective in vitro growth of T lymphocytes from normal human bone marrows. *Science* **1976**, *193*, 1007–1008. [CrossRef] [PubMed]
156. Donohue, J.H.; Rosenstein, M.; Chang, A.E.; Lotze, M.T.; Robb, R.J.; Rosenberg, S.A. The systemic administration of purified interleukin 2 enhances the ability of sensitized murine lymphocytes to cure a disseminated syngeneic lymphoma. *J. Immunol.* **1984**, *132*, 2123–2128. [PubMed]
157. Muul, L.M.; Spiess, P.J.; Director, E.P.; Rosenberg, S.A. Identification of specific cytolytic immune responses against autologous tumor in humans bearing malignant melanoma. *J. Immunol.* **1987**, *138*, 989–995. [PubMed]
158. Rosenberg, S.A.; Spiess, P.; Lafreniere, R. A new approach to the adoptive immunotherapy of cancer with tumor-infiltrating lymphocytes. *Science* **1986**, *233*, 1318–1321. [CrossRef]
159. Rosenberg, S.A.; Packard, B.S.; Aebersold, P.M.; Solomon, D.; Topalian, S.L.; Toy, S.T.; Simon, P.; Lotze, M.T.; Yang, J.C.; Seipp, C.A. Use of tumor-infiltrating lymphocytes and interleukin-2 in the immunotherapy of patients with metastatic melanoma. A preliminary report. *N. Engl. J. Med.* **1988**, *319*, 1676–1680. [CrossRef]
160. Slavin, S.; Nagler, A.; Naparstek, E.; Kapelushnik, Y.; Aker, M.; Cividalli, G.; Varadi, G.; Kirschbaum, M.; Ackerstein, A.; Samuel, S.; et al. Nonmyeloablative stem cell transplantation and cell therapy as an alternative to conventional bone marrow transplantation with lethal cytoreduction for the treatment of malignant and nonmalignant hematologic diseases. *Blood* **1998**, *91*, 756–763. [CrossRef]
161. Dudley, M.E.; Wunderlich, J.R.; Yang, J.C. A phase I study of nonmyeloablative chemotherapy and adoptive transfer of autologous tumor antigen-specific T lymphocytes in patients with metastatic melanoma. *J. Immunother.* **2002**, *25*, 243. [CrossRef]
162. Dudley, M.E.; Wunderlich, J.R.; Robbins, P.F.; Yang, J.C.; Hwu, P.; Schwartzentruber, D.J.; Topalian, S.L.; Sherry, R.; Restifo, N.P.; Hubicki, A.M.; et al. Cancer regression and autoimmunity in patients after clonal repopulation with antitumor lymphocytes. *Science* **2002**, *298*, 850–854. [CrossRef]
163. Morgan, R.A.; Dudley, M.E.; Wunderlich, J.R.; Hughes, M.S.; Yang, J.C.; Sherry, R.M.; Royal, R.E.; Topalian, S.L.; Kammula, U.S.; Restifo, N.P.; et al. Cancer regression in patients after transfer of genetically engineered lymphocytes. *Science* **2006**, *314*, 126–129. [CrossRef]
164. Johnson, L.A.; Morgan, R.A.; Dudley, M.E.; Cassard, L.; Yang, J.C.; Hughes, M.S.; Kammula, U.S.; Royal, R.E.; Sherry, R.M.; Wunderlich, J.R.; et al. Gene therapy with human and mouse T-cell receptors mediates cancer regression and targets normal tissues expressing cognate antigen. *Blood* **2009**, *114*, 535–546. [CrossRef]
165. Robbins, P.F.; Morgan, R.A.; Feldman, S.A.; Yang, J.C.; Sherry, R.M.; Dudley, M.E.; Wunderlich, J.R.; Nahvi, A.V.; Helman, L.J.; Mackall, C.L.; et al. Tumor regression in patients with metastatic synovial cell sarcoma and melanoma using genetically engineered lymphocytes reactive with NY-ESO-1. *J. Clin. Oncol.* **2011**, *29*, 917–924. [CrossRef]
166. Pule, M.A.; Savoldo, B.; Myers, G.D.; Rossig, C.; Russell, H.V.; Dotti, G.; Huls, M.H.; Liu, E.; Gee, A.P.; Mei, Z.; et al. Virus-specific T cells engineered to coexpress tumor-specific receptors: Persistence and antitumor activity in individuals with neuroblastoma. *Nat. Med.* **2008**, *14*, 1264–1270. [CrossRef]
167. Parkhurst, M.R.; Yang, J.C.; Langan, R.C.; Dudley, M.E.; Nathan, D.-A.N.; Feldman, S.A.; Davis, J.L.; Morgan, R.A.; Merino, M.J.; Sherry, R.M.; et al. T cells targeting carcinoembryonic antigen can mediate regression of metastatic colorectal cancer but induce severe transient colitis. *Mol. Ther.* **2011**, *19*, 620–626. [CrossRef]
168. Robbins, P.F.; Lu, Y.-C.; El-Gamil, M.; Li, Y.F.; Gross, C.; Gartner, J.; Lin, J.C.; Teer, J.K.; Cliften, P.; Tycksen, E.; et al. Mining exomic sequencing data to identify mutated antigens recognized by adoptively transferred tumor-reactive T cells. *Nat. Med.* **2013**, *19*, 747–752. [CrossRef]
169. Tran, E.; Turcotte, S.; Gros, A.; Robbins, P.F.; Lu, Y.-C.; Dudley, M.E.; Wunderlich, J.R.; Somerville, R.P.; Hogan, K.; Hinrichs, C.S.; et al. Cancer immunotherapy based on mutation-specific CD4+ T cells in a patient with epithelial cancer. *Science* **2014**, *344*, 641–645. [CrossRef]
170. Chandran, S.S.; Somerville, R.P.T.; Yang, J.C.; Sherry, R.M.; Klebanoff, C.A.; Goff, S.L.; Wunderlich, J.R.; Danforth, D.N.; Zlott, D.; Paria, B.C.; et al. Treatment of metastatic uveal melanoma with adoptive transfer of tumour-infiltrating lymphocytes: A single-centre, two-stage, single-arm, phase 2 study. *Lancet Oncol.* **2017**, *18*, 792–802. [CrossRef]

171. Lo, W.; Parkhurst, M.; Robbins, P.F.; Tran, E.; Lu, Y.-C.; Jia, L.; Gartner, J.J.; Pasetto, A.; Deniger, D.; Malekzadeh, P.; et al. Immunologic Recognition of a Shared p53 Mutated Neoantigen in a Patient with Metastatic Colorectal Cancer. *Cancer Immunol. Res.* **2019**, *7*, 534–543. [CrossRef]
172. Dudley, M.E.; Rosenberg, S.A. Adoptive cell transfer therapy. *Semin. Oncol.* **2007**, *34*, 524–531. [CrossRef]
173. Hakomori, S. Aberrant glycosylation in tumors and tumor-associated carbohydrate antigens. *Adv. Cancer Res.* **1989**, *52*, 257–331.
174. Werdelin, O.; Meldal, M.; Jensen, T. Processing of glycans on glycoprotein and glycopeptide antigens in antigen-presenting cells. *Proc. Natl. Acad. Sci. USA* **2002**, *99*, 9611–9613. [CrossRef]
175. Garrido, F.; Aptsiauri, N.; Doorduijn, E.M.; Garcia Lora, A.M.; van Hall, T. The urgent need to recover MHC class I in cancers for effective immunotherapy. *Curr. Opin. Immunol.* **2016**, *39*, 44–51. [CrossRef]
176. Gross, G.; Waks, T.; Eshhar, Z. Expression of immunoglobulin-T-cell receptor chimeric molecules as functional receptors with antibody-type specificity. *Proc. Natl. Acad. Sci. USA* **1989**, *86*, 10024–10028. [CrossRef]
177. Stancovski, I.; Schindler, D.G.; Waks, T.; Yarden, Y.; Sela, M.; Eshhar, Z. Targeting of T lymphocytes to Neu/HER2-expressing cells using chimeric single chain Fv receptors. *J. Immunol.* **1993**, *151*, 6577–6582. [PubMed]
178. Hwu, P.; Shafer, G.E.; Treisman, J.; Schindler, D.G.; Gross, G.; Cowherd, R.; Rosenberg, S.A.; Eshhar, Z. Lysis of ovarian cancer cells by human lymphocytes redirected with a chimeric gene composed of an antibody variable region and the Fc receptor gamma chain. *J. Exp. Med.* **1993**, *178*, 361–366. [CrossRef] [PubMed]
179. Krause, A.; Guo, H.F.; Latouche, J.B.; Tan, C.; Cheung, N.K.; Sadelain, M. Antigen-dependent CD28 signaling selectively enhances survival and proliferation in genetically modified activated human primary T lymphocytes. *J. Exp. Med.* **1998**, *188*, 619–626. [CrossRef]
180. Finney, H.M.; Lawson, A.D.; Bebbington, C.R.; Weir, A.N. Chimeric receptors providing both primary and costimulatory signaling in T cells from a single gene product. *J. Immunol.* **1998**, *161*, 2791–2797. [PubMed]
181. Haynes, N.M.; Trapani, J.A.; Teng, M.W.L.; Jackson, J.T.; Cerruti, L.; Jane, S.M.; Kershaw, M.H.; Smyth, M.J.; Darcy, P.K. Single-chain antigen recognition receptors that costimulate potent rejection of established experimental tumors. *Blood* **2002**, *100*, 3155–3163. [CrossRef]
182. Lamers, C.H.J.; Sleijfer, S.; Vulto, A.G.; Kruit, W.H.J.; Kliffen, M.; Debets, R.; Gratama, J.W.; Stoter, G.; Oosterwijk, E. Treatment of metastatic renal cell carcinoma with autologous T-lymphocytes genetically retargeted against carbonic anhydrase IX: First clinical experience. *J. Clin. Oncol.* **2006**, *24*, e20-2. [CrossRef]
183. Kershaw, M.H.; Westwood, J.A.; Parker, L.L.; Wang, G.; Eshhar, Z.; Mavroukakis, S.A.; White, D.E.; Wunderlich, J.R.; Canevari, S.; Rogers-Freezer, L.; et al. A phase I study on adoptive immunotherapy using gene-modified T cells for ovarian cancer. *Clin. Cancer Res.* **2006**, *12*, 6106–6115. [CrossRef]
184. Till, B.G.; Jensen, M.C.; Wang, J.; Chen, E.Y.; Wood, B.L.; Greisman, H.A.; Qian, X.; James, S.E.; Raubitschek, A.; Forman, S.J.; et al. Adoptive immunotherapy for indolent non-Hodgkin lymphoma and mantle cell lymphoma using genetically modified autologous CD20-specific T cells. *Blood* **2008**, *112*, 2261–2271. [CrossRef]
185. Hollyman, D.; Stefanski, J.; Przybylowski, M.; Bartido, S.; Borquez-Ojeda, O.; Taylor, C.; Yeh, R.; Capacio, V.; Olszewska, M.; Hosey, J.; et al. Manufacturing validation of biologically functional T cells targeted to CD19 antigen for autologous adoptive cell therapy. *J. Immunother* **2009**, *32*, 169–180. [CrossRef]
186. Kochenderfer, J.N.; Wilson, W.H.; Janik, J.E.; Dudley, M.E.; Stetler-Stevenson, M.; Feldman, S.A.; Maric, I.; Raffeld, M.; Nathan, D.-A.N.; Lanier, B.J.; et al. Eradication of B-lineage cells and regression of lymphoma in a patient treated with autologous T cells genetically engineered to recognize CD19. *Blood* **2010**, *116*, 4099–4102. [CrossRef]
187. Kalos, M.; Levine, B.L.; Porter, D.L.; Katz, S.; Grupp, S.A.; Bagg, A.; June, C.H. T cells with chimeric antigen receptors have potent antitumor effects and can establish memory in patients with advanced leukemia. *Sci. Transl. Med.* **2011**, *3*, 95ra73. [CrossRef]
188. Porter, D.L.; Levine, B.L.; Kalos, M.; Bagg, A.; June, C.H. Chimeric antigen receptor-modified T cells in chronic lymphoid leukemia. *N. Engl. J. Med.* **2011**, *365*, 725–733. [CrossRef]
189. Milone, M.C.; Fish, J.D.; Carpenito, C.; Carroll, R.G.; Binder, G.K.; Teachey, D.; Samanta, M.; Lakhal, M.; Gloss, B.; Danet-Desnoyers, G.; et al. Chimeric receptors containing CD137 signal transduction domains mediate enhanced survival of T cells and increased antileukemic efficacy in vivo. *Mol. Ther.* **2009**, *17*, 1453–1464. [CrossRef]

190. Shimabukuro-Vornhagen, A.; Gödel, P.; Subklewe, M.; Stemmler, H.J.; Schlößer, H.A.; Schlaak, M.; Kochanek, M.; Böll, B.; von Bergwelt-Baildon, M.S. Cytokine release syndrome. *J. Immunother. Cancer* **2018**, *6*, 56. [CrossRef]
191. Kochenderfer, J.N.; Dudley, M.E.; Feldman, S.A.; Wilson, W.H.; Spaner, D.E.; Maric, I.; Stetler-Stevenson, M.; Phan, G.Q.; Hughes, M.S.; Sherry, R.M.; et al. B-cell depletion and remissions of malignancy along with cytokine-associated toxicity in a clinical trial of anti-CD19 chimeric-antigen-receptor-transduced T cells. *Blood* **2012**, *119*, 2709–2720. [CrossRef]
192. Kochenderfer, J.N.; Dudley, M.E.; Kassim, S.H.; Somerville, R.P.T.; Carpenter, R.O.; Stetler-Stevenson, M.; Yang, J.C.; Phan, G.Q.; Hughes, M.S.; Sherry, R.M.; et al. Chemotherapy-refractory diffuse large B-cell lymphoma and indolent B-cell malignancies can be effectively treated with autologous T cells expressing an anti-CD19 chimeric antigen receptor. *J. Clin. Oncol.* **2015**, *33*, 540–549. [CrossRef]
193. Maus, M.V.; Grupp, S.A.; Porter, D.L.; June, C.H. Antibody-modified T cells: CARs take the front seat for hematologic malignancies. *Blood* **2014**, *123*, 2625–2635. [CrossRef]
194. Grupp, S.A.; Kalos, M.; Barrett, D.; Aplenc, R.; Porter, D.L.; Rheingold, S.R.; Teachey, D.T.; Chew, A.; Hauck, B.; Wright, J.F.; et al. Chimeric antigen receptor-modified T cells for acute lymphoid leukemia. *N. Engl. J. Med.* **2013**, *368*, 1509–1518. [CrossRef]
195. Lee, D.W.; Gardner, R.; Porter, D.L.; Louis, C.U.; Ahmed, N.; Jensen, M.; Grupp, S.A.; Mackall, C.L. Current concepts in the diagnosis and management of cytokine release syndrome. *Blood* **2014**, *124*, 188–195. [CrossRef]
196. Yeku, O.; Li, X.; Brentjens, R.J. Adoptive T-Cell Therapy for Solid Tumors. *Am. Soc. Clin. Oncol. Educ. Book* **2017**, *37*, 193–204. [CrossRef] [PubMed]
197. Baybutt, T.R.; Flickinger, J.C.; Caparosa, E.M.; Snook, A.E. Advances in Chimeric Antigen Receptor T-Cell Therapies for Solid Tumors. *Clin. Pharmacol. Ther.* **2019**, *105*, 71–78. [CrossRef] [PubMed]
198. Mukherjee, S. Genomics-Guided Immunotherapy for Precision Medicine in Cancer. *Cancer Biother. Radiopharm.* **2019**. [CrossRef]

5

Understanding the Effects of Radiotherapy on the Tumour Immune Microenvironment to Identify Potential Prognostic and Predictive Biomarkers of Radiotherapy Response

Shuhui Cheng [1], Eleanor J. Cheadle [1] and Timothy M. Illidge [1,2,*]

1 Manchester Academic Health Science Centre, Manchester NIHR Biomedical Research Centre, Division of Cancer Sciences, Faculty of Biology, Medicine and Health, University of Manchester, Manchester M13 9PL, UK; shuhui.cheng@postgrad.manchester.ac.uk (S.C.); Eleanor.J.Cheadle@manchester.ac.uk (E.J.C.)

2 The Christie NHS Foundation Trust, Manchester M20 4BX, UK

* Correspondence: tim.illidge@manchester.ac.uk

Simple Summary: Around 50% of all cancer patients receive radiotherapy as part of their treatment. Recently immunotherapy has shown promising results and become established as an effective treatment for some cancers. Combining radiotherapy and immunotherapy is a novel approach to further increase the number of patients responding to immunotherapy. Biological markers of response (biomarkers) are urgently required to hasten the clinical translation and improve outcomes further. Radiotherapy can both stimulate and inhibit the immune system and understanding the immune effects of radiotherapy on the tumour and surrounding cells may lead to the identification of predictive and prognostic biomarkers to help make more individualized treatment decisions, when combining radiotherapy with immunotherapy. This review summarizes the immune effects of radiotherapy and biomarkers of response identified to date; providing new perspectives for future research which may facilitate the development of novel radiotherapy immunotherapy combinations based on tumour immunology and biomarker identification.

Abstract: Radiotherapy (RT) is a highly effective anti-cancer treatment. Immunotherapy using immune checkpoint blockade (ICI) has emerged as a new and robust pillar in cancer therapy; however, the response rate to single agent ICI is low whilst toxicity remains. Radiotherapy has been shown to have local and systemic immunomodulatory effects. Therefore, combining RT and immunotherapy is a rational approach to enhance anti-tumour immune responses. However, the immunomodulatory effects of RT can be both immunostimulatory or immunosuppressive and may be different across different tumour types and patients. Therefore, there is an urgent medical need to establish biomarkers to guide clinical decision making in predicting responses or in patient selection for RT-based combination treatments. In this review, we summarize the immunological effects of RT on the tumour microenvironment and emerging biomarkers to help better understand the implications of these immunological changes, and we provide new insights into the potential for combination therapies with RT and immunotherapy.

Keywords: radiotherapy; immunotherapy; tumour microenvironment; biomarker

---

1. Introduction

Radiotherapy (RT) is a highly effective anti-cancer treatment delivered to between 50% and 60% of all cancer patients as part of either curative treatment or for palliation of their disease [1].

Following the breakthrough of immune checkpoint inhibitors (ICI), immunotherapy has now become established as an important component of cancer therapy. However, the response rate to single agent ICI in most solid tumours is low, at approximately 20% to 30%, and further developments are ongoing to improve response rates and outcomes further. RT has long since been known to be highly effective at inducing DNA damage and in recent years has been shown to have local and systemic immunomodulatory effects. Therefore, combining RT and immunotherapy is a logical approach to enhance anti-tumour immune responses. However, the immunomodulatory effects of RT can be both immunostimulatory and immunosuppressive, which may be different across different tumour types and patients. This potential diversity in the immune response to RT adds complexity to the interpretation of how the immune landscape in the tumour microenvironment (TME) might respond in patients receiving RT. The nature of the immune response to RT and whether this is immunostimulatory or immunosuppressive further highlights the importance of identifying immunological biomarkers to assess treatment responses in patients undergoing RT. In this review, the effects of RT on the tumour microenvironment, candidate immune targets, emerging biomarkers and the related cutting-edge technologies for analysis of immune biomarkers will be outlined. Finally, the implications of these immunological consequences on the potential for combination therapy with RT and immunotherapy will be discussed.

2. The Tumour Immune Microenvironment

2.1. The Components and Classification of TME

The term "tumour microenvironment" (TME) refers to an "ecological niche" which affects tumour growth and progression and is characterized by complex biological interactions between the tumour and the stroma [2,3]. The TME encompasses cancer cells, stromal cells (such as fibroblasts), a diversity of resident and infiltrating immune cells and soluble messengers [2]. The constituent cell types in the TME vary from T cells, dendritic cells (DCs), tumour-associated macrophages (TAMs), myeloid-derived suppressor cells (MDSCs), mast cells, to natural killer (NK) cells, which secrete a variety of factors (chemokines, cytokines and enzymes) that directly or indirectly participate in immune responses. The composition and the interplay of the components within the TME may have a critical role in the outcome of tumour evolution and treatment response [2].

There are certain cell types in the TME that play an essential role in immune surveillance, such as DCs, cytotoxic T cells and NK cells. Among these, the T cell infiltrates are potentially some of the most important immune effector cells populations which have been investigated extensively. One such investigation is the immunoscore, which refers to the density of two different lymphocyte populations (CD3+, CD8+ or CD45RO+ cells) quantified in the tumour core and the invasive margin, which was first shown to correlate with outcome in colorectal cancer (CRC) [4]. The prognostic power of the immunoscore is also being investigated and validated in other cancer types including melanoma and breast cancer [5].

The TME can however become highly immunosuppressive as a result of the infiltration and interaction of a multitude of immune effector cells which act to suppress immune responses, including MDSCs, regulatory T cells (Tregs) and TAMs. Tregs play a significant role in facilitating immune escape and promoting tumour progression. A low number of Tregs before treatment was found to be correlated with active immune responses and favourable clinical outcome in breast cancer patients following surgery and RT [6]. In terms of TAM, the TME encourages the switch from a tumour-killing M1-TAM to a tumour-promoting M2-TAM type. MDSCs are a heterogeneous population of myeloid cells [7] and have been demonstrated to be associated with a poor prognosis in pancreatic, oesophageal and gastric cancers, which suggests their potential as an important prognostic biomarker [7].

It is increasingly recognized that tumour responses to treatments to some extent depend on the microenvironment. Therefore, it is important to understand how immunostimulatory and suppressive effects are reflected and balanced in the TME, thereby hopefully tailoring the treatment according to the TME landscape.

2.2. *The Effects of RT on the Tumour Microenvironment*

RT has been widely used to eradicate cancer with its direct tumour-killing effects [8]; however, increasing evidence shows that RT can cause tumour rejection by enhancing local anti-tumour immune responses that can lead to a distant systemic immune response called the "abscopal effect", where the tumour regresses outside the irradiated site [9]. However, it is increasingly understood that RT has both immunostimulatory and immunosuppressive effects. In order to utilize RT to enhance the immunostimulatory effects and overcome intrinsic immunosuppression within the TME, a greater understanding of RT-induced immune effects is required.

2.2.1. RT-Induced Immunostimulation

RT is well documented to initiate tumour rejection by enhancing anti-tumour immune responses, although mostly in murine tumours [10–16]. The phenomenon "abscopal effect", which refers to a tumour in a non-irradiated site regressing after RT [17], offers further evidence of the ability of RT to induce immunological responses. RT can mediate these effects in several ways including immunogenic effects on tumour cells and immunostimulatory effects on the immune system.

RT can increase the antigenicity of tumour cells by inducing or upregulating the release of tumour-associated antigen (TAA) through induction of tumour cell death and increasing the expression of MHC class I molecules that are expressed on the surface of tumour cells. RT can also greatly alter the repertoire of MHC class I restricted peptides [18].

It has been shown that RT is able to induce immunogenic cell death (ICD), whereby tumour cells dying after RT undergo a form of cellular death induced by a cascade of complex reactions which can elicit immune responses [19] (Figure 1).

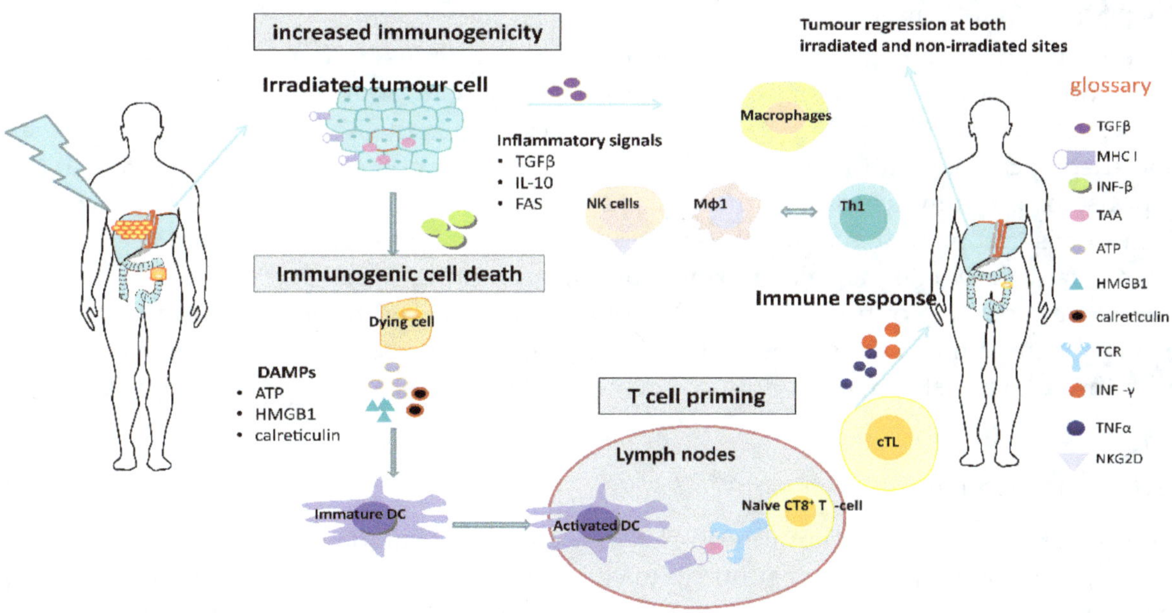

Figure 1. Immunostimulatory effects of radiotherapy. Radiotherapy can enhance the antigenicity of tumour cells by stimulating the induction of immunogenic cell death mediated by damage-associated molecular pattern molecules (DAMPs), which contributes to DC maturation and T cell priming. Activated cytotoxic T cells (cTL) in the blood can cause systemic immune responses, potentially resulting in tumour regression outside the irradiated field. DC, dendritic cell; Mφ1 cells, macrophage type-1 cell; Th1 cell, T helper type 1 cell.

After irradiation, tumour cells can undergo a form of cell death known as immunogenic cell death and express damage-associated molecule patterns (DAMP) or "danger signals", which includes exposure of calreticulin, the extracellular release of ATP and high mobility group box 1 (HMGB1) and uric acid. Calreticulin is a protein that can serve as an "eat me" signal, stimulating the engulfment of dying tumour cells and their apoptotic debris by macrophages and immature DCs [19,20]. ATP can be a potent signal for activating myeloid cells including monocytes/macrophages and immature DCs. HMGB1 is a factor that can be released by dead cells and can interact with several distinct pattern recognition receptors, including toll-like receptor 4 (TLR4). These DAMPs, induced by RT, may potentially play an important role in promoting the recruitment, differentiation and effective acquisition, processing and presentation of TAA by stimulating dendritic cell (DC) maturation within TME [21].

Additionally, there are other potential immunological mechanisms through which RT can increase the susceptibility to anti-tumour immune surveillance. These include the multiple death receptors induced by RT expressed on the surface of tumour cells, including FAS (also known as CD95) and tumour necrosis factor-related apoptosis-inducing ligand (TRAIL) receptors 1 and 2 (TRAIL-R1 and TRAIL-R2), which can render the tumour cells more vulnerable to apoptosis [20].

In addition to these immunogenic and phenotypic changes, RT can stimulate immune responses via interactions with the immune system. Whilst the direct contribution of infiltrating versus resident T cells to overall tumour control remains to be clarified, the number and function of TILs have been shown to increase following single, ablative doses of RT. Likewise, both high single-dose and fractionated RT have been shown to increase T cell receptor (TCR) diversity and clonality, predominantly leading to the enrichment of T cell clones already resident within the TME [12,22].

RT can also upregulate MHC class I molecules, leading to enhanced recognition of tumour cells by cytotoxic T cells, and increased NKG2D expression may result in greater NK cell-mediated eradication of tumours [21,23].

Production of type I interferons due to RT-induced accumulation of cytosolic DNA and activation of the STING pathway [24] can also lead to increased expansion of tumour-specific T cells, as a consequence of enhanced cross-presentation of tumour antigens by dendritic cells. RT can trigger the production of pro-inflammatory chemokines including CXCL9, CXCL10 and CXCL16, resulting in the chemotactic recruitment of effector CD8+ T cells into the TME. Macrophages are another immune effector cell population in the TME which may have a potentially important role in dictating the response of the tumour to radiotherapy. Macrophages have been characterised into M1 and M2 phenotypes, although it is understood that there can be "plasticity" between such phenotypes. M1 macrophages mediate vascular normalization, promoting T cell recruitment and subsequent rejection of tumours. In contrast, the M2 phenotype is considered to promote immunosuppression. Interestingly, conventional lower doses of RT (2 Gy) frequently used in routine clinical practice have also been found to transform an immunosuppressive M2 TAM into a tumour-killing iNOS producing M1 TAM [25].

2.2.2. RT-Induced Immunosuppression

In contrast to the potential immunostimulatory effects, RT can have several immunosuppressive effects that may negatively impact or suppress the development of anti-cancer immunity. These negative effects of RT can be imposed directly on the TME, such as the RT-induced death of immune cells, or indirectly through modulation of stromal cells and tumour vasculature (Figure 2).

In addition to direct cytotoxic effects on immune cells, RT can lead to the production of pro-inflammatory cytokines and chemokines (such as TNF, interleukin and TGF-β) and the subsequent recruitment of suppressive immune cells such as MDSCs, TAMs and Tregs [26]. TGF-β is a potent immunosuppressive cytokine that inhibits cross-priming of T cells by damaging the antigen-presenting function of dendritic cells and the functional differentiation of T cells into effectors [27]. Infiltration of Tregs can lead to cytotoxic CD8+ T cell inactivation by expression of the checkpoint inhibitor molecule CTLA-4. Interestingly, on some occasions, these immunosuppressive reactions can be overcome by RT-induced immune stimulation, which is characterised by ICD induced antigen exposure, DC maturation, T cell recruitment and activation.

Irradiated normal tissue adjacent to tumour undergoes a process of inflammation, wound healing and fibrosis. This process involves the expansion of cancer-associated fibroblasts (CAFs) and extracellular matrix modelling, which leads to post-radiation tumour hardening and shrinkage, and ultimately facilitates tumour spread or recurrence [26]. CAFs are a heterogeneous cell population that constitute the majority of cells within the stroma in many carcinomas [28]. RT activates CAFs by causing DNA damage and production of ROS [29]. Irradiated CAFs can contribute to cancer progression via the transforming growth factor beta (TGF-β)-CXCL12 dependent pathway. However, whether CAFs play a tumour-killing or tumour-promoting role may vary depending on the type of signal [30]. RT-induced vascular damage is aggravated by tumour hypoxia through CXCL-12 and HIF-1α-mediated MDSC recruitment [31].

In hypoxic environments, RT-induced free radical production is reduced and consequently RT causes less DNA damage in hypoxic areas. A further potentially important mechanism for RT to induce immunosuppression in hypoxic areas may be increases in the production of vascular endothelial growth factor (VEGF), reactive oxygen species (ROS) and hypoxia-inducible factor-1α (HIF-1α) [26]. HIF-1α participates in several specific processes resulting in tumour vascularization and reoxygenation. Furthermore, it was found to be an independent predictor of poor prognosis after RT [26].

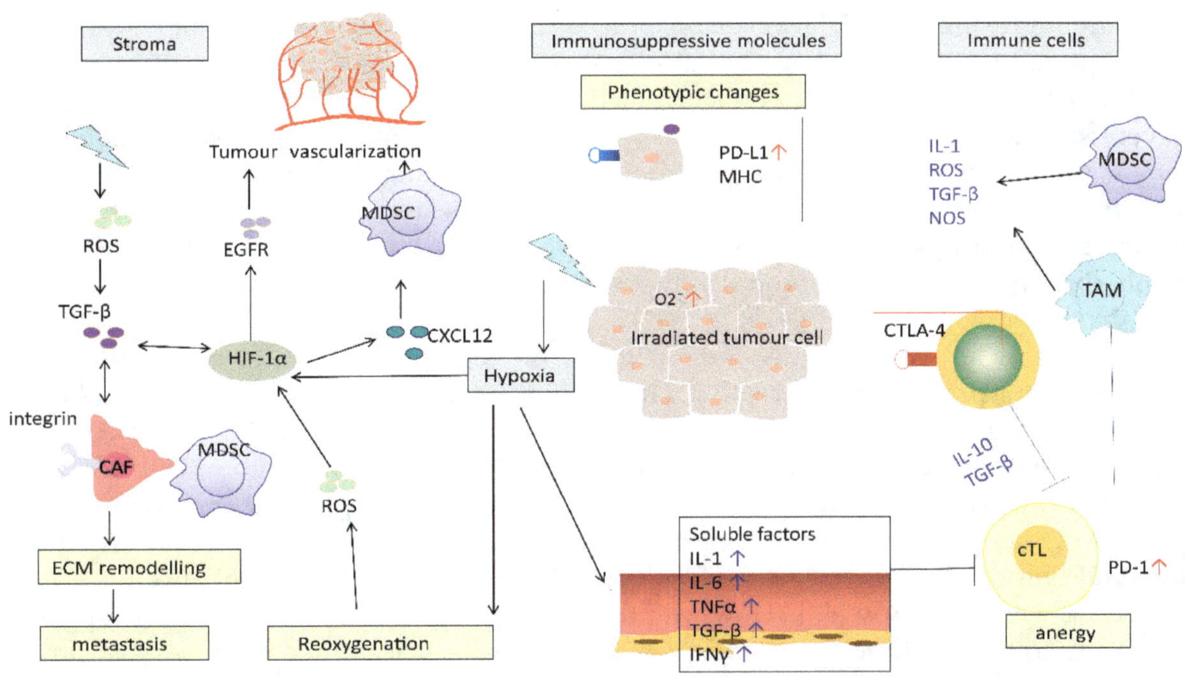

Figure 2. Potential mechanisms of RT-induced immunosuppression. RT causes a series of immunosuppressive processes: modifying tumour stromal environment, production of immunosuppressive molecules, recruiting immunosuppressive cells and impairing effective T cells. RT causes hypoxia, which induces HIF-1α and TGF-β. HIF-1α-activated CAFs mediated by TGF-β or directly by RT promote ECM re-modelling. These effects work in concert to promote cancer metastasis. CAF, cancer-associated fibroblasts; MDSC, myeloid-derived suppressor cell; cTL, cytotoxic T lymphocyte; TAM, tumour-associated macrophages; ECM, extracellular matrix; HIF-1α, hypoxia-inducible factor-1α; TGF-β, transforming growth factor beta.

2.2.3. RT and Cell Death

Tumour cells usually evolve to escape death by inactivating the cell death pathways commonly used to eliminate damaged and harmful cells [32]. This ability to avoid cell death may lead to resistance during treatment [33]. Therefore, it is necessary to have an overall understanding of the mechanisms of cell death induced by RT in order to develop new anti-tumour treatments.

For many years, apoptosis has been proposed as the principal cell death pathway induced by radiotherapy. Recently, non-apoptotic cell death morphologies or alternative death mechanisms have been discovered during radiation, including autophagy, necrosis, programmed necroptosis and ferroptosis, all of which will be summarised below. The mode of cell death induced by RT is of particular importance as certain modes of cell death will lead to the release of tumour antigens which are subsequently processed and presented on antigen-presenting cells [21].

Among all these cell death types, one particularly distinct type of "cell death" is radiation necrosis. Radiation necrosis is unprogrammed cell death and, for example, can occur as a rare late side effect following high-dose radiation (typically > 55 Gy) of both intracranial and extracranial tumours, such as nasopharyngeal carcinoma [34]. Unlike all other cell deaths, it has not been often reported to be associated with tumour suppression, but it presents similar imaging findings and symptoms to tumour recurrence, which can pose a challenge to differential diagnosis [35]. The aetiology of radiation necrosis is not yet clear. Possible histopathological changes might be radiation-induced vascular damage and the resultant ischemic necrosis, radiation-induced damage to oligodendrocytes and their precursors or impaired neurogenesis, implicating the vascular cells and/or oligodendrocytes as the targets of radiation injury [34].

Autophagy is a catabolic process whose activation acts as a pro-survival mechanism and can induce autophagic cell death in some circumstances [36]. Targeting autophagy has been proposed as a novel anti-tumour treatment [37]; however, it is still controversial as to whether autophagy stimulation or inhibition is better [38]. Autophagy has also been identified to play a dual role in the response of cancer cells to RT, with preclinical models showing that autophagy inhibition increases radiosensitivity in vitro yet reduces efficacy of radiotherapy in vivo due to deficient immunogenic signalling [39,40]. Inhibiting autophagy with chloroquine or hydroxychloroquine might improve the efficacy of several anticancer therapies in patients, and exploratory clinical studies are ongoing [41]. However, the results of trials using these drugs have been generally disappointing, with limited clinical efficacy [42,43]. In addition, some researchers have proposed that whether autophagy should be enhanced or inhibited is context-dependent [37,44].

Necroptosis is a caspase-independent form of regulated cell death executed by the receptor-interacting protein kinase 1 (RIP1), RIP3, and mixed lineage kinase domain-like protein (MLKL) [45], which can lead to DAMP release [46] and chronic inflammation associated with aging. Much of the tumour radioresistance and recurrence results from tumour cell repopulation after radiotherapy. A preclinical study showed that necroptosis-associated tumour repopulation after radiotherapy depended on activation of the RIP1/RIP3/MLKL/JNK/IL-8 pathway and this novel pathway could be a promising target for blocking tumour repopulation to enhance the efficacy of colorectal cancer radiotherapy [47]. However, there is still a long way to go for necroptosis-based cancer therapy to be developed as many questions are still unclear—for instance, the intrinsic or acquired defects of necroptotic machinery observed in many cancer cells [45].

Ferroptosis is a form of regulated cell death characterised by lipid peroxidation and was recently identified to be potentially tumour-suppressive. Ferroptotic cancer cells have modulatory effects on tumour immunity at many steps [48]; however, various putative signals released by ferroptotic cancer cells may lead to the stimulation or suppression of different immune cells. Triggering ferroptosis may be a novel approach in cancer therapy; several strategies to target ferroptosis have been investigated [48]. Although the link between RT and ferroptosis has not been experimentally addressed or widely proven, recent evidence suggests that radiotherapy induces ferroptosis in cancer patients [49], and increased ferroptosis was demonstrated to be associated with improved response to radiotherapy and better survival in oesophageal tumour samples [50].

3. Biomarkers

To date, there have been limited clinical studies addressing the RT-induced immunological changes in humans. Further preclinical and clinical investigations are needed to identify potential biomarkers of RT-induced immunological changes to guide decision-making in clinical practice, particularly when considering RT–IO agent combination therapies.

There is growing demand to develop predictive biomarkers which guide the development and delivery of tailored therapies, i.e., "right drug to the right patients", by predicting benefit to a medical intervention and prognostic biomarkers which are used to identify likelihood of a clinical event, disease recurrence or progression. Several diagnostic tumour markers are now included in routine clinical practice, such as PSA, CA125, β-HCG and AFP [51], but few biomarkers are currently validated for clinical practice in RT and none to guide RT in combination with IO agents. In addition to static biomarkers, dynamic biomarkers are proposed to investigate how treatments may influence key transitions and potentially identify responders and non-responders in a more timely fashion, sparing patients' toxicities from ineffective treatments and potentially guiding therapy decisions to more effective approaches. Such dynamic tumour biomarkers requiring serial sampling would facilitate real-time decision-making that has not been previously possible with pre-treatment biomarkers [52]. The process of developing biomarkers for patients undergoing RT is outlined below (Figure 3).

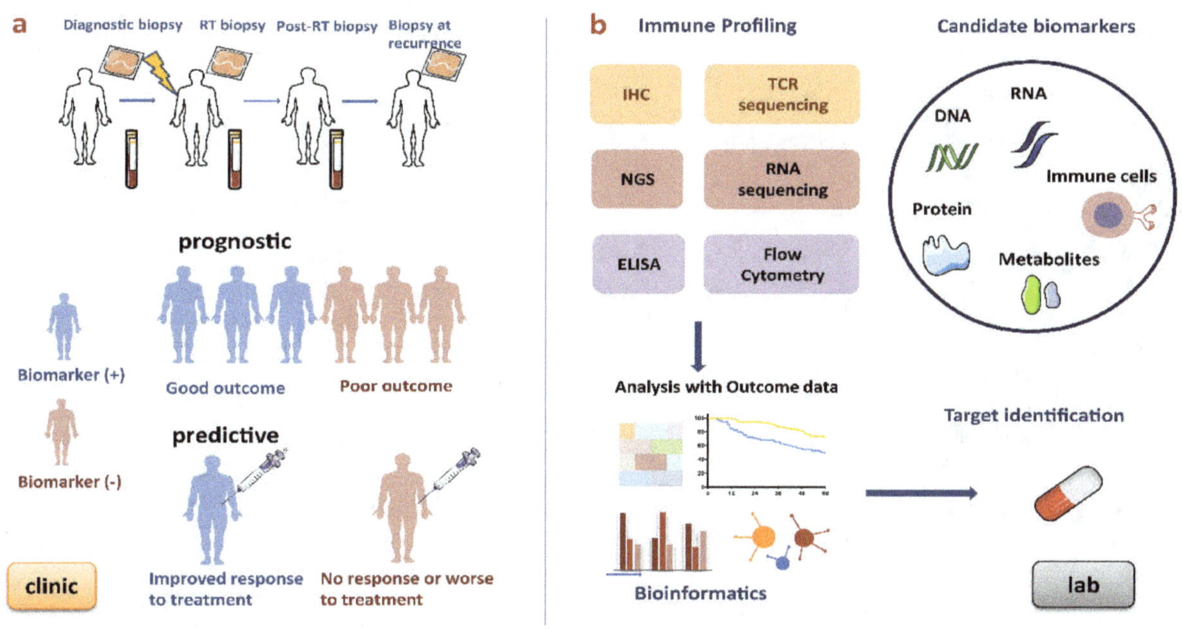

Figure 3. Process of developing biomarkers for patients undergoing radiotherapy. (**a**) Blood and tumour biopsies are taken at baseline, during RT, after RT and at recurrence to obtain dynamic immune profiling. This figure shows an ideal example of prognostic and predictive biomarkers. Prognostic biomarkers provide information on disease progression and outcomes, and predictive biomarkers indicate the response to a medical intervention. (**b**) In the lab, these biomarkers can be discovered by high-throughput gene technologies, immune-based technologies and analysed by bioinformatic approaches. RT, radiotherapy; IHC, immunohistochemistry; NGS, next-generation sequencing; TCR, T cell receptor; ELISA, enzyme-linked immunosorbent assay.

3.1. Radiotherapy-Related Biomarkers

It is important to note that the TME is dependent on many factors, such as patient age [53], treatment (chemotherapy, radiotherapy and immunotherapy), tumour type (e.g., solid or haematological) and whether the tumour is virally or hormonally driven. For virally driven tumours such as HNSCC, a recent study demonstrated that HPV-positivity correlated with increased immune cytolytic activity and a T-cell-inflamed gene expression profile, suggesting that HPV status can be used to predict the effectiveness of PD-1 inhibitors in HNSCC, independently of PD-L1 expression and TMB, and probably results from an inflamed TME induced by HPV infection and anti-tumour activity of HPV antigen-specific T cells [54]. For hormone dependent tumours such as breast cancer or prostate cancer, the TME may be affected by more complex regulation, such as oestrogen or testosterone signalling pathways [55,56]. Furthermore, it is difficult to delineate whether changes to the TME as a result of RT are due to a specific effect of RT or the change in tumour size as a result of RT, and serial biopsies allowing a thorough investigation into the dynamics and kinetics of changes are only possible in preclinical models. Here, we focus on the impact of RT on the TME, and some of the potential immune-related biomarkers of response to RT which have been identified to date are summarized below (Table 1). Whilst numerous biomarkers during RT are under investigation, there are few available to guide clinical decision-making in predicting responses or in patient selection for radiotherapy-based treatments. Furthermore, biomarker identification is in its infancy and it will be important to consider that any identified biomarker will need to be validated across factors such as different tumour types, age of patients and hormone or viral dependency of the tumour.

Table 1. Clinical studies on immune-related biomarkers in radiotherapy-based treatment.

Category	Sample Origin	Biomarker	Cancer Type	Treatment	Clinical Response	Reference
Circulating cells	Peripheral blood mononuclear cell	Lymphopenia	Cervical cancer	Definitive CRT	↓ OS, DFS	[57]
	Whole blood	↑ Myeloid-derived suppressor cell	HCC	RT	↓ OS	[58]
	Whole blood	↑ MDSCs + Tregs	Rectal cancer	Short-term pCRT + surgery	Early marker of response	[59]
Circulating cytokine	Plasma	VEGF, PIGF and IL-6	CRC	Neoadjuvant bevacizumab + CRT + surgery	Predictive of response	[60]
Immune Infiltrates	FFPE tissue	↑ CD3+, CD8+ TILs	HNSCC	Definitive CRT	↑ OS, PFS Predictive of CRT	[61]
	FFPE tissue, surgical specimens	↑ CD3+, CD8+ TILs	CRC	pCRT	Predictive of pathological downstaging	[62]
	FFPE tissue	↑ Ratio of PD-1+/CD8+ TILs	Extrahepatic cholangiocarcinoma	Adjuvant CRT	↓ OS	[63]
	FFPE tissue, surgical specimens	Immunoscore	CRC	pCRT	Predictive of downstaging after pCRT	[62]
	Surgical specimens	Immunoscore	Brain metastasis	Surgery + whole brain RT	Prognostic to OS	[62]
T-cell-related	FFPE tissue	PD-L1 (+) post RT	Cervical carcinoma	Carbon-ion	↑ PFS	[64]
	Plasma	↑ PD-L1	HCC	RT	↓ OS	[65]
	Plasma	T cell receptor repertoire and ↑ serum IFNβ	Lung cancer	RT + ipilimumab	Predictive of response to combination therapy	[66]
Gene expression profiling	FFPE tissue	High tumour mutational burden	HNSCC	Definitive CRT	↓ OS	[67]
	FFPE tissue	↑ IFN-γ signature	Bladder cancer	pCRT + surgery + CRT	↑ Disease-specific survival	[68]

CRT, chemoradiotherapy; RT, radiotherapy; HCC, hepatocellular carcinoma; pCRT, preoperative chemoradiotherapy; CRC, colorectal cancer; FFPE, formalin-fixed paraffin-embedded; HNSCC, head and neck squamous cell carcinoma; PD-L1, programmed death-ligand 1; OS, overall survival; PFS, progression-free survival; DFS, disease-free survival; ↑ increased; ↓ decreased.

3.1.1. PD-1/PD-L1 Expression

Engagement of PD-L1 with its receptor PD-1 results in the inactivation of T cells and NK cells, ultimately contributing to immune evasion [69]. Since Toplian and his colleagues first revealed that tumour PD-L1 expression reflects an immune-active microenvironment [70], several clinical trials have demonstrated that clinical responses to PD-1 blockade are correlated with PD-L1 expression in many cancer types [71–74].

The role of PD-L1 as a potential biomarker in patients treated with RT has emerged recently [64,75]. The PD-L1 expression after 12 Gy carbon-ion irradiation correlated with better progression-free survival in human uterine cervical adeno/adenosquamous carcinoma [64], while soluble PD-L1 was found to be correlated with worse survival in hepatocellular carcinoma [65]. Interestingly, both studies demonstrated that RT results in increased PD-L1 expression in vivo through interferon gamma production by T cells and that this appears to be an adaptive resistance pathway [10] that can be overcome by PD-L1-blockade [76]. Haematological malignancies such as Hodgkin lymphoma also show upregulation of PD-L1/PD-1 after chemotherapy/radiotherapy [77] and are known to be highly responsive to PD-1 blockade [78], and RT in combination with PD-1 blockade can induce abscopal responses [79]. The Pacific study showed that the addition of durvalumab (anti PD-L1) after consolidated chemoradiotherapy (CRT) enhanced both progression free survival (PFS) and overall survival (OS) of phase III unresectable non-small-cell lung carcinoma (NSCLC) patients; subgroup analysis showed that survival benefit was achieved in both PD-L1 positive and negative patients [76]. Long-term follow-up showed that the survival benefit of durvalumab was observed in subgroups with different PD-L1 levels, except patients with PD-L1 < 1% [80]. The findings from this study were disappointing regarding the potential utility of PD-L1 as a predictive biomarker, but since baseline PD-L1 level before CRT was not mandated and only measured where samples were available, it is currently unknown whether CRT changed the PD-L1 expression level and how it affected the results. Furthermore, durvalumab was given 2–42 days after CRT, which is a quite broad timespan; the optimal time for drug administration should be explored as well as how PD-L1 was affected by CRT dynamically.

In short, the level of PD-L1 within tumours has been suggested to be a promising prognostic biomarker in patients undergoing RT, but the role of PD-L1 as a predictive biomarker still needs further investigation. Ultimately, being able to clearly measure the number of cells expressing PD-L1 (reported as a percentage of stained cells) is critical. This issue is confounded by multiple unresolved problems: variable detection antibodies, differing IHC cut-off values, tissue preparation, processing variabilities, primary versus metastatic biopsies, oncogenic versus induced PD-L1 expression and staining of tumour versus immune cells [81,82]. The cut-off value constituting a positive or negative test result varies by both tumour type and by the antibody clone used to test the sample [83]. Moreover, there are several commercially available IHC assays to measure PD-L1 [83]. The measurement of PD-L1 requires standardization because the PD-L1 can be expressed on both lymphocytes and cancer cells, on both the cell membrane or in the cytoplasm. Recently, an IHC approach was approved by the US FDA as a companion diagnostic to make treatment recommendations for NSCLC patients using the anti-PD-1 agent pembrolizumab [83]. Three additional IHC assays have been approved as complementary diagnostics [84].

3.1.2. Immune Infiltrates

Immune infiltrates were proposed to be reflective of an adaptive anti-tumour response in the TME and may indicate a favourable response to RT. Data on the role of TILs in the context of RT are limited, with mixed findings. A retrospective single centre study examined pre-treatment specimens from 101 neck squamous cell carcinoma (HNSCC) patients before definitive CRT and reported that TILs are associated with favourable survival and are an independent prognostic factor to response to CRT [61]. However, the amount of CD8+ TIL infiltration alone is not always correlated with better clinical outcome. In patients with extrahepatic cholangiocarcinoma treated with adjuvant CRT, high expression of PD-1 on CD8+ TILs was strongly associated with inferior OS and the density of CD8+ TILs alone was not an independent prognostic factor for OS [63].

The presence of TILs can be measured by IHC, flow cytometry and droplet digital PCR technology. Moreover, there is an emerging novel technique of "immuno–positron emission tomography", which enables identification of CD8+ cells non-invasively and has been used in murine models of melanoma and breast cancer [85]. Whilst flow cytometry may enable quantification of a greater number of immune cells, issues around the requirement for fresh tumours mean that IHC of formalin-fixed tissue biopsies is currently the preferred method of choice for researchers.

3.1.3. Immunoscore

Given that the effect of TILs might be tumour-type-dependent, it is rational to develop combination analysis of different cell populations in immune infiltrates when exploring biomarkers for different cancers. For example, in a retrospective study of 166 CRC cancers with or without preoperative chemoradiation (pCRT), classification into one of five immunoscore groups significantly correlated with differences in disease free survival (DFS) and OS (all $p < 0.005$), with high infiltration of CD3+ and CD8+ lymphocytes in tumour biopsies associated with downstaging of the tumour after pCRT [62]. Currently, immune changes in the TME after CRT, including the value of immunoscore in response to chemoradiation, are mostly found in CRC patients [86]. This is possibly because the immunoscore was first validated and is most studied in CRC, perhaps due to the relatively easy opportunity to obtain biopsies to investigate the effects on the TME after RT and pCRT.

Another study took pre-treatment and post-treatment biopsies from 136 rectal cancer patients who underwent neoadjuvant RT, CT or CRT before radical resection and demonstrated that high levels of CD3+ and CD8+ TILs at baseline were correlated with better pathological responses (TRG $\geq$ 3) to neoadjuvant CRT and a favourable DFS and OS; in addition, CRT can enhance local immune response by increasing TIL infiltration [87]. One of the difficulties in the interpretation of this study is the diversity of treatment regimens used and the lack of matched immune blood markers to provide correlations with changes in TME. However, despite these caveats, changes in TILs after treatment were not associated with prognosis. Furthermore, Hagland et al. found a correlation between circulating T cells in pre-operative blood with intratumoural density and location of CD3+ and CD8+ T cells in colorectal cancer, suggestive of the potential for a liquid biopsy immunoscore [88]. However, this remains to be investigated for RT responses.

Brain metastases have also proven to be another good opportunity to study the effect of RT after whole brain radiotherapy (WBRT). Berghoff and colleagues investigated the influence of TIL and immunoscore on brain metastases [89]. Interestingly, despite the common preconception that the brain is an immune-privileged site, TIL infiltrates were detected in 115/116 (99.1%) brain metastasis biopsies. The density of CD3+, CD8+ and CD45RO+ TILs showed a significant correlation with favourable median OS. The immunoscore showed significant correlation with survival (27 vs. 10 mo; $p < 0.001$) and was established by multivariable analysis to be an independent prognostic factor (HR 0.612, $p < 0.001$). Interestingly, both the immunoscore and post-surgical WBRT showed an independent additive effect on OS. Considering that WBRT was delivered after surgery, the biopsy could not reflect the impact of RT on the TME; however, the immune infiltrates can serve as baseline data and may aid in patient selection for RT.

3.1.4. Gene Expression Profiling

Genetic mutation is one of the most significant hallmarks of cancer [2] and exists in metastatic settings across many cancer types, particularly frequently in cancers such as bladder cancer, melanoma, NSCLC, CRC and HNSCC [90]. Tumour mutational burden (TMB), which refers to the number of DNA mutations per megabase in a cancer cell, has previously been established as a prognostic biomarker and predictive factor of response to ICI across multiple tumour types [91,92]. The predictive value of gene expression profiling to evaluate the efficacy of RT currently remains unclear. A multicentre retrospective study from Germany developed a 327-gene panel to define TMB and then performed TMB analysis in 101 archival tumour samples from HNSCC patients treated with definitive CRT, aiming to assess the impact of TMB on prognosis. High TMB was demonstrated to be correlated with poor survival, which suggests that it may predict patients who might potentially benefit from CRT-ICI combinations [67]. Further research is needed to determine the value of TMB in response to RT alone.

Another retrospective study performed transcriptome-wide gene expression profiling of primary tumours from 136 muscle-invasive bladder cancer (MIBC) patients treated with bladder-sparing trimodality therapy (TMT) and compared to another cohort of 223 MIBC patients treated with neoadjuvant chemotherapy (NAC) and radical cystectomy (RC) in patients who had not received CRT. Results showed that signatures of T cell activation and IFN-γ signalling were associated with improved disease-specific survival (DSS) in the TMT cohort, but not in the NAC and RC cohort, whereas higher stromal infiltration was associated with shorter DSS after NAC and RC [68]. This suggests that gene expression profiling may be useful in developing predictive biomarkers to CRT but, given the limitations of this retrospective study, additional validation in larger prospective studies is required.

Currently, there is no uniform definition of a high TMB [93]. Standardization of the process of measuring TMB is required, including the method used, the ideal timing of TMB analysis (e.g., diagnostic biopsy or pre-treatment) and the ideal specimen (e.g., primary tumour versus metastasis). DNA next-generation sequencing approaches determining TMB include whole-exome sequencing (WES) and whole-genome sequencing (WGS). WES is considered to be the gold standard test as it generates a large amount of data and gives an overview of the gene mutation landscape; however, the fact that it is costly and requires more DNA may hinder its wider application. Targeted gene panels are unable to cover all the tumour mutations but offer reduced cost and requires less DNA, which enables easier integration into hospital labs.

3.1.5. Neoantigens

Neoantigens, as downstream products of TMB, are small peptide epitopes arising from tumour-specific mutations which are processed and presented on MHC molecules [94,95]. Unlike tumour-associated antigens (TAA) which are commonly shared by patients with the same tumour type, neoantigens are tumour-specific and are generally patient-specific. Recognition of neoantigens may be an important driver of the anti-immune responses to T cell targeting therapy including ICI [95–98]. One study demonstrated that clinical responses to ICIs mostly occur in patients with pre-existing neoantigen-specific T cells in tumours [99].

There is great interest in developing neoantigens as vaccines to induce immune responses [100]. Although it has been reported that neoantigens were generated in treatment with ICI alone [98] or combined with RT and may be a biomarker of response [66,79], there are some barriers even at the experimental stage. For example, approximately only 1% of all tumour mutations generate a neoantigen with sufficient affinity for MHC to prime T cell responses; therefore, determining how to define a high-quality neoantigen which can trigger robust immune responses still presents a significant challenge. With the development of bioinformatics tools, several findings have emerged. Łuksza and colleagues proposed a neoantigen fitness model based on two main factors: the likelihood of neoantigen presentation on MHC and subsequent recognition by T cells [101]. Another study found that T cells targeting clonal mutations expressed by all tumour cells (trunk mutations) can achieve better anti-tumour immune responses than T cells targeting mutations expressed only in a proportion of tumour cells (subclonal branch mutations) in patients receiving ICI [98]. More work is needed to determine if the number of neoantigens or the frequency of neoantigen-specific T cells may be biomarkers of response to RT with or without ICI.

3.2. Imaging Biomarkers

In addition to the above blood-based biomarkers or tissue-based biomarkers, in recent years, non-invasive and clinically useful image-based techniques such as SPE-CT, PET-CT and MRI have been developed to evaluate the immune response to radiotherapy and/or immunotherapy [102]. These advanced imaging techniques may address the dilemma of patients unsuitable for biopisies or with multiple disease sites. A retrospective, European, multicentre cohort study examined tissue samples collected at diagnosis from 208 classical Hodgkin's lymphoma patients treated with two ABVD (doxorubicin, bleomycin, vinblastine and dacarbazine) courses with fluorodeoxyglucose (FDG)-PET and analysed baseline staging and interim restaging. They found that early-interim FDG-PET scan after two ABVD chemotherapy courses (PET-2) was the only factor able to predict both progression-free survival and overall survival. In PET-2 negative patients, expression of CD68 (≥25%) and PD1 (diffuse or rosetting pattern) in microenvironmental cells, and STAT1 negativity in Hodgkin Reed Sternberg cells, identified a subset of PET-2 negative patients with a 3-year progression-free survival significantly lower than that of the remaining PET-2 negative population [103]. This revealed the combined role of biomarkers and interim PET scan in prediction of treatment outcome and provided a new insight into developing immune cancer biomarkers.

Despite its role in staging being increasingly recognized in lymphoma and non-small cell lung cancer [104], ^{18}-FDG–PET has several major drawbacks for use in immune imaging. This is a particular problem when it comes to the phenomenon of pseudoprogression, where the increased immune activity in response to successful therapy is difficult to distinguish from increased tumour metabolism in response to therapeutic failure [105]. Additionally, other limitations of PET imaging are that it is costly and exposes patients to radiation, and these have hindered its wider application in the clinic.

3.3. Biomarkers for RT and ICI Combination Therapies

Since the emergence of ICIs as delivering durable anti-tumour responses in a range of cancer types, albeit in the minority of patients treated, the number of clinical trials evaluating immunotherapy alone or combined with conventional oncology treatments such as RT or chemotherapy has greatly increased, with thousands of clinical trials in progress or being developed [106]. Whilst a detailed list of the clinical trials combining RT with immuno-oncology agents is beyond the scope of this review, the synergistic anti-tumour effects of RT and ICI has been investigated in many clinical studies and there are significant numbers of RT and ICI combination trials registered on clinicaltrials.gov [107].

One prospective trial investigated the efficacy of RT plus the anti-CTLA-4 ICI Ipilimumab in relapsed non-small-cell lung cancer. Twenty one of thirty nine enrolled patients completed the treatment protocol, with an overall objective response rate of 18%. Of the 20 evaluable patients, an increased serum IFN-β after RT and early dynamic changes in T cell clones appeared to be the strongest predictive biomarkers of response. Interestingly, T cells targeting a neoantigen controlled by a gene upregulated by RT were identified in one responding patient whose samples were analysed in more detail [66], but this "in-depth analysis" was only performed in one responding patient. Similarly, another study analysed three patients with refractory Hodgkin's lymphoma treated with a combination of radiation and nivolumab; results showed that all three patients achieved durable complete local and abscopal responses. Further analysis found high PD-L1 expression in all three patient tumours, a mutation in the STAT6 gene, amplification of a "neoantigen" Erb-B2 receptor tyrosine kinase 2 (ERBB2) along with DNA damage response in patient 2 and an intermediate tumour mutation burden (TMB) with 8.15 mutations per megabase in patient 3. This suggested that the expression of PD-L1, DNA damage response and TMB might be potential biomarkers of response [79]. Due to the limitation of a small sample size and the retrospective nature of the study, these findings require validation in larger patient groups.

4. Conclusions and Future Directions

Tumours have been broadly divided into immunologically "hot", characterised by high numbers of tumour-infiltrating T cells, and "cold", characterised by low numbers of T cells [108]. What is currently less well characterised is how RT interacts with such "hot" or "cold" tumours to induce immune changes in human tumours. RT may well be immunostimulatory and potentially further enhance "hot" tumours and increase the number and diversity of T cell clones or potentially convert a "cold' tumour to a "hot" tumour with an increase in T cell infiltration. In contrast, RT could be immunosuppressive and convert a "hot" tumour to a "cold" tumour or make the tumour microenvironment of an already "cold" tumour even more immunosuppressive by inducing the cytokines that lead to infiltration of immunosuppressive immune effector cells. An enhanced understanding of how RT affects the TME in "real time" as the patient is receiving RT will be extremely informative but requires a huge effort for serial tumour biopsies with the development of dynamic tumour biomarkers. Only when such data are available can we realistically begin to potentially implement different strategies to potentially enhance or modulate the RT-induced immune response and move towards a more personalized treatment approach for patients.

Currently, preclinical data are emerging which suggest that such a strategy of selecting an IO agent to combine with RT to improve outcomes may be possible at least for the "hot" tumours. In some murine tumours, anti-PD1 (ICI) combined with RT may lead to the generation of systemic immunity and long-term tumour control [10,22]. In contrast, for "cold" tumours, which are normally poorly infiltrated by T cells and contain increased numbers of immunosuppressive myeloid cells, anti-PD1 and RT may be less effective. Therefore, combining RT with IO or immune-stimulatory agents which act to reprogramme myeloid cells and drive increased T cell infiltration into tumours (e.g., TLR agonists, anti-CD40 mAb, anti-OX40 mAb) may be required to overcome this immunosuppressive TME and improve tumour control and survival [109,110].

However, to date, there are still many unanswered questions and future work in both the preclinical and clinical settings is required to establish the optimal RT regimen and any potential biomarkers which may inform IO agent choice when trying to further enhance the synergy of RT in combination with different immunotherapy modalities. Firstly, current data on immune infiltrates and tumour cell PD-L1 expression come from pre-treatment biopsies or surgery specimens, which mainly reflect the immune status at baseline, and there is limited information on changes in TME during or post-treatment. Additionally, few data exist on systemic immune biomarkers post-RT [57–59,111]. Therefore, there is an urgent unmet clinical need to collect tumour samples and matching bloods pre- and post-RT from patients undergoing routine RT to further understand the potentially diverse impact of RT between patients and tumour types.

Whilst changes in the TME are likely to be most reflective of immune changes induced by RT, investigations in peripheral blood may provide additional information to enable biomarker detection and surveillance during and after RT with less invasive sampling.

In addition, to identify whether a human tumour is immunologically "hot" or "cold", there are now many technologies available to analyse immunological markers in tumour and blood. IHC is often used to identify tumour immune contexture by analysing FFPE samples and platforms now exist to multiplex up to 40 different cell markers. RNA gene expression arrays can be used to profile changes in immune genes in greater depth and possible immune gene signatures may arise as potential biomarkers [112,113]. Systemic immune changes can be monitored by profiling of PBMC populations through flow cytometry or mass spectrometry, TCR sequencing to investigate T cell clonality and analysis of serum cytokines and chemokines though multiplex bead-based assays or ELISAs. A thorough investigation of RT-induced changes in the immune TME and in the systemic circulation is the first step to identifying potential biomarkers of immune responses post-RT and determining if these biomarkers are predictive, prognostic or dynamic.

There is still much work to be done to enhance our understanding in the development of biomarkers for RT and RT + immunotherapy combinations in the clinic. Although there are currently thousands of clinical trials evaluating IO agents alone or combined with conventional oncology treatments such as RT or chemotherapy [58], only the minority have translational immunological research that may provide mechanistic insights and help the development of immunological biomarkers. For RT and RT in combination with IO agents, this field is still in its infancy and requires the coordinated efforts of the pioneers to incorporate biomarker-driven research into their design. Only with this focus on translational research will progress be made and provide us with the possibility that tumours may be stratified for treatment according to immune biomarkers identified in the TME and/or the peripheral blood that will predict immune responses post-RT and may inform RT/IO combinations.

Author Contributions: All authors equally contributed to this review. All authors have read and agreed to the published version of the manuscript.

References

1. Herrera, F.G.; Bourhis, J.; Coukos, G. Radiotherapy combination opportunities leveraging immunity for the next oncology practice. *CA A Cancer J. Clin.* **2016**, *67*, 65–85. [CrossRef]
2. Hanahan, D.; Weinberg, R.A. Hallmarks of Cancer: The Next Generation. *Cell* **2011**, *144*, 646–674. [CrossRef] [PubMed]
3. Mantovani, A.; Ponzetta, A.; Inforzato, A.; Jaillon, S. Innate immunity, inflammation and tumour progression: Double-edged swords. *J. Intern. Med.* **2019**, *285*, 524–532. [CrossRef] [PubMed]
4. Pagès, F.; Kirilovsky, A.; Mlecnik, B.; Asslaber, M.; Tosolini, M.; Bindea, G.; Lagorce, C.; Wind, P.; Marliot, F.; Bruneval, P.; et al. In Situ Cytotoxic and Memory T Cells Predict Outcome in Patients With Early-Stage Colorectal Cancer. *J. Clin. Oncol.* **2009**, *27*, 5944–5951. [CrossRef]
5. Galon, J.; Pagès, F.; Marincola, F.M.; Angell, H.K.; Thurin, M.; Lugli, A.; Zlobec, I.; Berger, A.; Bifulco, C.B.; Botti, G.; et al. Cancer classification using the Immunoscore: A worldwide task force. *J. Transl. Med.* **2012**, *10*, 205. [CrossRef] [PubMed]
6. Chaudhary, B.; Elkord, E. Regulatory T Cells in the Tumor Microenvironment and Cancer Progression: Role and Therapeutic Targeting. *Vaccines* **2016**, *4*, 28. [CrossRef] [PubMed]
7. Lindau, D.; Gielen, P.; Kroesen, M.; Wesseling, P.; Adema, G.J. The immunosuppressive tumour network: Myeloid-derived suppressor cells, regulatory T cells and natural killer T cells. *Immunol.* **2013**, *138*, 105–115. [CrossRef]
8. Kim, W.; Lee, S.; Seo, D.; Kim, D.; Kim, K.; Kim, E.; Kang, J.; Seong, K.M.; Youn, H.; Youn, B. Cellular Stress Responses in Radiotherapy. *Cells* **2019**, *8*, 1105. [CrossRef]
9. Mole, R.H. Whole Body Irradiation—Radiobiology or Medicine? *Br. J. Radiol.* **1953**, *26*, 234–241. [CrossRef]
10. Dovedi, S.J.; Adlard, A.; Lipowska-Bhalla, G.; McKenna, C.; Jones, S.; Cheadle, E.J.; Stratford, I.J.; Poon, E.; Morrow, M.; Stewart, R.; et al. Acquired Resistance to Fractionated Radiotherapy Can Be Overcome by Concurrent PD-L1 Blockade. *Cancer Res.* **2014**, *74*, 5458–5468. [CrossRef]
11. Sharabi, A.B.; Nirschl, C.J.; Kochel, C.M.; Nirschl, T.R.; Francica, B.J.; Velarde, E.; Deweese, T.L.; Drake, C.G.; Francisca, B.J. Stereotactic Radiation Therapy Augments Antigen-Specific PD-1-Mediated Antitumor Immune Responses via Cross-Presentation of Tumor Antigen. *Cancer Immunol. Res.* **2014**, *3*, 345–355. [CrossRef] [PubMed]
12. Victor, C.T.-S.; Rech, A.J.; Maity, A.; Rengan, R.; Pauken, K.E.; Stelekati, E.; Benci, J.L.; Xu, B.; Dada, H.; Odorizzi, P.M.; et al. Radiation and dual checkpoint blockade activate non-redundant immune mechanisms in cancer. *Nature* **2015**, *520*, 373–377. [CrossRef] [PubMed]
13. Formenti, S.C.; DeMaria, S. Systemic effects of local radiotherapy. *Lancet Oncol.* **2009**, *10*, 718–726. [CrossRef]
14. Nesslinger, N.J.; Sahota, R.A.; Stone, B.; Johnson, K.; Chima, N.; King, C.; Rasmussen, D.; Bishop, D.; Rennie, P.S.; Gleave, M.; et al. Standard Treatments Induce Antigen-Specific Immune Responses in Prostate Cancer. *Clin. Cancer Res.* **2007**, *13*, 1493–1502. [CrossRef]
15. Schaue, D.; Comin-Anduix, B.; Ribas, A.; Zhang, L.; Goodglick, L.; Sayre, J.W.; Debucquoy, A.; Haustermans, K.; McBride, W.H. T-cell responses to survivin in cancer patients undergoing radiation therapy. *Clin. Cancer Res.* **2008**, *14*, 4883–4890. [CrossRef]
16. Reynders, K.; Illidge, T.; Siva, S.; Chang, J.Y.; De Ruysscher, D. The abscopal effect of local radiotherapy: Using immunotherapy to make a rare event clinically relevant. *Cancer Treat. Rev.* **2015**, *41*, 503–510. [CrossRef]
17. Postow, M.A.; Callahan, M.K.; Barker, C.A.; Yamada, Y.; Yuan, J.; Kitano, S.; Mu, Z.; Rasalan, T.; Adamow, M.; Ritter, E.; et al. Immunologic Correlates of the Abscopal Effect in a Patient with Melanoma. *N. Engl. J. Med.* **2012**, *366*, 925–931. [CrossRef]
18. Reits, E.A.; Hodge, J.W.; Herberts, C.A.; Groothuis, T.A.; Chakraborty, M.; K.Wansley, E.; Camphausen, K.; Luiten, R.M.; De Ru, A.H.; Neijssen, J.; et al. Radiation modulates the peptide repertoire, enhances MHC class I expression, and induces successful antitumor immunotherapy. *J. Exp. Med.* **2006**, *203*, 1259–1271. [CrossRef]

19. Obeid, M.; Tesniere, A.; Ghiringhelli, F.; Fimia, G.M.; Apetoh, L.; Perfettini, J.-L.; Castedo, M.; Mignot, G.; Panaretakis, T.; Casares, N.; et al. Calreticulin exposure dictates the immunogenicity of cancer cell death. *Nat. Med.* **2006**, *13*, 54–61. [CrossRef]
20. Kroemer, G.; Galluzzi, L.; Kepp, O.; Zitvogel, L. Immunogenic Cell Death in Cancer Therapy. *Annu. Rev. Immunol.* **2013**, *31*, 51–72. [CrossRef]
21. Honeychurch, J.; Illidge, T.M. The influence of radiation in the context of developing combination immunotherapies in cancer. *Ther. Adv. Vaccines Immunother.* **2018**, *5*, 115–122. [CrossRef] [PubMed]
22. Dovedi, S.J.; Cheadle, E.J.; Popple, A.; Poon, E.; Morrow, M.; Stewart, R.; Yusko, E.C.; Sanders, C.M.; Vignali, M.; Emerson, R.O.; et al. Fractionated Radiation Therapy Stimulates Antitumor Immunity Mediated by Both Resident and Infiltrating Polyclonal T-cell Populations when Combined with PD-1 Blockade. *Clin. Cancer Res.* **2017**, *23*, 5514–5526. [CrossRef] [PubMed]
23. Gasser, S.; Orsulic, S.; Brown, E.J.; Raulet, D.H. The DNA damage pathway regulates innate immune system ligands of the NKG2D receptor. *Nature* **2005**, *436*, 1186–1190. [CrossRef] [PubMed]
24. Durante, M.; Formenti, S.C. Radiation-Induced Chromosomal Aberrations and Immunotherapy: Micronuclei, Cytosolic DNA, and Interferon-Production Pathway. *Front. Oncol.* **2018**, *8*, 192. [CrossRef] [PubMed]
25. Klug, F.; Prakash, H.; Huber, P.E.; Seibel, T.; Bender, N.; Halama, N.; Pfirschke, C.; Voss, R.H.; Timke, C.; Umansky, L.; et al. Low-Dose Irradiation Programs Macrophage Differentiation to an iNOS+/M1 Phenotype that Orchestrates Effective T Cell Immunotherapy. *Cancer Cell* **2013**, *24*, 589–602. [CrossRef] [PubMed]
26. Barker, H.E.; Paget, J.T.E.; Khan, A.A.; Harrington, K.J. The tumour microenvironment after radiotherapy: Mechanisms of resistance and recurrence. *Nat. Rev. Cancer* **2015**, *15*, 409–425. [CrossRef]
27. Vanpouille-Box, C.; Diamond, J.M.; Pilones, K.A.; Zavadil, J.; Babb, J.S.; Formenti, S.C.; Barcellos-Hoff, M.H.; DeMaria, S. TGFβ Is a Master Regulator of Radiation Therapy-Induced Antitumor Immunity. *Cancer Res.* **2015**, *75*, 2232–2242. [CrossRef]
28. Yan, Y.; Chen, X.; Wang, X.; Zhao, Z.; Hu, W.; Zeng, S.; Wei, J.; Yang, X.; Qian, L.; Zhou, S.; et al. The effects and the mechanisms of autophagy on the cancer-associated fibroblasts in cancer. *J. Exp. Clin. Cancer Res.* **2019**, *38*, 171. [CrossRef]
29. Wang, Z.; Tang, Y.; Tan, Y.; Wei, Q.; Yu, W. Cancer-associated fibroblasts in radiotherapy: Challenges and new opportunities. *Cell Commun. Signal.* **2019**, *17*, 47. [CrossRef]
30. Augsten, M. Cancer-Associated Fibroblasts as Another Polarized Cell Type of the Tumor Microenvironment. *Front. Oncol.* **2014**, *4*, 62. [CrossRef]
31. Kioi, M.; Vogel, H.; Schultz, G.; Hoffman, R.M.; Harsh, G.R.; Brown, J.M. Inhibition of vasculogenesis, but not angiogenesis, prevents the recurrence of glioblastoma after irradiation in mice. *J. Clin. Investig.* **2010**, *120*, 694–705. [CrossRef]
32. Jäättelä, M. Multiple cell death pathways as regulators of tumour initiation and progression. *Oncogene* **2004**, *23*, 2746–2756. [CrossRef]
33. Long, J.S.; Ryan, K.M. New frontiers in promoting tumour cell death: Targeting apoptosis, necroptosis and autophagy. *Oncogene* **2012**, *31*, 5045–5060. [CrossRef]
34. Arrillaga-Romany, I.; Monje, M.; Wen, P.Y. Chapter 15—Neurologic Complications of Oncologic Therapy. In *Handbook of Neuro-Oncology Neuroimaging*, 2nd ed.; Newton, H.B., Ed.; Academic Press: San Diego, CA, USA, 2016; pp. 125–142.
35. Omay, S.B.; Atsina, K.K.; Baehring, J.M. Chapter 53—Nonneoplastic Mass Lesions of the Central Nervous System. In *Handbook of Neuro-Oncology Neuroimaging*, 2nd ed.; Newton, H.B., Ed.; Academic Press: San Diego, CA, USA, 2016; pp. 653–665.
36. Klionsky, D.J. Autophagy: From phenomenology to molecular understanding in less than a decade. *Nat. Rev. Mol. Cell Biol.* **2007**, *8*, 931–937. [CrossRef] [PubMed]
37. Levy, J.M.M.; Towers, C.G.; Thorburn, A. Targeting autophagy in cancer. *Nat. Rev. Cancer* **2017**, *17*, 528–542. [CrossRef] [PubMed]
38. Cirone, M.; Montani, M.S.G.; Granato, M.; Garufi, A.; Faggioni, A.; D'Orazi, G. Autophagy manipulation as a strategy for efficient anticancer therapies: Possible consequences. *J. Exp. Clin. Cancer Res.* **2019**, *38*, 262. [CrossRef] [PubMed]

39. Ko, A.; Kanehisa, A.; Martins, I.; Senovilla, L.; Chargari, C.; Dugue, D.; Mariño, G.; Kepp, O.; Michaud, M.; Perfettini, J.-L.; et al. Autophagy inhibition radiosensitizes in vitro, yet reduces radioresponses in vivo due to deficient immunogenic signalling. *Cell Death Differ.* **2013**, *21*, 92–99. [CrossRef] [PubMed]
40. Valkenburg, K.C.; De Groot, A.E.; Pienta, K.J. Targeting the tumour stroma to improve cancer therapy. *Nat. Rev. Clin. Oncol.* **2018**, *15*, 366–381. [CrossRef] [PubMed]
41. Chude, C.I.; Amaravadi, R.K. Targeting Autophagy in Cancer: Update on Clinical Trials and Novel Inhibitors. *Int. J. Mol. Sci.* **2017**, *18*, 1279. [CrossRef]
42. Rosenfeld, M.R.; Ye, X.; Supko, J.G.; Desideri, S.; Grossman, S.A.; Brem, S.; Mikkelson, T.; Wang, D.; Chang, Y.C.; Hu, J.; et al. A phase I/II trial of hydroxychloroquine in conjunction with radiation therapy and concurrent and adjuvant temozolomide in patients with newly diagnosed glioblastoma multiforme. *Autophagy* **2014**, *10*, 1359–1368. [CrossRef]
43. Rojas-Puentes, L.L.; González-Pinedo, M.; Crismatt, A.; Gómez, A.O.; Gamboa-Vignolle, C.; Núñez-Gómez, R.; Dorantes-Gallareta, Y.; Arce-Salinas, C.; Arrieta, O. Phase II randomized, double-blind, placebo-controlled study of whole-brain irradiation with concomitant chloroquine for brain metastases. *Radiat. Oncol.* **2013**, *8*, 209. [CrossRef] [PubMed]
44. Rubinsztein, D.C.; Codogno, P.; Levine, B. Autophagy modulation as a potential therapeutic target for diverse diseases. *Nat. Rev. Drug Discov.* **2012**, *11*, 709–730. [CrossRef] [PubMed]
45. Su, Z.; Yang, Z.; Xie, L.; DeWitt, J.P.; Chen, Y. Cancer therapy in the necroptosis era. *Cell Death Differ.* **2016**, *23*, 748–756. [CrossRef] [PubMed]
46. Royce, G.H.; Brown-Borg, H.M.; Deepa, S.S. The potential role of necroptosis in inflammaging and aging. *GeroScience* **2019**, *41*, 795–811. [CrossRef] [PubMed]
47. Wang, Y.; Zhao, M.; He, S.; Luo, Y.; Zhao, Y.; Cheng, J.; Gong, Y.; Xie, J.; Wang, Y.; Hu, B.; et al. Necroptosis regulates tumor repopulation after radiotherapy via RIP1/RIP3/MLKL/JNK/IL8 pathway. *J. Exp. Clin. Cancer Res.* **2019**, *38*, 1–16. [CrossRef]
48. Angeli, J.P.F.; Krysko, D.V.; Conrad, M. Ferroptosis at the crossroads of cancer-acquired drug resistance and immune evasion. *Nat. Rev. Cancer* **2019**, *19*, 405–414. [CrossRef]
49. Lang, X.; Green, M.D.; Wang, W.; Yu, J.; Choi, J.E.; Jiang, L.; Liao, P.; Zhou, J.; Zhang, Q.; Dow, A.; et al. Radiotherapy and Immunotherapy Promote Tumoral Lipid Oxidation and Ferroptosis via Synergistic Repression of SLC7A11. *Cancer Discov.* **2019**, *9*, 1673–1685. [CrossRef]
50. Lei, G.; Zhang, Y.; Koppula, P.; Liu, X.; Zhang, J.; Lin, S.H.; Ajani, J.A.; Xiao, Q.; Liao, Z.; Wang, H.; et al. The role of ferroptosis in ionizing radiation-induced cell death and tumor suppression. *Cell Res.* **2020**, *30*, 146–162. [CrossRef]
51. Gutman, S.; Kessler, L.G. The US Food and Drug Administration perspective on cancer biomarker development. *Nat. Rev. Cancer* **2006**, *6*, 565–571. [CrossRef]
52. Lesterhuis, W.J.; Bosco, A.; Millward, M.J.; Small, M.; Nowak, A.K.; Lake, R.A. Dynamic versus static biomarkers in cancer immune checkpoint blockade: Unravelling complexity. *Nat. Rev. Drug Discov.* **2017**, *16*, 264–272. [CrossRef]
53. Fane, M.; Weeraratna, A.T. How the ageing microenvironment influences tumour progression. *Nat. Rev. Cancer* **2019**, *20*, 89–106. [CrossRef] [PubMed]
54. Wang, J.; Sun, H.; Zeng, Q.; Guo, X.-J.; Wang, H.; Liu, H.-H.; Dong, Z.-Y. HPV-positive status associated with inflamed immune microenvironment and improved response to anti-PD-1 therapy in head and neck squamous cell carcinoma. *Sci. Rep.* **2019**, *9*, 13404. [CrossRef] [PubMed]
55. Stewart, G.D.; Ross, J.A.; McLaren, D.; Parker, C.C.; Habib, F.K.; Riddick, A.C. The relevance of a hypoxic tumour microenvironment in prostate cancer. *BJU Int.* **2010**, *105*, 8–13. [CrossRef]
56. Rothenberger, N.J.; Somasundaram, A.; Stabile, L.P. The Role of the Estrogen Pathway in the Tumor Microenvironment. *Int. J. Mol. Sci.* **2018**, *19*, 611. [CrossRef]
57. Onal, C.; Yildirim, B.A.; Guler, O.C.; Mertsoylu, H. The Utility of Pretreatment and Posttreatment Lymphopenia in Cervical Squamous Cell Carcinoma Patients Treated with Definitive Chemoradiotherapy. *Int. J. Gynecol. Cancer* **2018** *28*, 1553–1559. [CrossRef] [PubMed]
58. Wang, N.; An, G.; Xie, S.; Yao, Y.; Feng, G. The clinical and prognostic significance of CD14+HLA-DR−/low myeloid-derived suppressor cells in hepatocellular carcinoma patients receiving radiotherapy. *Tumor Biol.* **2016**, *37*, 10427–10433. [CrossRef]

59. Napolitano, M.; D'Alterio, C.; Cardone, E.; Trotta, A.; Pecori, B.; Rega, D.; Pace, U.; Scala, D.; Scognamiglio, G.; Tatangelo, F.; et al. Peripheral myeloid-derived suppressor and T regulatory PD-1 positive cells predict response to neoadjuvant short-course radiotherapy in rectal cancer patients. *Oncotarget* **2015**, *6*, 8261–8270. [CrossRef]
60. Willett, C.G.; Duda, D.G.; Di Tomaso, E.; Boucher, Y.; Ancukiewicz, M.; Sahani, D.V.; Lahdenranta, J.; Chung, D.C.; Fischman, A.J.; Lauwers, G.Y.; et al. Efficacy, Safety, and Biomarkers of Neoadjuvant Bevacizumab, Radiation Therapy, and Fluorouracil in Rectal Cancer: A Multidisciplinary Phase II Study. *J. Clin. Oncol.* **2009**, *27*, 3020–3026. [CrossRef]
61. Balermpas, P.; Michel, Y.; Wagenblast, J.; Seitz, O.; Weiss, C.; Rödel, F.; Rödel, C.; Fokas, E. Tumour-infiltrating lymphocytes predict response to definitive chemoradiotherapy in head and neck cancer. *Br. J. Cancer* **2013**, *110*, 501–509. [CrossRef]
62. Anitei, M.-G.; Zeitoun, G.; Mlecnik, B.; Marliot, F.; Haicheur, N.; Todosi, A.M.; Kirilovsky, A.; Lagorce, C.; Bindea, G.; Ferariu, D.; et al. Prognostic and Predictive Values of the Immunoscore in Patients with Rectal Cancer. *Clin. Cancer Res.* **2014**, *20*, 1891–1899. [CrossRef]
63. Lim, Y.J.; Koh, J.; Kim, K.; Chie, E.K.; Kim, B.; Lee, K.; Jang, J.-Y.; Kim, S.-W.; Oh, -Y.; Bang, Y.-J.; et al. High ratio of programmed cell death protein 1 (PD-1)+/CD8+ tumor-infiltrating lymphocytes identifies a poor prognostic subset of extrahepatic bile duct cancer undergoing surgery plus adjuvant chemoradiotherapy. *Radiother. Oncol.* **2015**, *117*, 165–170. [CrossRef] [PubMed]
64. Iijima, M.; Okonogi, N.; Nakajima, N.I.; Morokoshi, Y.; Kanda, H.; Yamada, T.; Kobayashi, Y.; Banno, K.; Wakatsuki, M.; Yamada, S.; et al. Significance of PD-L1 expression in carbon-ion radiotherapy for uterine cervical adeno/adenosquamous carcinoma. *J. Gynecol. Oncol.* **2020**, *31*, 19. [CrossRef] [PubMed]
65. Kim, H.J.; Park, S.; Kim, K.-J.; Seong, J. Clinical significance of soluble programmed cell death ligand-1 (sPD-L1) in hepatocellular carcinoma patients treated with radiotherapy. *Radiother. Oncol.* **2018**, *129*, 130–135. [CrossRef] [PubMed]
66. Formenti, S.C.; Rudqvist, N.-P.; Golden, E.; Cooper, B.T.; Wennerberg, E.; Lhuillier, C.; Vanpouille-Box, C.; Friedman, K.; De Andrade, L.F.; Wucherpfennig, K.W.; et al. Radiotherapy induces responses of lung cancer to CTLA-4 blockade. *Nat. Med.* **2018**, *24*, 1845–1851. [CrossRef]
67. Eder, T.; Hess, A.; Konschak, R.; Stromberger, C.; Jöhrens, K.; Fleischer, V.; Hummel, M.; Balermpas, P.; Von Der Grün, J.; Linge, A.; et al. Interference of tumour mutational burden with outcome of patients with head and neck cancer treated with definitive chemoradiation: A multicentre retrospective study of the German Cancer Consortium Radiation Oncology Group. *Eur. J. Cancer* **2019**, *116*, 67–76. [CrossRef]
68. Efstathiou, J.A.; Mouw, K.W.; Gibb, E.A.; Liu, Y.; Wu, C.-L.; Drumm, M.R.; Da Costa, J.B.; Du Plessis, M.; Wang, N.Q.; Davicioni, E.; et al. Impact of Immune and Stromal Infiltration on Outcomes Following Bladder-Sparing Trimodality Therapy for Muscle-Invasive Bladder Cancer. *Eur. Urol.* **2019**, *76*, 59–68. [CrossRef]
69. Pardoll, D.M. The blockade of immune checkpoints in cancer immunotherapy. *Nat. Rev. Cancer* **2012**, *12*, 252–264. [CrossRef]
70. Topalian, S.L.; Hodi, F.S.; Brahmer, J.R.; Gettinger, S.N.; Smith, D.C.; McDermott, D.F.; Powderly, J.D.; Carvajal, R.D.; Sosman, J.A.; Atkins, M.B.; et al. Safety, Activity, and Immune Correlates of Anti–PD-1 Antibody in Cancer. *N. Engl. J. Med.* **2012**, *366*, 2443–2454. [CrossRef]
71. Robert, C.; Long, G.; Brady, B.; Dutriaux, C.; Maio, M.; Mortier, L.; Hassel, J.C.; Rutkowski, P.; McNeil, C.; Kalinka-Warzocha, E.; et al. Nivolumab in Previously Untreated Melanoma without BRAF Mutation. *N. Engl. J. Med.* **2015**, *372*, 320–330. [CrossRef]
72. Larkin, J.; Hodi, F.S.; Wolchok, J.D.; E Valsecchi, M. Combined Nivolumab and Ipilimumab or Monotherapy in Untreated Melanoma. *N. Engl. J. Med.* **2015**, *373*, 23–34. [CrossRef]
73. Do, H.B.; Paz-Ares, L.; Horn, L.; Spigel, D.R.; Steins, M.; Ready, N.E.; Chow, L.Q.; Vokes, E.E.; Felip, E.; Holgado, E.; et al. Nivolumab versus Docetaxel in Advanced Nonsquamous Non-Small-Cell Lung Cancer. *N. Engl. J. Med.* **2015**, *373*, 1627–1639. [CrossRef]
74. Taube, J.M.; Klein, A.; Brahmer, J.R.; Xu, H.; Pan, X.; Kim, J.H.; Chen, L.; Pardoll, E.M.; Topalian, S.L.; Anders, R.A. Association of PD-1, PD-1 ligands, and other features of the tumor immune microenvironment with response to anti-PD-1 therapy. *Clin. Cancer Res.* **2014**, *20*, 5064–5074. [CrossRef] [PubMed]

75. Lee, V.H.F.; Lo, A.W.; Leung, C.-Y.; Shek, W.-H.; Kwong, R.L.W.; Lam, K.-O.; Tong, C.-C.; Sze, C.-K.; Leung, T.-W. Correlation of PD-L1 Expression of Tumor Cells with Survival Outcomes after Radical Intensity-Modulated Radiation Therapy for Non-Metastatic Nasopharyngeal Carcinoma. *PLoS ONE* **2016**, *11*, e0157969. [CrossRef] [PubMed]
76. Antonia, S.J.; Villegas, A.; Daniel, D.; Vicente, D.; Murakami, S.; Hui, R.; Yokoi, T.; Chiappori, A.; Lee, K.H.; de Wit, M.; et al. Durvalumab after Chemoradiotherapy in Stage III Non-Small-Cell Lung Cancer. *N. Engl. J. Med.* **2017**, *377*, 1919–1929. [CrossRef]
77. Hollander, P.; Amini, R.-M.; Ginman, B.; Molin, D.; Enblad, G.; Glimelius, I. Expression of PD-1 and PD-L1 increase in consecutive biopsies in patients with classical Hodgkin lymphoma. *PLoS ONE* **2018**, *13*, e0204870. [CrossRef]
78. De Re, V.; Caggiari, L.; Repetto, O.; Mussolin, L.; Mascarin, M.; Re, D. Classical Hodgkin's Lymphoma in the Era of Immune Checkpoint Inhibition. *J. Clin. Med.* **2019**, *8*, 1596. [CrossRef]
79. Qin, Q.; Nan, X.; Miller, T.; Fisher, R.; Teh, B.; Pandita, S.; Farach, A.M.; Pingali, S.R.; Pandita, R.K.; Butler, E.B.; et al. Complete Local and Abscopal Responses from a Combination of Radiation and Nivolumab in Refractory Hodgkin's Lymphoma. *Radiat. Res.* **2018**, *190*, 322–329. [CrossRef]
80. Antonia, S.J.; Villegas, A.; Daniel, D.; Vicente, D.; Murakami, S.; Hui, R.; Kurata, T.; Chiappori, A.; Lee, K.H.; De Wit, M.; et al. Overall Survival with Durvalumab after Chemoradiotherapy in Stage III NSCLC. *N. Engl. J. Med.* **2018**, *379*, 2342–2350. [CrossRef]
81. Popple, A.; Illidge, T. Harmonization of programmed cell death ligand-1 diagnostic assays in non-small cell lung cancer. *Transl. Cancer Res.* **2017**, *6*, S553–S556. [CrossRef]
82. Patel, S.P.; Kurzrock, R. PD-L1 Expression as a Predictive Biomarker in Cancer Immunotherapy. *Mol. Cancer Ther.* **2015**, *14*, 847–856. [CrossRef]
83. Rimm, D.L.; Han, G.; Taube, J.M.; Yi, E.S.; Bridge, J.A.; Flieder, U.B.; Homer, R.; West, W.W.; Wu, H.; Roden, A.C.; et al. A Prospective, Multi-institutional, Pathologist-Based Assessment of 4 Immunohistochemistry Assays for PD-L1 Expression in Non-Small Cell Lung Cancer. *JAMA Oncol.* **2017**, *3*, 1051–1058. [CrossRef] [PubMed]
84. FDA Nods for Atezolizumab and Nivolumab. *Cancer Discov.* **2016**, *6*, 811. [CrossRef] [PubMed]
85. Rashidian, M.; Ingram, J.R.; Dougan, M.; Dongre, A.; Whang, K.A.; Le Gall, C.; Cragnolini, J.J.; Bierie, B.; Gostissa, M.; Gorman, J.; et al. Predicting the response to CTLA-4 blockade by longitudinal noninvasive monitoring of CD8 T cells. *J. Exp. Med.* **2017**, *214*, 2243–2255. [CrossRef] [PubMed]
86. Huang, A.; Xiao, Y.; Peng, C.; Liu, T.; Lin, Z.; Yang, Q.; Zhang, T.; Liu, J.; Ma, H. 53BP1 expression and immunoscore are associated with the efficacy of neoadjuvant chemoradiotherapy for rectal cancer. *Strahlenther. Onkol.* **2019**, *196*, 465–473. [CrossRef]
87. Teng, F.; Mu, D.; Meng, X.; Kong, L.; Zhu, H.; Liu, S.; Zhang, J.; Yu, J. Tumor infiltrating lymphocytes (TILs) before and after neoadjuvant chemoradiotherapy and its clinical utility for rectal cancer. *Am. J. Cancer Res.* **2015**, *5*, 2064–2074.
88. Hagland, H.; Lea, D.; Watson, M.; Søreide, K. Correlation of circulating T-cells in pre-operative blood to intratumoral density and location of CD3+ and CD8+ T-cells in colorectal cancer: A potential for an immunoscore by liquid biopsy? *Eur. J. Cancer* **2017**, *72*, S49–S50. [CrossRef]
89. Berghoff, A.S.; Fuchs, E.; Ricken, G.; Mlecnik, B.; Bindea, G.; Spanberger, T.; Hackl, M.; Widhalm, G.; Dieckmann, K.; Prayer, D.; et al. Density of tumor-infiltrating lymphocytes correlates with extent of brain edema and overall survival time in patients with brain metastases. *OncoImmunology* **2015**, *5*, e1057388. [CrossRef]
90. Zehir, A.; Benayed, R.; Shah, R.; Syed, A.; Middha, S.; Kim, H.R.; Srinivasan, P.; Gao, J.; Chakravarty, D.; Devlin, S.M.; et al. Mutational landscape of metastatic cancer revealed from prospective clinical sequencing of 10,000 patients. *Nat. Med.* **2017**, *23*, 703–713. [CrossRef]
91. Snyder, A.; Makarov, V.; Merghoub, T.; Yuan, J.; Zaretsky, J.M.; Desrichard, A.; Walsh, L.A.; Postow, M.A.; Wong, P.; Ho, T.S.; et al. Genetic Basis for Clinical Response to CTLA-4 Blockade in Melanoma. *N. Engl. J. Med.* **2014**, *371*, 2189–2199. [CrossRef]

92. Rizvi, N.A.; Hellmann, M.D.; Snyder, A.; Kvistborg, P.; Makarov, V.; Havel, J.J.; Lee, W.; Yuan, J.; Wong, P.; Ho, T.S.; et al. Mutational landscape determines sensitivity to PD-1 blockade in non–small cell lung cancer. *Science* **2015**, *348*, 124–128. [CrossRef]
93. Samstein, R.M.; Lee, C.-H.; Shoushtari, A.; Hellmann, M.D.; Shen, R.; Janjigian, Y.Y.; Barron, D.A.; Zehir, A.; Jordan, E.J.; Omuro, A.; et al. Tumor mutational load predicts survival after immunotherapy across multiple cancer types. *Nat. Genet.* **2019**, *51*, 202–206. [CrossRef] [PubMed]
94. Efremova, M.; Finotello, F.; Rieder, D.; Trajanoski, Z. Neoantigens Generated by Individual Mutations and Their Role in Cancer Immunity and Immunotherapy. *Front. Immunol.* **2017**, *8*, 1679. [CrossRef] [PubMed]
95. Schumacher, T.N.; Scheper, W.; Kvistborg, P. Cancer Neoantigens. *Annu. Rev. Immunol.* **2019**, *37*, 173–200. [CrossRef] [PubMed]
96. Yarchoan, M.; Johnson, B.A.; Lutz, E.R.; Laheru, D.A.; Jaffee, E.M. Targeting neoantigens to augment antitumour immunity. *Nat. Rev. Cancer* **2017**, *17*, 209–222. [CrossRef]
97. Schumacher, T.N.; Schreiber, R.D. Neoantigens in cancer immunotherapy. *Science* **2015**, *348*, 69–74. [CrossRef]
98. McGranahan, N.; Furness, A.J.S.; Rosenthal, R.; Ramskov, S.; Lyngaa, R.; Saini, S.K.; Jamal-Hanjani, M.; Wilson, G.A.; Birkbak, N.J.; Hiley, C.; et al. Clonal neoantigens elicit T cell immunoreactivity and sensitivity to immune checkpoint blockade. *Science* **2016**, *351*, 1463–1469. [CrossRef]
99. Tumeh, P.C.; Harview, C.L.; Yearley, J.H.; Shintaku, I.P.; Taylor, E.J.M.; Robert, L.; Chmielowski, B.; Spasić, M.; Henry, G.; Ciobanu, V.; et al. PD-1 blockade induces responses by inhibiting adaptive immune resistance. *Nature* **2014**, *515*, 568–571. [CrossRef]
100. Peng, M.; Mo, Y.; Wang, Y.; Wu, P.; Zhang, Y.; Xiong, F.; Guo, C.; Wu, X.; Li, Y.; Li, X.; et al. Neoantigen vaccine: An emerging tumor immunotherapy. *Mol. Cancer* **2019**, *18*, 1–14. [CrossRef]
101. Łuksza, M.; Riaz, N.; Makarov, V.; Balachandran, V.P.; Hellmann, M.D.; Solovyov, A.; Rizvi, N.A.; Merghoub, T.; Levine, A.J.; Chan, T.A.; et al. A neoantigen fitness model predicts tumour response to checkpoint blockade immunotherapy. *Nature* **2017**, *551*, 517–520. [CrossRef]
102. Grassberger, C.; Ellsworth, S.G.; Wilks, M.Q.; Keane, F.K.; Loeffler, J.S. Assessing the interactions between radiotherapy and antitumour immunity. *Nat. Rev. Clin. Oncol.* **2019**, *16*, 729–745. [CrossRef]
103. Agostinelli, C.; Gallamini, A.; Stracqualursi, L.; Agati, P.; Tripodo, C.; Fuligni, F.; Sista, M.T.; Fanti, S.; Biggi, A.; Vitolo, U.; et al. The combined role of biomarkers and interim PET scan in prediction of treatment outcome in classical Hodgkin's lymphoma: A retrospective, European, multicentre cohort study. *Lancet Haematol.* **2016**, *3*, e467–e479. [CrossRef]
104. Fischer, B.M.; Lassen, U.; Mortensen, J.; Larsen, S.; Loft, A.; Bertelsen, A.; Ravn, J.; Clementsen, P.; Høgholm, A.; Larsen, K.; et al. Preoperative Staging of Lung Cancer with Combined PET–CT. *N. Engl. J. Med.* **2009**, *361*, 32–39. [CrossRef] [PubMed]
105. Chiou, V.L.; Burotto, M. Pseudoprogression and Immune-Related Response in Solid Tumors. *J. Clin. Oncol.* **2015**, *33*, 3541–3543. [CrossRef] [PubMed]
106. Kang, J.; DeMaria, S.; Formenti, S.C. Current clinical trials testing the combination of immunotherapy with radiotherapy. *J. Immunother. Cancer* **2016**, *4*, 51. [CrossRef]
107. Liu, Y.; Dong, Y.; Kong, L.; Shi, F.; Zhu, H.; Yu, J. Abscopal effect of radiotherapy combined with immune checkpoint inhibitors. *J. Hematol. Oncol.* **2018**, *11*, 104. [CrossRef] [PubMed]
108. Galon, J.; Bruni, D. Approaches to treat immune hot, altered and cold tumours with combination immunotherapies. *Nat. Rev. Drug Discov.* **2019**, *18*, 197–218. [CrossRef]
109. Aguilera, T.; Elghonaimy, E.A.; Shehade, H.; Rafat, M.; Castellini, L.; Jiang, D.; Kariolis, M.; Koong, A.C.; Le, Q.-T.; Ellies, L.G.; et al. Induced Tumor Heterogeneity Reveals Factors Informing Radiation and Immunotherapy Combinations. *Clin. Cancer Res.* **2020**, *26*, 2972–2985. [CrossRef]
110. Schölch, S.; Rauber, C.; Tietz, A.; Rahbari, N.N.; Bork, U.; Schmidt, T.; Kahlert, C.; Haberkorn, U.; Tomai, M.A.; Lipson, K.E.; et al. Radiotherapy combined with TLR7/8 activation induces strong immune responses against gastrointestinal tumors. *Oncotarget* **2014**, *6*, 4663–4676. [CrossRef]
111. Brøndum, L.; Eriksen, J.G.; Sørensen, B.S.; Mortensen, L.S.; Toustrup, K.; Overgaard, J.; Alsner, J. Plasma proteins as prognostic biomarkers in radiotherapy treated head and neck cancer patients. *Clin. Transl. Radiat. Oncol.* **2017**, *2*, 46–52. [CrossRef]

112. Ayers, M.; Lunceford, J.K.; Nebozhyn, M.V.; Murphy, E.; Loboda, A.; Kaufman, D.R.; Albright, A.; Cheng, J.D.; Kang, S.P.; Shankaran, V.; et al. IFN-γ-related mRNA profile predicts clinical response to PD-1 blockade. *J. Clin. Investig.* **2017**, *127*, 2930–2940. [CrossRef]

113. Karachaliou, N.; González-Cao, M.; Crespo, G.; Drozdowskyj, A.; Aldeguer, E.; Giménez-Capitán, A.; Teixido, C.; Molina-Vila, M.Á.; Viteri, S.; De Los Llanos Gil, M.; et al. Interferon gamma, an important marker of response to immune checkpoint blockade in non-small cell lung cancer and melanoma patients. *Ther. Adv. Med. Oncol.* **2018**, *10*. [CrossRef] [PubMed]

6

Botulinum Neurotoxins and Cancer

Shivam O. Mittal [1] **and Bahman Jabbari** [2,*]

1 Head, Section for Parkinson's Disease and Movement Disorders, Cleveland Clinic Abu Dhabi, Abu Dhabi 112412, UAE; shivamommittal@gmail.com
2 Department of Neurology, Yale University School of Medicine, New Haven, CT 06519, USA
* Correspondence: bahman.jabbari@yale.edu

Abstract: Botulinum neurotoxins (BoNT) possess an analgesic effect through several mechanisms including an inhibition of acetylcholine release from the neuromuscular junction as well as an inhibition of specific pain transmitters and mediators. Animal studies have shown that a peripheral injection of BoNTs impairs the release of major pain transmitters such as substance P, calcitonin gene related peptide (CGRP) and glutamate from peripheral nerve endings as well as peripheral and central neurons (dorsal root ganglia and spinal cord). These effects lead to pain relief via the reduction of peripheral and central sensitization both of which reflect important mechanisms of pain chronicity. This review provides updated information about the effect of botulinum toxin injection on local pain caused by cancer, painful muscle spasms from a remote cancer, and pain at the site of cancer surgery and radiation. The data from the literature suggests that the local injection of BoNTs improves muscle spasms caused by cancerous mass lesions and alleviates the post-operative neuropathic pain at the site of surgery and radiation. It also helps repair the parotid damage (fistula, sialocele) caused by facial surgery and radiation and improves post-parotidectomy gustatory hyperhidrosis. The limited literature that suggests adding botulinum toxins to cell culture slows/halts the growth of certain cancer cells is also reviewed and discussed.

Keywords: botulinum toxin; botulinum neurotoxin; cancer; cancer cells; neuropathic pain; post-surgical pain; parotid gland; submaxillary gland; gustatory hyperhidrosis; sialocele; parotid fistula

Key Contribution: This review demonstrates that local injection of botulinum toxins can alleviate neuropathic pain experienced at the site of surgery and radiation in cancer patients. Local injection of botulinum neurotoxins can also heal fistula and sialocele in the parotid gland of cancer patients damaged by surgical trauma and radiation.

---

1. Introduction

Currently, there are vast indications for the use of botulinum neurotoxins (BoNT) type A and B in clinical medicine. Their specific inhibitory action on cholinergic synapses makes them desirable for the treatment of several hyperkinetic movement disorders as well as symptoms caused by glandular hyperactivity (sialorrhea and hyperhidrosis) and bladder dysfunction [1]. Disease-oriented reviews indicate that these agents are frequently used for the treatment of spasticity in several common disease conditions such as stroke, cerebral palsy, multiple sclerosis, cerebral, and spinal cord injury [2]. The efficacy of BoNT therapy in migraine headaches, predicted by early investigators [3], has been proven via two large, multicenter clinical trials leading to the approval of onabotulinumtoxinA for the treatment of chronic migraine [4]. Animal and human studies have shown that the local injection of botulinum toxins has an analgesic effect and can relieve several forms of neuropathic pain [5–7].

The data indicate an analgesic activity for BoNTs in a wide range of pain disorders that include both neuropathic and non-neuropathic pain.

In recent years, several publications have drawn attention to the utility of BoNT injections in cancer-related pain syndromes arising either by direct pressure from a neoplastic mass or from neuropathic pain at the site of cancer surgery or radiation [8]. Aside from pain, BoNT injection into parotid or submaxillary glands has been shown to reduce symptoms such as sialorrhea resulting from gland injury as well as healing surgical complications such as fistula and sialocele [9]. BoNT injections have been reported to relieve gustatory hyperhidrosis resulting from parotid and oral surgery in cancer patients [10]. The limited literature also suggests that adding BoNT to the culture of cancer cell lines slows growth and mitotic activity of certain cancer cells and promotes apoptosis [11].

This review is based on a literature search using the search engines of Pub Med, Ovid embrace, and Google Scholar from 1989 to 1 September 2019. The terms botulinum toxin, botulinum neurotoxin, onabotulinumtoxinA, incobotulinumtoxinA, abobotulinumtoxinA, and rimabotulinumtoxinB were crossed with cancer pain, postsurgical cancer pain, post-radiation cancer pain, salivary glands, sialorrhea, gustatory sweating, cancer cells, and cancer cell line. Book chapters that were written over the past 10 years focusing on the subject of botulinum toxin therapy in cancer patients were also reviewed. The inclusion criteria encompassed all articles found via those three afore-mentioned search engines using the above-mentioned search words. Inclusion required that the manuscript's abstract contain both words cancer (or neoplasm) and botulinum toxin (or botulinum neurotoxin) therapy. Manuscripts that did not have both cancer and botulinum toxin therapy noted in the abstract were excluded. Manuscripts with benign mass lesions were also excluded.

2. Results

The search identified 746 manuscripts from which 76 were relevant to the subject of botulinum toxins and cancer (see flow chart in Figure 1). After eliminating 12 duplications (due to an overlap between MedLine and Google Scholar), 64 manuscripts remained for final analysis. The collected data can be classified under 3 categories: (1) The role of botulinum toxins in post-radiation and post-surgical cancer pain; (2) the repairing and healing function of BoNT injections upon parotid gland damaged by radiation or surgery; and (3) the effect of botulinum toxins on cancer cell line, cell growth, and apoptosis.

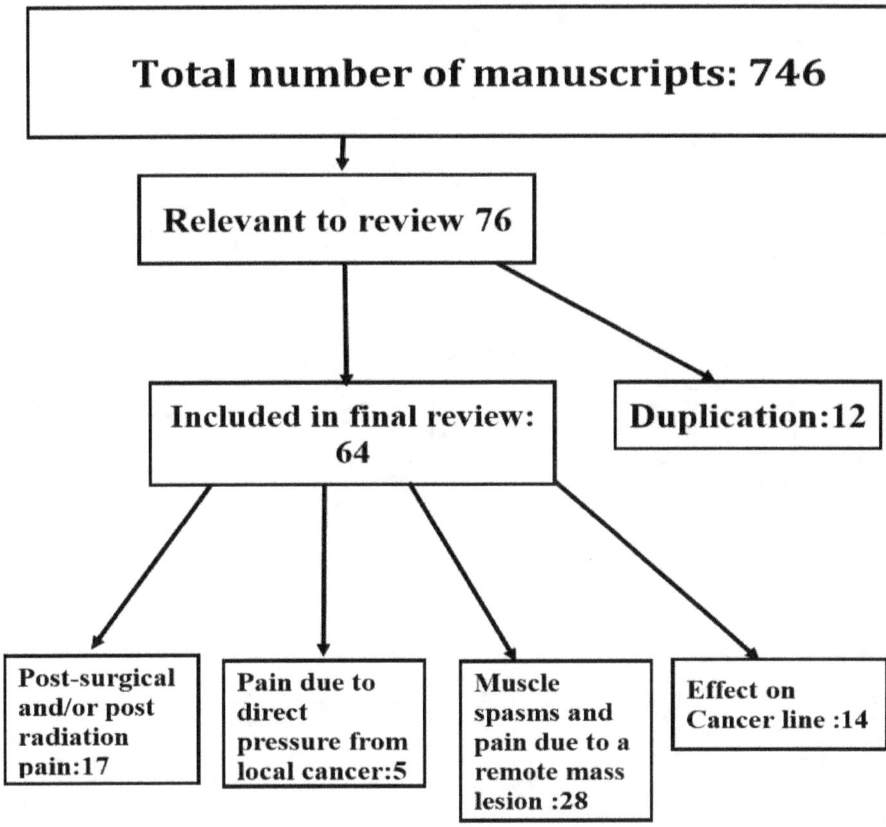

Figure 1. Flow chart of the reviewed manuscripts on cancer and botulinum neurotoxin therapy.

2.1. Botulinum Neurotoxins Therapy for Post-Radiation And/Or Post-Surgical Cancer Pain

This heading includes six prospective clinical trials, four retrospective studies, one double blind placebo-controlled study, and six single case reports (Table 1). A majority of patients had burning and searing pain along the region of fibrosis and keloid formation (neuropathic pain). Some also experienced additional local muscle spasms close to the scarred tissue affecting the neck and shoulder muscles. The most affected muscles were sternocleidomastoid, splenius capitus, trapezius, and levator scapulae. Injections were either subcutaneous (close or at the area of keloid and post-surgical scars, see Figure 2) or both subcutaneous and intramuscular.

Table 1. Published studies on the effect of botulinum neurotoxins (BoNT) on local pain resulting from radiation and/or surgery *.

Authors	Pts Study	Toxin	Dose Units	Treatment	Location of Cancer	Primary Outcome	Result
Van Daele et al., 2002 [12]	6 Retro	OnaA	20–25	Radiation chemotherapy	Head and neck	Pain VAS	Complete pain relief in four of six patients. Significant improvement of quality of life using SF36, EQ-5D scales
Layeeque et al., 2004 [13]	48 Pro	OnaA	100	Mastectomy, assessed for pain after expander placement	Breast	(1) Pain assessed by VAS (2) Narcotic use	Less pain in BoNT group ($p < 0.00001$) Less narcotic use in BoNT group ($p < 0.0001$)
Vasan et al., 2004 [14]	16 Pro	AboA	100 to 320	Surgery	Head and neck	Pain (VAS- days 3 and 4 weeks), global. Quality of life	Significant pain reduction ($p = 0.05$); Quality of life improved ($p = 0.7$)
Wittekindt et al., 2006 [15]	23 Pro	OnaA	60–120 160–240	Radiation; surgery	Head and neck	Pain VAS: 28 weeks	Significant reduction of pain (<0.05)
Hartl et al., 2008 [16]	19 Pro	OnaA AboA	50 250	Chemotherapy; radiation	Head and neck	Pain: (VAS) Function: At 4 weeks	Improved pain ($p = 0.02$) Function ($p = 0.04$)
Stubblefield et al., 2008 [17]	23 Retro	OnaA	25–200	Radiation; surgery	Head, neck, breast	Pain (VAS)	Pain improved in Improved in 85% of patients
Mittal et al., 2012 [18]	7 Retro	OnaA	100	Radiation; surgery	Head, neck, breast	Pain (VAS) PGIC At 4 weeks	VAS: Six of seven patients improved: $p < 0.05$ PGIC: Six of seven, very satisfied QoL: Six of seven improved ($p < 0.05$)
Bach et al., 2012 [19]	9 Pro	OnaA	100–400	Radiation and surgery	Head and neck	Pain (VAS) and FDSNP at 4 weeks	Both pain and FDSNP improved ($p < 0.01$)
Rostami et al., 2014 [20]	12 Pro	IncoA	100	Radiation and surgery	Head neck breast	Pain (VAS) and PGIC at week 6	VAS improved ($p < 0.05$) PGIC: Very satisfied QoL improved in 38% of patients ($p < 0.05$)
De Groef et al. 2018 [21]	50 DBPC	onaA	100	Surgery	Breast	Pain measured by VAS	Pain reduction 60% in the BoNT and 40% in saline group (statistically ns)
Mailly et al., 2019 [22]	16 Retro	incoA aboA	20 40	Radiation and surgery	Head and neck	Pain (VAS)	VAS improved $p < 0.01$

* Case reports are not included. onaA: OnabotulinumtoxinA; aboA: AbobotulinumtoxinA; incoA: IncobotulinumtoxinA; VAS: Visual Analogue Scale; PGIC: Patient Global Impression of Change; FDSNP: Functional Disability Scale for Neck Pain; Pro: Prospective; Retro: Retrospective; DBPC: double-blind, placebo-controlled; QoL: Quality of Life.

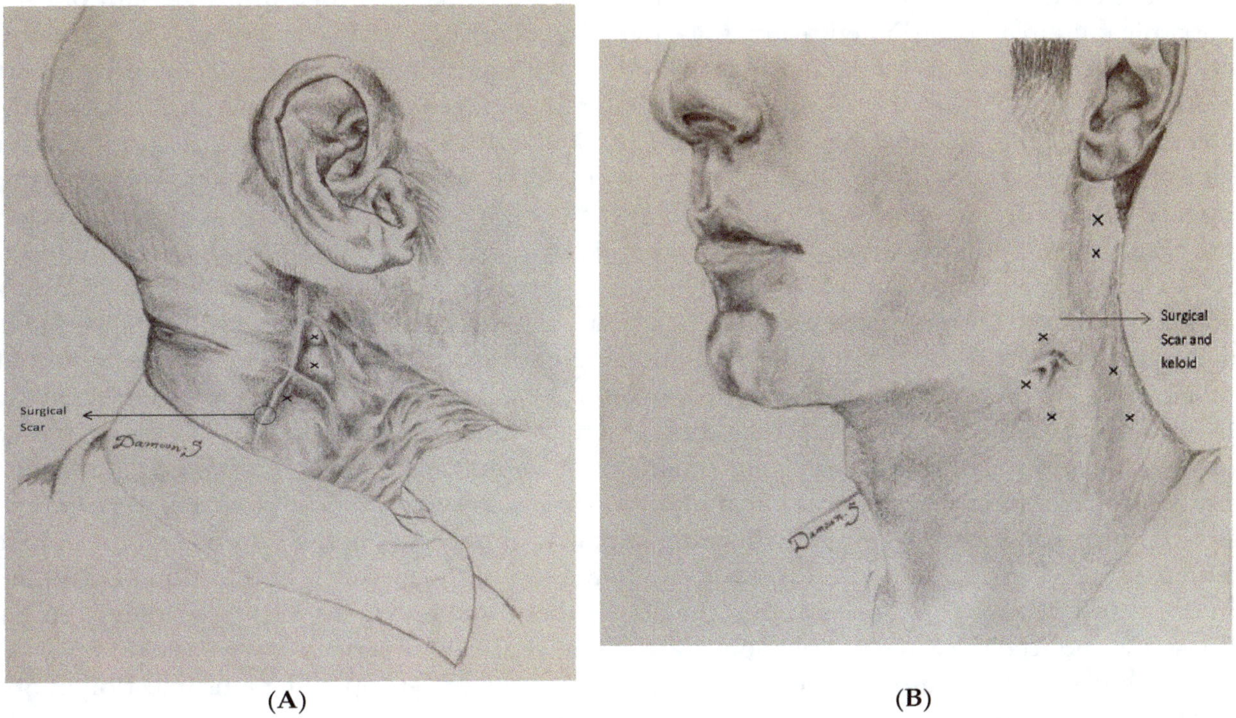

Figure 2. Post-surgical and post-radiation pain treated with BoNT. Example of two patients. From Jabbari B. Botulinum Toxin Treatment in Pain Disorders. Springer, New York 2015. Printed with permission from the publisher. (**A**) A 47-year-old man had undergone right neck dissection and radiotherapy for cancer of the tongue and cervical adenopathy 6 years prior to visiting the Yale clinic. A year following surgery and radiotherapy, severe pain (VAS 9–10, both sharp and deep) developed over the right side of the neck which was mostly felt below the mandible and anterior to the angle of the jaw. Injecting onabotulinumtoxinA into the areas designated by X on the figure, (30, 30, and 20 units) reduced the pain significantly (VAS 1) within a week after injection. He remained responsive and satisfied (assessed by PGIC) receiving injections every 4–6 months over 7 years of follow-up. (**B**) A 48-year old man with squamous cell carcinoma of piriform sinus had supraglottic laryngectomy. Two years following neck dissection and radiotherapy, he developed severe pain (VAS 9) over the left side of the neck. The pain was deep as well as sharp and superficial. Injection of onabotulinumtoxinA, 20 units into each superficial pain region (Xs around the jaw) and 30 units into nearby posteriorly located muscles (splenius and trapezius) designated by X reduced the pain to VAS 0–1 level. The total dose was 200 units. The patient enjoyed pain relief with repeat injections over the 3 years of follow-up. Drawings courtesy of Damoun Safarpour M.D.

A total of 10 of 11 studies used a standardized scale for pain measurement (Visual Analogue Scale: VAS) which in 9 of 10 demonstrated statistically significant improvement of local pain at 4–8 post-injection weeks compared to baseline ($p < 0.05$) (Table 1). Two studies included patient global impression of change (PGIC) in the evaluation, using a 7-grade scale ranging from "very unsatisfied" to "very satisfied". In both studies, patients expressed significant satisfaction with the results [18,20]. Four studies used a scale for evaluating quality of life. Three of 4 demonstrated significant improvement of quality of life after BoNT-A (onaA and incoA) injection therapy [14,18,20]. One study demonstrated significant reduction of daily opioid use after BoNT therapy [13]. One prospective study provided long-term follow up of up to 82 months [20]. Side effects consisted mainly of transient pain at the site of injection(s) and minor local bleeding. None of the 229 patients, reported in Table 1, demonstrated any serious side effect following BoNT injections.

Clinical data from case reports includes six single case reports. One publication reported a 50 year-old man with adenocarcinoma of the soft palate, who following radiotherapy, developed trismus and myokymia of the masseter muscles. Trismus and myokymia improved after injection of 25 units of onaA into each masseter muscle [23]. Two other manuscripts described improvement of central neuropathic pain in association with a mass lesion. One described a 55 year-women who developed severe burning pain and allodynia in the distribution of T1 dermatomes bilaterally following partial resection of an angioma at the C7–C8 region. Subcutaneous injection of onaA at 25 sites into T1 dermatomes (100 units on each sides) resulted in a marked reduction of neuropathic pain and allodynia. This effect was sustained with repeated injections over a follow up period of three years [24]. A similar experience with central pain was reported by Nam et al. [25], in a 62-year old man who had developed severe allodynia and neuropathic pain over the posterior aspect of the left thigh contralateral to a frontal lobe malignant brain tumor. A subcutaneous injection of onaA with a total dose of 100 units at 16 sites substantially improved the patient's neuropathic pain and allodynia over the affected region. In another patient, radiation of a left submandibular chondrosarcoma resulted in hyperactivity of the spinal accessory nerve and gradual painful hypertrophy of the left trapezius muscle. An injection of 90 units of onaA resulted in a substantial reduction of left shoulder pain and diminished the involuntary myokymic movements of the left trapezius muscle [26]. Boukovalas et al. [27] reported a patient with squamous cell carcinoma of the anterior mandible who, following mandibulectomy, bilateral neck dissection, and radiotherapy, gradually developed pain and tightness of the sternocleidomastoid and platysmal muscles associated with Raynaud phenomenon of the lower face. Injection of botulinum toxin (type and dose not mentioned) into the above-mentioned muscles improved painful muscle tightness and reduced the Raynaud phenomena. Schuler et al. [28] described a 47-year old female who, at the scarred skin site of resected melanoma, developed severe neuropathic pain. Injection of onaA, 50 units in a grid-like pattern (injection sites were 1.5 cm apart), resulted in 50% reduction of pain four weeks after BoNT injection.

The duration of action of BoNT injections for pain relief in the above-mentioned studies was 3–6 months (mean 3.9 month). In most studies, the follow up was short term, not exceeding 6–12 months. In some cases, however, patients were followed-up for years with repeated injections. Two patients described in Figure 1 were followed-up for 3 and 7 years (see figure legend). Nine of 11 studies reported no side effects. One study reported increased pain for a few days at the site of injection in one patient, which was followed by baseline pain improvement [14]. One study reported the occurrence of a diffuse maculo-papular rash in one patient 2–3 days after the botulinum neurotoxin injection after which the rash disappeared over a month [20].

2.2. Botulinum Neurotoxins Therapy for Post-Radiation or Postsurgical Damage to Parotid Gland

This category includes six prospective clinical trials, 10 retrospective studies, and 12 single case reports (Table 2). All prospective studies are open label. Botulinum toxin treatment was used for the remedy of post-parotidectomy complications such as gustatory hyperhidrosis (GH), post-parotidectomy sialorrhea, fistula, and sialocele formation.

Table 2. BoNT therapy for post-parotidectomy gustatory hyperhidrosis, fistula, sialocele formation, and for post-parotidectomy sialorrhea.

Authors	Design	Pts #	Clinical Problem	Injection Site	Toxin and Dose	Result
Laskawi et al., 2013 [29]	R	10	Post-parotidectomy fistula	Parotid gland	OnaA 30–50 units	Treated within 6 weeks of surgery: Fistulas healed in 9 of 10 patients
Marchese-Ragona et al., 2006 [30]	R	3	Post-parotidectomy fistula	Parotid gland	OnaA 15–20 units	Complete healing of fistula with follow ups 12,18, and 14 months
Nolte et al., 2004 [31]	P	20	Gustatory sweating after parotidectomy	Facial skin	OnaA 3 units/cm	Complete loss of sweating for 12 months

Table 2. *Cont.*

Authors	Design	Pts #	Clinical Problem	Injection Site	Toxin and Dose	Result
Kuttner et al., 2001 [32]	R	8	GH after parotidectomy	Face	BoNT-A 0.5 units/cm	Stopped facial sweating within one week
Vargas et al., 2000 [33]	P	4	Post-parotidectomy sialocele-pain	Parotid gland	OnaA 30–50 units	Total resolution in 4 weeks in all patients
Steffen et al., 2014 [34]	R	25	Head and neck cancer FHS: (19) Fistula (6)	Parotid gland	OnaA and incoA: Par: 30 U SM: 20 U	FHS: 11 of 19 improved. Fistula: 4 of 6 improved
Machese et al., 2008 [35]	R	8	Head and neck cancer sialorrhea: 6, fistula: 1, and sialocele: 1	Parotid gland	AboA: 100 U	Fistulas healed. Sialorrhea stopped
Eckardt et al., 2003 [36]	R	33	GH after parotidectomy	Face	OnaA 16 to 80 units	Facial sweating disappeared within a week after injections
Cantarella and Barbieri [37]	R	7	GH after parotidectomy	Face	RimaB 2200 units	Cessation of sweating in 6 of 7 patients 4 weeks after injection
Matos Dias et al., 2008 [38]	R	10	GH after parotidectomy	Face	Ona-A 38 units	Sweating stopped
Hatrl et al., 2008 [39]	R	7	GH after parotidectomy	Face	BoNT-A	Sweating and quality of life improved
Pomprasit et al., 2007 [40]	P	9	GH after Parotidectomy	Face	Ona-A 10.6 units	Sweating stopped in 5 and reduced in 4
Cavalot et al., 2000 [41]	P	40	GH after parotidectomy	Face	Ona-A, 2.5/cm^2	100% response in severe group, 72% response in moderate group
Von Lindern et al., 2000 [42]	R	7	GH after parotidectomy	Face	Ona-A	Sweating stopped after BoNT injection
Laccourreye et al., 1998 [43]	P	14	GH after parotidectomy	Face	Ona-A	All showed total cessation of sweating
Bjerkhoel et al., 1997 [44]	P	15	GH after parotidectomy	Face	Ona-A	Total cessation of facial sweating in 13 patients

Case reports are not included for salivary gland problems related to cancer surgery or cancer irradiation. R: Retrospective; P: Prospective; onaA: OnabotulinumtoxinA; incoA: IncobotulinumtoxinA; aboA: AbobotulinumtoxinA; FHS: Functional hypersalivation; Par: Parotid, SM: Submandibular.

The positive information of these studies has been supported by several case reports [45–56]. Among these 12 case reports, six described healing of post-parotidectomy fistula and four reported on healing of sialocele. One case reported improvement of gustatory hyperhidrosis and another one reported improvement of post-parotidectomy sialorrhea. A total of 11 studies had used type-A and one had used type B toxin.

In these 11 studies, no serious side effects were reported. One study reported a patient on anticoagulation in whom a small hematoma developed at the site of injection [34]. One study reported dry mouth as the only side effect [38]. One study cited non-specified, minor issues limited to the site of injection [41]. One study mentioned mild transient weakness of the upper lip in two patients [43] and another study described transient weakness of orbicularis oris muscle in one patient [44].

The clinical studies cited above investigating the analgesic effect of BoNTs in patients after surgery or radiation therapy and BoNT's healing effect on parotid glands injured by surgery or radiation strongly suggest the efficacy of BoNTs in cancer patients affected by surgical and radiation side effects. All three type-A FDA approved BoNTs seem to have analgesic effect in post-surgical and post-radiation pain. In case of parotid injury, at least one study (Table 2) suggests that type B is also effective. Although anecdotal observations have demonstrated safety over 3 to 7 years of treatment (cases presented in Figure 1), the long term safety of BoNT therapy in cancer patients needs to be further investigated through controlled, prospective clinical trials.

2.3. The Effects of Botulinum Neurotoxins Injections on Malignant Tumors and Cancer Cell Line

This category includes 14 studies. In three studies, investigators injected BoNT into a malignant tumor and demonstrated cellular apoptosis and reduction of tumor size [57–59] (Table 3). In another six studies, adding BoNT-A to cancer cell cultures reduced cell growth, induced apoptosis, and inhibited mitosis in various cancer cell lines: Prostate, breast, colon, and pancreatic tumors [60–65]. In one study, transfection of insulin secreting cells by BoNT-A reduced insulin secretion, suggesting a potential for treatment of insulinomas [66]. In another study, the addition of BoNT-A to Her2 positive breast cancer cell line increased Herceptin efficacy [67]. In one study, authors reported no effect on prostate tumor growth and LNCaP and PC3 cancer cells after exposure to BoNT [68]. In one study, increased tumor oxygenation after the injection of BoNT-A into hepatic sarcoma and fibrosarcoma suggested that the BoNT injection potentially made these tumors more susceptible to chemotherapy [69]. In another study, the injection of onaA into one side of cancerous human prostate increased apoptosis on the injected side (compare to saline injected into other side) [70].

Table 3. In vivo and in vitro effects of BoNT injection on malignant tumors and cancer cell lines.

Authors	Study Type	Type of Cells or Tissue	Study Design	Results
Vezdrevanis 2011 [57]	In vivo	Prostatic cancer	Injected BoNT into prostate	Tumor size reduction
Ulloa et al., 2015 [58]	In vivo	Glioblastoma cells	Cells with or without transfection by BoNT-C1 injected into mice striatum	By BoNT-C1 blocks the growth of Glioblastoma cells via blocking Syntaxin1
He et al., 2016 [59]	In vivo	Mice with pancreatic tumor	Injected onaA or saline into tumor	Reduced tumor size; increased apoptosis
Karsenty et al., 2009 [60]	In vitro	Prostate LNCaP and PC-3 cell lines	LNCaP and PC-3 cell lines were exposed to onaA	OnaA inhibited LNCasP cell proliferation; had no effect on PC-3 cell
Nam et al., 2012 [61]	In vitro	Breast and colorectal cancer	PLC-γl-transformed cells were exposed to BoNT-A (difficile)	Caused apoptosis and mitotic inhibition
Proietti et al., 2012 [62]	In vitro	Prostate LNCaP and PC-3 cell lines	Prostate cancer cell lines were exposed to incoA	Tumor cell growth slowed down probably due to toxin effect on SV2 receptors
Bandala et al., 2013 [63]	In vitro	Breast T47D cancer cells	Breast T47D cancer cells were exposed to diverse dilutions of BoNT	BoNT via caspase 3, slow down the growth of T47d cells and caused apoptosis
Bandala et al., 2015 [64]	In vitro	Breast cancer cell line	Added BoNT-A to breast cancer cell line	BoNT-A diminished SV2 protein on the surface of breast cancer cells
Rust et al., 2016 [65]	In vitro	Human neuroblastoma cells	Added BoNT-C to human neuroblastoma cell culture	Apoptosis of neuroblastoma cells
Huang et al., 1998 [66]	Invitro	Insulin secreting HIT-T15 cells	Insulin secreting cells were transfected by BoNT-A	Marked reduction of insulin secretion-potential to treat insulinoma
Hajighasemlou et al., 2015 [67]	In vitro	Her2 positive breast cancer cell line	Assessed the effect of BoNT-A on Her2 positive cells responsive to Herceptin	Herceptin efficacy significantly improved
Cheng et al., 2013 [68]	In vitro and in vivo	Prostate cancer cell line in Mice	LNCaP and PC3 cancer cells were exposed to 1 to 10 units of onaA	No effect on tumor growth in LNCaP and PC3 cancer cells
Ansiaux et al., 2006 [69]	In vivo	Fibrosarcoma, hepatosarcoma	BoNT-A injected into the tumor	Increased oxygenation of the tumor and made it more susceptible to chemo and radiotherapy
Coarfa et al., 2017 [70]	In vivo	Prostate of 250 nude mice Four human cancerous prostates	Effect of onaA versus saline injection into cancer cells implanted into rodent's prostate Assessed the effect of onaA versus saline injection in cancerous prostate before prostatectomy	Increased apoptosis; slowed cancer progression Increased apoptosis in ona-A injected side of prostate

OnaA: OnabotulinumtoxinA (Botox). IncoA: IncobotulinumtoxinA (Xeomin).

3. Discussion

Botulinum neurotoxins exert their analgesic effect through two known mechanisms. The inhibitory effect of the BoNTs upon the release of acetylcholine at the neuromuscular junction is mostly responsible for the relief of pain caused by muscle spasms. In the case of neuropathic pain, it is currently believed that the analgesic effect of botulinum injections predominantly results from inhibition of pain neurotransmitters both at peripheral and at central sensory levels [5,6,71,72]. The peripheral injection of botulinum toxin-A into the muscle or close to peripheral nerve endings reduces the release of calcitonin gene related peptide, a major pain transmitter from trigeminal ganglion [73]. Direct exposure of dorsal root ganglia to botulinum toxin-A significantly reduces the thermal sensitivity in the animal model of thermal pain [74]. In the formalin pain model, injection botulinum toxin B into the rat's paw reduced substance P release from ipsilateral sensory spinal neurons and prevented spinal sensory neuron activation (c-Fos) which occurred after formalin injection [75]. Injection of botulinum toxins into mice hind paw reduces glutamate release from spinal sensory neurons [76]. Intra-articular injection of botulinum toxin in animal models of pain reduces upregulation of transient receptor potential cation channel subfamily V member 1 (TrpV1), a protein closely associated with pain pathophysiology [77]. A central analgesic function for botulinum toxins has been suggested by studies that have shown the presence of cleaved SNAP-25 in medullary and midbrain sensory regions following the peripheral injection of botulinum toxins [78,79]. Further suggestion for central effects of BoNTs comes from the studies that have demonstrated bilateral improvement of pain sensations after the unilateral injection of botulinum toxin in animal models of diabetic neuropathy and acidic saline injection [80,81]. The analgesic effect of BoNTs results from their direct and indirect effects since patients experience analgesia prior to the muscle relaxation [82].

Pain is a common symptom in cancer patients and when present often impairs the patient's quality of life [83]. Approximately 20–60% of the patients with breast cancer and 30% of the patients with head and neck cancer experience chronic pain localized to the site of radiation or surgery [84]. Post-radiation/surgical pain may be treated with the topical application of a hyaluronic acid, calendula officinalis, trolamine, and lidocaine patch [85,86]. However, sustained relief from pain happens only in 25% of the patients using these remedies [87]. Potent systemic analgesic agents such as opioids provide pain relief in many patients but the development of undesirable side effects including nausea, somnolence, constipation, and addiction complicates their use [88]. Botulinum toxin treatment has two major advantages over these pharmacological remedies. Firstly, the effects of the BoNT-A and B injection lasts 3–6 months. Secondly, the BoNT injection has fewer side effects and is safer when compared to potent analgesic agents. Lack of any serious side effect in the studies cited above supports this statement.

Gustatory hyperhidrosis (Frey syndrome) can be congenital or acquired. Acquired gustatory hyperhidrosis results from injury to the parotid gland or face as well as conditions such as diabetic autonomic neuropathy. Gustatory hyperhidrosis after parotidectomy results from the aberrant innervation of sweat glands from parasympathetic nerves of the parotid region. Facial sweating during chewing and eating is often a cause of social embarrassment. Gustatory hyperhidrosis (GH) is common after parotidectomy and about half of the patients complained of this symptom after surgery [89]. Botulinum neurotoxins via blocking acetylcholine release at autonomic synapses are highly effective in treatment of autonomic dysfunctions such as sialorrhea and hyperhidrosis [90]. In a meta-analysis of literature on Frey syndrome (multiple etiologies) treated with BoNTs, Xie et al. found the effectiveness of BoNT therapy to be present in 98% of the patients [10].

Fistula with sialorrhea and sialocele (entrapped saliva with cyst formation) are two common complications of parotidectomy. Treatment of post-parotidectomy fistula consist of pressure dressing, systemic anticholinergic drugs, suction drain insertion, tympanic neurectomy, and surgery [91]. Overall, the results of the above mentioned surgical and medical strategies in the treatment of parotid fistula is disappointing [92]. Furthermore, side effects of anticholinergic therapy such as memory loss, blurring of vision, dryness of the mouth, and urinary dysfunction are not well tolerated, especially in the elderly. Botulinum toxin injections provides a safe and effective way to suppress sialorrhea and to help heal the fistula.

4. Conclusions

The studies of botulinum toxins in post-surgical and post-radiation pain indicated that the local injection of BoNT improved neuropathic pain and local muscle spasm at/or close to the site of surgery and radiation. The proof of efficacy of botulinum toxin therapy in this form of cancer-related pain, however, awaits the results of blinded and placebo-controlled studies. The same conclusion applies to the use of botulinum neurotoxins in gustatory hyperhidrosis and in the management of post-parotidectomy fistula and sialocele where all open-label studies suggest efficacy. The positive effect of BoNTs on different cancer cell lines and their direct effects upon certain cancerous tumors is encouraging. More studies are necessary to verify these results and if verified to devise a methodology through which BoNT injections can safely be used for the treatment of certain human cancers.

References

1. Jankovic, J. Botulinum toxin: State of the Art. *Mov. Disord.* **2017**, *32*, 1131–1138. [CrossRef]
2. Jabbari, B. (Ed.) A disease- oriented approach. In *Botulinum Toxin Treatment in Clinical Medicine*; Springer: New York, NY, USA, 2018.
3. Aoki, K.R. Evidence for antinociceptive activity of botulinum toxin type A in pain management. *Headache* **2003**, *43* (Suppl. S1), 9–15. [CrossRef] [PubMed]
4. Dodick, D.W.; Turkel, C.C.; DeGryse, R.E.; Aurora, S.K.; Silberstein, S.D.; Lipton, R.B.; Diener, H.C.; Brin, M.F. OnabotulinumtoxinA for treatment of chronic migraine: Pooled results from the double-blind, randomized, placebo-controlled phases of the PREEMPT clinical program. *Headache* **2010**, *50*, 921–936. [CrossRef] [PubMed]
5. Oh, H.M.; Chung, M.E. Botulinum Toxin for Neuropathic Pain: A Review of the Literature. *Toxins* **2015**, *7*, 3127–3154. [CrossRef] [PubMed]
6. Park, J.; Park, H.J. Botulinum Toxin for the Treatment of Neuropathic Pain. *Toxins* **2017**, *9*, 260. [CrossRef] [PubMed]
7. Safarpour, Y.; Jabbari, B. Botulinum toxin treatment of pain syndromes—An evidence based review. *Toxicon* **2018**, *147*, 120–128. [CrossRef]
8. Shaw, L.; Bazzell, A.F.; Dains, J.E. Botulinum Toxin for Side-Effect Management and Prevention of Surgical Complications in Patients Treated for Head and Neck Cancers and Esophageal Cancer. *J. Adv. Pract. Oncol.* **2019**, *10*, 40–52. [PubMed]
9. Melville, J.C.; Stackowicz, D.J.; Jundt, J.S.; Shum, J.W. Use of Botox (OnabotulinumtoxinA) for the Treatment of Parotid Sialocele and Fistula After Extirpation of Buccal Squamous Cell Carcinoma with Immediate Reconstruction Using Microvascular Free Flap: A Report of 3 Cases. *J. Oral Maxillofac. Surg.* **2016**, *74*, 1678–1686. [CrossRef]
10. Xie, S.; Wang, K.; Xu, T.; Guo, X.S.; Shan, X.F.; Cai, Z.G. Efficacy and safety of botulinum toxin type A for treatment of Frey's syndrome: Evidence from 22 published articles. *Cancer Med.* **2015**, *4*, 1639–1650. [CrossRef]
11. Matak, I.; Lacković, Z. Botulinum neurotoxin type A: Actions beyond SNAP-25? *Toxicology* **2015**, *335*, 79–84. [CrossRef]
12. Van Daele, D.J.; Finnegan, E.M.; Rodnitzky, R.L.; Zhen, W.; McCulloch, T.M.; Hoffman, H.T. Head and neck muscle spasm after radiotherapy: Management with botulinum toxin A injection. *Arch. Otolaryngol. Head Neck Surg.* **2002**, *128*, 956–959. [CrossRef]
13. Layeeque, R.; Hochberg, J.; Siegel, E.; Kunkel, K.; Kepple, J.; Henry-Tillman, R.S.; Dunlap, M.; Seibert, J.; Klimberg, V.S. Botulinum toxin infiltration for pain control after mastectomy and expander reconstruction. *Ann. Surg.* **2004**, *240*, 608–613. [CrossRef] [PubMed]
14. Vasan, C.W.; Liu, W.C.; Klussmann, J.P.; Guntinas-Lichius, O. Botulinum toxin type A for the treatment of chronic neck pain after neck dissection. *Head Neck* **2004**, *26*, 39–45. [CrossRef] [PubMed]
15. Wittekindt, C.; Liu, W.C.; Preuss, S.F.; Guntinas-Lichius, O. Botulinum toxin A for neuropathic pain after neck dissection: A dose-finding study. *Laryngoscope* **2006**, *116*, 1168–1171. [CrossRef] [PubMed]
16. Hartl, D.M.; Cohen, M.; Juliéron, M.; Marandas, P.; Janot, F.; Bourhis, J. Botulinum toxin for radiation-induced facial pain and trismus. *Otolaryngol. Head Neck Surg.* **2008**, *138*, 459–463. [PubMed]

17. Stubblefield, M.D.; Levine, A.; Custodio, C.M.; Fitzpatrick, T. The role of botulinum toxin type A in the radiation fibrosis syndrome: A preliminary report. *Arch. Phys. Med. Rehabil.* **2008**, *89*, 417–421. [CrossRef]
18. Mittal, S.; Machado, D.G.; Jabbari, B. OnabotulinumtoxinA for treatment of focal cancer pain after surgery and/or radiation. *Pain Med.* **2012**, *13*, 1029–1033. [CrossRef]
19. Bach, C.A.; Wagner, I.; Lachiver, X.; Baujat, B.; Chabolle, F. Botulinum toxin in the treatment of post-radiosurgical neck contracture in head and neck cancer: A novel approach. *Eur. Ann. Otorhinolaryngol. Head Neck Dis.* **2012**, *129*, 6–10. [CrossRef]
20. Rostami, R.; Mittal, S.O.; Radmand, R.; Jabbari, B. Incobotulinum Toxin-A Improves Post-Surgical and Post-Radiation Pain in Cancer Patients. *Toxins* **2016**, *8*, 22. [CrossRef]
21. De Groef, A.; Devoogdt, N.; Van Kampen, M.; Nevelsteen, I.; Smeets, A.; Neven, P.; Geraerts, I.; Dams, L.; Van der Gucht, E.; Debeer, P. Effectiveness of Botulinum Toxin A for Persistent Upper Limb Pain After Breast Cancer Treatment: A Double-Blinded Randomized Controlled Trial. *Arch. Phys. Med. Rehabil.* **2018**, *99*, 1342–1351. [CrossRef]
22. Mailly, M.; Benzakin, S.; Chauvin, A.; Brasnu, D.; Ayache, D. Douleurs post-radiques après radiothérapie pour cancer des voies aérodigestives superieures: Traitement par injections de toxine botulique A [Radiation-induced head and neck pain: Management with botulinum toxin a injections]. *Cancer Radiother.* **2019**, *23*, 312–315. [CrossRef] [PubMed]
23. Lou, J.S.; Pleninger, P.; Kurlan, R. Botulinum toxin A is effective in treating trismus associated with postradiation myokymia and muscle spasm. *Mov. Disord.* **1995**, *10*, 680–681. [CrossRef] [PubMed]
24. Jabbari, B.; Maher, N.; Difazio, M.P. Botulinum toxin a improved pain and allodynia in two patients with intracranial pathology. *Pain Med.* **2003**, *4*, 206–210. [CrossRef] [PubMed]
25. Nam, K.E.; Kim, J.S.; Hong, B.Y. Botulinum Toxin Type A Injection for Neuropathic Pain in a Patient With a Brain Tumor: A Case Report. *Ann. Rehabil. Med.* **2017**, *41*, 1088. [CrossRef]
26. Filippakis, A.; Ho, D.T.; Small, J.E.; Small, K.M.; Ensrud, E.R. Radiation-induced painful neurogenic hypertrophy Treated with Botulinum Toxin, A. *J. Clin. Neuromuscul. Dis.* **2018**, *19*, 135–137. [CrossRef]
27. Boukovalas, S.; Mays, A.C.; Selber, J.C. Botulinum Toxin Injection for Lower Face and Oral Cavity Raynaud Phenomenon after Mandibulectomy, Free Fibula Reconstruction, and Radiation Therapy. *Ann. Plast. Surg.* **2019**, *82*, 53–54. [CrossRef]
28. Schuler, A.; Veenstra, J.; Ozog, D. Battling Neuropathic Scar Pain with Botulinum Toxin. *J. Drugs Dermatol.* **2019**, *18*, 937–938.
29. Laskawi, R.; Winterhoff, J.; Köhler, S.; Kottwitz, L.; Matthias, C. Botulinum toxin treatment of salivary fistulas following parotidectomy: Follow-up results. *Oral Maxillofac. Surg.* **2013**, *17*, 281–285. [CrossRef]
30. Marchese-Ragona, R.; Marioni, G.; Restivo, D.A.; Staffieri, A. The role of botulinum toxin in postparotidectomy fistula treatment. A technical note. *Am. J. Otolaryngol.* **2006**, *27*, 221–224. [CrossRef]
31. Nolte, D.; Gollmitzer, I.; Loeffelbein, D.J.; Hölzle, F.; Wolff, K.D. Botulinumtoxin zur Behandlung des gustatorischen Schwitzens. Eine prospektive randomisierte Therapiestudie [Botulinum toxin for treatment of gustatory sweating. A prospective randomized study]. *Mund Kiefer Gesichtschir.* **2004**, *8*, 369–375. [CrossRef]
32. Kuttner, C.; Tröger, M.; Dempf, R.; Eckardt, A. Effektivität von Botulinumtoxin A in der Behandlung des gustatorischen Schwitzens [Effectiveness of botulinum toxin A in the treatment of gustatory sweating]. *Nervenarzt* **2001**, *72*, 787–790. [CrossRef] [PubMed]
33. Vargas, H.; Galati, L.T.; Parnes, S.M. A pilot study evaluating the treatment of postparotidectomy sialoceles with botulinum toxin type A. *Arch. Otolaryngol. Head Neck Surg.* **2000**, *126*, 421–424. [CrossRef] [PubMed]
34. Steffen, A.; Hasselbacher, K.; Heinrichs, S.; Wollenberg, B. Botulinum toxin for salivary disorders in the treatment of head and neck cancer. *Anticancer Res.* **2014**, *34*, 6627–6632. [PubMed]
35. Marchese, M.R.; Almadori, G.; Giorgio, A.; Paludetti, G. Post-surgical role of botulinum toxin-A injection in patients with head and neck cancer: Personal experience. *Acta Otorhinolaryngol. Ital.* **2008**, *28*, 13–16. [PubMed]
36. Eckardt, A.; Kuettner, C. Treatment of gustatory sweating (Frey's syndrome) with botulinum toxin A. *Head Neck* **2003**, *25*, 624–628. [CrossRef] [PubMed]
37. Cantarella, G.; Berlusconi, A.; Mele, V.; Cogiamanian, F.; Barbieri, S. Treatment of Frey's syndrome with botulinum toxin type B. *Otolaryngol. Head Neck Surg.* **2010**, *143*, 214–218. [CrossRef]

38. Martos Díaz, P.; Bances del Castillo, R.; Mancha de la Plata, M.; Gías, L.; Nieto, C.M.; Lee, G.Y.; Guerra, M.M. Clinical results in the management of Frey's syndrome with injections of Botulinum toxin. *Med. Oral Patol. Oral Cir. Bucal* **2008**, *13*, E248–E252.
39. Hartl, D.M.; Julieron, M.; LeRidant, A.M.; Janot, F.; Marandas, P.; Travagli, J.P. Botulinum toxin A for quality of life improvement in post-parotidectomy gustatory sweating (Frey's syndrome). *J. Laryngol. Otol.* **2008**, *122*, 1100–1104. [CrossRef]
40. Pomprasit, M.; Chintrakarn, C. Treatment of Frey's syndrome with botulinum toxin. *J. Med. Assoc. Thail.* **2007**, *90*, 2397–2402.
41. Cavalot, A.L.; Palonta, F.; Preti, G.; Nazionale, G.; Ricci, E.; Staffieri, A.; Di Girolamo, S.; Cortesina, G. Sindrome di Frey post parotidectomia. Trattamento con tossina botulinica di tipo A [Post-parotidectomy Frey's syndrome. Treatment with botulinum toxin type A]. *Acta Otorhinolaryngol. Ital.* **2000**, *20*, 187–191.
42. Von Lindern, J.J.; Niederhagen, B.; Bergé, S.; Hägler, G.; Reich, R.H. Frey syndrome: Treatment with type A botulinum toxin. *Cancer* **2000**, *89*, 1659–1663. [CrossRef]
43. Laccourreye, O.; Muscatelo, L.; Naude, C.; Bonan, B.; Brasnu, D. Botulinum toxin type A for Frey's syndrome: A preliminary prospective study. *Ann. Otol. Rhinol. Laryngol.* **1998**, *107*, 52–55. [CrossRef] [PubMed]
44. Bjerkhoel, A.; Trobbe, O. Frey's syndrome: Treatment with botulinum toxin. *J. Laryngol. Otol.* **1997**, *111*, 839–844. [CrossRef] [PubMed]
45. Ferron, C.; Cernea, S.S.; Almeida, A.R.T.; Cesar, D.V.G. Primary treatment of early fistula of parotid duct with botulinum toxin type A injection. *An. Bras. Dermatol.* **2017**, *92*, 864–866. [CrossRef] [PubMed]
46. Philouze, P.; Vertu, D.; Ceruse, P. Bilateral gustatory sweating in the submandibular region after bilateral neck dissection successfully treated with botulinum toxin. *Br. J. Oral Maxillofac. Surg.* **2014**, *52*, 761–763. [CrossRef] [PubMed]
47. Ihler, F.; Laskawi, R.; Matthias, C.; Rustenbeck, H.H.; Canis, M. Botulinumtoxin A gegen Hypersalivation. Einsatz bei Wundheilung nach Resektion eines Zungenkarzinoms [Botulinum toxin A after microvascular ALT flap in a patient with (corrected) squamous cell carcinoma of the tongue] [published correction appears in HNO. 2012 Oct; 60, 905]. *HNO* **2012**, *60*, 524–527. [CrossRef]
48. Pantel, M.; Volk, G.F.; Guntinas-Lichius, O.; Wittekindt, C. Botulinum toxin type b for the treatment of a sialocele after parotidectomy. *Head Neck* **2013**, *35*, E11–E12. [CrossRef]
49. Steffen, A.; Wollenberg, B.; Schönweiler, R.; Brüggemann, N.; Meyners, T. Drooling nach Strahlentherapie. Botulinumtoxin als erfolgreiches Therapieverfahren [Drooling following radiation. Botulinum toxin as a successful treatment modality]. *HNO* **2011**, *59*, 115–117. [CrossRef]
50. Hill, S.E.; Mortimer, N.J.; Hitchcock, B.; Salmon, P.J. Parotid fistula complicating surgical excision of a basal cell carcinoma: Successful treatment with botulinum toxin type A. *Dermatol. Surg.* **2007**, *33*, 1365–1367. [CrossRef]
51. Kizilay, A.; Aladağ, I.; Ozturan, O. Parotidektomi sonrasi gelişen tükürük fistülünün botulinum toksini ile iyileşmesi [Successful use of botulinum toxin injection in the treatment of salivary fistula following parotidectomy]. *Kulak Burun Bogaz Ihtis Derg.* **2003**, *10*, 78–81.
52. Guntinas-Lichius, O.; Sittel, C. Treatment of postparotidectomy salivary fistula with botulinum toxin. *Ann. Otol. Rhinol. Laryngol.* **2001**, *110*, 1162–1164. [CrossRef] [PubMed]
53. Marchese Ragona, R.; Blotta, P.; Pastore, A.; Tugnoli, V.; Eleopra, R.; De Grandis, D. Management of parotid sialocele with botulinum toxin. *Laryngoscope* **1999**, *109*, 1344–1346. [CrossRef] [PubMed]
54. Báez, A.; Paleari, J.; Durán, M.N.; Rudy, T.; Califano, I.; Barbosa, N.; Casas Parera, I. Síndrome de Frey por submaxilectomía y tratamiento con toxina botulínica [Frey syndrome secondary to submaxillectomy and botulinic treatment]. *Medicina (B Aires)* **2007**, *67*, 478–480.
55. Hatzis, G.P.; Finn, R. Using botox to treat a mohs defect repair complicated by a parotid fistula. *J. Oral Maxillofac. Surg.* **2007**, *65*, 2357–2360. [CrossRef]
56. Birch, J.F.; Varma, S.K.; Narula, A.A. Botulinum toxoid in the management of gustatory sweating (Frey's syndrome) after superficial parotidectomy. *Br. J. Plast. Surg.* **1999**, *52*, 230–231. [CrossRef]
57. Vezdrevanis, K. Prostatic carcinoma shrunk after intraprostatic injection of botulinum toxin. *Urol. J.* **2011**, *8*, 239–241.

58. Ulloa, F.; Gonzàlez-Juncà, A.; Meffre, D.; Barrecheguren, P.J.; Martínez-Mármol, R.; Pazos, I.; Olivé, N.; Cotrufo, T.; Seoane, J.; Soriano, E. Blockade of the SNARE protein syntaxin 1 inhibits glioblastoma tumor growth. *PLoS ONE* **2015**, *10*, e0119707. [CrossRef]
59. He, D.; Manzoni, A.; Florentin, D.; Fisher, W.; Ding, Y.; Lee, M.; Ayala, G. Biologic effect of neurogenesis in pancreatic cancer. *Hum. Pathol.* **2016**, *52*, 182–189. [CrossRef]
60. Karsenty, G.; Rocha, J.; Chevalier, S.; Scarlata, E.; Andrieu, C.; Zouanat, F.Z.; Rocchi, P.; Giusiano, S.; Elzayat, E.A.; Corcos, J. Botulinum toxin type A inhibits the growth of LNCaP human prostate cancer cells in vitro and in vivo. *Prostate* **2009**, *69*, 1143–1150. [CrossRef]
61. Nam, H.J.; Kang, J.K.; Chang, J.S.; Lee, M.S.; Nam, S.T.; Jung, H.W.; Kim, S.K.; Ha, E.M.; Seok, H.; Son, S.W.; et al. Cells transformed by PLC-gamma 1 overexpression are highly sensitive to clostridium difficile toxin A-induced apoptosis and mitotic inhibition. *J. Microbiol. Biotechnol.* **2012**, *22*, 50–57. [CrossRef]
62. Proietti, S.; Nardicchi, V.; Porena, M.; Giannantoni, A. Attività della tossina botulinica A in linee cellulari di cancro prostatico [Botulinum toxin type-A toxin activity on prostate cancer cell lines]. *Urologia* **2012**, *79*, 135–141. [CrossRef] [PubMed]
63. Bandala, C.; Perez-Santos, J.L.; Lara-Padilla, E.; Delgado Lopez, G.; Anaya-Ruiz, M. Effect of botulinum toxin A on proliferation and apoptosis in the T47D breast cancer cell line. *Asian Pac. J. Cancer Prev.* **2013**, *14*, 891–894. [CrossRef] [PubMed]
64. Bandala, C.; Cortés-Algara, A.L.; Mejía-Barradas, C.M.; Ilizaliturri-Flores, I.; Dominguez-Rubio, R.; Bazán-Méndez, C.I.; Floriano-Sánchez, E.; Luna-Arias, J.P.; Anaya-Ruiz, M.; Lara-Padilla, E.; et al. Botulinum neurotoxin type A inhibits synaptic vesicle 2 expression in breast cancer cell lines. *Int. J. Clin. Exp. Pathol.* **2015**, *8*, 8411–8418. [PubMed]
65. Rust, A.; Leese, C.; Binz, T.; Davletov, B. Botulinum neurotoxin type C protease induces apoptosis in differentiated human neuroblastoma cells. *Oncotarget* **2016**, *7*, 33220–33228. [CrossRef]
66. Huang, X.; Wheeler, M.B.; Kang, Y.H.; Sheu, L.; Lukacs, G.L.; Trimble, W.S.; Gaisano, H.Y. Truncated SNAP-25 (1-197), like botulinum neurotoxin A, can inhibit insulin secretion from HIT-T15 insulinoma cells. *Mol. Endocrinol.* **1998**, *12*, 1060–1070. [CrossRef]
67. Hajighasemlou, S.; Alebouyeh, M.; Rastegar, H.; Manzari, M.T.; Mirmoghtadaei, M.; Moayedi, B.; Ahmadzadeh, M.; Parvizpour, F.; Johari, B.; Naeini, M.M.; et al. Preparation of Immunotoxin Herceptin-Botulinum and Killing Effects on Two Breast Cancer Cell Lines. *Asian Pac. J. Cancer Prev.* **2015**, *16*, 5977–5981. [CrossRef]
68. Cheng, Y.T.; Chung, Y.H.; Kang, H.Y.; Tai, M.H.; Chancellor, M.B.; Chuang, Y.C. OnobotulinumtoxinA Has No Effects on Growth of LNCaP and PC3 Human Prostate Cancer Cells. *Low. Urin. Tract Symptoms* **2013**, *5*, 168–172. [CrossRef]
69. Ansiaux, R.; Gallez, B. Use of botulinum toxins in cancer therapy. *Expert Opin. Investig. Drugs* **2007**, *16*, 209–218. [CrossRef]
70. Coarfa, C.; Florentin, D.; Putluri, N.; Ding, Y.; Au, J.; He, D.; Ragheb, A.; Frolov, A.; Michailidis, G.; Lee, M.; et al. Influence of the neural microenvironment on prostate cancer. *Prostate* **2018**, *78*, 128–139. [CrossRef]
71. Matak, I.; Bölcskei, K.; Bach-Rojecky, L.; Helyes, Z. Mechanisms of Botulinum Toxin Type A Action on Pain. *Toxins* **2019**, *11*, 459. [CrossRef]
72. Mittal, S.O.; Safarpour, D.; Jabbari, B. Botulinum Toxin Treatment of Neuropathic Pain. *Semin. Neurol.* **2016**, *36*, 73–83. [CrossRef] [PubMed]
73. Kitamura, Y.; Matsuka, Y.; Spigelman, I.; Ishihara, Y.; Yamamoto, Y.; Sonoyama, W.; Kamioka, H.; Yamashiro, T.; Kuboki, T.; Oguma, K. Botulinum toxin type a (150 kDa) decreases exaggerated neurotransmitter release from trigeminal ganglion neurons and relieves neuropathy behaviors induced by infraorbital nerve constriction. *Neuroscience* **2009**, *159*, 1422–1429. [CrossRef] [PubMed]
74. Omoto, K.; Maruhama, K.; Terayama, R.; Yamamoto, Y.; Matsushita, O.; Sugimoto, T.; Oguma, K.; Matsuka, Y. Cross-Excitation in Peripheral Sensory Ganglia Associated with Pain Transmission. *Toxins* **2015**, *7*, 2906–2917. [CrossRef] [PubMed]
75. Marino, M.J.; Terashima, T.; Steinauer, J.J.; Eddinger, K.A.; Yaksh, T.L.; Xu, Q. Botulinum toxin B in the sensory afferent: Transmitter release, spinal activation, and pain behavior. *Pain* **2014**, *155*, 674–684. [CrossRef] [PubMed]

76. Hong, B.; Yao, L.; Ni, L.; Wang, L.; Hu, X. Antinociceptive effect of botulinum toxin A involves alterations in AMPA receptor expression and glutamate release in spinal dorsal horn neurons. *Neuroscience* **2017**, *357*, 197–207. [CrossRef] [PubMed]
77. Fan, C.; Chu, X.; Wang, L.; Shi, H.; Li, T. Botulinum toxin type A reduces TRPV1 expression in the dorsal root ganglion in rats with adjuvant-arthritis pain. *Toxicon* **2017**, *133*, 116–122. [CrossRef]
78. Restani, L.; Antonucci, F.; Gianfranceschi, L.; Rossi, C.; Rossetto, O.; Caleo, M. Evidence for anterograde transport and transcytosis of botulinum neurotoxin A (BoNT/A). *J. Neurosci.* **2011**, *31*, 15650–15659. [CrossRef]
79. Matak, I.; Bach-Rojecky, L.; Filipović, B.; Lacković, Z. Behavioral and immunohistochemical evidence for central antinociceptive activity of botulinum toxin A. *Neuroscience* **2011**, *186*, 201–207. [CrossRef]
80. Bach-Rojecky, L.; Salković-Petrisić, M.; Lacković, Z. Botulinum toxin type A reduces pain supersensitivity in experimental diabetic neuropathy: Bilateral effect after unilateral injection. *Eur. J. Pharmacol.* **2010**, *633*, 10–14. [CrossRef]
81. Bach-Rojecky, L.; Lacković, Z. Central origin of the antinociceptive action of botulinum toxin type A. *Pharmacol. Biochem. Behav.* **2009**, *94*, 234–238. [CrossRef]
82. Arezzo, J.C. Possible mechanisms for the effects of botulinum toxin on pain. *Clin. J. Pain.* **2002**, *18* (Suppl. S6), S125–S132. [CrossRef]
83. Neufeld, N.J.; Elnahal, S.M.; Alvarez, R.H. Cancer pain: A review of epidemiology, clinical quality and value impact. *Future Oncol.* **2017**, *13*, 833–841. [CrossRef] [PubMed]
84. Schreiber, K.L.; Kehlet, H.; Belfer, I.; Edwards, R.R. Predicting, preventing and managing persistent pain after breast cancer surgery: The importance of psychosocial factors. *Pain Manag.* **2014**, *4*, 445–459. [CrossRef] [PubMed]
85. Fisher, J.; Scott, C.; Stevens, R.; Marconi, B.; Champion, L.; Freedman, G.M.; Asrari, F.; Pilepich, M.V.; Gagnon, J.D.; Wong, G. Randomized phase III study comparing best supportive care to Biafine as a prophylactic agent for radiation-induced skin toxicity for women undergoing breast irradiation: Radiation Therapy Oncology Group [RTOG] 97–13. *Int. J. Radiat. Oncol. Biol. Phys.* **2000**, *48*, 1307–1310. [CrossRef]
86. Chargari, C.; Fromantin, I.; Kirova, Y.M. Importance of local skin treatments during radiotherapy for prevention and treatment of radio-induced epithelitis. *Cancer Radiother.* **2009**, *13*, 259–266. [CrossRef] [PubMed]
87. Kirova, Y.M.; Fromantin, I.; De Rycke, Y.; Fourquet, A.; Morvan, E.; Padiglione, S.; Falcou, M.C.; Campana, F.; Bollet, M.A. Can we decrease the skin reaction in breast cancer patients using hyaluronic acid during radiation therapy-results of phase III randomised trial. *Radiother. Oncol.* **2011**, *100*, 205–209. [CrossRef]
88. Fleming, J.A.; O'Connor, B.D. Use of lidocaine patches for neuropathic pain in a comprehensive cancer center. *Pain Res. Manag.* **2009**, *14*, 381–388. [CrossRef]
89. Wiffen, P.J.; Derry, S.; Moore, R.A. Impact of morphine, fentanyl, oxycodone or codeine on patient consciousness, appetite and thirst when used to treat cancer pain. *Cochrane Database Syst. Rev.* **2014**, *5*, CD011056.
90. Lakraje, A.A.; Moghimi, N.; Jabbari, B. Sialorrhea, anatomy, physiology and treatment with emphasis on the role of botulinum toxins. *Toxins* **2013**, *5*, 1010–1031. [CrossRef]
91. Schindel, J.; Markowicz, H.; Levie, B. Combined surgical-radiological treatment of parotid gland fistulae. *J. Laryngol. Otol.* **1968**, *82*, 867–870. [CrossRef]
92. Lovato, A.; Restivo, D.A.; Ottaviano, G.; Marioni, G.; Marchese-Ragona, R. Botulinum toxin therapy: Functional silencing of salivary disorders. Terapia con tossina botulinica: Silenziamento funzionale dei disordini salivari. *Acta Otorhinolaryngol. Ital.* **2017**, *37*, 168–171. [CrossRef] [PubMed]

7

Pro-Inflammatory Cytokines in the Formation of the Pre-Metastatic Niche

Ru Li, Annie Wen and Jun Lin *

Department of Anesthesiology, Stony Brook University Health Sciences Center,
Stony Brook, NY 11794-8480, USA; ru.li@stonybrookmedicine.edu (R.L.); annie.wen@stonybrook.edu (A.W.)
* Correspondence: jun.lin@stonybrookmedicine.edu

Simple Summary: The formation of the pre-metastatic niche, a favorable microenvironment in an organ distant from a primary tumor, is critical for tumor metastasis. We review the role of a key player, a class of proteins named pro-inflammatory cytokines secreted from both tumor cells and other cells in tissues, in helping to build the pre-metastatic niche. Various drugs have been developed to target pro-inflammatory cytokines, and their effects on tumor metastases are under investigation. Future clinical studies should focus on combining those drugs and applying them during cancer surgery, a critical moment for the establishment of the pre-metastatic niche.

Abstract: In the presence of a primary tumor, the pre-metastatic niche is established in secondary organs as a favorable microenvironment for subsequent tumor metastases. This process is orchestrated by bone marrow-derived cells, primary tumor-derived factors, and extracellular matrix. In this review, we summarize the role of pro-inflammatory cytokines including interleukin (IL)-6, IL-1β, CC-chemokine ligand 2 (CCL2), granulocyte-colony stimulating factor (G-CSF), granulocyte–macrophage colony-stimulating factor (GM-CSF), stromal cell-derived factor (SDF)-1, macrophage migration inhibitory factor (MIF), and Chemokine (C–X–C motif) ligand 1 (CXCL1) in the formation of the pre-metastatic niche according to the most recent studies. Pro-inflammatory cytokines released from tumor cells or stromal cells act in both autocrine and paracrine manners to induce phenotype changes in tumor cells, recruit bone marrow-derived cells, and form an inflammatory milieu, all of which prime a secondary organ's microenvironment for metastatic cell colonization. Considering the active involvement of pro-inflammatory cytokines in niche formation, clinical strategies targeting them offer ways to inhibit the establishment of the pre-metastatic niche and therefore attenuate metastatic progression. We review clinical trials targeting different inflammatory cytokines in patients with metastatic cancers. Due to the pleiotropy and redundancy of pro-inflammatory cytokines, combined therapies should be designed in the future.

Keywords: pre-metastatic niche; pro-inflammatory cytokines; clinical trials

---

1. Introduction

Tumor metastasis is the main cause of therapeutic failure and mortality, with few effective treatment options. It has been suggested that the tumor microenvironment plays a prominent role in the formation of metastasis, collaborating with genetic and epigenetic networks in cancer cells [1,2]. A key step for the formation of tumor metastases is the extravasation of circulating tumor cells into distant organs and their adaption to new environments. Therefore, the reciprocal interactions between to the disseminated cancer cells and the microenvironment in distant organs are imperative to successful metastasis. Primary tumor cells orchestrate the metastasis process through secreting a variety of molecules which promote the mobilization and recruitment of various types of cells to the premetastatic sites and alter the expression of matrix proteins and the properties of the extracellular matrix (ECM) in secondary organs. All these events help create the so-called pre-metastatic niche (PMN), suitable for the engraftment of metastasizing tumor cells. The concept of PMN was first proposed by Dr. David Lyden in 2005 [3]. Since then, targeting the PMN to prevent metastasis has become a promising strategy for cancer treatment. However, much remains to be revealed about the factors that facilitate the establishment of the implantation site for tumor metastasis.

Priming of the organ-specific premetastatic sites is an important yet incompletely understood step during metastasis formation. Bone marrow-derived cells (BMDCs) and tumor-derived secreted factors are the two crucial components for pre-metastatic niche formation. The main type of BMDCs accumulated in the pre-metastatic niche is myeloid-derived suppressor cells (MDSCs). When infections and tissue injuries occur, the myeloid lineage is promptly expanded, and myeloid leukocytes in the bone marrow perform a protective role in host defense against such stresses and traumas. However, chronic inflammation associated with cancer induces the expression of pro-inflammatory cytokines that drive the differentiation of myeloid cells towards MDSCs. MDSCs are a heterogeneous population of immature myeloid cells including macrophages, granulocytes, neutrophiles, and dendritic cells. They accumulate in the circulation of cancer patients and are recruited to peripheral lymphoid organs and tumor sites by growth factors released by cancer cells. Within the tumor microenvironment, MDSC were shown to inhibit the proliferation and activity of killer T cells, promote angiogenesis, and improve tumor cells survival, thereby promoting tumor invasion and metastasis [4]. Besides the recruited MDSCs, the host stromal environment of the PMN also includes fibroblast, endothelial cells, and ECM.

Tumor-derived secreted factors play important roles in preparing distant organs for pre-metastatic niche formation. Tumor-derived secreted factors include cytokines, chemokines, growth factors, and extracellular vesicles (EV). Cytokines are a diverse family of small proteins secreted by cells, predominantly by helper T cells and macrophages for cell-to-cell communication. Cytokines could act on the cells releasing them (autocrine action), on nearby cells (paracrine action), or on distant cells (endocrine action) and are often produced in a cascade, as one cytokine stimulates its target cells to produce additional cytokines. The major subgroups of cytokines include interleukins, interferons, colony-stimulating factors, chemokines, and tumor necrosis factors. Cytokines exert their effects through binding to cytokine receptors on target cells, which activates a sequence of downstream proteins for the desired responses. It should be noted that the effects of different cytokines are sometimes redundant, with different cytokines eliciting similar responses [5,6]. Cytokines play a key role in tumor progression and metastasis by either directly regulating tumor growth, invasiveness, and metastasis or indirectly affecting stromal cells and immune cells [7]. Accumulating evidence suggests that pro-inflammatory cytokines are pivotal in the formation of the pre-metastatic niche. Tumor cell-derived pro-inflammatory cytokines and chemokines recruit a variety of regulatory and suppressive immune cells into distant sites to prime the local environment. The proliferative and invasive abilities of disseminated cancer cells are enhanced by proinflammatory cytokines from the surrounding microenvironment as paracrine signals. Thus, cancer cells can undergo epithelial-to-mesenchymal transition (EMT) to grow in distant tissues. In this review, we focus on the role of important pro-inflammatory cytokines in the establishment of the PMN and highlight the underlying mechanisms of PMN formation in various organs based on the most recent studies (Figure 1).

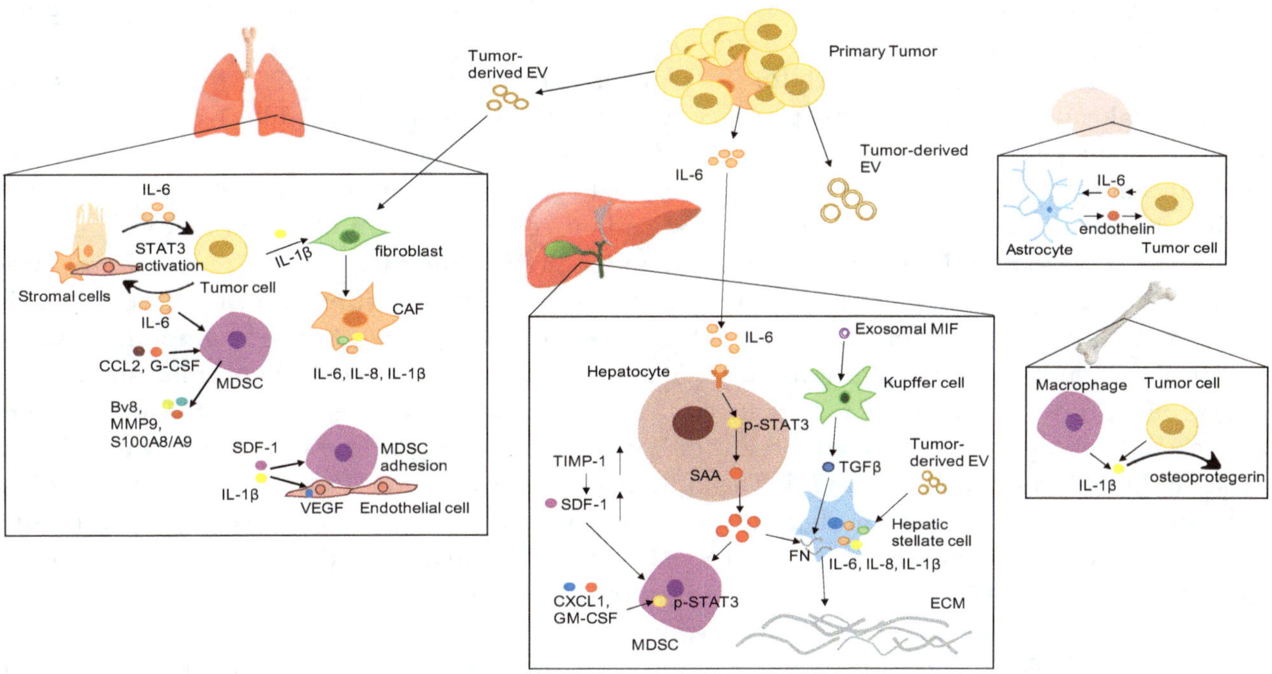

Figure 1. Proposed mechanisms by which various pro-inflammatory cytokines promote the formation of the pre-metastatic niche in different organs. Abbreviation: EV: extracellular vesicles; IL-6: interleukin 6; IL-1β: interleukin-1β; SDF-1 α: stromal cell-derived factor 1; IL-8: interleukin 8; VEGF: vascular endothelial growth factor; G-CSF: granulocyte-colony stimulating factor; CCL2: CC-chemokine ligand 2; CXCL1: C-X-C motif ligan 1; MIF: macrophage migration inhibitory factor; TIMP-1: tissue inhibitor of metalloproteinases 1; GM-CSF: granulocyte-macrophage colony-stimulating factor; SAA: serum amyloid A; TGF-β: transforming growth factor beta; FN: fibronectin; ECM: extracellular matrix; STAT3: signal transducer and activator of transcription 3; CAF: cancer associated fibroblast; MDSC: myeloid-derived suppressor cells.

2. Interleukin 6

Interleukin 6 (IL-6) is recognized as a potent inflammatory cytokine that is widely expressed in a variety of immune cells and malignant tumors. IL-6 binds to its receptor to form a binary complex, which further dimerizes with its coreceptor glycoprotein 130 (GP130). Subsequently, GP130 activates Janus kinase (JAK), which then induces the phosphorylation of signal transducer and activator of transcription 3 (STAT3) [8]. The elevated IL-6 level and hyperactivation of the JAK/STAT3 pathway are often associated with poor patient outcomes [9–12]. JAK-mediated STAT3 tyrosine phosphorylation not only drives malignant cell proliferation, survival, and invasiveness, but also strongly compromises antitumor immunity in the tumor microenvironment [13–15]. In parallel, activated STAT3 can also promote IL-6 gene expression, resulting in a feed-forward autocrine loop. In the tumor microenvironment, the IL-6 signaling pathway affects a variety of stromal cells, including endothelial cells, fibroblasts, and cells of the immune system, which are active participants in angiogenesis and inflammatory and immune-suppressive responses [16].

During tumor progression, the induction of EMT is a key step for the transition from a quiescent to a metastatic tumor. In colorectal cancer cells, IL-6 activated STAT3 to suppress the MIR34A gene via a conserved STAT3-binding site in the first intron and further promoted EMT and invasion. Members of the miR-34 family are induced by tumor suppressor p53 and are known to suppress the early phases of metastasis through inhibiting EMT. They also directly target IL-6R and downregulate it. The IL6/STAT3/miR-34a feedback loop appears essential for EMT, invasion, and metastasis of colorectal, breast, and prostate cancer cells [17]. In addition to miR-34a, other microRNAs in EV profoundly affect the establishment of the PMN through various mechanisms including angiogenesis, EMT, metastatic colonization, as reviewed [18,19]. In breast cancer, adipocytes from the tumor microenvironment could produce IL-6, which then activates STAT3 in cancer cells and induces the EMT phenotype by increasing the expression of PLOD2, which is important for matrix remodeling [20,21].

Liver metastases develop in nearly 25% of patients with colorectal cancer [22]. Ji et al. have shown in a colorectal cancer model that the primary tumor released integrin beta-like 1-rich extracellular vesicles to lungs and liver, which converted resident fibroblasts to cancer-associated fibroblast (CAF) in the lungs and activated hepatic stellate cells in the liver by stimulating TNFAIP3-mediated NF-κB signaling pathway [23]. As one of the most abundant cell types in the tumor microenvironment, the activated CAFs modulate the inflammatory microenvironment by secreting pro-inflammatory cytokines including IL-6, IL-8, and IL-1β and play a key role in depositing and the ECM. CAFs also produce high levels of transforming growth factor beta (TGF-β), α-SMA, and chemokine CXCL12, transforming fibroblasts into myofibroblasts. The interaction between CAFs and metastatic tumor cells has been studied extensively (as reviewed [24]). Pancreatic cancer also frequently spreads to the liver. Lee and colleagues investigated the role of IL-6 in forming the pre-metastatic niche in the liver in mouse models of pancreatic cancer [25]. The authors demonstrated that IL-6 derived from fibroblasts in a primary pancreatic tumor binds to its receptor on hepatocytes, the main cell type in the liver, and drives the expression and activation of STAT3. Subsequently, the activated hepatocytes secrete serum amyloid A1 (SAA1) and SAA2, which then attract myeloid cells into the liver. The accumulation of myeloid cells dampens immune surveillance by releasing cytokines that inhibit cancer-killing T cells. The activation of STAT3 also drives the deposition of extracellular matrix, which contributes to the initial anchoring and sustenance of metastatic cancer cells. All these events prepare the liver for the influx of cancer cells.

The lung is one of the most common sites of cancer metastasis, partially due to its efficiency at arresting circulating tumor cells because of the reduced capillary size. In experimental metastasis models, pre-metastatic events, including BMDC mobilization and the activation of inflammatory pathways, have been suggested to modify the lungs in order to facilitate the development of a pre-metastatic environment for circulating tumor cells [3,26,27]. Chang et al. showed that IL-6 derived from invasive breast cancer cells at advanced stages activated STAT3 through JAK in both the tumor itself and the surrounding stromal cells. It also regulated MDSC (CD11b+/Gr1+) expansion and macrophage (CD11b+/F480+) infiltration in distant organs like the lungs, leading to the establishment of an inflammatory microenvironment in pre-metastatic sites [28]. A recently published study investigated inter-lung metastasis of lung cancer. In lung tissue, GPRC5A (G-protein-coupled receptor, family C, member 5A) is predominately expressed and acts as a lung tumor suppressor gene [29]. The suppression of GPRC5A contributes to lung cancer development with chronic inflammation. The study showed that depletion of the upregulated IL-6 in GPRC5A knockout (Gprc5a-ko) mice almost completely eliminated lung metastasis. Dysregulated IL-6 signaling is intrinsically linked to the stem-like and immunosuppressive features of the metastatic tumor. IL-6 also induced recruitment of MDSCs and macrophage polarization, which inhibits host immunity. All these pieces of evidence indicated that IL-6 in Gprc5a-ko mouse lungs is essential for pre-metastatic niche formation [30]. IL-6/STAT3 signaling in tumor-containing lung tissue is activated via reciprocal interactions between metastatic tumor cells and stromal cells. Blockade of STAT3 signaling in lung cancer cells prevented lung metastasis in immune-competent syngeneic mice, but not in immune-deficient nude mice, which implies that STAT3-mediated immunosuppressive traits in tumor cells are functionally critical for lung metastasis in vivo [30]. Moreover, lymphatic endothelial cells of stromal lymphatic vessels in the pre-metastatic niche also contribute to metastasis. Primary tumor-secreted IL-6 activated STAT3 in lymphatic endothelial cells, which then induced the expression of hypoxia-inducible factor 1 (HIF-1), vascular endothelial growth factor (VEGF), and chemokine ligand 5 (CCL5). Tumor-conditioned lymphatic endothelial cells directed disseminated tumor cells into lungs and lymph nodes, promoted angiogenesis in distant organs, and allowed tumor extravasation and colonization [25].

Brain metastases of breast cancer, mostly in patients with HER2+ or triple-negative tumors, have exceeded the incident rate of 30% in metastatic breast cancer patients [31] and confer a poor prognosis, with extremely short survival despite treatment [32]. Current systemic treatments include surgery and radiotherapy but have inadequate effects due to the enhanced resistance of metastatic tumor cells in the brain and limited access of drug to the brain because of the blood–brain barrier (BBB). It has been shown that the interaction between astrocyte and MDA-MB-231 cells induced the production of IL-6 and IL-8 by cancer cells. Cancer cell-derived IL-6 and IL-8 upregulated endothelin receptor expression on cancer cells and the production of endothelin from astrocytes. The endothelin axis then activated protein kinase B (AKT) and mitogen-activated protein kinase (MAPK) signaling pathways in MDA-MB-231 cells and protected the cancer cells from chemotherapeutic agents [33].

Through all these pre-clinical studies, we can conclude that IL-6 is a potent inflammatory cytokines and activator of STAT3, produced not only by tumor cells but also by cells in the PMN (Figure 1). It would suggest that tumor cells and stromal cells interdependently regulate IL-6 expression in cancers, which may account for the localized activation of the IL-6/STAT3 pathway. Although all these studies differed in murine models and cancer cells used, the therapeutic paradigm of targeting IL-6 pathway at the early stages of metastasis formation is promising. These discoveries should be investigated further, especially in aggressive tumors such as triple-negative breast cancer, pancreatic cancer, colorectal cancer, and lung cancer.

3. Interleukin-1β

Interleukin-1β (IL-1β) is a pleiotropic cytokine that affects inflammatory responses, immune reactivity, and hemopoiesis in broad paracrine and endocrine manners. The potency of IL-1β originates from its ability to induce the secretion of a network of proinflammatory molecules and the expression of adhesion molecules in diverse cells, thereby amplifying and sustaining its responses. As a mature secreted molecule, IL-1β is one of the most potent pro-inflammatory cytokines abundant in primary tumor sites and in the tumor microenvironment in distant organs, which controls local proinflammatory cascades and thereby also affects the balance between antitumor cell immunity and destructive inflammation [34–36]. The local expression of IL-1β in tumor sites has been correlated with increased invasiveness in experimental tumors and in cancer patients and is associated with a bad prognosis [34,37]. Neutralizing IL-1β or blocking its receptor represents a direct targeted approach. Nowadays, several mediators blocking or neutralizing the IL-1 pathway such as antibodies and small-molecule inhibitors are in use or being tested for cancer treatment [38,39]. In this review, we will focus on the effect of IL-1β on the establishment of pre-metastatic niches.

In breast cancer metastasis, Schmid and colleague found that IL-1β was highly expressed in the microenvironment of murine lung, pancreatic, and breast tumors and was produced only by tumor-associated granulocytes and macrophage. The recruitment of myeloid cells induces inflammation in the premetastatic niche. IL-1β works together with SDF-1α to stimulate the adhesion of myeloid cells to the endothelium by activating integrin α4β1 [40]. Furthermore, IL-1β has been demonstrated to induce the expression and the release of IL-17 in γδ T cells (γδ T cells are a small subset of T cells that express heterodimeric T cell receptors composed of γ and δ chains) that led to the expansion and polarization of granulocyte-colony stimulating factor (G-CSF)-dependent neutrophils in mammary tumor-bearing mice. The accumulation of neutrophils and γδ T cells in turn suppressed $CD8^+$ T lymphocytes and allowed for pulmonary and lymph node metastasis formation [41]. A recent study showed that CXCR3-postive metastatic MDA-MB-231 cells (MDA-MB-231 cells expressing the chemokine receptor CXCR3) expressed high levels of IL-1α/β via JNK signaling to evoke phenotypic changes in lung fibroblasts. Those fibroblasts in an inflammatory state produced the chemokines CXCL9 and CXCL10 through NF-κB signaling, supporting the formation of the metastatic niche. CXCR3 is the only receptor known to bind and be activated by CXCL9 and CXCL10. Meanwhile, knockdown of IL-1β was shown to limit the capability of cancer cells to colonize the lungs, demonstrating that IL-1β is needed for lung metastasis formation and growth [42].

The poor prognosis of advance breast cancer patients with bone metastasis urges new therapeutic approaches. Knowledge of the molecular mechanism of breast cancer colonization of the bone microenvironment is imperative for the development of future diagnostic and curative therapies. In breast cancer bone metastasis, it was suggested that IL-1β contributed to the osteotropic nature of breast cancer cells. The analysis of tumor tissues from advanced-stage breast cancer patients demonstrated an increase in the likelihood of developing bone metastases in patients with IL-1β-positive primary tumors compared to patients with IL-1β-negative tumors. Based on that observation, Nutter and colleagues developed a bone-homing clone of the triple-negative breast cancer cells MDA-MB-231 and found that it had increased expression of IL-1β and decreased expression of the cell adhesion molecule fibronectin and of the calcium-binding proteins S100A4 [43]. Besides the autocrine mechanism of breast-cancer derived IL-1β in driving the cancer cell bone-seeking behavior, it was observed that MDA-MB-231 cells migrated to and colonized human bone tissue-conditioned medium that contained high levels of IL-1β, which indicates that IL-1β derived from the bone tissue microenvironment may also support the osteotropic breast cancer cell behavior [44]. Moreover, IL-1β from macrophages or breast cancer cells themselves has been shown to induce the secretion of osteoprotegerin, a secreted member of the TNF receptor family involved in bone resorption, in breast cancer via the p38 and p42/22 MAPK signaling pathways. Inhibition of osteoprotegerin limits tumor invasion and metastasis, suggesting that osteoprotegerin and IL-1β play a role in mediating breast cancer metastasis [45].

Another significant effect of IL-1β promoting tumor metastasis is its ability to potentiate tumor angiogenesis. Carmi and colleague found that the cross-talk between IL-1β and VEGF regulated the early angiogenic response, which procured a microenvironment suitable for angiogenesis and tumor development. VEGFR1^{+}/IL-1R1^{+} immature myeloid cells produce IL-1β along with other inflammatory chemokines and cytokines that enable endothelial cells to produce VEGF and other proangiogenic factors. In fact, IL-1β appeared essential for the in vivo response of endothelial cells that impaired IL-1β signaling and reduced the neo-angiogenic response in mice despite the presence of recombinant VEGF [46]. IL-1β was also found to upregulate the production of VEGF and its receptor on vascular smooth muscle cells, which activates p38 MAPK and MAPK-activated protein kinase 2 via IL-1R1, promoting cell migration and angiogenesis [47]. One study also noted an increased expression of IL-1β and E-selectin in premetastatic lungs in mice with melanoma, prior to the arrival of tumor cells. IL-1β was produced by monocytic MDSCs in the premetastatic lungs, promoted E-selectin expression, and led to tumor cell adhesion to the vascular endothelium [48].

In contrast to most of the available data, metastasis-inhibiting effects have also been described for IL-1β in breast cancer. Castano and colleague demonstrated that primary tumors elicited a response by innate immune cells that expressed IL-1β, which infiltrated metastatic microenvironments. At the metastatic site, IL-1β prevented metastatic cells from differentiating into highly proliferative E-cadherin-positive cells, which could form actively growing tumors. These authors also conducted a database analysis and revealed a beneficial effect of high primary tumor IL-1β expression on overall survival and distant metastasis-free survival in patients with lymph node-positive breast cancer [49].

The role of inflammatory IL-1β signaling in cancer is complex. Both pro-metastatic and anti-metastatic effects of IL-1 have been shown in mouse models, which are greatly dependent on the organ affected by cancer, cancer subtype, and the inflammatory background and stage of cancer. The source of IL-1β is also critical to determine its effect. The chronic low levels of IL-1β produced by the tumor itself may promote an immune-suppressive environment. On the other hand, exogenous administration of high levels of IL-1β might elicit an anti-tumorigenic effect.

4. Other Cytokines

Besides IL-6 and IL-1β, several other cytokine/chemokines are also studied in the PMN formation. CC-chemokine ligand 2 (CCL2), also known as monocyte chemotactic protein-1 (MCP-1), is a member of the CCβ cytokine family. Pollard and colleagues found that in the MMTV–PyMT mouse model of breast cancer, Gr1^{+} inflammatory monocytes expressing CCR2 (receptor for CCL2) were recruited to the premetastatic lung through CCL2 secreted by tumor and stromal cells and differentiated into tumor-associated macrophages (TAM) to promote the subsequent growth of metastatic cells.

Inhibition of CCL2 signaling or depletion of tumor cell-derived CCL2 diminished lung metastases in vivo [50]. However, monocytes are not the only population recruited to premetastatic lung by CCL2. Another study showed that tumor-entrained neutrophils also accumulated in the lungs via CCL2 and inhibited metastatic seeding in lungs by producing H_2O_2 [51]. Similar to IL-1β, both pro-metastatic and anti-metastatic effects have been reported for CCL2. To understand if CCL2 can be a clinical target, it is necessary to define how the pro- and anti-metastatic effects are concomitantly regulated and which effect is dominant at each stage of metastasis.

Kowanetz and colleagues have indicated that tumor-secreted G-CSF expanded and mobilized $Ly6G^+Ly6C^+$ granulocytes from the bone marrow. G-CSF-mobilized $Ly6G^+Ly6C^+$ cells produced a series of pro-metastatic proteins such as Bv8, matrix-degrading enzyme MMP-9, inflammatory chemoattractants S100A8/A9 [52]. In addition to G-CSF, primary tumor-derived TNF-α and TGFβ have also been implicated in the regulation of S100A8 and S100A9 expression in the pre-metastatic lungs, which were involved in the recruitment of MDSCs in distant organs [53]. Another colony-stimulating factor, tumor cell-secreted granulocyte–macrophage colony-stimulating factor (GM-CSF), has been shown to promote liver metastasis by inducing STAT3 phosphorylation in the liver MDSC. Activated STAT3 signaling promoted the expression of indoleamine 2,3-dioxygenase (IDO) and programmed death ligand 1 (PD-L1), both important mediators of T cell suppression. Inhibition of GM-CSF or GM-CSF-R markedly reduced IDO and PD-L1 expression in liver MDSCs, implicating tumor-derived GM-CSF in supporting the expression of immunoinhibitory molecules in MDSCs. Blockage of JAK2 and STAT3 also dramatically diminished IDO and PD-L1 expression in MDSCs, implying that STAT3 exerts transcriptional control over IDO and PD-L1 expression by binding to the *IDO1* and *PD-L1* promoters. All these results implicate GM-CSF and STAT3 as critical drivers of liver MDSC IDO/PD-L1 expression and potential mechanistic targets to enhance intrahepatic anti-tumor immunity [54].

One essential pathway governing tumor cell homing to the bone is the CXCL12–CXC chemokine receptor 4 (CXCR4) signaling axis. CXCL12 (stromal cell-derived factor 1, SDF-1) is a homeostatic chemokine predominantly produced by a diversity of stromal cells in the bone marrow including BM-MSCs, endothelial cells, CXCL12-abundant reticular (CAR) cells, and osteoblasts. Solid tumor cells overexpress the CXCL12 receptors CXCR4 and CXCR7 and migrate to CXCL12-expressing bone tissue via chemotaxis along a concentration gradient. In an experimental bone metastasis model of prostate cancer, prostate cancer cells target the hematopoietic stem cell (HSC) niche, use the CXCL12–CXCR4 axis to home to the niche, and compete with the HSC cells for niche support [55]. In colorectal cancer, a high systemic level of tissue inhibitor of metalloproteinases (TIMP)-1 led to increased hepatic SDF-1 level, which in turn promoted the recruitment of neutrophils to the liver. The activation of SDF-1 and the accumulation of neutrophils triggered the formation of a premetastatic niche and thus increased liver susceptibility towards metastasis. This promoted hepatic metastasis, independent of the origin or the intrinsic metastatic potential of tumor cells [56].

Macrophage migration inhibitory factor (MIF) is a well-known mediator of liver inflammation and fibrosis. For pancreatic cancer that metastasizes to the liver, exosomal MIF induced the release of TGFβ by Kupffer cells in the liver, which further induced the deposit of fibronectin in the ECM by hepatic stellate cells. Fibronectin deposition subsequently summoned BMDCs and triggered PMN formation [57].

Chemokine (C–X–C motif) ligand 1 (CXCL1) is a member of the CXCL class of chemokines with neutrophil chemotactic and angiogenic properties. In an orthotopic mouse model of colorectal cancer, VEGF secreted by colorectal tumor cells stimulated the production of CXCL1 from TAM. The increase of CXCL1 in the liver recruited CXCR2-positive (CXCL1 receptor) MDSCs and facilitated the establishment of PMN in the liver [58].

5. Clinical Trials Targeting Pro-Inflammatory Cytokines in Metastatic Cancer

Pro-inflammatory cytokines are key mediators of innate and adaptive immunity at the crossroad of diverse pathways shaping pre-metastatic niches. Nowadays, several agents targeting IL-6, IL-6 receptor,

JAKs, or STAT3 have been used in the treatment of myeloma and tested in patients with solid tumors [8,59]. There are two FDA-approved antibodies directly targeting IL-6: siltuximab, a chimeric anti-IL-6 antibody [60], and tocilizumab, a humanized monoclonal antibody against the IL-6 receptor. Various global clinical trials, series, and pilot studies of off-label use of siltuximab and tocilizumab provide strong indications [61] that the anti-IL-6 therapy may be used for the treatment of blood cancers such as multiple myeloma [62] and leukemia [63] and of solid tumors such as prostate cancer [64], breast cancer [65], and ovarian cancer [66]. However, two phase II trials which employed siltuximab as second-line therapy for patients with metastatic prostate cancer showed an increase in plasma IL-6 after treatment and confirmed the poor prognosis associated with elevated IL-6 [60,67]. Two clinical trials, one (NCT04191421) evaluating siltuximab in metastatic pancreatic cancer patients and the other (NCT03135171) evaluating tocilizumab in metastatic HER2-postive breast cancer patients are in progress (Table 1).

Downstream in the IL-6 signaling pathway, JAK is another important drug target for cancer treatment. Among various JAK inhibitors, ruxolitinib is the most extensively investigated for cancer treatment. Approved by the FDA in 2011 for the treatment of myelofibrosis and post-polycythemia vera, ruxolitinib is a potent and selective oral JAK1 and JAK2 inhibitor. Studies on the safety and effectiveness of ruxolitinib in cancer patients with solid tumors such as breast cancer (NCT01594216, lung cancer (NCT02145637), colorectal cancer (NCT04303403), pancreatic cancer (NCT04303403), and head and neck cancer (NCT03153982) are ongoing. Additional early-phase trials of ruxolitinib have been focused on cancer metastasis, including patients with metastatic prostate cancer and metastatic breast cancer, as listed in Table 1. However, two phase III trials (NCT02119663 and NCT02117479) of ruxolitinib with capecitabine in metastatic pancreatic cancer patients were terminated due to no additional benefit over capecitabine alone [68]. The same also occurred with a phase II trial of ruxolitinib with capecitabine in patients with metastatic HER2-postive breast cancer (NCT02120417). Besides ruxolitinib, itacitinib, a JAK1 specific inhibitor, has also been employed in a phase I trial of metastatic soft tissue sarcomas.

The third potential target in the IL-6 signaling pathway is STAT3, with several compounds inhibiting the function or expression of STATs in clinical trials for various solid tumors [69]. BBI608, an oral cancer stemness inhibitor that blocks STAT3-mediated transcription of cancer stemness genes in the β-catenin pathway, has reached Phase II and III to treat metastatic colorectal cancer (Table 1). WP1066, a novel STAT3 inhibitor first published in 2010 [70], is in phase I for malignant glioma, metastatic melanoma in the brain, and pediatric brain tumors (Table 1).

Similarly, IL-1-blocking therapies have also been implicated in cancer-related inflammation [38,39]. Currently, clinically available anti-IL-1 strategies include anakinra (IL-1 receptor antagonist), canakinumab (a human anti-IL-1β monoclonal antibody), CAN04 (an IL-1 receptor accessory protein binding protein), and isunakinra (a potent IL-1 receptor inhibitor). Accumulated evidence indicated that canakinumab is highly promising for the treatment of non-small-cell lung cancer, for which clinical trials are ongoing (NCT02090101, NCT01802970). Canakinumab is also being evaluated in metastatic pancreatic cancer, in a phase I clinical trial (Table 1). Another important anti-IL-1 drug for cancer treatment is anakinra, which is widely used to treat autoimmune and autoinflammatory diseases. It is also being tested as an adjunct therapy to reduce the inflammation associated with metastatic cancer, including colorectal cancer and breast cancer (Table 1).

In 2009, a phase II clinical trial has been conducted to test the effect of carlumab, a human mAb with high affinity and specificity for human CCL2, in patients with metastatic castration-resistant prostate cancer. In this trial, carlumab was unable to sustain a durable suppression of CCL2 and could not lead to meaningful clinical benefit responses (Table 1) [71]. Notably, the clinical application of CCL2 inhibitors for metastasis treatment requires a careful design.

Besides the extensively studied IL-6 and IL-1β, there are several early-phase clinical trials exploring the efficacy of targeting CSF, SDF-1, and MIF in the treatment of various metastatic tumors, as summarized in Table 1. The trials with SDF-1 and MIF have been completed, but no results have been reported yet.

Table 1. Registered clinical trials targeting pro-inflammatory cytokines in patients with cancer metastases.

Tested Drug	NCT Number	Title	Status	Conditions	Phases	Enrollment	Start Date	Completion Date
IL-6 pathway								
IL-6								
Siltuximab, anti-IL-6 chimeric monoclonal antibody	NCT00433446	S0354, Anti-IL-6 Chimeric Monoclonal Antibody in Patients with Metastatic Prostate Cancer That Did Not Respond to Hormone Therapy	Completed	Metastatic Prostate Cancer	Phase 2	62	2007	2011
	NCT00385827	A Safety and Efficacy Study of Siltuximab (CNTO 328) in Male Subjects with Metastatic Hormone-Refractory Prostate Cancer (HRPC)	Terminated	Metastatic Prostate Cancer	Phase 2	106	2017	2021
	NCT04191421	Siltuximab and Spartalizumab in Patients with Metastatic Pancreatic Cancer	Recruiting	Metastatic Stage IV Pancreatic Cancer	Phase 1|Phase 2	42	2020	2022
Tocilizumab, humanized monoclonal antibody against IL-6 receptor	NCT03135171	Trastuzumab and Pertuzumab in Combination with Tocilizumab in Subjects with Metastatic HER2-Positive Breast Cancer Resistant to Trastuzumab	Recruiting	HER2+ Breast Cancer	Phase 1	20	2017	2021
JAK								
Ruxolitinib, JAK1 and JAK2 inhibitor	NCT00638378	Study of Ruxolitinib (INCB018424) Administered Orally to Patients with Androgen-Independent Metastatic Prostate Cancer	Terminated	Prostate Cancer	Phase 2	22	2008	2009
	NCT01594216	Ruxolitinib in Estrogen Receptor-Positive Breast Cancer	Completed	Estrogen Receptor-Positive Invasive Metastatic Breast Cancer	Phase 2	29	2012	2016
	NCT02120417	A Study of Ruxolitinib in Combination with Capecitabine in Subjects with Advanced or Metastatic HER2-Negative Breast Cancer	Terminated	Breast Cancer	Phase 2	149	2014	2017
	NCT02041429	Ruxolitinib W/Preop Chemo for Triple-Negative Inflammatory Breast cancer	Active, not recruiting	Recurrent Breast Cancer|Metastatic Breast Cancer	Phase 1|Phase 2	24	2014	2021
	NCT02066532	Ruxolitinib in Combination with Trastuzumab in Metastatic HER2-Positive Breast Cancer	Active, not recruiting	Metastatic Breast Cancer|HER-2 Positive Breast Cancer	Phase 1|Phase 2	28	2014	2020

Table 1. *Cont.*

Tested Drug	NCT Number	Title	Status	Conditions	Phases	Enrollment	Start Date	Completion Date
	NCT03012230	Pembrolizumab and Ruxolitinib Phosphate in Treating Patients with Metastatic Stage IV Triple-Negative Breast Cancer	Recruiting	Metastatic Malignant Neoplasm in the Bone Stage IV Breast Cancer|Triple-Negative Breast Carcinoma	Phase 1	18	2017	2021
	NCT02876302	Study of Ruxolitinib (INCB018424) With Preoperative Chemotherapy for Triple-Negative Inflammatory Breast Cancer	Recruiting	Inflammatory Breast Cancer	Phase 2	64	2017	2024
Itacitinib, JAK1 inhibitor	NCT03670069	Itacitinib in Treating Patients with Refractory Metastatic/Advanced Soft Tissue Sarcomas	Recruiting	Metastatic Leiomyosarcoma|Metastatic Synovial Sarcoma	Phase 1	28	2019	2022
				STAT				
BBI608, STAT3 inhibitor	NCT03522649	A Phase III Clinical Study of Napabucasin (GB201) Plus FOLFIRI in Adult Patients with Metastatic Colorectal Cancer	Recruiting	Previously Treated Metastatic Colorectal Cancer	Phase 3	668	2018	2021
	NCT03647839	Modulation of The Tumor Microenvironment Using Either Vascular Disrupting Agents or STAT3 Inhibition in Order to Synergize With PD1 Inhibition in Microsatellite-Stable, Refractory Colorectal Cancer Patients	Active, not recruiting	Colorectal Cancer Metastatic	Phase 2	90	2018	2022
WP1066, JAK2/STAT3 inhibitor	NCT01904123	STAT3 Inhibitor WP1066 in Treating Patients with Recurrent Malignant Glioma or Progressive Metastatic Melanoma in the Brain	Recruiting	Metastatic Malignant Neoplasm in the Brain| Metastatic Melanoma	Phase 1	33	2018	2021
	NCT04334863	AflacST1901: Peds WP1066	Recruiting	Brain Tumor|Medulloblastoma| BrainMetastases	Phase 1	36	2020	2023
				IL-1				
Canakinumab, human anti-IL-1β monoclonal antibody	NCT03631199	Study of Efficacy and Safety of Pembrolizumab Plus Platinum-based Doublet Chemotherapy with or without Canakinumab in Previously Untreated Locally Advanced or Metastatic Non-Squamous and Squamous Non-Small Cell Lung Cancer (NSCLC) Subjects	Active, not recruiting	Non-Small Cell Lung Cancer	Phase 3	673	2018	2022

Table 1. *Cont.*

Tested Drug	NCT Number	Title	Status	Conditions	Phases	Enrollment	Start Date	Completion Date
	NCT04581343	A Phase 1B Study of Canakinumab, Spartalizumab, Nab-Paclitaxel, and Gemcitabine in Metastatic PC Patients	Recruiting	Metastatic Pancreatic Ductal Adenocarcinoma	Phase 1	10	2020	2022
Anakinra, human interleukin 1 receptor antagonist	NCT00072111	Anakinra in Treating Patients with Metastatic Cancer Expressing the Interleukin-1 Gene	Completed	Metastatic Cancer	Phase 1		2003	2015
	NCT02090101	Study Evaluating the Influence of LV5FU2 Bevacizumab Plus Anakinra Association on Metastatic Colorectal Cancer	Completed	Metastatic Colorectal Cancer	Phase 2	32	2014	2017
	NCT01802970	Safety and Blood Immune Cell Study of Anakinra Plus Physician's Chemotherapy Choice in Metastatic Breast Cancer Patients	Completed	Metastatic Breast Cancer	Phase 1	10	2012	2017
	NCT01624766	Everolimus and Anakinra or Denosumab in Treating Participants with Relapsed or Refractory Advanced Cancers	Active, not recruiting	Advanced Malignant Neoplasm|Metastatic Malignant Neoplasm|Recurrent Malignant Neoplasm|Refractory Malignant Neoplasm	Phase 1	57	2012	2020
CCL2								
Carlumab	NCT00992186	A Study of the Safety and Efficacy of Single-Agent Carlumab (an Anti-Chemokine Ligand 2 [CCL2]) in Participants with Metastatic Castrate-Resistant Prostate Cancer	Completed	Prostate cancer	Phase 2	46	2009	2011
CSF								
SNDX-6352, CSF receptor inhibitor	NCT03238027	A Phase 1 Study to Investigate SNDX-6352 Alone or in Combination With Durvalumab in Patients With Solid Tumors	Active, not recruiting	Solid Tumor|Metastatic Tumor	Phase 1	45	2017	2021
SDF-1								
Olaptesed, binding to SDF-1	NCT03168139	Olaptesed (NOX-A12) Alone and in Combination with Pembrolizumab in Colorectal and Pancreatic Cancer Patients	Completed	Metastatic Colorectal Cancer|Metastatic Pancreatic Cancer	Phase 1|Phase 2	20	2017	2020
MIF								
Anti-MIF antibody	NCT01765790	Phase 1 Study of Anti-Macrophage Migration Inhibitory Factor (Anti-MIF) Antibody in Solid Tumors	Completed	Metastatic Adenocarcinoma of the Colon or Rectum	Phase 1	68	2012	2016

6. Conclusions

Cancer metastasis poses significant challenges to the development of curative therapies due to insufficient knowledge of the mechanisms governing this process. Targeting the molecular interactions that build the PMN has the potential to prevent and eradicate metastases before they manifest. It would be most useful to block the signaling systems that promote the establishment of the PMN right after dissecting a primary tumor, i.e., in the critical post-operative window when no visible metastases are observed but PMN formation is probably ongoing. Compelling evidence implies the rise of pro-inflammatory cytokines and the suppression of the immune function during the peri-operative and post-operative periods [72,73], which all contribute to PMN formation. However, the combination of pro-inflammatory cytokines in the PMN is still under investigation and may vary in different types of cancer or even in individual patients. The advanced 'omics' technology could help design more precise and individualized therapeutic approaches in future clinical trials. Admittedly, some clinical trials targeting IL-6 or IL-1 have failed in preventing metastasis. Human solid tumors are more complex than mouse models, and the heterogeneity of cancer cells could be a factor affecting treatment efficacy. Thus, monotherapy to inhibit a single cytokine may not be sufficient to treat advanced tumors. Taking in consideration the pleiotropy and redundancy of pro-inflammatory cytokines, further in vitro and in vivo studies should be designed to determine the joint power of pro-inflammatory cytokines in PMN formation, as well as to analyze their combined targeting in cancer metastasis.

Author Contributions: Literature search, R.L. and A.W.; IL-6 writing, R.L.; IL-1 writing, A.W.; original draft preparation, R.L.; writing—review and editing, J.L.; supervision, J.L. All authors have read and agreed to the published version of the manuscript.

List of Abbreviations

ECM:	extracellular matrix
PMN:	pre-metastatic niche
BMDC:	bone marrow-derived cells
MDSC:	myeloid-derived suppressor cells
TAM:	tumor-associated macrophage
EV:	extracellular vesicles
EMT:	epithelial-to-mesenchymal transition
CAF:	cancer associated fibroblast
HSC:	hematopoietic stem cell
BBB:	blood–brain barrier
IL-6:	interleukin 6
IL-1β:	interleukin-1β
CXCL12/SDF-1 α:	stromal cell-derived factor 1
IL-8:	interleukin 8
VEGF:	vascular endothelial growth factor
G-CSF:	granulocyte-colony stimulating factor
MIF:	macrophage migration inhibitory factor
TIMP-1:	tissue inhibitor of metalloproteinases 1
GM-CSF:	granulocyte–macrophage colony-stimulating factor
SAA:	serum amyloid A
TGF-β:	transforming growth factor beta
HIF-1:	hypoxia-inducible factor 1
CCL2:	CC-chemokine ligand 2
CCL5:	chemokine ligand 5

CXCL1: C–X–C motif ligand 1
JAK: Janus kinase
STAT3: signal transducer and activator of transcription 3
AKT: protein kinase B
MAPK: mitogen-activated protein kinase
IDO: indoleamine 2,3-dioxygenase
PD-L1: programmed death ligand 1

References

1. Vanharanta, S.; Massagué, J. Origins of metastatic traits. *Cancer Cell* **2013**, *24*, 410–421. [CrossRef] [PubMed]
2. Joyce, J.A.; Pollard, J.W. Microenvironmental regulation of metastasis. *Nat. Rev. Cancer* **2009**, *9*, 239–252. [CrossRef] [PubMed]
3. Kaplan, R.N.; Riba, R.D.; Zacharoulis, S.; Bramley, A.H.; Vincent, L.; Costa, C.; MacDonald, D.D.; Jin, D.K.; Shido, K.; Kerns, S.A.; et al. VEGFR1-positive haematopoietic bone marrow progenitors initiate the pre-metastatic niche. *Nature* **2005**, *438*, 820–827. [CrossRef]
4. Law, A.M.K.; Valdes-Mora, F.; Gallego-Ortega, D. Myeloid-Derived Suppressor Cells as a Therapeutic Target for Cancer. *Cells* **2020**, *9*, 561. [CrossRef] [PubMed]
5. Ozaki, K.; Leonard, W.J. Cytokine and cytokine receptor pleiotropy and redundancy. *J. Biol. Chem.* **2002**, *277*, 29355–29358. [CrossRef]
6. Altan-Bonnet, G.; Mukherjee, R. Cytokine-mediated communication: A quantitative appraisal of immune complexity. *Nat. Rev. Immunol.* **2019**, *19*, 205–217. [CrossRef]
7. Dranoff, G. Cytokines in cancer pathogenesis and cancer therapy. *Nat. Rev. Cancer* **2004**, *4*, 11–22. [CrossRef]
8. Johnson, D.E.; O'Keefe, R.A.; Grandis, J.R. Targeting the IL-6/JAK/STAT3 signalling axis in cancer. *Nat. Rev. Clin. Oncol.* **2018**, *15*, 234. [CrossRef]
9. Ludwig, H.; Nachbaur, D.M.; Fritz, E.; Krainer, M.; Huber, H. Interleukin-6 is a prognostic factor in multiple myeloma. *Blood* **1991**, *77*, 2794–2795. [CrossRef]
10. Macha, M.A.; Matta, A.; Kaur, J.; Chauhan, S.S.; Thakar, A.; Shukla, N.K.; Gupta, S.D.; Ralhan, R. Prognostic significance of nuclear pSTAT3 in oral cancer. *Head Neck* **2011**, *33*, 482–489. [CrossRef]
11. Chen, Y.; Wang, J.; Wang, X.; Liu, X.; Li, H.; Lv, Q.; Zhu, J.; Wei, B.; Tang, Y. STAT3, a Poor Survival Predicator, Is Associated with Lymph Node Metastasis from Breast Cancer. *J. Breast Cancer* **2013**, *16*, 40–49. [CrossRef] [PubMed]
12. Kusaba, T.; Nakayama, T.; Yamazumi, K.; Yakata, Y.; Yoshizaki, A.; Inoue, K.; Nagayasu, T.; Sekine, I. Activation of STAT3 is a marker of poor prognosis in human colorectal cancer. *Oncol. Rep.* **2006**, *15*, 1445–1451. [CrossRef] [PubMed]
13. Yu, H.; Kortylewski, M.; Pardoll, D. Crosstalk between cancer and immune cells: Role of STAT3 in the tumour microenvironment. *Nat. Rev. Immunol.* **2007**, *7*, 41. [CrossRef] [PubMed]
14. Yu, H.; Lee, H.; Herrmann, A.; Buettner, R.; Jove, R. Revisiting STAT3 signalling in cancer: New and unexpected biological functions. *Nat. Rev. Cancer* **2014**, *14*, 736. [CrossRef]
15. Kortylewski, M.; Kujawski, M.; Wang, T.; Wei, S.; Zhang, S.; Pilon-Thomas, S.; Niu, G.; Kay, H.; Mule, J.; Kerr, W.G.; et al. Inhibiting Stat3 signaling in the hematopoietic system elicits multicomponent antitumor immunity. *Nat. Med.* **2005**, *11*, 1314–1321. [CrossRef]
16. Jones, S.A.; Jenkins, B.J. Recent insights into targeting the IL-6 cytokine family in inflammatory diseases and cancer. *Nat. Rev. Immunol.* **2018**, *18*, 773–789. [CrossRef]
17. Rokavec, M.; Oner, M.G.; Li, H.; Jackstadt, R.; Jiang, L.; Lodygin, D.; Kaller, M.; Horst, D.; Ziegler, P.K.; Schwitalla, S.; et al. IL-6R/STAT3/miR-34a feedback loop promotes EMT-mediated colorectal cancer invasion and metastasis. *J. Clin. Investig.* **2014**, *124*, 1853–1867. [CrossRef]
18. Leone, P.; Buonavoglia, A.; Fasano, R.; Solimando, A.G.; De Re, V.; Cicco, S.; Vacca, A.; Racanelli, V. Insights into the Regulation of Tumor Angiogenesis by Micro-RNAs. *J. Clin. Med.* **2019**, *8*, 2030. [CrossRef]
19. Kim, J.; Yao, F.; Xiao, Z.; Sun, Y.; Ma, L. MicroRNAs and metastasis: Small RNAs play big roles. *Cancer Metastasis Rev.* **2018**, *37*, 5–15. [CrossRef]
20. Gyamfi, J.; Lee, Y.-H.; Eom, M.; Choi, J. Interleukin-6/STAT3 signalling regulates adipocyte induced epithelial-mesenchymal transition in breast cancer cells. *Sci. Rep.* **2018**, *8*, 8859. [CrossRef]

21. He, J.Y.; Wei, X.H.; Li, S.J.; Liu, Y.; Hu, H.L.; Li, Z.Z.; Kuang, X.H.; Wang, L.; Shi, X.; Yuan, S.T.; et al. Adipocyte-derived IL-6 and leptin promote breast Cancer metastasis via upregulation of Lysyl Hydroxylase-2 expression. *Cell Commun. Signal.* **2018**, *16*, 100. [CrossRef] [PubMed]
22. Abbruzzese, J.L.; Abbruzzese, M.C.; Lenzi, R.; Hess, K.R.; Raber, M.N. Analysis of a diagnostic strategy for patients with suspected tumors of unknown origin. *J. Clin. Oncol.* **1995**, *13*, 2094–2103. [CrossRef] [PubMed]
23. Ji, Q.; Zhou, L.; Sui, H.; Yang, L.; Wu, X.; Song, Q.; Jia, R.; Li, R.; Sun, J.; Wang, Z.; et al. Primary tumors release ITGBL1-rich extracellular vesicles to promote distal metastatic tumor growth through fibroblast-niche formation. *Nat. Commun.* **2020**, *11*, 1211. [CrossRef] [PubMed]
24. Erdogan, B.; Webb, D.J. Cancer-associated fibroblasts modulate growth factor signaling and extracellular matrix remodeling to regulate tumor metastasis. *Biochem. Soc. Trans.* **2017**, *45*, 229–236. [CrossRef]
25. Lee, E.; Fertig, E.J.; Jin, K.; Sukumar, S.; Pandey, N.B.; Popel, A.S. Breast cancer cells condition lymphatic endothelial cells within pre-metastatic niches to promote metastasis. *Nat. Commun.* **2014**, *5*, 4715. [CrossRef]
26. Huang, Y.; Song, N.; Ding, Y.; Yuan, S.; Li, X.; Cai, H.; Shi, H.; Luo, Y. Pulmonary vascular destabilization in the premetastatic phase facilitates lung metastasis. *Cancer Res.* **2009**, *69*, 7529–7537. [CrossRef]
27. Hiratsuka, S.; Ishibashi, S.; Tomita, T.; Watanabe, A.; Akashi-Takamura, S.; Murakami, M.; Kijima, H.; Miyake, K.; Aburatani, H.; Maru, Y. Primary tumours modulate innate immune signalling to create pre-metastatic vascular hyperpermeability foci. *Nat. Commun.* **2013**, *4*, 1853. [CrossRef]
28. Chang, Q.; Bournazou, E.; Sansone, P.; Berishaj, M.; Gao, S.P.; Daly, L.; Wels, J.; Theilen, T.; Granitto, S.; Zhang, X.; et al. The IL-6/JAK/Stat3 feed-forward loop drives tumorigenesis and metastasis. *Neoplasia* **2013**, *15*, 848–862. [CrossRef]
29. Tao, Q.; Fujimoto, J.; Men, T.; Ye, X.; Deng, J.; Lacroix, L.; Clifford, J.L.; Mao, L.; Van Pelt, C.S.; Lee, J.J.; et al. Identification of the retinoic acid-inducible Gprc5a as a new lung tumor suppressor gene. *J. Natl. Cancer Inst.* **2007**, *99*, 1668–1682. [CrossRef]
30. Jing, B.; Wang, T.; Sun, B.; Xu, J.; Xu, D.; Liao, Y.; Song, H.; Guo, W.; Li, K.; Hu, M.; et al. IL6/STAT3 Signaling Orchestrates Premetastatic Niche Formation and Immunosuppressive Traits in Lung. *Cancer Res.* **2020**, *80*, 784–797. [CrossRef]
31. Tabouret, E.; Chinot, O.; Metellus, P.; Tallet, A.; Viens, P.; Goncalves, A. Recent trends in epidemiology of brain metastases: An overview. *Anticancer Res.* **2012**, *32*, 4655–4662. [PubMed]
32. Witzel, I.; Laakmann, E.; Weide, R.; Neunhöffer, T.; Park-Simon, T.J.; Schmidt, M.; Fasching, P.A.; Hesse, T.; Polasik, A.; Mohrmann, S.; et al. Treatment and outcomes of patients in the Brain Metastases in Breast Cancer Network Registry. *Eur. J. Cancer* **2018**, *102*, 1–9. [CrossRef] [PubMed]
33. Kim, S.W.; Choi, H.J.; Lee, H.J.; He, J.; Wu, Q.; Langley, R.R.; Fidler, I.J.; Kim, S.J. Role of the endothelin axis in astrocyte- and endothelial cell-mediated chemoprotection of cancer cells. *Neuro Oncol.* **2014**, *16*, 1585–1598. [CrossRef] [PubMed]
34. Apte, R.N.; Voronov, E. Interleukin-1–a major pleiotropic cytokine in tumor-host interactions. *Semin. Cancer Biol.* **2002**, *12*, 277–290. [CrossRef]
35. Dinarello, C.A. Overview of the IL-1 family in innate inflammation and acquired immunity. *Immunol. Rev.* **2018**, *281*, 8–27. [CrossRef] [PubMed]
36. Bent, R.; Moll, L.; Grabbe, S.; Bros, M. Interleukin-1 Beta-A Friend or Foe in Malignancies? *Int. J. Mol. Sci.* **2018**, *19*, 2155. [CrossRef]
37. Krelin, Y.; Voronov, E.; Dotan, S.; Elkabets, M.; Reich, E.; Fogel, M.; Huszar, M.; Iwakura, Y.; Segal, S.; Dinarello, C.A.; et al. Interleukin-1beta-driven inflammation promotes the development and invasiveness of chemical carcinogen-induced tumors. *Cancer Res.* **2007**, *67*, 1062–1071. [CrossRef]
38. Dinarello, C.A.; Simon, A.; van der Meer, J.W. Treating inflammation by blocking interleukin-1 in a broad spectrum of diseases. *Nat. Rev. Drug Discov.* **2012**, *11*, 633–652. [CrossRef]
39. Molgora, M.; Supino, D.; Mantovani, A.; Garlanda, C. Tuning inflammation and immunity by the negative regulators IL-1R2 and IL-1R8. *Immunol. Rev.* **2018**, *281*, 233–247. [CrossRef]
40. Schmid, M.C.; Avraamides, C.J.; Foubert, P.; Shaked, Y.; Kang, S.W.; Kerbel, R.S.; Varner, J.A. Combined blockade of integrin-alpha4beta1 plus cytokines SDF-1alpha or IL-1beta potently inhibits tumor inflammation and growth. *Cancer Res.* **2011**, *71*, 6965–6975. [CrossRef]
41. Coffelt, S.B.; Kersten, K.; Doornebal, C.W.; Weiden, J.; Vrijland, K.; Hau, C.S.; Verstegen, N.J.M.; Ciampricotti, M.; Hawinkels, L.; Jonkers, J.; et al. IL-17-producing gammadelta T cells and neutrophils conspire to promote breast cancer metastasis. *Nature* **2015**, *522*, 345–348. [CrossRef] [PubMed]

42. Pein, M.; Insua-Rodriguez, J.; Hongu, T.; Riedel, A.; Meier, J.; Wiedmann, L.; Decker, K.; Essers, M.A.G.; Sinn, H.P.; Spaich, S.; et al. Metastasis-initiating cells induce and exploit a fibroblast niche to fuel malignant colonization of the lungs. *Nat. Commun.* **2020**, *11*, 1494. [CrossRef] [PubMed]
43. Nutter, F.; Holen, I.; Brown, H.K.; Cross, S.S.; Evans, C.A.; Walker, M.; Coleman, R.E.; Westbrook, J.A.; Selby, P.J.; Brown, J.E.; et al. Different molecular profiles are associated with breast cancer cell homing compared with colonisation of bone: Evidence using a novel bone-seeking cell line. *Endocr. Relat. Cancer* **2014**, *21*, 327–341. [CrossRef] [PubMed]
44. Templeton, Z.S.; Lie, W.R.; Wang, W.; Rosenberg-Hasson, Y.; Alluri, R.V.; Tamaresis, J.S.; Bachmann, M.H.; Lee, K.; Maloney, W.J.; Contag, C.H.; et al. Breast Cancer Cell Colonization of the Human Bone Marrow Adipose Tissue Niche. *Neoplasia* **2015**, *17*, 849–861. [CrossRef]
45. Chung, S.T.; Geerts, D.; Roseman, K.; Renaud, A.; Connelly, L. Osteoprotegerin mediates tumor-promoting effects of Interleukin-1beta in breast cancer cells. *Mol. Cancer* **2017**, *16*, 27. [CrossRef]
46. Carmi, Y.; Dotan, S.; Rider, P.; Kaplanov, I.; White, M.R.; Baron, R.; Abutbul, S.; Huszar, M.; Dinarello, C.A.; Apte, R.N.; et al. The role of IL-1β in the early tumor cell-induced angiogenic response. *J. Immunol.* **2013**, *190*, 3500–3509. [CrossRef]
47. Jung, Y.D.; Liu, W.; Reinmuth, N.; Ahmad, S.A.; Fan, F.; Gallick, G.E.; Ellis, L.M. Vascular endothelial growth factor is upregulated by interleukin-1 beta in human vascular smooth muscle cells via the P38 mitogen-activated protein kinase pathway. *Angiogenesis* **2001**, *4*, 155–162. [CrossRef]
48. Shi, H.; Zhang, J.; Han, X.; Li, H.; Xie, M.; Sun, Y.; Liu, W.; Ba, X.; Zeng, X. Recruited monocytic myeloid-derived suppressor cells promote the arrest of tumor cells in the premetastatic niche through an IL-1β-mediated increase in E-selectin expression. *Int. J. Cancer* **2017**, *140*, 1370–1383. [CrossRef]
49. Castaño, Z.; San Juan, B.P.; Spiegel, A.; Pant, A.; DeCristo, M.J.; Laszewski, T.; Ubellacker, J.M.; Janssen, S.R.; Dongre, A.; Reinhardt, F.; et al. IL-1β inflammatory response driven by primary breast cancer prevents metastasis-initiating cell colonization. *Nat. Cell Biol.* **2018**, *20*, 1084–1097. [CrossRef]
50. Qian, B.Z.; Li, J.; Zhang, H.; Kitamura, T.; Zhang, J.; Campion, L.R.; Kaiser, E.A.; Snyder, L.A.; Pollard, J.W. CCL2 recruits inflammatory monocytes to facilitate breast-tumour metastasis. *Nature* **2011**, *475*, 222–225. [CrossRef]
51. Granot, Z.; Henke, E.; Comen, E.A.; King, T.A.; Norton, L.; Benezra, R. Tumor entrained neutrophils inhibit seeding in the premetastatic lung. *Cancer Cell* **2011**, *20*, 300–314. [CrossRef] [PubMed]
52. Kowanetz, M.; Wu, X.; Lee, J.; Tan, M.; Hagenbeek, T.; Qu, X.; Yu, L.; Ross, J.; Korsisaari, N.; Cao, T.; et al. Granulocyte-colony stimulating factor promotes lung metastasis through mobilization of Ly6G+Ly6C+ granulocytes. *Proc. Natl. Acad. Sci. USA* **2010**, *107*, 21248–21255. [CrossRef] [PubMed]
53. Hiratsuka, S.; Watanabe, A.; Aburatani, H.; Maru, Y. Tumour-mediated upregulation of chemoattractants and recruitment of myeloid cells predetermines lung metastasis. *Nat. Cell Biol.* **2006**, *8*, 1369–1375. [CrossRef] [PubMed]
54. Thorn, M.; Guha, P.; Cunetta, M.; Espat, N.J.; Miller, G.; Junghans, R.P.; Katz, S.C. Tumor-associated GM-CSF overexpression induces immunoinhibitory molecules via STAT3 in myeloid-suppressor cells infiltrating liver metastases. *Cancer Gene Ther.* **2016**, *23*, 188–198. [CrossRef]
55. Shiozawa, Y.; Pedersen, E.A.; Havens, A.M.; Jung, Y.; Mishra, A.; Joseph, J.; Kim, J.K.; Patel, L.R.; Ying, C.; Ziegler, A.M.; et al. Human prostate cancer metastases target the hematopoietic stem cell niche to establish footholds in mouse bone marrow. *J. Clin. Investig.* **2001**, *121*, 1298–1312. [CrossRef]
56. Seubert, B.; Grünwald, B.; Kobuch, J.; Cui, H.; Schelter, F.; Schaten, S.; Siveke, J.T.; Lim, N.H.; Nagase, H.; Simonavicius, N.; et al. Tissue inhibitor of metalloproteinases (TIMP)-1 creates a premetastatic niche in the liver through SDF-1/CXCR4-dependent neutrophil recruitment in mice. *Hepatology* **2015**, *61*, 238–248. [CrossRef]
57. Costa-Silva, B.; Aiello, N.M.; Ocean, A.J.; Singh, S.; Zhang, H.; Thakur, B.K.; Becker, A.; Hoshino, A.; Mark, M.T.; Molina, H.; et al. Pancreatic cancer exosomes initiate pre-metastatic niche formation in the liver. *Nat. Cell Biol.* **2015**, *17*, 816–826. [CrossRef]
58. Wang, D.; Sun, H.; Wei, J.; Cen, B.; DuBois, R.N. CXCL1 Is Critical for Premetastatic Niche Formation and Metastasis in Colorectal Cancer. *Cancer Res.* **2017**, *77*, 3655–3665. [CrossRef]
59. Sansone, P.; Bromberg, J. Targeting the interleukin-6/Jak/stat pathway in human malignancies. *J. Clin. Oncol.* **2012**, *30*, 1005–1014. [CrossRef]

60. Dorff, T.B.; Goldman, B.; Pinski, J.K.; Mack, P.C.; Lara, P.N., Jr.; Van Veldhuizen, P.J., Jr.; Quinn, D.I.; Vogelzang, N.J.; Thompson, I.M., Jr.; Hussain, M.H. Clinical and correlative results of SWOG S0354: A phase II trial of CNTO328 (siltuximab), a monoclonal antibody against interleukin-6, in chemotherapy-pretreated patients with castration-resistant prostate cancer. *Clin. Cancer Res.* **2010**, *16*, 3028–3034. [CrossRef]
61. Kampan, N.C.; Xiang, S.D.; McNally, O.M.; Stephens, A.N.; Quinn, M.A.; Plebanski, M. Immunotherapeutic Interleukin-6 or Interleukin-6 Receptor Blockade in Cancer: Challenges and Opportunities. *Curr. Med. Chem.* **2018**, *25*, 4785–4806. [CrossRef] [PubMed]
62. Iftikhar, A.; Hassan, H.; Iftikhar, N.; Mushtaq, A.; Sohail, A.; Rosko, N.; Chakraborty, R.; Razzaq, F.; Sandeep, S.; Valent, J.N.; et al. Investigational Monoclonal Antibodies in the Treatment of Multiple Myeloma: A Systematic Review of Agents under Clinical Development. *Antibodies* **2019**, *8*, 34. [CrossRef]
63. Riegler, L.L.; Jones, G.P.; Lee, D.W. Current approaches in the grading and management of cytokine release syndrome after chimeric antigen receptor T-cell therapy. *Ther. Clin. Risk Manag.* **2019**, *15*, 323–335. [CrossRef] [PubMed]
64. Culig, Z.; Puhr, M. Interleukin-6 and prostate cancer: Current developments and unsolved questions. *Mol. Cell. Endocrinol.* **2018**, *462*, 25–30. [CrossRef] [PubMed]
65. Masjedi, A.; Hashemi, V.; Hojjat-Farsangi, M.; Ghalamfarsa, G.; Azizi, G.; Yousefi, M.; Jadidi-Niaragh, F. The significant role of interleukin-6 and its signaling pathway in the immunopathogenesis and treatment of breast cancer. *Biomed. Pharmacother.* **2018**, *108*, 1415–1424. [CrossRef] [PubMed]
66. Angevin, E.; Tabernero, J.; Elez, E.; Cohen, S.J.; Bahleda, R.; van Laethem, J.L.; Ottensmeier, C.; Lopez-Martin, J.A.; Clive, S.; Joly, F.; et al. A phase I/II, multiple-dose, dose-escalation study of siltuximab, an anti-interleukin-6 monoclonal antibody, in patients with advanced solid tumors. *Clin. Cancer Res.* **2014**, *20*, 2192–2204. [CrossRef] [PubMed]
67. Fizazi, K.; De Bono, J.S.; Flechon, A.; Heidenreich, A.; Voog, E.; Davis, N.B.; Qi, M.; Bandekar, R.; Vermeulen, J.T.; Cornfeld, M.; et al. Randomised phase II study of siltuximab (CNTO 328), an anti-IL-6 monoclonal antibody, in combination with mitoxantrone/prednisone versus mitoxantrone/prednisone alone in metastatic castration-resistant prostate cancer. *Eur. J. Cancer* **2012**, *48*, 85–93. [CrossRef]
68. Giaccone, G.; Sanborn, R.E.; Waqar, S.N.; Martinez-Marti, A.; Ponce, S.; Zhen, H.; Kennealey, G.; Erickson-Viitanen, S.; Schaefer, E. A Placebo-Controlled Phase II Study of Ruxolitinib in Combination With Pemetrexed and Cisplatin for First-Line Treatment of Patients With Advanced Nonsquamous Non-Small-Cell Lung Cancer and Systemic Inflammation. *Clin. Lung Cancer* **2018**, *19*, e567–e574. [CrossRef]
69. Zou, S.; Tong, Q.; Liu, B.; Huang, W.; Tian, Y.; Fu, X. Targeting STAT3 in Cancer Immunotherapy. *Mol. Cancer* **2020**, *19*, 145. [CrossRef]
70. Horiguchi, A.; Asano, T.; Kuroda, K.; Sato, A.; Asakuma, J.; Ito, K.; Hayakawa, M.; Sumitomo, M.; Asano, T. STAT3 inhibitor WP1066 as a novel therapeutic agent for renal cell carcinoma. *Br. J. Cancer* **2010**, *102*, 1592–1599. [CrossRef]
71. Pienta, K.J.; Machiels, J.P.; Schrijvers, D.; Alekseev, B.; Shkolnik, M.; Crabb, S.J.; Li, S.; Seetharam, S.; Puchalski, T.A.; Takimoto, C.; et al. Phase 2 study of carlumab (CNTO 888), a human monoclonal antibody against CC-chemokine ligand 2 (CCL2), in metastatic castration-resistant prostate cancer. *Investig. New Drugs* **2013**, *31*, 760–768. [CrossRef] [PubMed]
72. Li, R.; Huang, Y.; Lin, J. Distinct effects of general anesthetics on lung metastasis mediated by IL-6/JAK/STAT3 pathway in mouse models. *Nat. Commun.* **2020**, *11*, 642. [CrossRef] [PubMed]
73. Hiller, J.G.; Perry, N.J.; Poulogiannis, G.; Riedel, B.; Sloan, E.K. Perioperative events influence cancer recurrence risk after surgery. *Nat. Rev. Clin. Oncol.* **2018**, *15*, 205–218. [CrossRef] [PubMed]

8

Cnf1 Variants Endowed with the Ability to Cross the Blood–Brain Barrier: A New Potential Therapeutic Strategy for Glioblastoma

Andrea Colarusso [1], Zaira Maroccia [2], Ermenegilda Parrilli [1], Elena Angela Pia Germinario [2], Andrea Fortuna [2], Stefano Loizzo [2], Laura Ricceri [2], Maria Luisa Tutino [1], Carla Fiorentini [2,3] and Alessia Fabbri [2,*]

1 Department of Chemical Sciences, University of Naples Federico II, Complesso Universitario M. S. Angelo, Via Cintia, 80126 Napoli, Italy; andrea.colarusso@unina.it (A.C.); erparril@unina.it (E.P.); tutino@unina.it (M.L.T.)

2 Istituto Superiore di Sanità, Viale Regina Elena 299, 00161 Rome, Italy; zaira.maroccia@iss.it (Z.M.); elena.germinario@iss.it (E.A.P.G.); andrea.fortuna@iss.it (A.F.); stefano.loizzo@iss.it (S.L.); laura.ricceri@iss.it (L.R.); carla.fiorentini@iss.it (C.F.)

3 Association for Research on Integrative Oncological Therapies (ARTOI), 00165 Rome, Italy

* Correspondence: alessia.fabbri@iss.it

Abstract: Among gliomas, primary tumors originating from glial cells, glioblastoma (GBM) identified as WHO grade IV glioma, is the most common and aggressive malignant brain tumor. We have previously shown that the *Escherichia coli* protein toxin cytotoxic necrotizing factor 1 (CNF1) is remarkably effective as an anti-neoplastic agent in a mouse model of glioma, reducing the tumor volume, increasing survival, and maintaining the functional properties of peritumoral neurons. However, being unable to cross the blood–brain barrier (BBB), CNF1 requires injection directly into the brain, which is a very invasive administration route. Thus, to overcome this pitfall, we designed a CNF1 variant characterized by the presence of an N-terminal BBB-crossing tag. The variant was produced and we verified whether its activity was comparable to that of wild-type CNF1 in GBM cells. We investigated the signaling pathways engaged in the cell response to CNF1 variants to provide preliminary data to the subsequent studies in experimental animals. CNF1 may represent a novel avenue for GBM therapy, particularly because, besides blocking tumor growth, it also preserves the healthy surrounding tissue, maintaining its architecture and functionality. This renders CNF1 the most interesting candidate for the treatment of brain tumors, among other potentially effective bacterial toxins.

Keywords: glioblastoma; drug discovery; cytotoxic necrotizing factor type 1; protein purification; recombinant protein production

Key Contribution: We designed and produced the CNF1 variant An2-CNF1-H8 that might be endowed with the ability to cross the blood–brain barrier when intravenously injected. We characterized its cellular activity and demonstrated that the An2-CNF1-H8 variant preserves the same original activity profile of the wild-type CNF1 in different cell types, thus representing a promising therapeutic strategy for glioblastoma, also considering its beneficial effects on surrounding tissues.

1. Introduction

Gliomas are primary tumors occurring in the central nervous system (CNS) that arise from glial cells. Glioblastoma (GBM; World Health Organization grade IV glioma) [1] represents the most malignant form, being highly invasive and not responsive to standard treatments that include surgical resection of the tumoral mass followed by combined radio- and chemo-therapy. Therefore, the life expectancy after diagnosis is very poor [2].

We have previously shown that the *Escherichia coli* protein toxin cytotoxic necrotizing factor 1 (CNF1) is remarkably effective as an anti-neoplastic agent in a mouse model of glioma, reducing the tumoral mass, increasing the survival, and maintaining the functional properties of peritumoral neurons [3,4]. CNF1 specifically modulates Rho GTPases, thus affecting fundamental cellular processes that may induce different outcomes in different cell types. In fact, besides triggering an epithelial-mesenchymal transition in transformed epithelial cells where the movement and proliferating activity of the toxin are increased [3], CNF1 inhibits the growth of glioma cells that finally undergo death. Its detrimental activity on GBM cells is probably due to its ability to block cytodieresis in proliferating cells, leading them to senescence and death, whereas the beneficial activity on peritumoral neurons is still under investigation but seems to rely on the enhancement of synaptic plasticity and the preservation of functional attributes. These abilities point at CNF1 as a possible new strategy for the treatment of brain tumors.

However, being unable to cross the blood–brain barrier (BBB), CNF1 requires an intracerebral injection, as evidenced in all studies so far conducted using CNF1 on mouse models for CNS pathologies, including Rett syndrome (RTT) [5–7], Alzheimer's disease [8], epilepsy [9] as well as GBM [4,10,11]. Therefore, considering the invasive route of administration, the difficulty to propose the toxin as an innovative therapy prompted us to seek more tolerable delivery systems. To address this point, we have designed and produced a CNF1 variant that might be endowed with the ability to cross the BBB when intravenously (*iv*) injected (An2-CNF1-H8). Its main feature consists of the addition of an N-terminal Angiopep-2 (An2) peptide which should promote receptor-mediated transcytosis [12]. The recombinant protein was completed by the addition of a C-terminal His-tag (H8) to be used for the recombinant toxin purification. The demonstration that An2-CNF1-H8 preserves the original activity profile of the wild-type (*wt*) protein in different cell types, would also reinforce the hypothesis of CNF1 as a new candidate drug for the treatment of other disorders, such as RTT and mitochondrial encephalomyopathies. In particular, GBM cells have been the recipient for a more accurate investigation, propaedeutic to in vivo studies.

2. Results

2.1. Design and Production of a CNF1 Variant Bearing the Potentiality to Cross the BBB When Peripherally Injected

We have previously demonstrated that a carboxy terminally his-tagged version of CNF1 (CNF1-H8) can be efficiently expressed in and purified from recombinant *E. coli* BL21(DE3) cells [13]. In this study, we attempted the production of a slightly modified version of the same toxin harboring an N-terminal peptide, named Angiopep-2 (An2), and capable of interacting with low-density lipoprotein receptor-related protein-1 (LRP1). This receptor is known to be involved in the transcytosis of the brain delivery vector An2 [12]. This new version of the protein was named An2-CNF1-H8, as it still possessed a C-terminal polyhistidine tag (Figure 1A). The recombinant expressions of both CNF1-H8 and An2-CNF1-H8 were carried out at a low temperature of 15 °C, as previously reported [13]. The analysis of total cellular extracts obtained at the end of the bacterial growths indicated that an overexpression was clearly visible for both the constructs via SDS- polyacrylamide gel electrophoresis (PAGE) (Figure 1(B1)) and western blot (Figure 1(B2)). It is worth noting that the addition of the N-terminal An2 peptide led to a significantly higher production of the protein in comparison with the CNF1-H8 (Figure 1B). This outcome might be due to either a more efficient translation initiation or an increased half-life of the protein. Nevertheless, in terms of recombinant production of An2-CNF1-H8, this boost proved to be unfruitful, as the protein mainly accumulated as insoluble aggregates. This result is depicted in Figure 1C, where soluble (S) and insoluble (P) fractions, collected after cellular disruption, were analyzed via SDS-PAGE (Figure 1(C1,C3)) and western blot (Figure 1(C2,C4)). In the case of CNF1-H8 bearing bacteria, the recombinant product mainly accumulated as a soluble protein, as observable in the left part of Figure 1C. Conversely, *E. coli* synthesizing An2-CNF1-H8 suffered from the formation of inclusion bodies, distinguishable both in the Coomassie-stained gel and in western blot in the right part of Figure 1C. Despite a considerable loss of An2-CNF1-H8 as insoluble aggregates, its recovery in the cellular soluble fraction was still feasible using a previously established procedure [13].

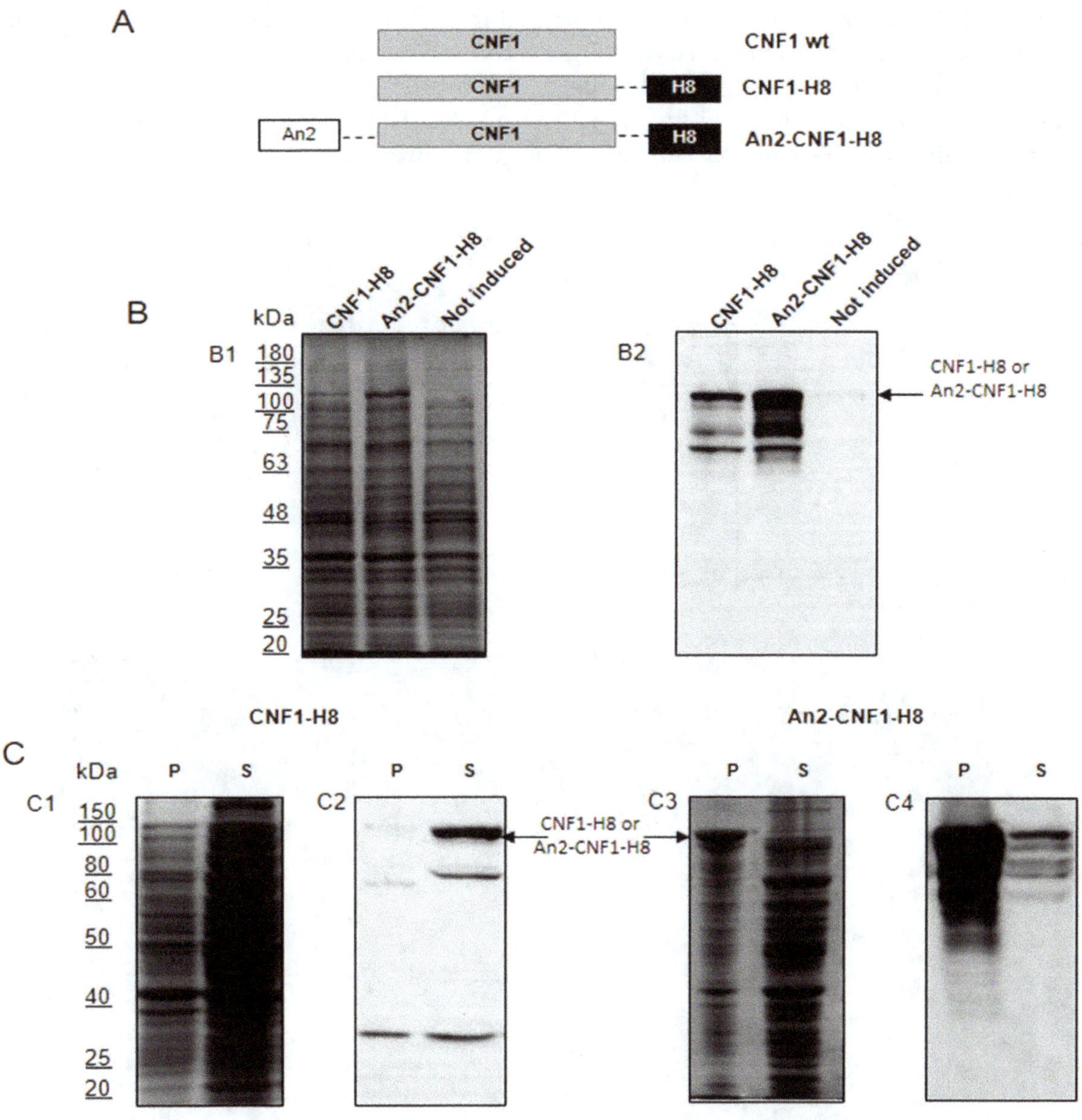

Figure 1. Design, expression, and solubility of cytotoxic necrotizing factor 1 (CNF1) variants. (**A**) Scheme of engineered CNF1 constructs presenting the following N-terminal and C-terminal tags: Angiopep-2 (An2), spaced by the GGSSRSS linker; 8xHis fused to a Tobacco Etch Virus recognition site (H8). (**B**) Recombinant protein expression levels in *E. coli* BL21 (DE3). Total cellular extracts obtained at 15 °C after 18 h induction with 0.5 mM IPTG were separated by 10% SDS-PAGE and analyzed either by Coomassie staining (**B1**) or western blot (**B2**) using a monoclonal anti-CNF1 antibody (NG8). Induced cells expressing CNF1-H8; induced cells expressing An2-CNF1-H8; not induced recombinant cells harboring pET40b-*cnf1-h8*. (**C**) Evaluation of CNF1 solubility in *E. coli* extracts. After cellular lysis, insoluble (P) and soluble (S) fractions were analyzed. The first two panels are relative to the solubility assay concerning CNF1-H8 expression carried out using SDS-PAGE (**C1** and **C3**) and western blot (**C2** and **C4**). The third and fourth images represent the SDS-PAGE and western blot relative to An2-CNF1-H8 solubility, respectively.

2.2. *The An2-CNF1-H8 Variant Preserves the Original Activity Profile of wt CNF1 in HEp-2 Cells*

The activity of the An2-CNF1-H8 variant was first tested on HEp-2 cells. The first set of experiments was carried out to verify whether the An2-CNF1-H8 variant could act in the same vein of CNF1. Therefore, to address this point, we used HEp-2 cells, the best characterized and responsive cell model for CNF1. CNF1-H8, and *wt* CNF1 were employed as controls in all the experiments. Once assessed that the An2-CNF1-H8 sample was more concentrated than *wt* CNF1 and CNF1-H8, as evidenced by polyacrylamide gel and western blot analysis (Figure 2A), we performed a titration experiment to find the lowest concentration inducing CNF1-like effects, i.e., multinucleation and ruffling (Figure S1). We found that the morphological effects induced by the An2-CNF1-H8 variant were comparable to that of *wt* CNF1 and obtained in the same concentration range (Figure 2B).

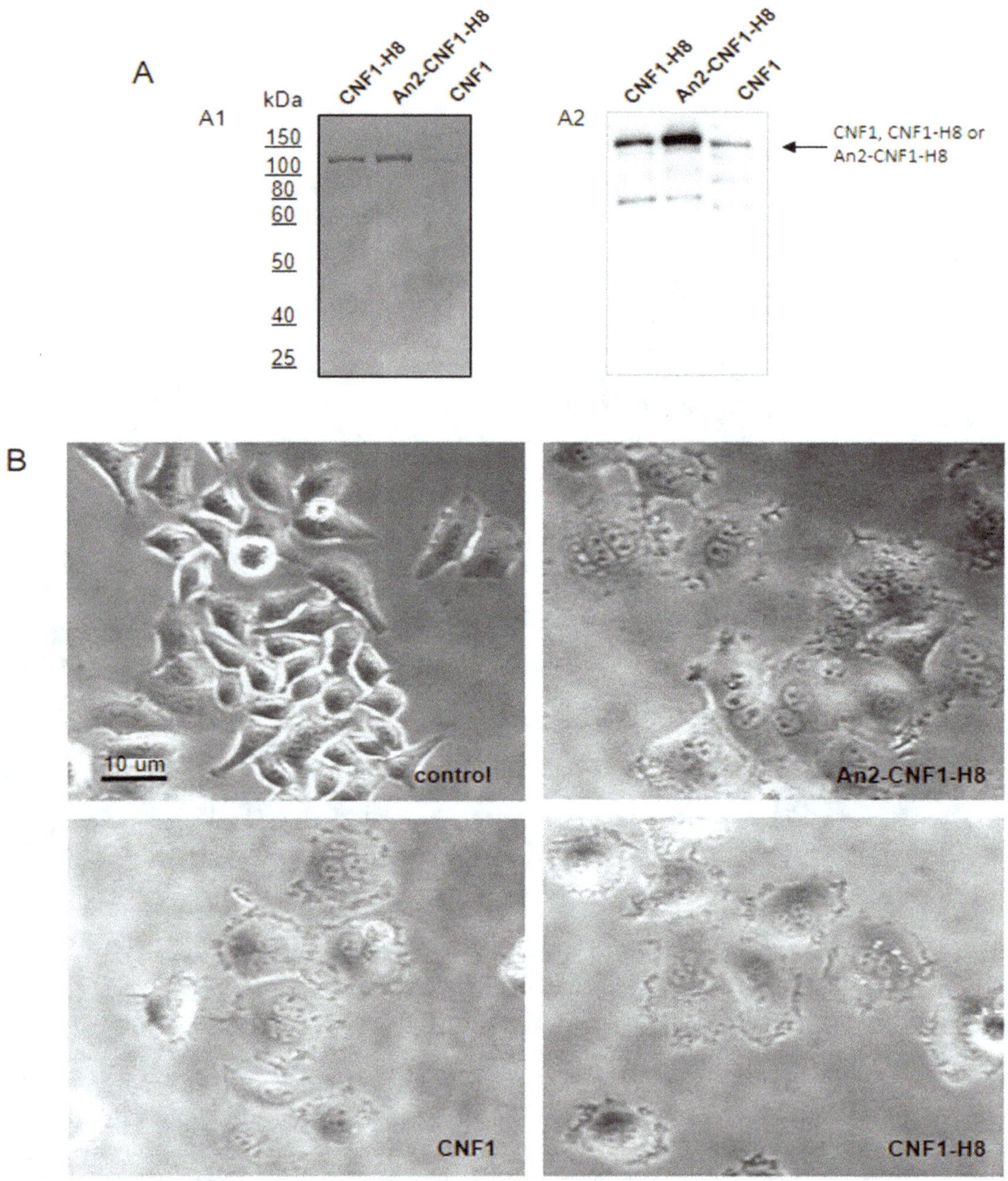

Figure 2. CNF1 variants activity. (**A**) SDS-polyacrylamide gel (**A1**) and western blot (**A2**) of CNF1 variants. (**B**) Phase-contrast micrographs of HEp-2 cells treated with CNF1 variants, showing the multinucleating/ruffling effects. Scale bar: 10 μm.

2.3. *The An2-CNF1-H8 Variant Enters the Cells in the Same Vein of wt CNF1*

To investigate whether the An2-CNF1-H8 variant binds to the same receptor engaged by the *wt* CNF1 or if it can enter via alternative pathways or receptors, we performed experiments in which we challenged the non-catalytic mutant CNF1-C866S (mCNF1, which maintains the ability to bind to the receptor but does not possess the enzymatic activity) with the CNF1 variant. As shown in Figure 3A, as the dose of mCNF1 increases, the An2-CNF1-H8 variant is inhibited, i.e., the percentage of multinucleated cells is decreased to zero, proving the engagement of the same receptor used by *wt* CNF1, at least in HEp-2 cells.

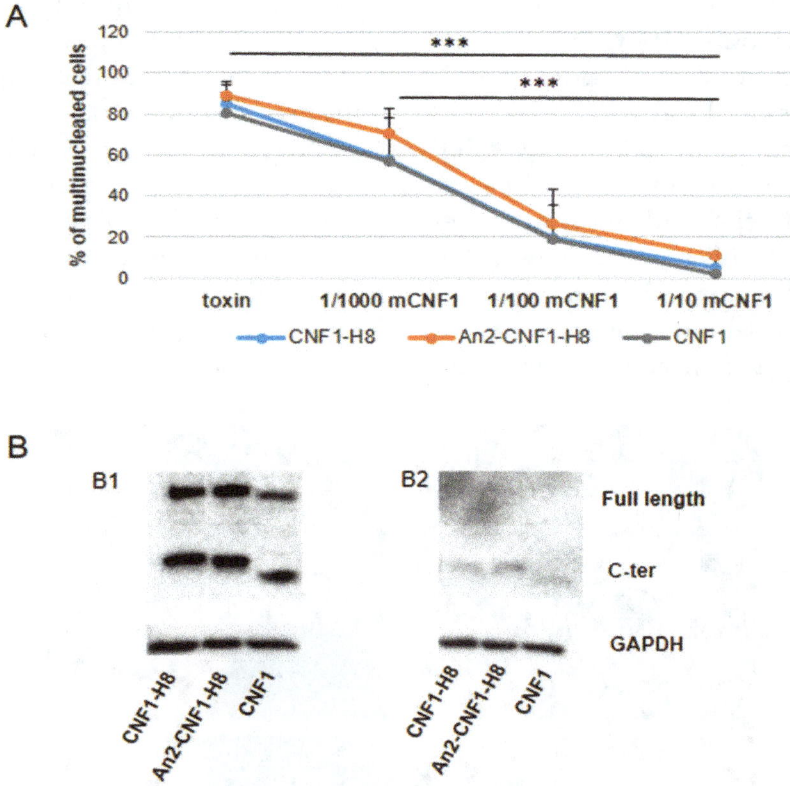

Figure 3. Entry of CNF1 variants into HEp-2 cells. (**A**) Graph showing the inhibition of variants entry by mCNF1. (**B**) Western blot analysis of HEp-2 cells treated with An2-CNF1-H8 and its controls (CNF1-H8 and *wt* CNF1) and stained with an antibody against CNF1, normalized as a function of GAPDH. Note that all the toxins are found as full length and 55 kDa C-ter portions after 24 h treatment (**B1**). Over a longer period of time, that is 48 h of treatment, washing to eliminate any remaining molecules in the culture medium, and further culture for 24 h, the full-length portions completely disappeared while the 55 kDa C-ter portions were present at a much lower concentration (**B2**). All in all, these results point at the fact that An2-CNF1-H8 follows the same route of entry of *wt* CNF1. Variants and *wt* CNF1 were used at 10^{-10} M. Data on the graph represent the mean ± SEM from at least three independent experiments. *** $p < 0.001$.

Then, to verify if the variant enters the cells via the canonical pathway of CNF1 endocytosis, being processed to release the C-terminal catalytic fragment (CNF1-C-ter) into the cytoplasm, HEp-2 cells were treated with An2-CNF1-H8 at the concentration of 10^{-9} M and lysed after 24 h. As evidenced in Figure 3(B1), the CNF1-C-ter portion of the variant was present in the cytoplasm, proving the entry through the classical CNF1 pathway. At the same time, we checked if all the administrated toxin was internalized over a longer period of time. To address this last question, we washed the cells with fresh medium after 48 h of treatment, to eliminate any remaining molecules left in the culture medium. The cells were then cultured for further 24 h before being lysed and subjected to western blot using the anti-CNF1 against the CNF1-C-ter. It should be noted that in these conditions (Figure 3(B2)) the whole CNF1 completely disappeared and the C-ter parts were present at a much lower concentration if compared to cells exposed for 24 h only. This indicates that, not only all the proteins are processed by freeing the toxin C-ter portion in the cytoplasm, but also that an amount of C-ter portion undergoes an elimination process.

2.4. *Activities of the An2-CNF1-H8 Variant on the Human Brain Endothelial Cell Line HBEC-5i*

The variants were built to find an inoculation system less invasive than the intracerebroventricular injection, such as the *iv* administration. Since *iv*-injected toxins need to act on endothelial cells in order to cross the BBB, we verified the activity of the CNF1 variant on the human brain endothelial cell line HBEC-5i. Interestingly, HBEC-5i cells highly express the LRP1 receptor for An2 and, therefore, we analyzed whether the variant could enter in this cellular system more easily than in the others. As reported in Figure 4, the An2-CNF1-H8 variant induces modification of the actin architecture on HBEC-5i cells comparable to that of *wt* CNF1, also in terms of fluorescence intensity (Figure S2). Moreover, competition experiments with the mutant CNF1 C866S were carried out in this endothelial cell line as in HEp-2 cells, and the results were overlapping (not shown). Therefore, our results demonstrate that An2-CNF1-H8 behaves as the *wt* CNF1 even in HBEC-5i cells. On the other hand, our preliminary in vivo experiments show that when mice were *iv* inoculated with the An2-CNF1-H8 variant, spinophilin amount increased in the hippocampus after 4 h (data not shown) as well as 7 days from inoculation (Figure S3), suggesting that the variant could pass the BBB.

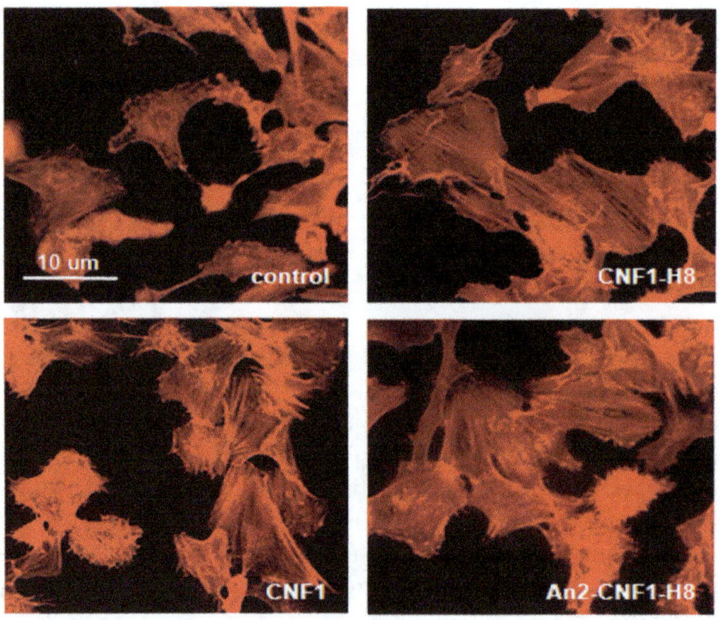

Figure 4. An2-CNF1-H8 activity on endothelial cells. Fluorescence micrographs of HBEC-5i cells treated with the An2-CNF1-H8 variant and its controls. Note the same actin architecture in cells exposed to the *wt* CNF1 and to the variants, indicating the same activity. Scale bar: 10 μm.

2.5. *Activities of the An2-CNF1-H8 Variant on the Human GBM Cells*

Since CNF1 has been reported to be remarkably effective as an antineoplastic agent in a mouse model of GBM, and to induce toxicity in GBM cells obtained from surgical specimens (WHO grade IV) [4,10,11], we verified whether the An2-CNF1-H8 variant could be effective on a human GBM cell line, the U87MG cells. We performed a cell growth analysis and, as shown in Figure 5A, whereas control cells underwent an increase in cell number over time, although characterized by a biphasic growth possibly due to depletion of some rate-limiting resource, cells treated with different concentrations of An2-CNF1-H8 stopped growing, starting from 24 h of exposure. The same result was obtained with the *wt* CNF1 (Figure 5B). A morphological analysis showed that the An2-CNF1-H8 variant could induce F-actin modification, in term of stress fibers and ruffles, and multinucleation. Interestingly, it caused an increase in the number of mitochondria but a reduction in their size, with respect to controls (Figure 6A). Western blot analysis showed that Tom20, a component of the translocase of the outer mitochondrial membrane (Tom), the main mitochondrial entry gate for nuclear-encoded proteins, was transiently increased following treatment with An2-CNF1-H8, with the maximum increment at 24 h. After 48 h of An2-CNF1-H8 treatment, Tom20 expression returned similar to the control level (Figure 6B). The amount of OPA-1 protein, involved in mitochondrial fusion, was not modified by the variant An2-CNF1-H8 (Figure 6B), as reported for *wt* CNF1 in other model systems [9,14]. We wondered whether the An2-CNF1-H8 variant stimulates senescence or apoptosis to cause cell number reduction. We then analyzed Bax, a pro-apoptotic protein, and found that An2-CNF1-H8 variant treatment induced an increase in Bax concentration starting from 24 h of exposure (Figure 6C), thus suggesting an involvement of apoptosis in the variant killing activity. However, we failed to observe the activation of caspase-3 (data not shown). On the other hand, western blot analysis of the senescence-associated beta-galactosidase (beta-gal) showed no significant differences (Figure 6C).

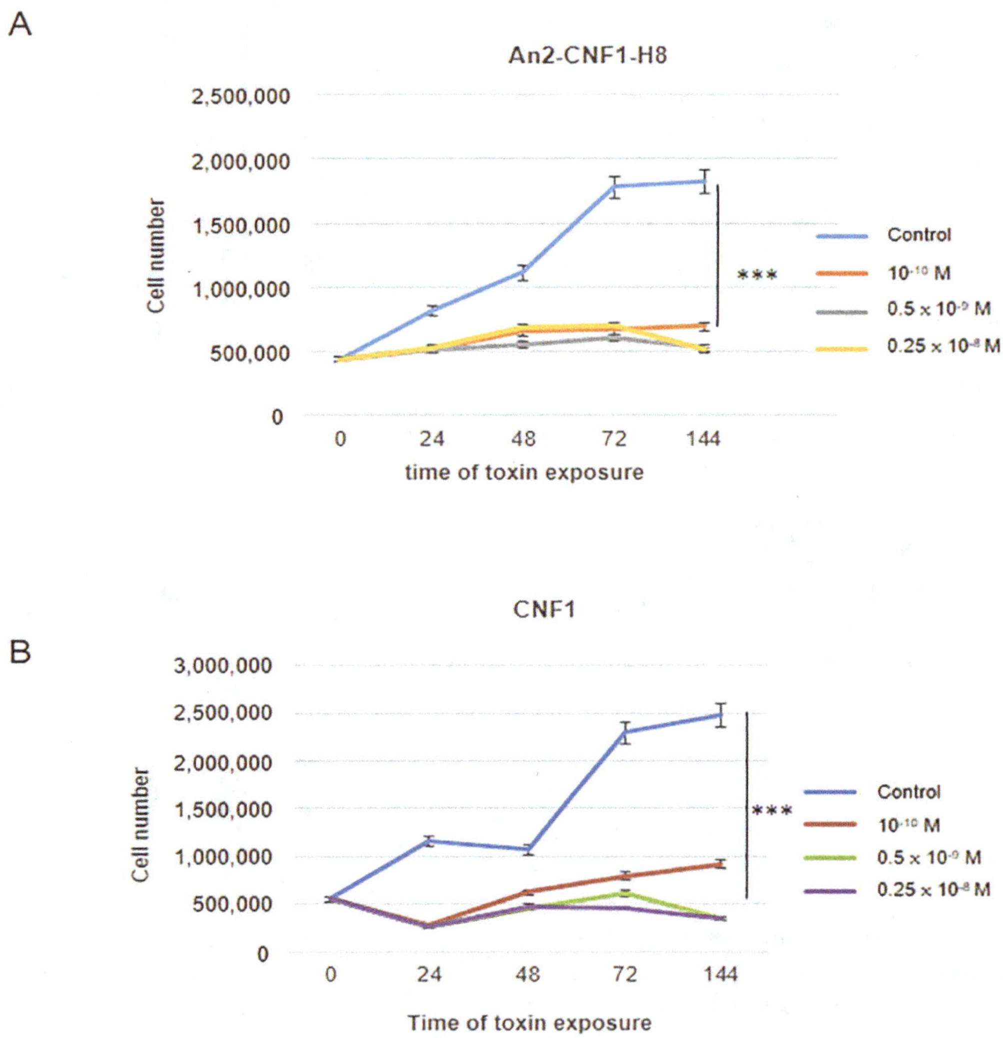

Figure 5. An2-CNF1-H8 impairs growth in U87MG GBM cells. (**A** and **B**) Graphs showing cell growth impairment by An2-CNF1-H8 (**A**) and CNF1 (**B**) on U87MG GBM cells. Note that, whereas controls cells increase in cell number in the function of time, cells treated with An2-CNF1-H8 and CNF1 stopped growing. Data on the graph represent the mean ± SEM from at least three independent experiments. *** $p < 0.001$.

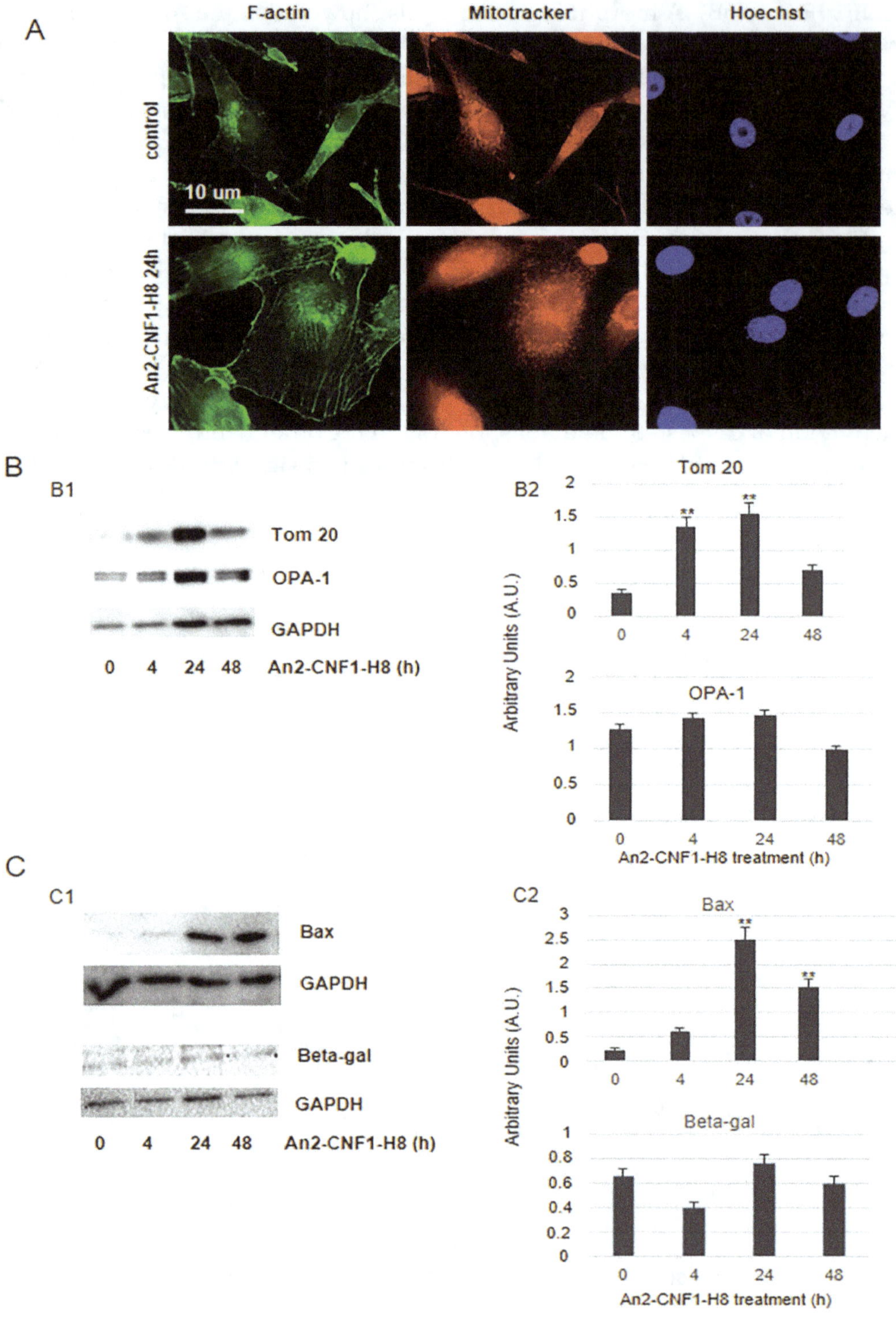

Figure 6. Mitochondrial impact and toxicity of An2-CNF1-H8 on U87MG cells. (**A**) Fluorescence micrographs of U87MG cells treated with An2-CNF1-H8 and stained with phalloidin, to detect F-actin, Mitotracker, to detect mitochondria and Hoechst 33342 to stain nuclei. Note that the variant impacts on mitochondria that appear slightly fragmented and scattered throughout the cell body with respect to controls. (**B** and **C**) Western blot of U87MG cells treated with An2-CNF1-H8 and graph analyses, showing that (**B1** and **B2**) Tom20 was transiently increased, whereas OPA-1 protein was not modified by the An2-CNF1-H8; (**C1** and **C2**) the pro-apoptotic Bax protein, involved in mitochondrial outer membrane permeabilization, was increased whereas the senescence marker beta-gal remained unvaried. Proteins were normalized as a function of GAPDH. ** $p < 0.01$. Scale bar: 10 μm.

3. Discussion

We previously reported an efficient strategy for the production and purification of the CNF1 toxin as a his-tagged recombinant protein (CNF1-H8) from *E. coli* extracts [13]. In the present manuscript, we describe the production and purification of the An2-CNF1-H8 variant, a CNF1 variant displaying an N-terminal Angiopep tag potentially endowed with the ability to allow BBB crossing.

The recombinant production of the An2-CNF1-H8 variant was approached following the protocol optimized for CNF1-H8. It turned out that the amount of recombinant An2-CNF1-H8 variant was significantly higher, but it largely accumulated as inclusion bodies, although the production was carried out at 15 °C by using only 0.5 mM inducer. Lowering of the production temperature can be a successful approach to get the soluble product when the protein has the tendency to accumulate as inclusion bodies, as in the case of CNF1-H8 [13]. However, the higher production yields achieved for An2-CNF1-H8 shifted the equilibrium towards the formation of insoluble aggregates. Nevertheless, its purification from the soluble extracts in native conditions was still feasible. Once purified, the cellular activity of the An2-CNF1-H8 variant was compared to that of *wt* CNF1 and it turned out that cellular effects completely overlapped, causing multinucleation and actin cytoskeleton changes in the same concentration ranges.

It is interesting to note that the route of entry into cells followed by the An2-CNF1-H8 variant is the same used by the *wt* CNF1. It is known that CNF1 binds to its receptor [15,16], enters endocytic vesicles by receptor-mediated endocytosis and is routed to the endosomal compartment [17] where its catalytic domain (55-kDa fragment) is transferred into the cytosol [18]. The mutant toxin CNF1 C866S, herein indicated as mCNF1, devoid of enzymatic activity [19] was able to compete for the binding to the receptor with the An2-CNF1-H8 variant inhibiting its multinucleating activity. Besides, a 55-kDa fragment was recorded into the cytosol. All these findings indicate that the variant behaves in the same way of *wt* CNF1, demonstrating that the addition of An2 and H8 at the N- and C-terminal end, respectively, did not compromise its activity on epithelial cells, although further studies on neuronal cell models should also be performed. When endothelial cells were exposed to An2-CNF1-H8, a typical CNF1-induced actin rearrangement was observed, indicating that the variant entered into this cell line and exerted its action. Since HBEC-5i cells highly express the LRP1 receptor for An2, we were expecting a better efficiency of An2-CNF1-H8 in its entry into this cell type with a consequent major effect on the targets. The observed actin rearrangement, however, was in line with what so far documented in other cell systems, underlying the necessity of further experiments to verify our hypothesis. It is interesting to note that *iv* inoculation of the An2-CNF1-H8 variant in mice can increase the amount of spinophilin in the hippocampus. This result, besides suggesting the ability of the variant to link its LRP1 receptor, represents an important step forward the demonstration of the An2-CNF1-H8 ability to cross the BBB. Further studies are needed, however, to confirm that An2-CNF1-H8 can actually pass through the barrier.

Our previous studies disclosed the potentiality of CNF1 as a novel therapeutic strategy for the treatment of CNS tumors. Vannini and coworkers reported that CNF1 possesses a cytotoxic effect on a GBM cell line as well as on primary human GBM cells, also permitting a long-term survival in a murine GBM model [10]. Besides, CNF1 reduces GBM growth and saves the function and structure of neurons [4]. Our results demonstrate that the An2-CNF1-H8 variant exerts a cell growth arrest of U87MG GBM cells in the same vein of CNF1. From a morphological point of view, it is interesting to note that An2-CNF1-H8, although inducing typical CNF1 effects consisting of F-actin polymerization and multinucleation [20], impacts on mitochondria in a different way in comparison to data reported so far. On epithelial cells and fibroblasts, CNF1 induces mitochondria elongation [21,22] due, at least in epithelial cells, to inhibition of mitochondrial fission [14]. Here, we report that, in U87MG GBM cells, both the An2-CNF1-H8 variant and CNF1 (data not shown), induced fragmentation of mitochondria and did not vary the amount of OPA1 protein, involved in mitochondria fusion. However, the number of mitochondria seems to be increased in cells challenged with the variant with respect to control cells, as also suggested by the transient increase in Tom20, a component of the outer mitochondrial membrane [23]. The dynamic of mitochondria allows the cell to respond to its ever-changing physiological conditions and in this context, fragmented mitochondria can be found in damaged or quiescent cells, associated with functional defects or early in the apoptotic pathway [24]. For this reason, we analyzed some proteins of the apoptotic as well as of the senescence pathway. Our results demonstrate that the An2-CNF1-H8 variant increased the amount of the pro-apoptotic protein Bax, although we failed to find a concomitant activation of caspase-3. On the other hand, the level of the senescence-associated marker beta-gal was almost unchanged with respect to control cells. Further studies are needed to dissect the cellular pathway engaged by the An2-CNF1-H8 variant to arrest cell growth of GBM cells. In fact, senescence may be a late phenomenon, as reported by Vannini and coworkers [10] whereas caspases may be activated later in our model. Besides, we cannot rule out the hypothesis that necroptosis can occur in U87MG GBM cells exposed to the An2-CNF1-H8 variant [24]. It is worth noting that CNF1 is being increasingly recognized as a pro-carcinogenic agent in the intestine [3,25], indicating that the toxin behaves in two different manners in the intestine and in the brain. This is not surprising since bacterial toxins, by acting as signaling modifying agents, are profoundly influenced by several factors such as, for example, different environmental and cellular/tissue conditions. In this context, it is well established that CNF1 exerts beneficial effects in mice models of Rett Syndrome and Alzheimer once injected in the brain [6,8]. On the other hand, we have very recently reported that the CNF1 ability to promote carcinogenic traits in epithelial cells is dramatically influenced by the surrounding microenvironment as well as by the cell type [3]. In all the cell types studied so far, CNF1 causes mitochondrial elongation whereas we herein report that the CNF1 variant causes mitochondria fragmentation in GBM cells, reinforcing the emerging hypothesis that the target cell type plays a pivotal role in the response to an infectious agent [26]. This last finding on mitochondria highlights a new perspective for the understanding of CNF1 activity on GBM cells.

Altogether, our results point at the An2-CNF1-H8 variant as a promising tool against GBM, preserving the same cytotoxic activities of CNF1 but being characterized by the potential ability to cross the BBB.

4. Materials and Methods

4.1. Production and Purification of CNF1 and CNF1 Variants

cnf1-h8 and *an2-cnf1-h8* genes were expressed using pET40b plasmid. The preparation of pET40b-*cnf1-h8* has been previously described [13]. For the development of pET40-*an2-cnf1-h8*, the 5′ extremity of *cnf1-h8* was replaced with a newly synthesized one using NdeI/BglII double digestion. The new DNA fragment of 188 bp was purchased from Thermo Fisher Scientific (Thermo Fisher Scientific, Waltham, MA, USA) and encodes the An2 peptide (MGTFFYGGSRGKRNNFKTEEY) coupled to a linker (GGSSRSSS) that has already been used for the production of a GFP variant fused to An2 [27].

Both An2-CNF1-H8 and CNF1-H8 were produced in *E. coli* BL21(DE3) and purified using two chromatographic steps as reported [13]. For preliminary solubility analysis, the recombinant cellular pellets were re-suspended in 5 mL/g wet cell weight of Lysis buffer (50 mM TrisHCl pH 8.0, 150 mM NaCl, 20 mM Imidazole, 15% v/v glycerol) supplemented with the complete EDTA-free protease inhibitor cocktail (Roche, Basel, Switzerland). Afterward, the suspensions were sonicated (30 s cycles, 25% amplitude with 30 sec pauses between each cycle for a total process of 20 min at 4 °C) and the soluble and insoluble fractions were separated by centrifugation (13,000 g, 4 °C, 45 min). Then, the insoluble fractions were re-suspended in an equal volume of Lysis buffer as its relative soluble fraction and the total protein profiles were studied using 10% SDS-PAGE. For western blot analysis, an anti-CNF1 antibody (NG8, Santa Cruz Biotechnology, Dallas, TX, USA, diluted 1:1000) was used following the manufacturer's instructions.

CNF1 *wt* was obtained from the *E. coli* pISS392 strain (kindly provided by V. Falbo, Istituto Superiore di Sanità, Rome, Italy), and the plasmid coding for the recombinant protein CNF1 C866S, in which the enzymatic activity on Rho GTPases is abrogated by a change of cysteine with serine at position 866 [28], was kindly provided by E. Lemichez (U627 INSERM, Nice, France). Both toxins were purified essentially as described [29], with some modifications in the procedure. All dilutions were prepared with 20 mM Tris, pH 7.4.

4.2. Cell Cultures

HEp-2 laryngeal carcinoma cells and U87MG human GBM cells were grown in Dulbecco's Modified Eagle's Medium (D-MEM, EuroClone S.p.A., Pero, Italy) enriched with 10% fetal bovine serum (FBS, EuroClone), 100 U/l mL of penicillin and 100 µg/mL of streptomycin. The cells were grown in a controlled atmosphere incubator (5% CO2, 90% humidity, temperature 37 °C). For the various steps, cells were detached with 10 mM EDTA and 0.25% trypsin in PBS, without calcium and magnesium, at pH 7.4. All treatments were performed in a microbiological safety cabinet.

For all experiments, the cells were seeded in Petri dishes or in 24-well plates, depending on the type of assay: (i) 24-well plates for all titration, inhibition, and competition experiments; (ii) 60 mm Petri dishes for western blot. Cells were seeded at a density of 2×10^4 cm^2 cells. Twenty-four h after seeding, cells were treated with the An2-CNF1-H8, CNF1-H8 and *wt* CNF1 for different times depending on the experiment considered.

HBEC-5i cerebral microvascular endothelium cells (ATCC® CRL3245™) were grown in 1% gelatin-coated culture flasks using DMEM:F12 with FBS 10% and 40 µg/mL endothelial growth supplement (Sigma–Aldrich, St. Louis, MO, USA).

4.3. CNF1 Variant Titration

Each variant was added by making successive dilutions in the culture medium, starting from a concentration of 10^{-7} M up to 10^{-14} M. After 24 h, HEp-2 cell multinucleation was estimated under a phase contrast microscope. At least 100 cells for each variant and for each dilution were counted, and the percentage of multinucleation was calculated. For HBEC-5i, since multinucleation is not evident, the cells were fixed in paraformaldehyde and labeled to highlight F-actin, which is significantly modified by CNF1, in terms of stress fibers and ruffles. All the toxins showed a similar activity ranging around 10^{-10} M.

4.4. Competition Experiments with CNF1 C866S

HEp-2 cells were put on ice for 20 min. CNF1 C866S was added to the dilutions of 1:10, 1:100, 1:1000 for 10 min on ice. An2-CNF1-H8, CNF1-H8, and *wt* CNF1 were added at 10^{-10} M. After 30 min on ice, cells were washed 3 times with fresh medium before being placed in an incubator at 37 °C for 24 h. Finally, for both HEp-2 and HBEC-5i cells, the effect of the variants was measured.

4.5. Protein Extraction of Polyacrylamide and Western Blot Gel

One or 5 µL of the different variants were run on 8% or 12% polyacrylamide gel. After the run, the proteins were stained using the brilliant blue Comassie followed by discoloration. For western blot, proteins separated by polyacrylamide gel were transferred onto Polyvinylidene Fluoride (PVDF) membrane (Bio-Rad Laboratories, Inc., Hercules, CA, USA) and an anti-CNF1 antibody recognizing the C-terminal was used. For western blot, cells were washed twice with cold PBS and then lysed with a denaturing pad composed of 50 mmol/L Tris-HCl, pH 7.5, 2 mmol/L EDTA, 100 mmol/L NaCl, 1 mmol/L Na3Vo4, 1% Nonidet P-40, 10 g/mL leupeptin, 5 g/mL aprotinin, and 10 g/mL phenyl-methyl-sulfonyl fluoride for 10 min. The lysed cells were collected with a scraper, placed in the Eppendorf, and centrifuged for 5 min at 1200 rpm. The protein concentration of the supernatants was determined with the "Bio-Rad Protein Dc" assay (Bio-Rad Laboratories). Regards in vivo experiments, tissues were lysed in the same buffer, clarified and quantified as above described. Ten µg of protein per sample were taken and subsequently solubilized by boiling in "Laemmli Sample Buffer" (Sigma–Aldrich). The proteins were separated on SDS-PAGE polyacrylamide gel [30], and subsequently electrically transferred onto a PVDF membrane (Bio-Rad Laboratories) using a Semi-dry system (Bio-Rad Laboratories). According to this procedure, the membrane in contact with the gel is placed between two absorbent paper sheets damped with the Semi-dry buffer inside the transfer apparatus. After saturating the free membrane sites with Tris-buffered saline-tween 20 (TBS-T) (20 mM Tris-HCl pH 7.5, 150 mM NaCl, 0.02% Tween 20) containing 5% skimmed milk, the same membrane was incubated overnight at 4 °C with the following antigen-specific antibodies diluted in TBS-T containing 5% skimmed milk: anti-CNF1-NG8 (Abcam, Cambridge, UK, mouse monoclonal, diluted 1:1000); anti-GAPDH (Santa Cruz, mouse monoclonal antibody, diluted 1:2000); anti-Tom20 and anti-beta-gal (Cell Signaling Technology, Inc., Danvers, MA, USA, diluted 1:1000); anti-OPA-1 (BD bioscience, diluted 1:1000); anti-Bax (Cell Signaling, diluted 1:1000); anti-spinophilin (Upstate, Lake Placid, NY, USA, diluted 1:1000).

Following washings in TBS-T, membranes were incubated with the species-specific HRP-conjugated secondary antibodies (Jackson ImmunoResearch, Ely, UK) and immune complexes were detected by chemiluminescent HRP substrates (Immobilion Western, Millipore, Burlington, MA, USA). The images were acquired through ChemiDoc (Bio-Rad Laboratories).

4.6. Cell Growth Experiments

U87MG cells were grown in 60 mm Petri dishes. Twenty-four h after seeding, cells were treated with the An2-CNF1-H8 and *wt* CNF1 at 3 different concentrations (10^{-10} M, 0.5×10^{-9}, 0.25×10^{-8}). At different time points, An2-CNF1-H8 and CNF1-treated cells were detached from the culture dish with 10 mM EDTA and 0.25% trypsin in PBS and counted by using a Neubauer chamber. Cell counts were conducted five times and at least three separate experiments were carried out.

4.7. Mouse Studies

C57BL6/J male mice (Charles River Italia), were housed under standard conditions (21/23 °C, 40/50% humidity, 12 h light-dark cycle, food and water ad libitum). All procedures were carried out in accordance with the European and National Legislation (63/2010 EU, DL 26/2014, respectively) and approved by the Italian Ministry of Health (n.469/2018-PR). Mice were treated by tail vein injection with An2-H8, CNF1-H8 (0.5×10^{-10} M in a final volume of 175 μL) or Tris. General health and behavior of each mouse were monitored for 10 days following *iv* injection. Then, mice were sacrificed, brain extracted from the skull, and brain regions rapidly dissected and frozen for further biochemical analyses.

4.8. Fluorescence Microscopy

U87MG control and treated cells were fixed and processed as previously described [21]. Fitc-phalloidin (Sigma–Aldrich) was used to stain F-actin and Mitotracker (Molecular Probes, Eugene, OR, USA) was used to stain mitochondria. Nuclei were stained with Hoechst 33258 (Sigma–Aldrich). Glass coverslips were observed with a fluorescence optical microscope Olympus BX51/BX52 and images were acquired using the program IAS 2000 (Delta System, Rome, Italy).

4.9. Statistical Analysis

Data are presented as mean ± sem. Statistical analysis was performed by one-way ANOVA. When a significant main effect was detected, Tukey's test for post-hoc comparisons was performed, with $p < 0.05$ as a threshold for significant differences.

Author Contributions: Conceptualization, A.F. (Alessia Fabbri) and C.F.; Software, Z.M.; Investigation, A.C., A.F. (Andrea Fortuna), S.L., L.R., and E.A.P.G.; Formal analysis, A.F. (Alessia Fabbri), S.L., L.R., M.L.T., and C.F.; Data Curation, A.F. (Alessia Fabbri); Writing—Original Draft Preparation, A.F. (Alessia Fabbri); Writing—Review & Editing, A.C., Z.M., E.P., E.A.P.G., M.L.T., C.F., and A.F. (Alessia Fabbri); Visualization, Z.M.; Funding Acquisition, M.L.T. and A.F. (Alessia Fabbri). All authors have read and agreed to the published version of the manuscript.

Acknowledgments: The authors thank Rossella Di Nallo (ISS) for invaluable technical support.

References

1. Louis, D.N.; Perry, A.; Reifenberger, G.; von Deimling, A.; Figarella-Branger, D.; Cavenee, W.K.; Ohgaki, H.; Wiestler, O.D.; Kleihues, P.; Ellison, D.W. The 2016 world health organization classification of tumors of the central nervous system: A summary. *Acta Neuropathol.* **2016**, *131*, 803–820. [CrossRef] [PubMed]
2. Yang, K.; Niu, L.; Bai, Y.; Le, W. Glioblastoma: Targeting the autophagy in tumorigenesis. *Brain Res. Bull.* **2019**, *153*, 334–340. [CrossRef] [PubMed]
3. Fabbri, A.; Travaglione, S.; Rosadi, F.; Ballan, G.; Maroccia, Z.; Giambenedetti, M.; Guidotti, M.; Ødum, N.; Krejsgaard, T.; Fiorentini, C. The Escherichia coli protein toxin cytotoxic necrotizing factor 1 induces epithelial mesenchymal transition. *Cell. Microbiol.* **2019**, *22*, e13138. [CrossRef] [PubMed]
4. Vannini, E.; Olimpico, F.; Middei, S.; Ammassari-Teule, M.; de Graaf, E.L.; McDonnell, L.; Schmidt, G.; Fabbri, A.; Fiorentini, C.; Baroncelli, L.; et al. Electrophysiology of glioma: A Rho GTPase-activating protein reduces tumor growth and spares neuron structure and function. *Neuro. Oncol.* **2016**, *18*, 1634–1643. [CrossRef]
5. De Filippis, B.; Valenti, D.; de Bari, L.; De Rasmo, D.; Musto, M.; Fabbri, A.; Ricceri, L.; Fiorentini, C.; Laviola, G.; Vacca, R.A. Mitochondrial free radical overproduction due to respiratory chain impairment in the brain of a mouse model of Rett syndrome: Protective effect of CNF1. *Free Radic. Biol. Med.* **2015**, *83*, 167–177. [CrossRef]
6. De Filippis, B.; Fabbri, A.; Simone, D.; Canese, R.; Ricceri, L.; Malchiodi-Albedi, F.; Laviola, G.; Fiorentini, C. Modulation of RhoGTPases Improves the Behavioral Phenotype and Reverses Astrocytic Deficits in a Mouse Model of Rett Syndrome. *Neuropsychopharmacology* **2012**, *37*, 1152–1163. [CrossRef]
7. De Filippis, B.; Valenti, D.; Chiodi, V.; Ferrante, A.; de Bari, L.; Fiorentini, C.; Domenici, M.R.; Ricceri, L.; Vacca, R.A.; Fabbri, A.; et al. Modulation of Rho GTPases rescues brain mitochondrial dysfunction, cognitive deficits and aberrant synaptic plasticity in female mice modeling Rett syndrome. *Eur. Neuropsychopharmacol.* **2015**, *25*, 889–901. [CrossRef]
8. Loizzo, S.; Rimondini, R.; Travaglione, S.; Fabbri, A.; Guidotti, M.; Ferri, A.; Campana, G.; Fiorentini, C. CNF1 Increases Brain Energy Level, Counteracts Neuroinflammatory Markers and Rescues Cognitive Deficits in a Murine Model of Alzheimer's Disease. *PLoS ONE* **2013**, *8*, e65898. [CrossRef]
9. Travaglione, S.; Ballan, G.; Fortuna, A.; Ferri, A.; Guidotti, M.; Campana, G.; Fiorentini, C.; Loizzo, S. CNF1 enhances brain energy content and counteracts spontaneous epileptiform phenomena in aged DBA/2J mice. *PLoS ONE* **2015**, *10*, e0140495. [CrossRef]
10. Vannini, E.; Panighini, A.; Cerri, C.; Fabbri, A.; Lisi, S.; Pracucci, E.; Benedetto, N.; Vannozzi, R.; Fiorentini, C.; Caleo, M.; et al. The bacterial protein toxin, cytotoxic necrotizing factor 1 (CNF1) provides long-term survival in a murine glioma model. *BMC Cancer* **2014**, *14*, 449. [CrossRef]
11. Vannini, E.; Maltese, F.; Olimpico, F.; Fabbri, A.; Costa, M.; Caleo, M.; Baroncelli, L. Progression of motor deficits in glioma-bearing mice: Impact of CNF1 therapy at symptomatic stages. *Oncotarget* **2017**, *8*, 23539–23550. [CrossRef] [PubMed]
12. Demeule, M.; Currie, J.C.; Bertrand, Y.; Ché, C.; Nguyen, T.; Régina, A.; Gabathuler, R.; Castaigne, J.P.; Béliveau, R. Involvement of the low-density lipoprotein receptor-related protein in the transcytosis of the brain delivery vector Angiopep-2. *J. Neurochem.* **2008**, *106*, 1534–1544. [CrossRef] [PubMed]
13. Colarusso, A.; Caterino, M.; Fabbri, A.; Fiorentini, C.; Vergara, A.; Sica, F.; Parrilli, E.; Tutino, M.L. High yield purification and first structural characterization of the full-length bacterial toxin CNF1. *Biotechnol. Prog.* **2018**, *34*, 150–159. [CrossRef] [PubMed]
14. Travaglione, S.; Loizzo, S.; Rizza, T.; Del Brocco, A.; Ballan, G.; Guidotti, M.; Vona, R.; Di Nottia, M.; Torraco, A.; Carrozzo, R.; et al. Enhancement of mitochondrial ATP production by the *Escherichia coli* cytotoxic necrotizing factor 1. *FEBS J.* **2014**, *281*, 3473–3488. [CrossRef] [PubMed]
15. Kim, K.J.; Chung, J.W.; Kim, K.S. 67-kDa laminin receptor promotes internalization of cytotoxic necrotizing factor 1-expressing Escherichia coli K1 into human brain microvascular endothelial cells. *J. Biol. Chem.* **2005**, *280*, 1360–1368. [CrossRef] [PubMed]
16. Chung, J.W.; Hong, S.J.; Kim, K.J.; Goti, D.; Stins, M.F.; Shin, S.; Dawson, V.L.; Dawson, T.M.; Kim, K.S. 37-kDa laminin receptor precursor modulates cytotoxic necrotizing factor 1-mediated RhoA activation and bacterial uptake. *J. Biol. Chem.* **2003**, *278*, 16857–16862. [CrossRef]

17. Contamin, S.; Galmiche, A.; Doye, A.; Flatau, G.; Benmerah, A.; Boquet, P. The p21 Rho-activating toxin cytotoxic necrotizing factor 1 is endocytosed by a clathrin-independent mechanism and enters the cytosol by an acidic-dependent membrane translocation step. *Mol. Biol. Cell* **2000**, *11*, 1775–1787. [CrossRef]
18. Knust, Z.; Blumenthal, B.; Aktories, K.; Schmidt, G. Cleavage of escherichia coli cytotoxic necrotizing factor 1 is required for full biologic activity. *Infect. Immun.* **2009**, *77*, 1835–1841. [CrossRef]
19. Lerm, M.; Schmidt, G.; Goehring, U.M.; Schirmer, J.; Aktories, K. Identification of the region of Rho involved in substrate recognition by Escherichia coli cytotoxic necrotizing factor 1 (CNF1). *J. Biol. Chem.* **1999**, *274*, 28999–29004. [CrossRef]
20. Fabbri, A.; Travaglione, S.; Fiorentini, C. Escherichia coli cytotoxic necrotizing factor 1 (CNF1): Toxin biology, in vivo applications and therapeutic potential. *Toxins (Basel)* **2010**, *2*, 283–296. [CrossRef]
21. Giamboi-Miraglia, A.; Travaglione, S.; Filippini, P.; Fabbri, A.; Fiorentini, C.; Falzano, L. A multinucleating Escherichia coli cytotoxin perturbs cell cycle in cultured epithelial cells. *Toxicol. In Vitro* **2007**, *21*, 235–239. [CrossRef] [PubMed]
22. Fabbri, A.; Travaglione, S.; Maroccia, Z.; Guidotti, M.; Pierri, C.; Primiano, G.; Servidei, S.; Loizzo, S.; Fiorentini, C. The Bacterial Protein CNF1 as a Potential Therapeutic Strategy against Mitochondrial Diseases: A Pilot Study. *Int. J. Mol. Sci.* **2018**, *19*, 1825. [CrossRef] [PubMed]
23. Johnson, A.E.; Jensen, R.E. Barreling through the membrane. *Nat. Struct. Mol. Biol.* **2004**, *11*, 113–114. [CrossRef] [PubMed]
24. Westermann, B. Mitochondrial fusion and fission in cell life and death. *Nat. Rev. Mol. Cell Biol.* **2010**, *11*, 872–884. [CrossRef]
25. Buc, E.; Dubois, D.; Sauvanet, P.; Raisch, J.; Delmas, J.; Darfeuille-Michaud, A.; Pezet, D.; Bonnet, R. High Prevalence of mucosa-associated *E. coli* producing cyclomodulin and genotoxin in colon cancer. *PLoS ONE* **2013**, *8*, e56964. [CrossRef]
26. Keener, A.B. Host with the most: Targeting host cells instead of pathogens to fight infectious disease. *Nat. Med.* **2017**, *23*, 528–531. [CrossRef]
27. Serna, N.; Céspedes, M.V.; Saccardo, P.; Xu, Z.; Unzueta, U.; Álamo, P.; Pesarrodona, M.; Sánchez-Chardi, A.; Roldán, M.; Mangues, R.; et al. Rational engineering of single-chain polypeptides into protein-only, BBB-targeted nanoparticles. *Nanomedicine* **2016**, *12*, 1241–1251. [CrossRef]
28. Schmidt, G.; Selzer, J.; Lerm, M.; Aktories, K. The Rho-deamidating cytotoxic necrotizing factor 1 from Escherichia coli possesses transglutaminase activity. Cysteine 866 and histidine 881 are essential for enzyme activity. *J. Biol. Chem.* **1998**, *273*, 13669–13674. [CrossRef]
29. Falzano, L.; Fiorentini, C.; Donelli, G.; Michel, E.; Kocks, C.; Cossart, P.; Cabanié, L.; Oswald, E.; Boquet, P. Induction of phagocytic behaviour in human epithelial cells by Escherichia coli cytotoxic necrotizing factor type 1. *Mol. Microbiol.* **1993**, *9*, 1247–1254. [CrossRef]
30. Laemmli, U.K. Cleavage of structural proteins during the assembly of the head of bacteriophage T4. *Nature* **1970**, *227*, 680–685. [CrossRef]

Investigating Radiotherapy Response in a Novel Syngeneic Model of Prostate Cancer

Charles M. Haughey [1,2,†], Debayan Mukherjee [3,†], Rebecca E. Steele [1,4], Amy Popple [3], Lara Dura-Perez [1], Adam Pickard [1,5], Mehjabin Patel [3], Suneil Jain [1], Paul B. Mullan [1], Rich Williams [1], Pedro Oliveira [6], Niamh E. Buckley [1,7], Jamie Honeychurch [3], Simon S. McDade [1], Timothy Illidge [3,6,*], Ian G. Mills [1,2,*] and Sharon L. Eddie [1,*]

1 Patrick G Johnston Centre for Cancer Research, Queen's University, Belfast BT9 7AE, UK; charles.haughey@nds.ox.ac.uk (C.M.H.); rebecca.steele@icr.ac.uk (R.E.S.); laraduraperez@gmail.com (L.D.-P.); adam.pickard@manchester.ac.uk (A.P.); s.jain@qub.ac.uk (S.J.); P.Mullan@qub.ac.uk (P.B.M.); rich.williams@qub.ac.uk (R.W.); n.obrien@qub.ac.uk (N.E.B.); S.McDade@qub.ac.uk (S.S.M.)

2 Nuffield Department of Surgical Sciences, John Radcliffe Hospital, University of Oxford, Oxford OX3 9DU, UK

3 Targeted Therapy Group, Division of Cancer Sciences, Faculty of Biology Medicine and Health, The University of Manchester, Manchester M13 9PL, UK; debayan.mukherjee@manchester.ac.uk (D.M.); apopple@microbiotica.com (A.P.); mehjabinpatel94@hotmail.com (M.P.); Jamie.Honeychurch@manchester.ac.uk (J.H.)

4 The Breast Cancer Now Toby Robins Breast Cancer Research Centre, The Institute of Cancer Research, London SM2 5NG, UK

5 Wellcome Centre for Cell Matrix Research, University of Manchester, Manchester M13 9PL, UK

6 The Christie Hospital Foundation Trust, Manchester M20 4BX, UK; Pedro.Oliveira@christie.nhs.uk

7 School of Pharmacy, Queen's University Belfast, Belfast BT9 7BL, UK

* Correspondence: tim.illidge@manchester.ac.uk (T.I.); ian.mills@nds.ox.ac.uk (I.G.M.); s.eddie@qub.ac.uk (S.L.E.)

† Joint first authorship—These authors contributed equally to this work.

Simple Summary: Pre-clinical models are required to develop new therapeutics to improve patient care. In the prostate cancer field, significant progress has been made in the development of in vivo models but with a predominant focus on transgenics, which are time and cost prohibitive. Conversely, other available models do not closely resemble patient disease and tumour immune microenvironment. In this study, a new graft-based model is described, using a cell-line derived from a transgenic: the DVL3 model. Grafts using the DVL3 cells retain the pathological and immunological features of localized clinical disease, whilst genetically the model is sustained by poor prognosis drivers of disease progression. Irradiating tumours post-engraftment leads to remodeling of the tumour immune microenvironment and increased expression of genes associated with nucleic acid sensing pathways and the type I interferon response. This paper establishes this model as resource for the pre-clinical characterization of new prostate cancer therapies and biological responses to treatment.

Abstract: The prostate cancer (PCa) field lacks clinically relevant, syngeneic mouse models which retain the tumour microenvironment observed in PCa patients. This study establishes a cell line from prostate tumour tissue derived from the *Pten*$^{-/-}$/*trp53*$^{-/-}$ mouse, termed DVL3 which when subcutaneously implanted in immunocompetent C57BL/6 mice, forms tumours with distinct glandular morphology, strong cytokeratin 8 and androgen receptor expression, recapitulating high-risk localised human PCa. Compared to the commonly used TRAMP C1 model, generated with SV40 large T-antigen, DVL3 tumours are immunologically cold, with a lower proportion of CD8+ T-cells, and high proportion of immunosuppressive myeloid derived suppressor cells (MDSCs), thus resembling high-risk PCa. Furthermore, DVL3 tumours are responsive to fractionated RT, a standard treatment for localised and metastatic PCa, compared to the TRAMP C1 model. RNA-sequencing of irradiated DVL3 tumours identified upregulation of type-1 interferon and STING pathways, as well as transcripts associated with MDSCs. Upregulation of STING expression in tumour epithelium and the recruitment of MDSCs following irradiation was confirmed by immunohistochemistry. The DVL3 syngeneic model represents substantial progress in preclinical PCa modelling, displaying pathological, micro-environmental and treatment responses observed in molecular high-risk disease. Our study supports using this model for development and validation of treatments targeting PCa, especially novel immune therapeutic agents.

Keywords: tumour microenvironment; syngeneic model; prostate cancer; radiotherapy; preclinical modelling; myeloid-derived suppressor cells

---

1. Introduction

Prostate cancer (PCa) is the most common cancer in men and the fifth leading cause of cancer deaths [1]. It is estimated that 1.3 million new cases of PCa were diagnosed worldwide in 2018 alone [1]. The vast majority of PCa (91%) is localised disease at diagnosis [2], and can be treated with a range of therapeutic modalities including surgery, androgen-deprivation therapy (ADT) and radiotherapy (RT). Unfortunately, roughly 30% of high-risk localised PCa will develop into aggressive metastatic disease [3], with limited treatment options. The current standard of care for these patients is ADT, but this has many adverse side effects and has a median relapse rate of only 11 months [4].

As a result, efforts have focused on the use of RT, as it can be utilised to treat both localised and metastatic disease, with comparable patient outcomes to radical prostatectomy [5]. However, one major challenge in enhancing RT response, by combining this modality with other treatments, is the paucity of appropriate preclinical PCa models in which to test these combinations. Immune comprised mice are required for xenograft models, thus failing to recapitulate the patient tumour microenvironment (TME) and the critical role the immune component plays in both therapeutic response and relapse of disease.

The most commonly used immune-competent model is the TRAMP C1 murine cell line, which can be syngenically, subcutaneously grafted to generate more uniform, accessible prostate tumours [6]. The TRAMP C1 model was generated by engineered expression of viral SV40 large T-antigen. Unfortunately, TRAMP C1 allografts develop neuroendocrine tumours which are rare clinically, rather than adenocarcinomas which are most often seen in PCa patients [7].

Consequently, novel PCa models that more accurately recapitulate human tumours and the surrounding TME are urgently required, in order to continue to develop and improve PCa treatment. *PTEN* deletion occurs in ~20% of localized PCa, and is implicated in RT failure [8,9], however, an engraftable mouse syngeneic model with *Pten* deletion, which can be utilised to investigate host response to radiotherapy has long been lacking. In this study we have developed a syngenic model from the *Pten*$^{-/-}$/*trp53*$^{-/-}$ transgenic mouse tumour [10]; the DVL3 cell line (derived from tumour formed from the dorsal, ventral and lateral prostate lobes. These lobes are most similar to the peripheral zone of the human prostate where 75–85% of adenocarcinomas originate [11]; whereas, the anterior lobe of the mouse prostate is considered analogous to the central zone which rarely develops cancer in the human prostate [12].

DVL3 cells develop tumours in immune competent, C57BL/6 mice that retain morphological, lineage and immune characteristics of localised, high-risk PCa. These tumours respond to RT, retain androgen receptor (AR) expression and sensitivity to androgens, and display an immune 'cold' phenotype with tumours being poorly infiltrated by T-cells, and heavily infiltrated with myeloid cells, which is primarily driven by *Pten* loss [13]. Clinically, human prostate cancers are broadly classified as non-T-cell inflamed/ 'cold' tumours [14], and PTEN deficiency is associated with an immunosuppressive TME [15]. The DVL3 model accurately mimics both patient disease and TME and is therefore ideal for future pre-clinical evaluation of novel treatment combinations including immune therapeutic agents.

2. Results

2.1. DVL3 Cell Engraftment in Immunocompetent Mice Results in Tumour Formation, which Accurately Models Human Prostate Adenocarcinoma

Murine cell lines were generated via spontaneous immortalisation of normal prostate epithelium (mPECs) and prostate tumours (DVL3) (Supplementary Figure S1). To establish tumorigenic potential, both mPEC and the DVL3 cells were subcutaneously implanted into wild-type C57BL/6 male mice, as all cell lines were originally generated from the C57BL/6 strain. Engrafted tumour growth rate was compared to the established TRAMP C1 model. Mice engrafted with mPEC cells did not develop any sign of disease after 12 weeks (data not shown), consistent with their status as untransformed, but spontaneously immortalised wild-type prostate epithelial cells. DVL3 tumours grew at a similar rate to the TRAMP C1 model, with measurable tumour established after 4 weeks post-inoculation (Figure 1A). DVL3 tumours displayed heterogeneous pathology with neoplastic, glandular structures akin to human acinar adenocarcinoma (Figure 1B, Supplementary Figure S2A). Some regions of adenosarcoma were observed in larger, terminal endpoint tumours as previously reported arising from *Pten*$^{-/-}$/*trp53*$^{-/-}$ Pb-Cre4 mice [10]. In contrast, TRAMP C1 tumours were uniformly undifferentiated and lacked glandular morphology (Figure 1B).

PCa arises from glandular epithelium of the prostate, and retains expression of classical prostate markers including cytokeratins 5 and 8 (CK5 and CK8, basal and luminal epithelial markers respectively) [16]. Immunohistochemical staining revealed that the DVL3 tumours highly expressed CK8 throughout the entire tumour, particularly in the cells surrounding the lumen of glandular structures (representative images in Figure 1B,C with further images in Supplementary Figure S3). DVL3 tumours also had regions of CK5 positivity, with varied expression between the tumours. In comparison the TRAMP C1 tumours lacked the expression of both CK8 and CK5 (Figure 1B,C).

Androgen receptor (AR) was present in the nucleus of cells throughout DVL3 tumours but was most abundant in clustered regions lining the lumen of glandular structures. Conversely, TRAMP C1 tumours had notably less AR staining likely due to fewer glandular structures, with some tumours lacking AR expression entirely (Figure 1B,C, Supplementary Figures S2 and S3). To investigate if AR within the tumours was active, a downstream target of the AR, NKX3.1 expression was evaluated. NKX3.1 is prostate-specific protein, and thus used to identify PCa metastatic disease and is also known to be lost in castrate-resistant PCa [17,18]. Both the DVL3 and the TRAMP C1 tumours were positive for NKX3.1 throughout the tumour section (Supplementary Figures S2B and S3). Expression of CD34, which highlights endothelial cells, was also investigated, with no notable differences observed in staining intensity between the models (Supplementary Figure S2B).

Characterisation of mPEC and DVL3 cell lines was also performed to establish expression in serially passaged cell lines in vitro. qRT-PCR revealed significantly higher mRNA expression of CK5 and CK8 in mPEC and DVL3 cells compared to the TRAMP C1 cells (Figure 1D). Protein expression of CK8 was also notably higher in mPEC and DVL3 cells compared to TRAMP C1 and the DVL3 cells did not express Pten, in keeping with their origin (Figure 1E, densitometry provided in Supplementary Figure S4). All models expressed AR at both the mRNA and protein level (Supplementary Figures S2C,D and S4). Although expression of AR was higher in TRAMP C1 cells, DVL3 responded similarly to the AR antagonist (enzalutamide), as demonstrated in vitro using cell viability assay (Supplementary Figure S2E). The expression of CK8 and AR was also validated using immunofluorescence staining (Figure 1F). Interestingly, CK5 protein expression was not detectable in any of the prostate cell models when examined via immunocytochemistry (Figure 1F).

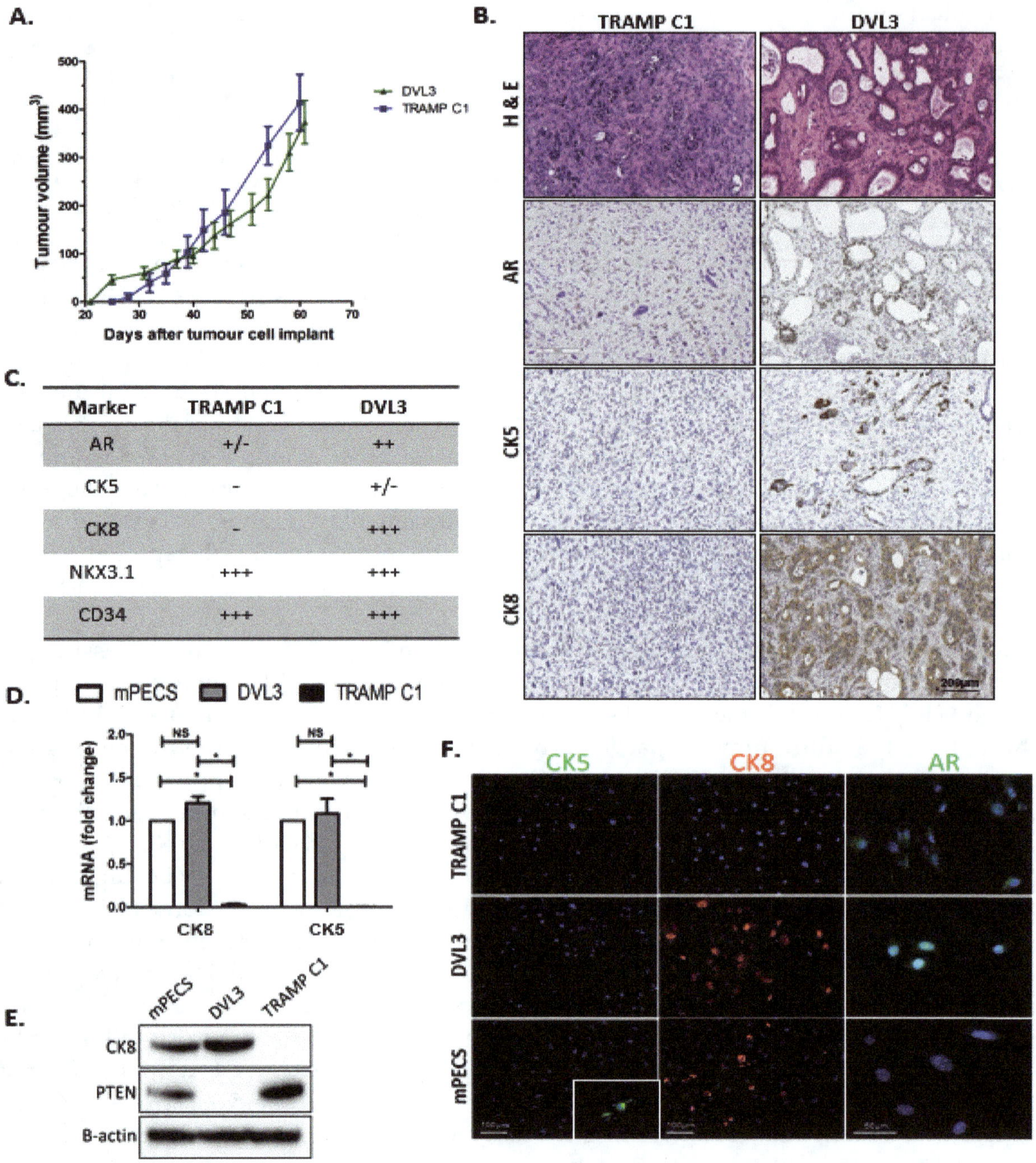

Figure 1. DVL3 syngeneic tumours replicate patient disease. (**A**) DVL3 tumour growth (Green) is comparable to TRAMP C1 (Blue), n = 5–8 mice per group. Both models take ~4 weeks to generate substantial tumours. The mPEC model of normal prostate epithelium did not generate tumours (data not shown) (**B**) DVL3 tumours develop heterogeneous glandular morphology graded at Gleason 7, whereas TRAMP C1 tumours were undifferentiated with neuroendocrine features (H&E). DVL3 also expressed clinical prostate cancer markers; androgen receptor (AR), cytokeratin 5 (CK5) and cytokeratin 8 (CK8). TRAMP C1 expressed no CK8 or CK5 and less AR than DVL3 tumours, with complete absence of AR noted in some tumours. (**C**) Summary of histological evaluation of prostate specific markers in DVL3 and TRAMP C1 prostate tumours (– indicates absence, +/– presence in only some of tumour samples, and + indicates the level of positive expression). Both DVL3 and TRAMP C1 express NKX3.1 and CD34 (Supplementary Figure S2). (**D**) Both novel cell models (mPEC and DVL3) express CK5 and CK8 mRNA at significantly higher levels than TRAMP C1 cells, as analysed via qRT-PCR (n = 3 biological replicates per cell type). mRNA expression was normalised to β-actin expression and shown as a fold change relative to

mPECs transcript levels. (**E**) Expression of CK8 (luminal marker, 60 kDa) was also evident at the protein level. Importantly, DVL3 cells demonstrate loss of the clinically relevant tumour suppressor, Pten (55 kDA). B-actin provided as a loading control (47 kDa). (**F**) Immunocytochemical staining was consistent with qRT-PCR and western blotting results for CK8 (Red) and AR (Green). CK5 protein (Green) was not detectable in any of the models (MCF7 cells provided as a positive control, inset). Dapi (Blue) used as a counterstain. Data represents mean ± SEM. * denotes $p \leq 0.05$, NS denotes non-significant, as determined by Student's *t*-test. Immunohistochemistry and western blotting are representative of $n = 3$ biological replicates.

2.2. DVL3 Tumours Have Immunosuppressive Microenvironment Similar to Human Prostate Adenocarcinomas

Human prostate cancers are broadly classified as non-T-cell inflamed/'cold' tumours with dysfunctional or suppressed tumour infiltrating lymphocytes (TILs) [14]. Pten deficient prostate cancers are also associated with an immunosuppressive TME [15]. Having established that DVL3 tumours ($Pten^{-/-}/trp53^{-/-}$) retained expression of several key markers of human disease, the immunological characteristic of the TME were assessed compared to the TRAMP-C1. Flow cytometry was performed for T cells (CD4+, CD8+), macrophages (F4/80), and myeloid-derived suppressor cells (MDSC), identified as dual (Gr1+/CD11b+) cells in dissociated DVL3 and TRAMP C1 (gating strategy demonstrated in Supplementary Figure S5), at similar size/ tumor volume for baseline immune profiling (Supplementary Figure S6A). The DVL3 tumours have a lower proportion of both cytotoxic CD8 + T-cells (0.187% vs. 2.05%, $p = 0.01$) and CD4 + T-cells (0.36% vs. 4.31%, $p = 0.01$) compared to the TRAMP C1 tumours (Figure 2A,B). In contrast, both tumour lines have comparable level of macrophage (F4/80+) cells (Figure 2C). The DVL3 tumours have a higher proportion of MDSCs (CD11b+/ Gr1+), compared to the TRAMP C1 tumour (16.90% vs 6.61%, $p = 0.04$, Figure 2D).

Interestingly, the DVL3 tumours have higher proportion of MDSCs (CD11b+/Gr1+ cells) compared to other syngeneic mouse models, such as 4T1 (breast cancer) CT26 (colorectal cancer) and 4434 ($BRAF^{V600E}$ melanoma) models ($p = 0.003$. 0.01, and 0.01 respectively, Supplementary Figure S6B,C). Comparison to other syngeneic models was performed using tumours that had reached terminal endpoint and thus were larger in volume. Notably, these data suggest that in the DVL3 model, irrespective of the tumour size, the relative ratio of (CD11b +/Gr1 +) cells within the leukocyte compartment is significantly higher and increases over time or as the tumour develops.

We also evaluated the CD8+ T cell using immunohistochemistry in DVL3 tumours compared to the 4434 melanoma model, which are immunologically active, 'hot' tumours [19] (Figure 2E). In agreement with the flow cytometry data (Figure 2A), immunohistochemistry demonstrates the DVL3 tumours are immunologically 'cold' having very few basal CD8+ T cells, that were sparsely distributed primarily around the tumour edge, but absent in the centre or around the tumour epithelium/ glandular structures.

In comparison the syngeneic murine melanoma 4434 ($BRAF^{V600E}$) model had a greater proportion of CD8 + T-cells ($p < 0.001$), which were uniformly distributed, including in the central region of the tumour (Figure 2E,F). These data demonstrate that murine DVL3 prostate tumours have immunologically inactive/ non-inflamed phenotype, with the TME primarily compromising of myeloid cells, but, lacking TILs population similar to the advanced human disease.

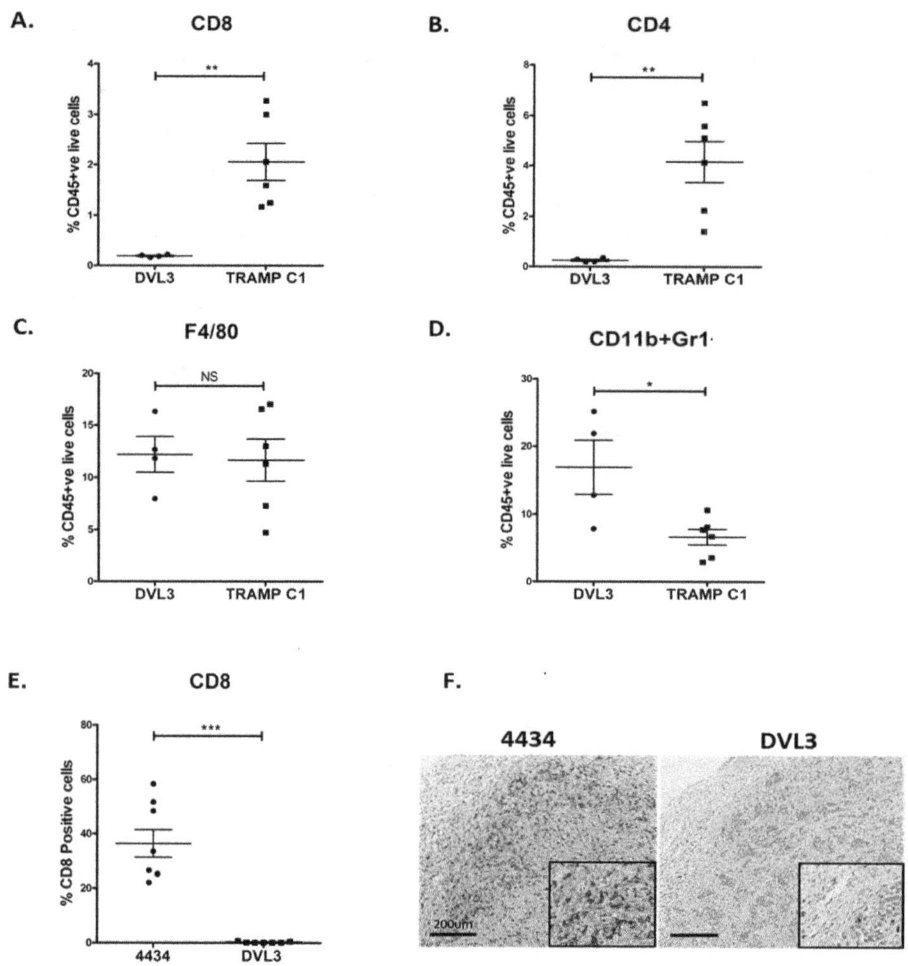

Figure 2. The DVL3 model generates immunosuppressive, 'cold' tumours similar to the TME seen clinically in prostate cancer. Flow cytometry was performed on DVL3 and TRAMP-C1 subcutaneous, syngeneic tumours taken 4-6 weeks post engraftment or when they reached the treatment size (100–200 mm^3). DVL3 tumours had significantly fewer (**A**) cytotoxic (CD8+) and (**B**) helper T cells (CD4+) when compared with the TRAMP-C1 model. (**C**) There was no difference in the proportion of macrophages (F4/80) between the two models. (**D**) However, the population of myeloid derived suppressor cells (MDSCs, CD11b+Gr1+) was significantly increased in the DVL3 compared to TRAMP-C1 tumours. (**E**) Quantification of immunohistochemical staining for CD8+ T-cells in inflamed syngeneic murine (4434 Braf^{4006E}) melanoma model compared to the non-immunogenic DVL3 murine prostate cancer model shown as a percentage of total cells as quantified by haematoxylin. (**F**) Representative IHC staining comparing 4434 (Braf^{4006E}) melanoma vs DVL3 prostate tumour demonstrating lack of CD8+T-cells within the tumour microenvironment in the DVL3 tumours. In 4434 (Braf^{4006E}) melanoma model CD8+ T-cells are uniformly distributed, including the central of the tumour. Data represents mean ± SEM of $n = 4$–9 independent murine tumors as indicated by points on each graph. * denotes $p \leq 0.05$, ** denotes $p \leq 0.01$, *** denotes $p < 0.001$ as determined by Mann-Whitney, non-parametric testing.

2.3. Fractionated Radiotherapy Leads to Marginal Growth Delay and Alters the Local Tumour Immune Microenvironment

RT is a radical primary treatment administered to patients with high-risk localised PCa, and also to patients with metastatic PCa. Therefore, therapeutic response to RT was evaluated in the DVL3 model and compared to the TRAMP C1 model. Established tumours (100–200 mm^3) were assigned to treatment groups. The mice received either a single high dose of 8 Gy, which is often prescribed to treat PCa patients with metastatic disease; or conventional fractionated RT of 2 Gy administered over 5-consecutive days, which is similar to that used to treat localised disease (Figure 3A). Both single high dose (8 Gy) and fractioned RT (5 × 2 Gy) exhibited a growth delay compared to non-treated controls (0 Gy, $p = 0.02$, Figure 3B) and this improved survival of mice with engrafted DVL3 tumour cells ($p = 0.03$ and 0.02 respectively, Figure 3C). Conversely, neither the TRAMP C1 tumour size nor survival was significantly affected by either RT regime (Figure 3D,E). This demonstrates DVL3 allograft tumours are responsive to RT, including fractionated RT, whilst TRAMP C1 do not, as previously described (summarized in Figure 3F) [20].

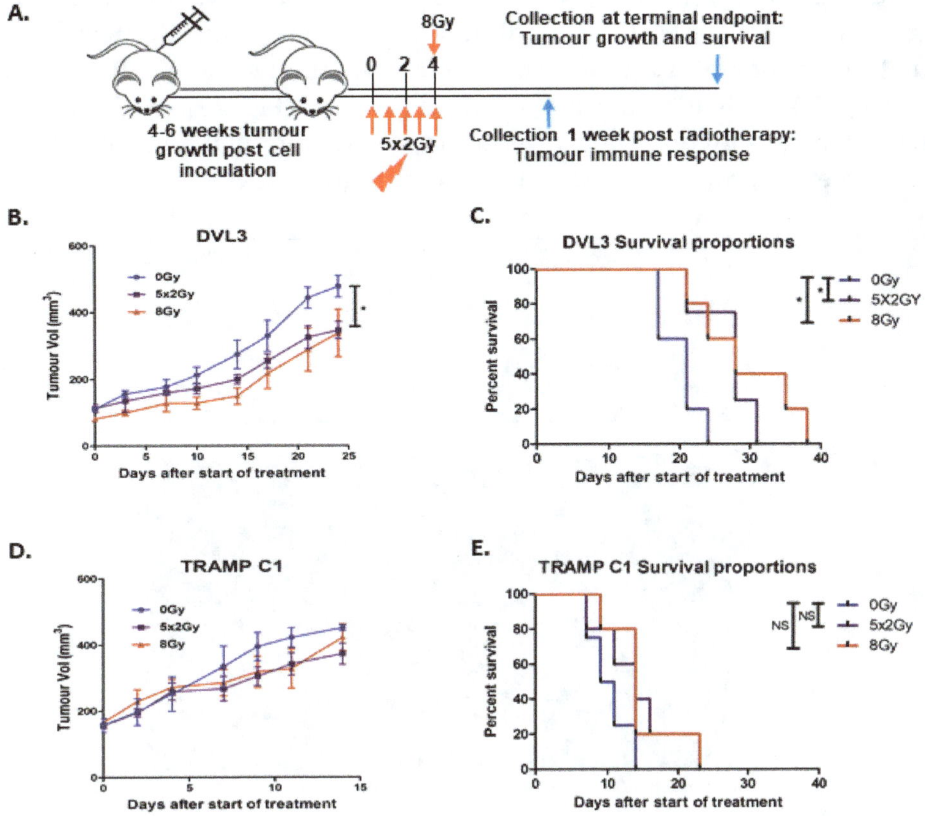

F.

Radiation dose	DVL3 Median survival (Days)	TRAMP C1 Median survival (Days)
0Gy	21 (±4)	10 (±4)
5x2Gy	28 (±7)	14 (±9)
8Gy	28 (±10)	14 (±9)

Figure 3. DVL3 tumours respond and are more sensitive to radiotherapy than the resistant TRAMP C1 model. (**A**) DVL3 or TRAMP C1 cells were engrafted into immune competent mice and allowed to reach a tumour volume of 100–200 mm^3. Mice were randomly assigned to no treatment (0 Gy) (Blue), fractionated dose (5 × 2 Gy) (Purple) or single high dose (8 Gy) (Red) radiotherapy (RT) group. A cohort of mice were sacrificed one week after radiotherapy to examine immune response and a further cohort was left to terminal endpoint to examine tumour growth (Figure 1A) and survival. (**B**) DVL3 tumours were sensitive to fractionated RT but no difference was seen with single high dose RT. (**C**) Kaplan Meier curves showing survival in mice engrafted with DVL3 tumour cells was improved for both treatment regimens (5 × 2 Gy and 8 Gy) compared to for mice treated with 0 Gy (5 × 2 Gy $p = 0.0255$ and 8 Gy $p = 0.0386$). (**D**) TRAMP C1 tumours did not respond to radiotherapy. (**E**) There was no change in survival with radiation in the mice engrafted with TRAMP C1 cells treated with RT. (**F**) Summary of timeline for DVL3 and TRAMP C1 tumours treated with RT, demonstrating DVL3 tumours are more radiosensitive. Data represents mean ± SEM of n = 5–8 mice per treatment group. * denotes $p \leq 0.05$, NS denotes non-significant, as determined by Student's t-test or log Mantel-cox tests on Kaplan-Meier plots.

2.4. Fractionated Radiotherapy Differentially Upregulated Genes Associated with STING/Type-1 Interferon Signalling and Myeloid Signatures

RT induces immunological changes in tumour cells and can re-calibrate the immune contexture of the tumour microenvironment [21]. In order to establish how fractionated (5 × 2 Gy) RT altered the tumour immune microenvironment, RNA sequencing analysis was performed on DVL3 tumours excised a week after final dose of RT (Figure 3A). Interestingly, ENRICHR pathway analysis on differentially expressed genes highlighted an enrichment for pathways involved in interferon alpha/beta (IFN-b) signalling ($p < 0.001$), IRF3 mediated activation of type-1 Interferon (IFN) pathway ($p = 0.02$), regulation of innate immune responses to cystolic DNA ($p < 0.05$), and stimulator of interferon genes (STING) mediated immune response ($p < 0.05$, Figure 4A). RT also led to significant downregulation of pathways involved in extra cellular matrix remodelling, collagen degradation and activation of matrix metalloproteinases (Supplementary Figure S7A).

A.

Reactome 2016 *in vivo* Pathway - Upregulated	Adjusted p-value
Interferon Alpha/Beta Signalling	<0.001
Interferon Signalling	0.002
IRF3 Mediated Activation of Type 1 IFN	0.020
Cytokine Signalling in Immune System	0.022
IRF3-mediated induction of Type I IFN	0.023
Regulation of Innate Immune Responses to Cytosolic DNA	0.023
STING mediated induction of Host Immune Responses	0.023

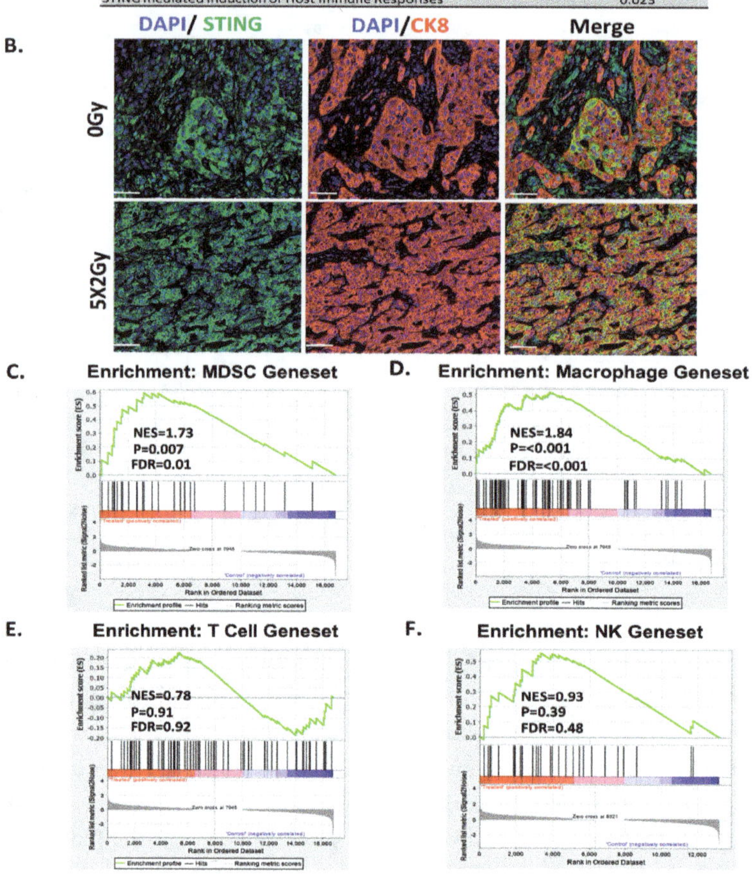

Figure 4. DVL3 immunosuppressive microenvironment enhanced by radiotherapy treatment. (**A**) Pathway enrichment analysis was performed using the online software Enricher for differential gene expression comparing the fractionated (5 × 2 Gy) syngeneic tumours to non-irradiated control ($n = 3$ samples per group). Upregulated pathways enrichment in the Reactome 2016 for transcripts with a significance of greater than 0.05 and fold increase of ≥1. Upregulated pathways include interferon signalling and immune response. (**B**) In keeping with RNA sequencing analysis, STING immunohistochemical analysis (Green) revealed a significant upregulation of expression in response to

RT primarily within glandular epithelium as demonstrated via co-localisation with CK8 (Red). DAPI nuclear counterstain shown in blue. Scale bar equals 50 μm. Image representative of $n = 3$ independent tumour samples. GSEA enrichment analysis of tumours treated with fractionated (5 × 2 Gy) radiotherapy demonstrates an upregulation of (**C**) MDSC and (**D**) macrophage and signatures, but no enrichment of (**E**) T-cell or (**F**) NK cell signatures when compared with non-irradiated tumours. NES: normalized enrichment score, FDR: false discovery rate.

In order to establish phenotypic significance of the activation of type-1 IFN-pathway, the expression of STING was evaluated via immunohistochemistry in the irradiated DVL3 tumours. Fractionated RT led to a substantial, but non-significant increase in STING expression compared to non-treated controls (Supplementary Figure S7B). The increase in STING expression was primarily expressed by tumour epithelium in glandular structures. This was confirmed by multiplex immunohistochemistry, demonstrating STING co-localisation primarily in CK8+ tumour cells (Figure 4B, Supplementary Figure S8). Although STING expression was highest in tumour epithelium, this was not exclusive, as STING was also observed in the stromal and other cellular compartments (defined here as CK8 negative areas). Taken together with the RNA seq analysis, our data indicates towards a global upregulation of STING, and associated pathways within the tumour.

STING-dependent cytosolic DNA sensing promotes type-1 interferon response which is critical for activation and influx of MDSC population after radiation [22], and it is well documented that it can also enhance both T-and NK cell activation [23,24]. Therefore, Gene Set Enrichment Analysis (GSEA) was performed using the published gene set for MDSCs signature [25]. In the irradiated DVL3 tumours there was enrichment of the MDSC gene signature (Figure 4C; $p = 0.007$). We also performed GSEA analysis for gene signatures associated with activated macrophages, T-cells and NK cells, however, interestingly our data showed only upregulation of transcripts associated with activated macrophages (Figure 4D; $p < 0.001$), but not the cytotoxic T-cells (CD8) nor the natural killer T-cells or any other associated pathways (Figure 4E,F).

2.5. Fractionated Radiotherapy Resulted in an Increase in Infiltration of Myeloid Cells, but no Changes Were Observed in T-Cell Infiltrates

In order to establish how RT induces phenotypic changes in the immune cell infiltrates in our novel syngeneic tumour model, immunohistochemical staining was performed for T cells and myeloid cells. A marginal increase in natural killer T cells was observed in a portion of irradiated tumours, which predominantly localised around the necrotic areas, defined by morphological assessment and cleaved caspase-3 staining (NKp46, Figure 5A,C, Supplementary Figure S9A). Fractionated RT did not result in a significant change to the macrophage population (F4/80, Figure 5A,D).

Using multiplex immunohistochemistry, T-cell (CD4, CD8) and myeloid cell (CD11b) expression were investigated in excised tumours (Figure 5B). RT did not result in an increase in either CD8+ or CD4+ T cells (Figure 5E,F). However, RT lead to an increase in myeloid cell infiltration (CD11b+) in the irradiated tumours compared to non-treated tumours (23.32% vs. 15.15%, $p = 0.04$. Figure 5G). As the F4/80 macrophage numbers showed no difference after administration of fractionated RT, the increase in CD11b myeloid cells could be due to an increase in either granulocytic and/or monocytic MDSCs.

Next, the expression of program cell-death ligand 1 (PD-L1) was investigated in the irradiated DVL3 tumours [26]. We have previously demonstrated that IFN-γ produced by CD8+ T-cells can cause adaptive upregulation of PD-L1 on tumour cells after delivery of low dose fractionated radiotherapy [27]. RT can also lead to increase in expression of PD-L1 on MDSCs and macrophages as demonstrated previously in a range of tumour models at higher doses [24]. Interestingly, in the DVL3 tumours, fractionated RT had no impact on PD-L1 expression measured as median fluorescence intensity on the surface of tumour cells, MDSCs cell or the macrophages (Supplementary Figure S9B–D).

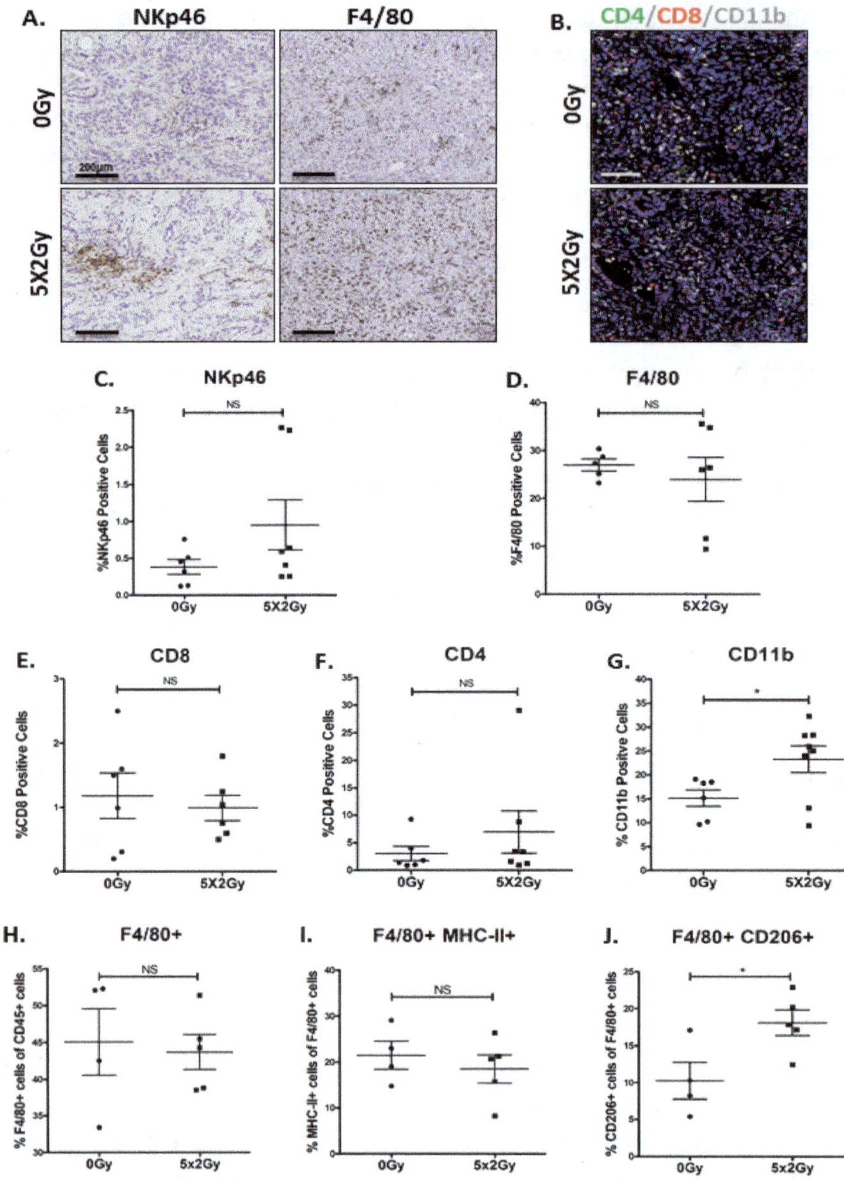

Figure 5. Radiotherapy resulted in an increase in immunosuppressive myeloid cells infiltrates and macrophages acquiring an M2 phenotype in the DVL3 tumours. (**A**) Representative immunohistochemical staining for natural killer T-cells (Nkp46) and macrophages (F/480) in DVL3 tumours. Nkp46 staining was sparse and mainly localised around the necrotic areas within the tumour. (**B**). Representative multiplex staining images for CD4 (green), CD8 (red) and CD11b (white) in the DVL3 tumours revealing an increase in CD11b staining in the irradiated tumours. Quantification of immunohistochemical staining comparing untreated (0 Gy) and tumours treated with fractionated radiotherapy (5×2 Gy) showed no significant difference in (**C**) NK-T-cells (NKp46), (**D**) macrophages (F4/80), (**E**) cytotoxic T cells (CD8), or (**F**) helper T cells (CD4). (**G**) However, radiotherapy treatment did induce a significant increase in myeloid cells (CD11b+) in the irradiated tumour. (**H**) Flow cytometry analysis for macrophages (gated as CD45+/F480+) cells showing no significant increase in proportion of cells in the irradiated tumours. (**I**) Flow cytometry analysis for MHC-II+ cells (M1 marker) on macrophages gated as (CD45+/F480+/ MHC-II+) in the irradiated tumours (**J**) Flow cytometry analysis for CD206 (Mannose receptor, an M2 marker) on macrophages gated as (CD45+/F480+/CD206+) revealing a significant increase in CD206+ staining in the irradiated tumours (gating strategy in Supplementary Figure S5). Data represents mean ± SEM of $n = 4$–8 independent murine tumors as indicated by points on each graph. * denotes $p \leq 0.05$, NS denotes non-significant, as determined by Student's t-test (immunohistochemistry) or Mann-Whitney, nonparametric testing (flow cytometry).

We also investigated whether RT had an impact on macrophage reprograming from M2 to M1 phenotype. Using flow cytometric analysis, we demonstrate that although there was no significant difference in either the macrophage numbers (Figure 5H) or in the proportion of macrophages expressing MHC-II (an M1 marker) in the irradiated tumour (Figure 5I). However, the macrophages were skewed towards an immunosuppressive M2 phenotype, defined as (F480+/CD206+) cells ($p = 0.03$; Figure 5J). These findings taken together with RNA sequencing data suggest that the activation of type-1 signaling in the irradiated DVL3 tumours could be due to influx of MDSCs and activation of myeloid innate immune response pathway, and not driven by T cells.

3. Discussion

Whilst significant progress has been made in the treatment of metastatic, castration-resistant prostate cancer (CRPC), the majority of these cancers remain incurable. In order to have greater impact, it is important to understand the involvement of the TME in PCa evolution and treatment resistance, so that more effective treatment combinations can be developed for molecular high risk disease. RT remains an important treatment for primary localized PCa, and is increasingly used for treatment for metastatic disease [28–32]. Although both *Pten* and *p53* loss have been implicated in treatment failure, the narrow range of PCa pre-clinical models limits therapeutic development. This study has developed two novel murine cell models; mPECs, which model normal prostate epithelium and the tumorigenic DVL3 cell line derived with genetically relevant drivers ($Pten^{-/-}/trp53^{-/-}$) which has been extensively characterized for sensitivity to RT and TME response. Additionally, the mPEC model serves as a normal epithelial control, but also provides a key model for further genetic manipulation to examine pathways thought to be important in tumour development or immune response in a syngeneic environment.

Transgenic tumours from which the DVL3 cells were generated, were derived via deletion of *Pten* and *trp53*, genes that are frequently mutated in human PCa and are implicated in aggressive forms of the disease [10]; thus, avoiding the introduction of tumorigenic viral proteins such as SV40 large T-antigen, which was used to generate the TRAMP C1 cell line [6]. Although the TRAMP C1 cell line has contributed significantly to PCa research, recent evidence indicates it generates neuroendocrine tumours, which clinically equates to only 0.5–2% of all PCa cases [7]. Furthermore, although other syngeneic PCa models exist [33,34] (e.g. MyC-CaP and Pten-CaP8), they have not been well characterized for their similarity to human disease, and immune microenvironment. The DVL3 cell line develops tumours that represent an adenocarcinoma phenotype much more akin to the majority of human PCa, and displays a similar TME to patient disease. The DVL3 model also sets itself apart, as it can be easily generated via subcutaneous allograft into immune-competent mice. As such, not only is it both time and cost beneficial compared with conventional GEM models, the tumours are easily accessible for therapeutic intervention, such as local delivery of RT and tumour assessment.

Transgenic models of PCa, and subsequent cell lines, generated from the $Pten^{-/-}/trp53^{-/-}$ model generate heterogeneous tumours, forming distinct glandular structures [10]. Arguably, heterogeneity is one of the greatest benefits of this model, as most cell-based models are thought to be clonally selected due to genetic drift. As PCa is a multifocal heterogeneous disease, the derivation of a bulk DVL3 population allows for research into PCa evolution and response to treatment [35]. Tumours formed by the DVL3 model maintained the heterogeneous CK8+/CK5+ glandular structures and regions of AR positivity, similar to the tumours from which they were derived. Additionally, unlike other $Pten^{-/-}/trp53^{-/-}$ murine cell lines, previously described in the literature, the DVL3 cells can be implanted in immune competent C57BL/6 mice, presenting with immunological cold tumour immune microenvironment, mirroring observations seen clinically [10,36].

Development of immune therapies as a method of harnessing the immune system's anti-tumour effects has recently gained traction [36]. Immune checkpoint inhibitors (ICI) have been used successfully to treat melanoma and lung cancers; however, their impact on PCa is more limited [37]. Unlike melanoma and lung cancer, PCa has low levels of infiltrating CD8+ T cells, high proportion of

MDSCs and tumour promoting M2 macrophages, therefore ICI are unlikely to work in majority of PCa patients [36,37]. Furthermore, variations in the PCa tumour microenvironment have been reported to correlate with PTEN-loss, defects in DNA repair pathways, low levels of tumour-associated antigens and differences in the immune function of patients [37]. PTEN loss occurs in 20% of primary PCa patients and has been associated with poorer overall survival [9,10,37]. Additionally, melanoma patients with PTEN loss also have lower levels of tumour infiltrating lymphocytes (TIL) [37]. We have confirmed that this is also true in the tumours resulting from DVL3 syngeneic engraftment, underscoring the more immuno-suppressed microenvironment of these tumours compared to the TRAMP C1 tumours.

Comparing the DVL3 allografts to published transgenic models driven by *Pten* deletion highlights other similarities and opportunities for future studies. For example *Pten* deletion is known to lead to the expansion and immunosuppressive activities of $Gr1^+/CD11b^+$ myeloid derived suppressor cells (MDSC) [13]. High numbers of MDSCs in a $Pten^{-/-}$ setting provide a protective effect on PCa cells from senescence, therefore sustaining tumour growth [13,38]. Mechanistically this has been observed to occur in CRPC patients and in transgenic prostate cancer models through the activation of AR signalling due to paracrine IL-23 secretion by MDSCs [39]. Furthermore, influx of tumour MDSCs has been detected following RT, an observation which has been previously associated with the RT-induced up-regulation of STING expression in tumour cells [22,40,41]. Targeting MDSC, through IL-23 inhibition, in combination with RT and ADT could therefore provide a survival benefit for PCa patients.

STING mediated type-1 IFN production can be an effective approach to cancer therapy, due to its role in T-cell priming and dendritic cell activation. Counterintuitively, STING activation can also be immunosuppressive as previously reported [24]. In the DVL3 model, RT mediated STING activation does not result in enrichment of T- or NK cell gene signatures, nor did it result in a significant increase in the proportion of T- or NK cells, suggesting dominant immunosuppressive effects in the TME. However, we did note aggregation of NK-cells in and around necrotic areas after RT [42]. Further studies using the DVL3 model are necessary to clarify the role of NK-cell mediated cell killing, which may have potential therapeutic implications. Interestingly, in spite of the IFN-type-1 pathway activation, no significant change in PD-L1 expression was observed either in the tumor or macrophages after RT. It has been demonstrated that the kinetics of PD-L1 expression can be transient, time, and radiation dose-dependent [27,43]. In this study, we investigated the expression of PD-L1 at a single time point (a week after RT), and after administration of low dose fractionated RT (5×2 Gy). As such, further investigations are required with high radiation dose and observation and differing time points to establish the kinetics of PD-L1 upregulation on tumour cells and macrophages. Furthermore, PD-L1 expression on MDSCs can be activated by type-1 IFN in an autocrine manner, which is partially controlled by IFNAR1 expression on MDSCs [44]. Our gene expression analysis demonstrated no significant change in the expression of IFNAR1 with RT (data not shown). This may partly explain our findings, however, we cannot fully rule out other environmental factors.

Overall, the DVL3 model recapitulates clinically relevant immune microenvironment features that have been previously observed in PCa transgenic models following RT or androgen deprivation therapy, such as influx of MDSC, M2 tumour promoting macrophages, and lack of cytotoxic T-cell priming [13,39,41]. Although similar models have previously been published upon [10,45,46], to our knowledge this is the first report of a model which has been proven to be syngeneically engraftable and is driven by relevant genetic drivers to prostate cancer (*Pten* and *trp53*), and mirrors clinical response. The genetic status of the model, resultant histological Gleason score, and immunological features suggest the DVL3 model is currently poised for extensive future work as a model of molecular high-risk localized disease, which is benefited by its cost and time effectiveness compared with other models, ease of accessibility and tumour tracking, and its accurate recapitulation of PCa patient disease. However, further characterization of the model is required to examine if it is also suitable as a model of metastatic disease via orthotopic engraftment to the prostate or bone.

4. Materials and Methods

4.1. Cell Line Derivation and Maintenance

Mouse prostate epithelial cells (mPEC) were generated from normal dorsal, ventral and lateral lobes of the prostate from Probasin Cre$^{-/-}$ (Pb-Cre4) mice. Murine prostate cancer cells (DVL3) were generated from tumours derived from the dorsal, ventral and lateral prostate lobes of a *Pten*$^{-/-}$/*trp53*$^{-/-}$ Pb-Cre4 mouse [10]. These lobes were specifically utilised for both models as they are morphologically more similar to the peripheral zone in the human prostate gland which generates adenocarcinoma [11] and these lobes are also those which generate adenocarcinoma in the *Pten*$^{-/-}$/*trp53*$^{-/-}$ Pb-Cre4 murine model. mPEC and DVL3 cell line generation is summarised in Supplemental Figure S1. Briefly, tissue fragments were collected in PBS and manually dissociated into 1 mm^3 fragments using a scalpel. The sample was centrifuged at 2000 rpm to remove extraneous blood and fat, and remaining tissue digested in 1 mg/mL collagenase/dispase in PBS for 30 min at 37 °C, after digestion the tissue was further disrupted via serological pippetting. The supernatant containing prostate cells was collected, and the collagnease/dispase inactivated with EDTA. The digestion process was repeated twice with remaining tissue fragments. Supernatant from the digestions was pooled and centrifuged at 2000 rpm and prostate cells were re-suspended in RPMI supplemented with 10% FBS, 1× penicillin/streptomycin, 100 nM DHT and 10 μmol/L ROCK inhibitor (Y-27632, Sigma, Gillingham, UK). These cells were then incubated for 10 min at 37 °C to allow for prostate fibroblasts to adhere to the tissue culture plastic. Remaining cell suspension, enriched for prostate epithelium was transferred to a new culture flask. This process of differential plating, allowing for initial adherence of fibroblasts and removal and retention of less adherent epithelial cells, was repeated for 10 passages, at which time use of the ROCK inhibitor (Y-27632, Sigma) was stopped and the population was characterised as epithelial. After isolation and initial 10 passages to reach a homogenous epithelial population, the mPEC and DVL3 cell lines were maintained in RPMI-media supplemented with 10% FBS, L-glutamine and 100 nM DHT.

The TRAMP C1 murine prostate carcinoma cells were purchased from ATCC (Manassas, VA, USA) and maintained in DMEM high glucose medium, supplemented with 4 mM L-glutamine, 5% FBS, 5% Nu Serum (Corning, Bedford, MA, USA), 0.005 mg/mL of bovine insulin, and 10 nM dehydroisoandrosterone (Sigma). CT26 murine colon carcinoma cells (ATCC) and 4434 cells isolated from BRAFV600E p16-/- mice (Richard Marias, Cancer Research UK Manchester Institute, Manchester, UK) were maintained in DMEM, and 4T1 triple-negative breast cancers (ATCC) maintained in RPMI-media supplemented with 10% FCS, 1% L-glutamine (Invitrogen, Paisley, UK).

4.2. Syngeneic Modelling

C57BL/6 and BALB/C male mice (8-weeks old) were obtained from Harlan (Derby, UK). All animal experiments were performed under United Kingdom Home Office Licenses held at Queen's University Belfast or the CRUK Manchester Institute, University of Manchester (PPL2775; PCC943F76 respectively). Prior to each in vivo experiment, cells were screened for mycoplasma contamination and mouse hepatitis virus (MHV). Mice were housed on a 12/12 light/dark cycle and were given filtered water and fed *ad libitum*. C57BL/6 male mice were inoculated subcutaneously with either 5×10^6 TRAMP C1, 1×10^6 DVL3 cells, 1×10^6 mPEC cells or 5×10^6 4434 cells; BALB/C mice were inoculated with 5×10^5 CT26 cells, 1×10^5 4T1 cells under light general anaesthetic using Isoflurane and oxygen gaseous mix in accordance with project license and home office regulations. Tumour volume was measured using calipers as length $\times$ (width)^2/2.

4.3. Sample Preparation

Tumour bearing mice were sacrificed at the indicated time points using standard schedule-1 procedure, and in accordance with current UK home office legislation. Tumour samples were cut into half and either fixed in 4% buffered formalin (Sigma Aldrich) for 24 h or collected in media for tumour disaggregation. The formalin fixed tumour samples were transferred to 70% ethanol and processed to FFPE blocks at the CRUK Manchester histology core facility. H&E slides obtained were evaluated by a dedicated uropathologist (PO) with the aim to compare with morphological features of human prostate cancer as well as estimate a Gleason pattern and score.

4.4. Immunohistochemistry

Briefly, the slides were deparaffinised in xylene followed by rehydration in ethanol. Antigen retrieval was performed using pH 6 citrate buffer, followed by 3% H_2O_2 block. Slides were incubated with 10% serum, prior to incubation with primary antibody overnight at 4° (Table S1). Primary antibody was detected with either HRP detection kit or biotinylated secondary antibody followed by ABC detection kit (Vector Labs, Burlingame, CA, USA). Slides were briefly incubated in DAB substrate (Vector Labs), washed in water, and counter-stained using haematoxylin. STING and cleaved Caspase-3 staining was performed on the BOND Rx automation system (Leica, Microsystems, Milton Keynes, UK) using standard protocol. For multiplex staining of mouse FFPE tumour sections, the opal TSA detection system (Opal 520®, 570® and 650®) were applied to sections following manufacturer's instruction and run on Leica BOND Rx automated system. The slides were counterstained with DAPI. Chromagen slides were scanned digitally using Leica SCN 4000 slide scanner (Leica Microsystems) VS-200 slide scanner (Olympus, Essex, UK), and the multiplex slides were scanned using Versa Slide scanner (Leica Microsystems) and VS-120 slide scanner (Olympus). Image analysis and quantification was performed using Definiens® Tissue Phenomics Software (Munich, Germany) or Halo® image analysis (Indica Labs, Albuquerque, NM, USA). Quantification of the percentage of positive cells was determined using either hematoxylin or DAPI staining to identify total cell count. Scoring of positive staining of chromogen slides (summarized in Figure 1C) was performed in a blinded fashion by two independent researchers. For quantification of co-localisation using Halo®; High plex FL Ver 3.1.0 module was used.

4.5. Immunocytochemistry

Cells were seeded onto glass slides pre-coated with collagen type II (BD Biosciences, San Jose, CA, USA) and left to adhere for 24 h before fixation with 4% paraformaldehyde at RT. Cells were permeabilised with 0.1% Triton X and blocked with 3% FBS-PBS. Primary antibody was added to slides and incubated for 1 h at RT followed by incubation in secondary antibody for 1 h at RT (Table S1). Coverslips were mounted onto glass slides using Mounting media (Invitrogen) containing Dapi and imaged.

4.6. RNA Isolation and cDNA Synthesis

Total RNA from cells was isolated using TriPure Isolation reagent (Roche, Mannheim, Germany) and phenol-chloroform extraction and cDNA synthesised using first strand cDNA (Roche) according to the respective manufacturer's instructions.

4.7. qRT-PCR

mRNA levels were determined by RT-PCR and measured on Roche LightCycler®480 II with SYBR Green I Master (Roche). All primers were obtained from Eurofins (Ebersberg, Germany) and sequences are detailed in (Table S2). mRNA expression was evaluated using β-actin and GAPDH housekeeping genes and is shown normalized to β-actin as a fold change relative to mPECs transcript levels.

4.8. Western Blotting

Cells were lysed with RIPA buffer (Sigma) supplemented with Protease Inhibitor Cocktail (Roche), centrifuged and supernatant containing protein analysed by SDS Page (Invitrogen). Proteins were transferred onto a nitrocellulose membrane, blocked for 1 h in 5% milk TBS-T prior to incubation with primary antibody at 4 °C overnight, concentrations are detailed in (Table S2). Complementary secondary antibodies were used at 1:3000. Membranes were visualised via chemiluminescence on a Syngene G:Box imager using reagent (Merck, Cambridge, UK).

4.9. Flow Cytometry on Cell Lines

Cells were incubated with primary antibody conjugated fluorophore for 30 min at 4 °C, washed with PBS and analysed on the Introducing the BD Accuri™ C6 Plus according to the manufacturer's instructions.

4.10. Radiotherapy

Upon tumour establishment (4–6 weeks post inoculation), mice were randomised to treatment groups. Irradiation was performed when the tumours were between (100–200 mm^3). The tumour bearing mice were placed in a lead jig with an opening for the tumour and shielding for the rest of the body. Radiotherapy was delivered using an AGO cell X-Ray unit and XSTRAHL (CIX3) in vivo irradiator at a dose rate of 2.086 Gy/min. Tumour bearing mice received either single dose of 8 Gy irradiation, or 5 fractions of 2 Gy delivered over 5 consecutive days (as shown in Figure 3A).

4.11. RNA Extraction for RNA Seq Analysis

RNA from FFPE mouse tumour tissue was extracted. Briefly, 2–4 (10 μM) sections were transferred into RNAase free microcentrifuge tube. The paraffin was removed by incubating in xylene and ethanol. For lysate and total RNA purification, digestion buffer and proteinase-K was added to the samples as per manufacturer's instructions (Norgen Kit, Ontario, Canada). The samples were spun briefly followed by transferring the supernatant to a new RNAase free microcentrifuge tube. The RNA containing tubes were incubated for 15 min at 80 °C. The lysates were then passed through RNA purification microcolumn and centrifuged for 1 min at 14,000 RPM. The microcolumns were washed according to manufacturer's instructions and the RNA eluted using the Elution solution (Norgen Kit).

4.12. RNA Library Preparation, Sequencing and Analysis

RNA libraries preparations were generated using the Quant-seq 3′ mRNA-Seq FWD kit (PART NO k15.96, Lexogen, Vienna, Austria) according to manufacturer's instructions, with 500ng input RNA. FFPE-derived RNA was prepared using the suggested manufacturer's instructions. Libraries were pooled and sequenced on the NextSeq 500 using the Queen's University Genomics Core Technology Unit, yielding an average of 10 million reads per sample. FASTQ files were aligned to the mm10 genomic reference using STAR aligner [47] and counts quantified at a gene level with HTseq-Counts [48] to yield 5-8M mapped reads per sample. Differential gene expression was performed between the irradiated and un-irradiated samples using the DESEQ 2. Differentially expressed genes were filtered; FDR adjusted—p Value < 0.05 and Log2 Fold-Change ≥ 1 (up-regulated) or ≤ -1 (down-regulated). Pathway analysis was performed on filtered genelists using the Reactome database [49] in Enrichr [50,51]. To identify enrichment of immune populations with the RT tumours vs untreated, enrichment analysis was performed using the open assess tool gene set enrichment analysis (GSEA) [52,53] with 1000 gene label permutations. Immune cell gene signatures for macrophages, NK cells, T-cells and MDSC were taken from previous published studies [25,54,55].

4.13. Flow Cytometry on Tumour Tissue

To obtain single cell suspensions, tumours were processed using a gentleMacs dissociator and a murine dissociation kit (Miltenyi Biotec, Surrey, UK). For staining of cells, non-specific binding was blocked with rat anti-CD16/CD32 Fc block on ice. Cells were incubated with Gr-1–FITC, CD11b–APC (eBioscience, Leicestershire, UK), washed in 1% FCS/PBS. For analysis, live cells were gated using vital dye exclusion (Invitrogen) and population phenotyped on FACs Canto (BD Bioscience) and analyzed using Flow Jo software. An example of the gating strategy employed is provided in Figure S5.

4.14. Statistical Analysis

Results were analysed using GraphPad Prism (v7.03, San Diego, CA, USA). Data was analysed via a Shapiro-Wilk normality test was first used to confirm that groups were distributed normally. When comparing two groups, if the data was normally distributed it was analysed by Student's *t*-test. Nonparametric data was analysed via Mann-Whitney testing. When comparing more than two groups a one-way analysis of variance (ANOVA) followed by a Tukey's multiple comparisons test was used to detect significant differences between means. The limit for significance was set at $p \leq 0.05$. Data are described with standard error of the mean (SEM). To compare survival curves from in vivo experiments, Log-Rank Mantel–Cox tests were performed on Kaplan–Meier plots.

5. Conclusions

This study highlights that the DVL3 model represents substantial progress in preclinical PCa modelling displaying similar molecular, histological, and microenvironmental features compared to alternative models. Furthermore, the DVL3 cells and subsequent tumours can be generated quickly and inexpensively compared to standard transgenic models, and tumours are readily accessible for therapeutic intervention. Importantly, DVL3 cells can be syngeneically engrafted into immune component hosts and respond to standard of care RT, with a similar immune influx, thus enabling future validation of novel therapeutics for PCa including immunomodulatory agents targeting MDSC, macrophages and agents that can prime T-cell responses either alone or in combination with standard of care RT or ADTs.

Author Contributions: Conceptualization, C.M.H., D.M., R.E.S., L.D.-P., A.P. (Adam Pickard), S.J., J.H., S.S.M., T.I., I.G.M., S.L.E.; Methodology, D.M., C.M.H., R.E.S., A.P. (Amy Popple), L.D.-P., A.P. (Adam Pickard), M.P., P.O., N.E.B., S.L.E.; Formal analysis, C.M.H., D.M., A.P. (Amy Popple), M.P., S.L.E.; Writing—original draft, C.M.H., D.M., S.L.E., I.G.M.; Writing—review/editing, C.M.H., D.M., R.E.S., A.P. (Amy Popple), L.D.-P., A.P. (Adam Pickard), S.J., P.O., N.E.B., P.B.M., R.W., J.H., S.S.M., T.I., I.G.M., S.L.E.; Funding acquisition, I.G.M., S.J., P.B.M., R.W., S.S.M., T.I. All authors have read and agreed to the published version of the manuscript.

Acknowledgments: We acknowledge the generous gift of mouse prostate tissue from the David Waugh laboratory from which the mPEC and DVL3 cell lines were generated. The authors thank the members of the Cancer Research UK Manchester Institute BRU core facility, Caron Behan and Garry Ashton from the Histology Core Facility for the technical expertise and help with staining, MBCF, Flow Cytometry Core Facilities and Alex Baker from Imaging Core facility for image analysis.

Ethical Approval: All procedures were performed in accordance with the Animal Scientific Procedures Act of 1986 (UK) (Project Licence Number PL2775 and PCC943F76) which was issued by the home office. Protocols were approved by the animal welfare and ethical review body at both Queen's University Belfast and the Cancer Research UK Manchester Institute. Animals were housed in individually ventilated cages on a 12:12 light: dark cycle and ad libitum access to food and filtered water. Prior to each in vivo experiment, cells were screened for mycoplasma and MHV contamination.

References

1. Bray, F.; Ferlay, J.; Soerjomataram, I.; Siegel, R.L.; Torre, L.A.; Jemal, A. Global cancer statistics 2018: GLOBOCAN estimates of incidence and mortality worldwide for 36 cancers in 185 countries. *CA A Cancer J. Clin.* **2018**, *68*, 394–424. [CrossRef]
2. Siegel, R.L.; Miller, K.D.; Jemal, A. Cancer statistics, 2018. *CA Cancer J Clin.* **2018**, *68*, 7–30. [CrossRef]
3. Jemal, A.; Siegel, R.; Xu, J.; Ward, E. Cancer statistics, 2010. *CA Cancer J Clin.* **2010**, *60*, 277–300. [CrossRef]
4. James, N.D.; Spears, M.R.; Clarke, N.W.; Dearnaley, D.P.; De Bono, J.S.; Gale, J.; Hetherington, J.; Hoskin, P.J.; Jones, R.; Laing, R.; et al. Survival with Newly Diagnosed Metastatic Prostate Cancer in the "Docetaxel Era": Data from 917 Patients in the Control Arm of the STAMPEDE Trial (MRC PR08, CRUK/06/019). *Eur. Urol.* **2015**, *67*, 1028–1038. [CrossRef]

5. Donovan, J.L.; Hamdy, F.C.; Lane, J.A.; Mason, M.; Metcalfe, C.; Walsh, E.; Blazeby, J.; Peters, T.J.; Holding, P.; Bonnington, S.; et al. Patient-Reported Outcomes after Monitoring, Surgery, or Radiotherapy for Prostate Cancer. *N. Engl. J. Med.* **2016**, *375*, 1425–1437. [CrossRef]
6. Foster, B.A.; Gingrich, J.R.; Kwon, E.D.; Madias, C.; Greenberg, N.M. Characterization of prostatic epithelial cell lines derived from transgenic adenocarcinoma of the mouse prostate (TRAMP) model. *Cancer Res.* **1997**, *57*, 3325–3330. [PubMed]
7. Berman-Booty, L.D.; Knudsen, K.E. Models of neuroendocrine prostate cancer. *Endocr.-Relat. Cancer* **2014**, *22*, R33–R49. [CrossRef] [PubMed]
8. Zafarana, G.; Ishkanian, A.S.; Malloff, C.A.; Locke, J.A.; Sykes, J.; Thoms, J.; Lam, W.L.; Squire, J.A.; Yoshimoto, M.; Ramnarine, V.R.; et al. Copy number alterations of c-MYC and PTEN are prognostic factors for relapse after prostate cancer radiotherapy. *Cancer* **2012**, *118*, 4053–4062. [CrossRef] [PubMed]
9. Geybels, M.S.; Fang, M.; Wright, J.L.; Qu, X.; Bibikova, M.; Klotzle, B.; Fan, J.-B.; Feng, Z.; Ostrander, E.A.; Nelson, P.S.; et al. PTEN loss is associated with prostate cancer recurrence and alterations in tumor DNA methylation profiles. *Oncotarget* **2017**, *8*, 84338–84348. [CrossRef]
10. Martin, P.; Liu, Y.-N.; Pierce, R.; Abou-Kheir, W.; Casey, O.; Seng, V.; Camacho, D.; Simpson, R.M.; Kelly, K. Prostate Epithelial Pten/TP53 Loss Leads to Transformation of Multipotential Progenitors and Epithelial to Mesenchymal Transition. *Am. J. Pathol.* **2011**, *179*, 422–435. [CrossRef]
11. Oliveira, D.S.M.; Dzinic, S.; Bonfil, A.I.; Saliganan, A.D.; Sheng, S.; Bonfil, R.D. The mouse prostate: A basic anatomical and histological guideline. *Bosn. J. Basic Med. Sci.* **2016**, *16*, 8–13. [CrossRef] [PubMed]
12. Roy-Burman, P.; Wu, H.; Powell, W.C.; Hagenkord, J.; Cohen, M.B. Genetically defined mouse models that mimic natural aspects of human prostate cancer development. *Endocr.-Relat. Cancer* **2004**, *11*, 225–254. [CrossRef] [PubMed]
13. Garcia, A.J.; Ruscetti, M.; Arenzana, T.L.; Tran, L.M.; Bianci-Frias, D.; Sybert, E.; Priceman, S.J.; Wu, L.; Nelson, P.S.; Smale, S.T.; et al. Pten Null Prostate Epithelium Promotes Localized Myeloid-Derived Suppressor Cell Expansion and Immune Suppression during Tumor Initiation and Progression. *Mol. Cell. Biol.* **2014**, *34*, 2017–2028. [CrossRef] [PubMed]
14. Sharma, P.; Hu-Lieskovan, S.; Wargo, J.A.; Ribas, A. Primary, Adaptive, and Acquired Resistance to Cancer Immunotherapy. *Cell* **2017**, *168*, 707–723. [CrossRef] [PubMed]
15. Vidotto, T.; Saggioro, F.P.; Jamaspishvili, T.; Chesca, D.L.; De Albuquerque, C.G.P.; Reis, R.B.; Graham, C.H.; Berman, D.M.; Siemens, D.R.; Squire, J.A.; et al. PTEN-deficient prostate cancer is associated with an immunosuppressive tumor microenvironment mediated by increased expression of IDO1 and infiltrating FoxP3+ T regulatory cells. *Prostate* **2019**, *79*, 969–979. [CrossRef]
16. Wang, Y.; Hayward, S.W.; Cao, M.; Thayer, K.A.; Cunha, G.R. Cell differentiation lineage in the prostate. *Differentiation* **2001**, *68*, 270–279. [CrossRef]
17. Bhatia-Gaur, R.; Donjacour, A.A.; Sciavolino, P.J.; Kim, M.; Desai, N.; Young, P.; Norton, C.R.; Gridley, T.; Cardiff, R.D.; Cunha, G.R.; et al. Roles for Nkx3.1 in prostate development and cancer. *Genes Dev.* **1999**, *13*, 966–977. [CrossRef]
18. Gurel, B.; Ali, T.Z.; Montgomery, E.A.; Begum, S.; Hicks, J.; Goggins, M.; Eberhart, C.G.; Clark, D.P.; Bieberich, C.J.; Epstein, J.I.; et al. NKX3.1 as a Marker of Prostatic Origin in Metastatic Tumors. *Am. J. Surg. Pathol.* **2010**, *34*, 1097–1105. [CrossRef]
19. Young, H.L.; Rowling, E.J.; Bugatti, M.; Giurisato, E.; Luheshi, N.; Arozarena, I.; Acosta, J.C.; Kamarashev, J.; Frederick, D.T.; Cooper, Z.; et al. An adaptive signaling network in melanoma inflammatory niches confers tolerance to MAPK signaling inhibition. *J. Exp. Med.* **2017**, *214*, 1691–1710. [CrossRef]
20. Chen, F.-H.; Chiang, C.-S.; Wang, C.-C.; Tsai, C.-S.; Jung, S.-M.; Lee, C.-C.; McBride, W.H.; Hong, J.-H. Radiotherapy decreases vascular density and causes hypoxia with macrophage aggregation in TRAMP-C1 prostate tumors. *Clin. Cancer Res.* **2009**, *15*, 1721–1729. [CrossRef]
21. Walshaw, R.C.; Honeychurch, J.; Illidge, T.; Choudhury, A. The anti-PD-1 era—An opportunity to enhance radiotherapy for patients with bladder cancer. *Nat. Rev. Urol.* **2017**, *15*, 251–259. [CrossRef] [PubMed]
22. Liang, H.; Deng, L.; Hou, Y.; Meng, X.; Huang, X.; Rao, E.; Zheng, W.; Mauceri, H.; Mack, M.; Xu, M.; et al. Host STING-dependent MDSC mobilization drives extrinsic radiation resistance. *Nat. Commun.* **2017**, *8*, 1736. [CrossRef] [PubMed]

23. Woo, S.-R.; Fuertes, M.B.; Corrales, L.; Spranger, S.; Furdyna, M.J.; Leung, M.Y.; Duggan, R.; Wang, Y.; Barber, G.N.; Fitzgerald, K.A.; et al. STING-dependent cytosolic DNA sensing mediates innate immune recognition of immunogenic tumors. *Immunity* **2014**, *41*, 830–842. [CrossRef] [PubMed]
24. Deng, L.; Liang, H.; Burnette, B.; Beckett, M.; Darga, T.; Weichselbaum, R.R.; Fu, Y.-X. Irradiation and anti-PD-L1 treatment synergistically promote antitumor immunity in mice. *J. Clin. Investig.* **2014**, *124*, 687–695. [CrossRef] [PubMed]
25. Wang, G.; Lü, X.; Dey, P.; Deng, P.; Wu, C.C.; Jiang, S.; Fang, Z.; Zhao, K.; Konaparthi, R.; Hua, S.; et al. Targeting YAP-Dependent MDSC Infiltration Impairs Tumor Progression. *Cancer Discov.* **2015**, *6*, 80–95. [CrossRef]
26. Ko, E.C.; Formenti, S.C. Radiotherapy and checkpoint inhibitors: A winning new combination? *Ther. Adv. Med. Oncol.* **2018**, *10*. [CrossRef]
27. Dovedi, S.J.; Adlard, A.; Lipowska-Bhalla, G.; McKenna, C.; Jones, S.; Cheadle, E.J.; Stratford, I.J.; Poon, E.; Morrow, M.; Stewart, R.; et al. Acquired Resistance to Fractionated Radiotherapy Can Be Overcome by Concurrent PD-L1 Blockade. *Cancer Res.* **2014**, *74*, 5458–5468. [CrossRef]
28. Brand, D.H.; Tree, A.C.; Ostler, P.; Van Der Voet, H.; Loblaw, A.; Chu, W.; Ford, D.; Tolan, S.; Jain, S.; Martin, A.; et al. Intensity-modulated fractionated radiotherapy versus stereotactic body radiotherapy for prostate cancer (PACE-B): Acute toxicity findings from an international, randomised, open-label, phase 3, non-inferiority trial. *Lancet Oncol.* **2019**, *20*, 1531–1543. [CrossRef]
29. Dearnaley, D.P.; Syndikus, I.; Mossop, H.; Khoo, V.; Birtle, A.; Bloomfield, D.; Graham, J.D.; Kirkbride, P.; Logue, J.; Malik, Z.; et al. Conventional versus hypofractionated high-dose intensity-modulated radiotherapy for prostate cancer: 5-year outcomes of the randomised, non-inferiority, phase 3 CHHiP trial. *Lancet Oncol.* **2016**, *17*, 1047–1060. [CrossRef]
30. Payne, H.; Mason, M. Androgen deprivation therapy as adjuvant/neoadjuvant to radiotherapy for high-risk localised and locally advanced prostate cancer: Recent developments. *Br. J. Cancer* **2011**, *105*, 1628–1634. [CrossRef]
31. Parker, C.; James, N.D.; Brawley, C.D.; Clarke, N.W.; Hoyle, A.P.; Ali, A.; Ritchie, A.W.S.; Attard, G.; Chowdhury, S.; Cross, W.; et al. Radiotherapy to the primary tumour for newly diagnosed, metastatic prostate cancer (STAMPEDE): A randomised controlled phase 3 trial. *Lancet* **2018**, *392*, 2353–2366. [CrossRef]
32. Weichselbaum, R.R. The 46th David A. Karnofsky Memorial Award Lecture: Oligometastasis—From Conception to Treatment. *J. Clin. Oncol.* **2018**, *36*, 3240–3250. [CrossRef] [PubMed]
33. Watson, P.A.; Ellwood-Yen, K.; King, J.C.; Wongvipat, J.; Lebeau, M.M.; Sawyers, C.L. Context-Dependent Hormone-Refractory Progression Revealed through Characterization of a Novel Murine Prostate Cancer Cell Line. *Cancer Res.* **2005**, *65*, 11565–11571. [CrossRef] [PubMed]
34. Jiao, J.; Wang, S.; Qiao, R.; Vivanco, I.; Watson, P.A.; Sawyers, C.L.; Wu, H. Murine Cell Lines Derived from Pten Null Prostate Cancer Show the Critical Role of PTEN in Hormone Refractory Prostate Cancer Development. *Cancer Res.* **2007**, *67*, 6083–6091. [CrossRef]
35. Carm, K.T.; Hoff, A.M.; Bakken, A.C.; Axcrona, U.; Axcrona, K.; Lothe, R.A.; Skotheim, R.I.; Løvf, M. Interfocal heterogeneity challenges the clinical usefulness of molecular classification of primary prostate cancer. *Sci. Rep.* **2019**, *9*, 13579–13586. [CrossRef]
36. Bilusic, M.; Madan, R.A.; Gulley, J.L. Immunotherapy of Prostate Cancer: Facts and Hopes. *Clin. Cancer Res.* **2017**, *23*, 6764–6770. [CrossRef]
37. Vitkin, N.; Nersesian, S.; Siemens, D.R.; Koti, M. The Tumor Immune Contexture of Prostate Cancer. *Front. Immunol.* **2019**, *10*. [CrossRef]
38. Di Mitri, D.; Toso, A.; Chen, J.; Sarti, M.; Pinton, S.; Jost, T.R.; D'Antuono, R.; Montani, E.; García-Escudero, R.; Guccini, I.; et al. Tumour-infiltrating Gr-1+ myeloid cells antagonize senescence in cancer. *Nature* **2014**, *515*, 134–137. [CrossRef]
39. Calcinotto, A.; Spataro, C.; Zagato, E.; Di Mitri, D.; Gil, V.; Crespo, M.; De Bernardis, G.; Losa, M.; Mirenda, M.; Pasquini, E.; et al. IL-23 secreted by myeloid cells drives castration-resistant prostate cancer. *Nature* **2018**, *559*, 363–369. [CrossRef]
40. Ostrand-Rosenberg, S.; Horn, L.A.; Ciavattone, N.G. Radiotherapy Both Promotes and Inhibits Myeloid-Derived Suppressor Cell Function: Novel Strategies for Preventing the Tumor-Protective Effects of Radiotherapy. *Front. Oncol.* **2019**, *9*. [CrossRef]

41. Vatner, R.E.; Formenti, S.C. Myeloid-Derived Cells in Tumors: Effects of Radiation. *Semin. Radiat. Oncol.* **2015**, *25*, 18–27. [CrossRef] [PubMed]
42. Pasero, C.; Gravis, G.; Guérin, M.; Granjeaud, S.; Piana, J.T.; Rocchi, P.; Paciencia-Gros, M.; Poizat, F.; Bentobji, M.; Azario-Cheillan, F.; et al. Inherent and Tumor-Driven Immune Tolerance in the Prostate Microenvironment Impairs Natural Killer Cell Antitumor Activity. *Cancer Res.* **2016**, *76*, 2153–2165. [CrossRef] [PubMed]
43. Vanpouille-Box, C.; Formenti, S.C.; Demaria, S. Toward precision radiotherapy for use with immune checkpoint blockers. *Clin. Cancer Res.* **2018**, *24*, 259–265. [CrossRef] [PubMed]
44. Xiao, W.; Klement, J.D.; Lu, C.; Ibrahim, M.L.; Liu, K. IFNAR1 Controls Autocrine Type I IFN Regulation of PD-L1 Expression in Myeloid-Derived Suppressor Cells. *J. Immunol.* **2018**, *201*, 264–277. [CrossRef]
45. Grabowska, M.M.; DeGraff, D.J.; Yu, X.; Jin, R.J.; Chen, Z.; Borowsky, A.D.; Matusik, R.J. Mouse models of prostate cancer: Picking the best model for the question. *Cancer Metastasis Rev.* **2014**, *33*, 377–397. [CrossRef] [PubMed]
46. Ittmann, M.M.; Huang, J.; Radaelli, E.; Martin, P.; Signoretti, S.; Sullivan, R.; Simons, B.W.; Ward, J.M.; Robinson, B.D.; Chu, G.C.; et al. Animal Models of Human Prostate Cancer: The Consensus Report of the New York Meeting of the Mouse Models of Human Cancers Consortium Prostate Pathology Committee. *Cancer Res.* **2013**, *73*, 2718–2736. [CrossRef]
47. Dobin, A.; Davis, C.A.; Schlesinger, F.; Drenkow, J.; Zaleski, C.; Jha, S.; Batut, P.; Chaisson, M.; Gingeras, T.R. STAR: Ultrafast universal RNA-seq aligner. *Bioinformatics* **2012**, *29*, 15–21. [CrossRef]
48. Anders, S.; Pyl, P.T.; Huber, W. HTSeq—A Python framework to work with high-throughput sequencing data. *Bioinformatics* **2014**, *31*, 166–169. [CrossRef]
49. Fabregat, A.; Jupe, S.; Matthews, L.; Sidiropoulos, K.; Gillespie, M.; Garapati, P.; Haw, R.; Jassal, B.; Korninger, F.; May, B.; et al. The Reactome Pathway Knowledgebase. *Nucleic Acids Res.* **2018**, *46*, D649–D655. [CrossRef]
50. Chen, E.Y.; Tan, C.M.; Kou, Y.; Duan, Q.; Wang, Z.; Meirelles, G.V.; Clark, N.R.; Ma'Ayan, A. Enrichr: Interactive and collaborative HTML5 gene list enrichment analysis tool. *BMC Bioinform.* **2013**, *14*, 128. [CrossRef]
51. Kuleshov, M.V.; Jones, M.R.; Rouillard, A.D.; Fernandez, N.F.; Duan, Q.; Wang, Z.; Koplev, S.; Jenkins, S.L.; Jagodnik, K.M.; Lachmann, A.; et al. Enrichr: A comprehensive gene set enrichment analysis web server 2016 update. *Nucleic Acids Res.* **2016**, *44*. [CrossRef] [PubMed]
52. Mootha, V.K.; Lindgren, C.M.; Eriksson, K.F.; Subramanian, A.; Sihag, S.; Lehar, J.; Puigserver, P.; Carlsson, E.; Laurila, E.; Tamayo, P.; et al. PGC-1α-responsive genes involved in oxidative phosphorylation are coordinately downregulated in human diabetes. *Nat Genet.* **2003**, *34*, 267–273. [CrossRef]
53. Subramanian, A.; Tamayo, P.; Mootha, V.K.; Mukherjee, S.; Ebert, B.L.; Gillette, M.A.; Paulovich, A.; Pomeroy, S.L.; Golub, T.R.; Lander, E.S.; et al. Gene set enrichment analysis: A knowledge-based approach for interpreting genome-wide expression profiles. *Proc. Natl. Acad. Sci. USA* **2005**, *102*. [CrossRef] [PubMed]
54. Nirmal, A.J.; Regan, T.; Shih, B.B.; Hume, D.A.; Sims, A.H.; Freeman, T. Immune Cell Gene Signatures for Profiling the Microenvironment of Solid Tumors. *Cancer Immunol. Res.* **2018**, *6*, 1388–1400. [CrossRef] [PubMed]
55. Cursons, J.; Souza-Fonseca-Guimaraes, F.; Foroutan, M.; Anderson, A.; Hollande, F.; Hediya-Zadeh, S.; Behren, A.; Huntington, N.; Davis, M.J. A gene signature predicting natural killer infiltration an dimproved survival in melanoma patients. *Cancer Immunol. Res* 2019. [CrossRef]

10

Inclusion of a Furin Cleavage Site Enhances Antitumor Efficacy against Colorectal Cancer Cells of Ribotoxin α-Sarcin- or RNase T1-Based Immunotoxins

Javier Ruiz-de-la-Herrán [1], Jaime Tomé-Amat [1,2], Rodrigo Lázaro-Gorines [1], José G. Gavilanes [1] and Javier Lacadena [1,*]

1 Departamento de Bioquímica y Biología Molecular, Facultad de Ciencias Químicas, Universidad Complutense de Madrid, Madrid 28040, Spain; chaosrorri@hotmail.com (J.R.-d.-l.-H.); jaime.tome@upm.es (J.T.-A.); rodrigolazarogorines@ucm.es (R.L.-G.); jggavila@ucm.es (J.G.G.)

2 Centre for Plant Biotechnology and Genomics (UPM-INIA), Universidad Politécnica de Madrid, Pozuelo de Alarcón, Madrid 28223, Spain

* Correspondence: jlacaden@ucm.es

Abstract: Immunotoxins are chimeric molecules that combine the specificity of an antibody to recognize and bind tumor antigens with the potency of the enzymatic activity of a toxin, thus, promoting the death of target cells. Among them, RNases-based immunotoxins have arisen as promising antitumor therapeutic agents. In this work, we describe the production and purification of two new immunoconjugates, based on RNase T1 and the fungal ribotoxin α-sarcin, with optimized properties for tumor treatment due to the inclusion of a furin cleavage site. Circular dichroism spectroscopy, ribonucleolytic activity studies, flow cytometry, fluorescence microscopy, and cell viability assays were carried out for structural and in vitro functional characterization. Our results confirm the enhanced antitumor efficiency showed by these furin-immunotoxin variants as a result of an improved release of their toxic domain to the cytosol, favoring the accessibility of both ribonucleases to their substrates. Overall, these results represent a step forward in the design of immunotoxins with optimized properties for potential therapeutic application in vivo.

Keywords: immunotoxin; ribotoxin; α-sarcin; RNase T1; furin; intracellular trafficking; colorectal cancer

Key Contribution: This work not only represents a step forward in optimizing the cytotoxic efficacy of immunotoxins based on RNase T1 and α-sarcin, but also highlights the development of an immunotoxin design platform based on these ribonucleases.

---

1. Introduction

Due to their high cytotoxicity, specificity, and effectivity, immunotoxins have arisen as potent and promising antitumor agents [1–3]. These chimeric proteins are composed of a target domain that specifically targets a tumor marker, fused to a toxic domain, responsible for the cytotoxicity [4,5]. Their mechanism of action involves, in a first step, high affinity binding to the tumor antigen by the targeting domain, followed by the internalization of the complex by endocytosis, and finally the release of the toxic domain promoting the death of target cells [6–8]. Over the last years, multiple evidences have been gathered demonstrating that the efficiency of immunotoxins depends on different aspects [9,10] such as the following: antibody functional affinity and specificity for the tumor antigen expressed on the cell surface, the complex internalization efficacy, the rate of the toxin release in its intracellular route, and its intrinsic specificity and potency.

Currently, most of the immunotoxins are designed as recombinant fusion proteins. Different antibody fragments and linkers have been used. Thus, immunotoxins have been engineered to achieve greater specificity and tumor labelling and enhanced antitumor efficacy by reducing size and improving tumor penetration. Regarding this field, antibody engineering has pursued the development of different new formats with improved properties that are being incorporated within immunotoxin constructs [11–14]. Furthermore, beyond antibodies, other specific molecules, such as interleukins and growth factors, have been employed as targeting domains, leading to the first FDA-approved immunotoxins indicated for the treatment of acute myeloid leukemia [15] or hairy cell leukemia [16].

Toxins from different origins, have also been employed such as *Pseudomonas* exotoxin A, Diphteria toxin, actinoporins, gelonin, and the plant toxin ricin, among others [17–26]. Interestingly, ribonucleases (RNases) have acquired a significant importance due to their ideal features for being included as immunotoxin toxic domains [27–32]. In particular, ribotoxins stand out within the family of extracellular fungal RNases, as part of the toxic domain of immunotoxins, due to their small size, high thermostability and resistance to proteases, poor immunogenicity, and especially because they are highly effective to inactivate ribosomes [33–38]. As proven by the previous results obtained within α-sarcin-based immunotoxins, α-sarcin arises as the most promising ribotoxin to be included in these antitumoral therapeutic designs [36,38–40]. Its specific ribonucleolytic activity against just one single rRNA phosphodiester bond, located at the sarcin-ricin loop (SRL) of the larger rRNA, causes protein biosynthesis inhibition and apoptosis [41–43].

Few studies, however, have been focused on improving the effectiveness of immunotoxins by modulating their intracellular pathway [44–46]. As a general mechanism, once the target domain binds to the tumor antigen and gets internalized, the antigen-immunotoxin complex is found in the early endosomes, where it can be later recycled and presented back into the cell membrane or finally degraded into lysosomes. Toxin release and endosomal escape depends then on its intrinsic features. The two main routes that are usually followed by toxins are the following: (1) the route via the Golgi apparatus or (2) direct translocation to the cytosol [1]. Therefore, intracellular toxin trafficking can be considered to be a key checkpoint for desired cytotoxic effects and regarding cytotoxic efficiency, toxin delivery to the cytosol appears as a well-stablished rate-limiting step [1,47].

In this sense, we have previously produced and characterized two immunoconjugates, IMTXA33αS and scFvA33T1, based in the ribotoxin α-sarcin or the nontoxic RNase T1, respectively, fused to the variable domains (scFv) of the monoclonal antibody A33, which recognize and bind specifically the tumor-associated antigen GPA33, overexpressed in most of colorectal cancers [30,36,48,49]. We have characterized in detail both immunoRNases, not only for their structural and functional features, but also as a model to evaluate the effect of the different toxic domains and the relationship between intracellular trafficking and immunotoxins cytotoxicity [39,40].

Briefly, the antitumoral activity differences observed between both constructs have been explained by two aspects. The exquisite specificity of the ribonucleolytic activity of α-sarcin against ribosomes [36,40] in comparison with that exhibited by RNase T1 [30,50] and the intracellular pathway followed by each toxic domain, being the latter extremely decisive [39]. On the one hand, regarding the enzymatic properties of RNase T1, it is a much less specific acid cyclizing ribonuclease, with preference for the hydrolysis of GpN bonds. Although it has the same catalytic mechanism as ribotoxins, the latter present structural differences and small modifications in their catalytic residues that make them highly specific in terms of their ribonucleolytic activity. On the other hand, α-sarcin release to the cytosol could be carried out directly from endosomes or from the retrograde pathway involving Golgi apparatus, due to its ability to interact with the acidic components of the endosomes and Golgi membranes. Conversely, RNase T1, a nontoxic RNase, with an acidic isoelectric point value (pI), is not able to interact with the acidic components of endosome or Golgi membranes. Therefore, its release into the cytosol is impaired, favoring its degradation in the lysosomes or its accumulation into the late Golgi apparatus (Figure 1) [39].

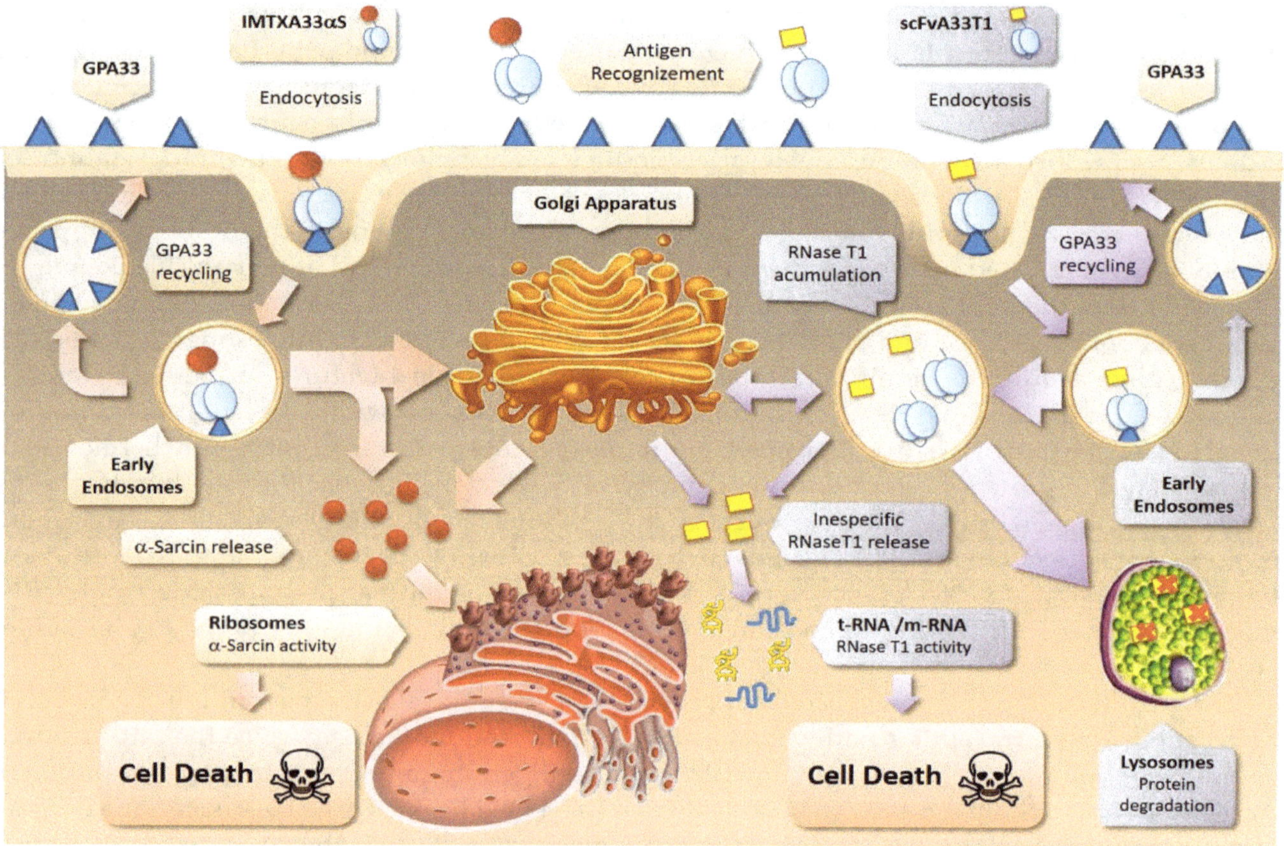

Figure 1. Scheme of the intracellular route followed by IMTXA33αS and scFvA33T1. As previously described [37], IMTXA33αS is internalized via early endosomes and follows the Golgi apparatus retrograde pathway, before α-sarcin release to the cytosol to exert its ribonucleolytic activity. Once internalized, scFvA33T1 appears also in the Golgi apparatus but mainly it is driven to lysosomes. These different pathways explain the more cytotoxic efficiency of IMTXA33αS.

In this context, some designs of immunotoxins with linkers including a specific furin cleavage site have been shown to be more cytotoxic [51–54]. This observation would confirm that intracellular processing and release of the toxic moiety is one of the key optimization spots for immunotoxin design [55–57]. Furin is a transmembrane enzyme present in the plasma membrane, the endosomes, and most notably in the trans-Golgi network [58]. It is a serine protease that belongs to the subtilisin family. Furin was known as the first mammalian proprotein-processing enzyme, exhibiting cleavage specificity for paired basic amino acid residues. Proteins were cleaved just downstream of the target sequence, canonically, Arg-X-(Arg/Lys)-Arg', with a minimal recognition cleavage site, described as Arg-X-X-Arg [59,60].

Within this idea, in this work we describe the production, purification, and in vitro functional characterization of two colorectal antitumor immunoRNases, including a furin cleavage site, based in the fungal ribotoxin α-sarcin and RNaseT1, IMTXA33furαS and scFvA33furT1, respectively (Figure 2). It is noted that our immunotoxins are usually produced in the heterologous system *P. pastoris*, a generally regarded as safe (GRAS) organism [61]. Thus, the immunotoxin secretion to the extracellular medium is driven by the α-factor signal peptide, which is finally released from the mature immunotoxin polypeptide chain by the action of Kex2 proteases. As furin belongs to this family and exhibits some of their recognition site characteristics, a minimum recognition sequence of furin has been used to avoid recognition by the Kex2 protease present in *P. pastoris* [62].

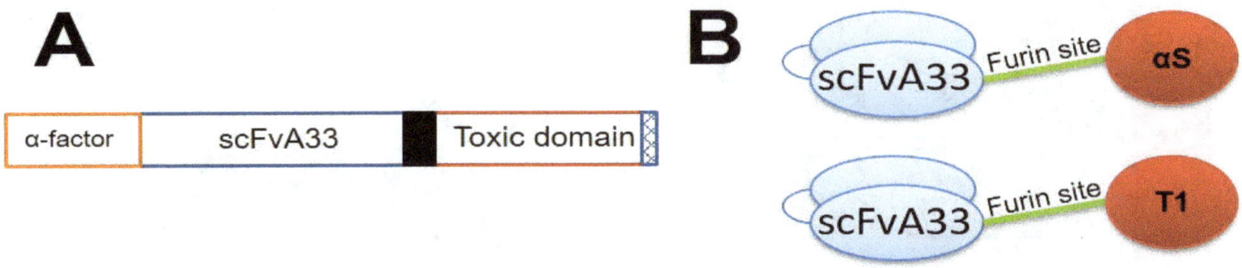

Figure 2. Schemes showing both genetic and domain structures of scFvA33-furin based immunotoxins. (**A**) Diagrammatic representation of gene construct. Both constructs include the α-factor signal peptide for secreted expression in *P. pastoris*, the anti-GPA33 scFvA33 gene (VH-linker-VL), a furin cleavage site linker (black box), the toxic domain, and the six His-tag (hatched box). The toxic domain was formed by ribotoxin α-sarcin or RNase T1. (**B**) Schematic model of the domain structure of scFvA33-furin based α-sarcin (upper) or RNase T1 (lower) immunotoxins.

2. Results

2.1. IMTXA33furαS and scFVA33furT1 Variants Were Purified as Fully Functional Immunoconjugates

Both IMTXA33furαS and scFVA33furT1 variants were successfully produced in the extracellular media of *P. pastoris* cultures after 48 h of methanol induction. Then both immunoconjugates were purified following dialysis and immobilized metal affinity chromatography (IMAC) (Figure 3A), as described in the Methods section. SDS-PAGE and western blot immunodetection, under reducing conditions, were carried out to analyze the identity and homogeneity of the purified proteins (Figure 3B). Bands of 42 and 45 kDa for scFvA33furT1 and IMTXA33furαS, respectively, corresponding to the expected theoretical molecular weight, were visualized by Coomassie blue staining and were also recognized by the anti-α-sarcin serum or anti-His-tag antibody. The final purification yield for both proteins was 1.5 and 3 mg per liter of induction medium for IMTXA33furαS and scFVA33furT1, respectively. The far-UV CD spectra for both IMTXA33furαS and scFvA33furT1 were coherent with those expected, according to the structural features of the domains that conform both immunoconjugates, and therefore compatible with water-soluble globular functional proteins. In this sense, a high content in beta sheet was observed that can be attributed to the folding described for the scFvA33, as well as to the contribution of RNase T1 and α-sarcin native conformation, which also present a high content of β-sheet and a small contribution of alpha helix [30,36] (Figure 3C).

To assess the correct functionality of these furin-variants immunoconjugates we first analyzed the ribonucleolytic activity of the two RNases included in their toxic domains. As expected, IMTXA33furαS was able to release the characteristic α-fragment, due to the specificity of its ribonucleolytic activity against the rRNA sarcin-ricin loop (SRL) present in the ribosomes (Figure 4A). Regarding scFvA33furT1, it exhibited nondistinguishable ribonucleolytic activity as compared with RNase T1 wild type or scFvA33T1 immunoconjugate when assayed in zymogram analysis against its typical substrate, poly(G), and in solution when *Torula* yeast RNA hydrolysis was measured (Figure 4B). The highly acidic feature of RNase T1 and its smaller size as compared with the immunoRNase, might explain the different intensities of the bands corresponding to scFvA33T1 and RNase T1. Thus, the incubations required to perform the assay would allow it to leak out of the gel. Both assays revealed proper functionality of the RNase moiety in the scFvA33furT1 variant. The ability of the targeting domain from both immunoconjugates to bind GPA33-positive cells SW1222 was also evaluated. As determined by flow cytometry results, both furin-variant constructs recognized GPA33-positive SW1222 cells (Figure 4C) as efficiently as IMTXA33αS and scFvA33T1, used as controls.

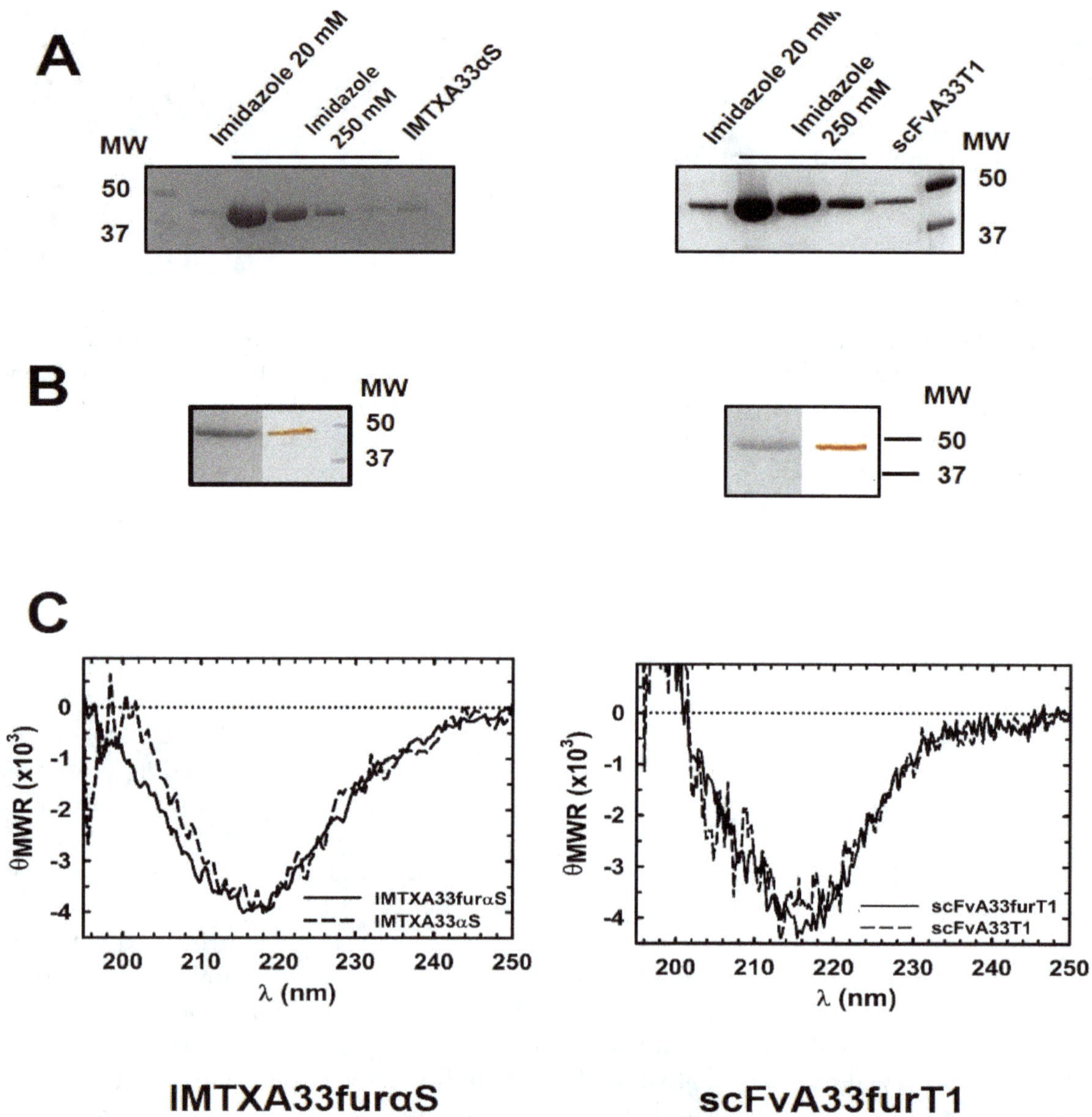

Figure 3. Production, purification, and structural characterization of furin-variant immunotoxins: IMTXA33furαS (left) or scFvA33furT1 (right). In both cases: (**A**) SDS-PAGE analysis of aliquots taken from IMAC performed to purify IMTXA33furαS or scFvA33furT1, visualized by Coomassie brilliant blue staining. (**B**) Purified IMTXA33furαS or scFvA33furT1 final fraction detection by Coomassie brilliant blue (left lane) or western blot (right lane). MW corresponds to prestained protein standards (Bio-Rad). (**C**) Far-UV circular dichroism spectra (θ_{MRW}, mean residue weight ellipticities were expressed as degree $\times$ cm^2 $\times$ dmol^{-1}) of: IMTXA33furαS (solid line) and IMTXA33αS (short dash line) (left); scFvA33furT1 (solid line) and scFvA33T1 (short dash line) (right).

Moreover, both constructs showed high structural stability and also maintained their functional integrity, when conditions mimicking a physiological context were assayed. In this sense, when purified proteins were incubated in media for at least 72 h at 37 °C, far-UV CD spectra showed that the full molecular folding of both immunotoxins were kept (Figure 5A,D). In addition, in the same conditions and for at least 72 h, the specific ribonucleolytic activity of α-sarcin (Figure 5B) and the specific antigen-binding ability of the target domain, in accordance with the flow cytometry analysis, were also preserved (Figure 5C,E).

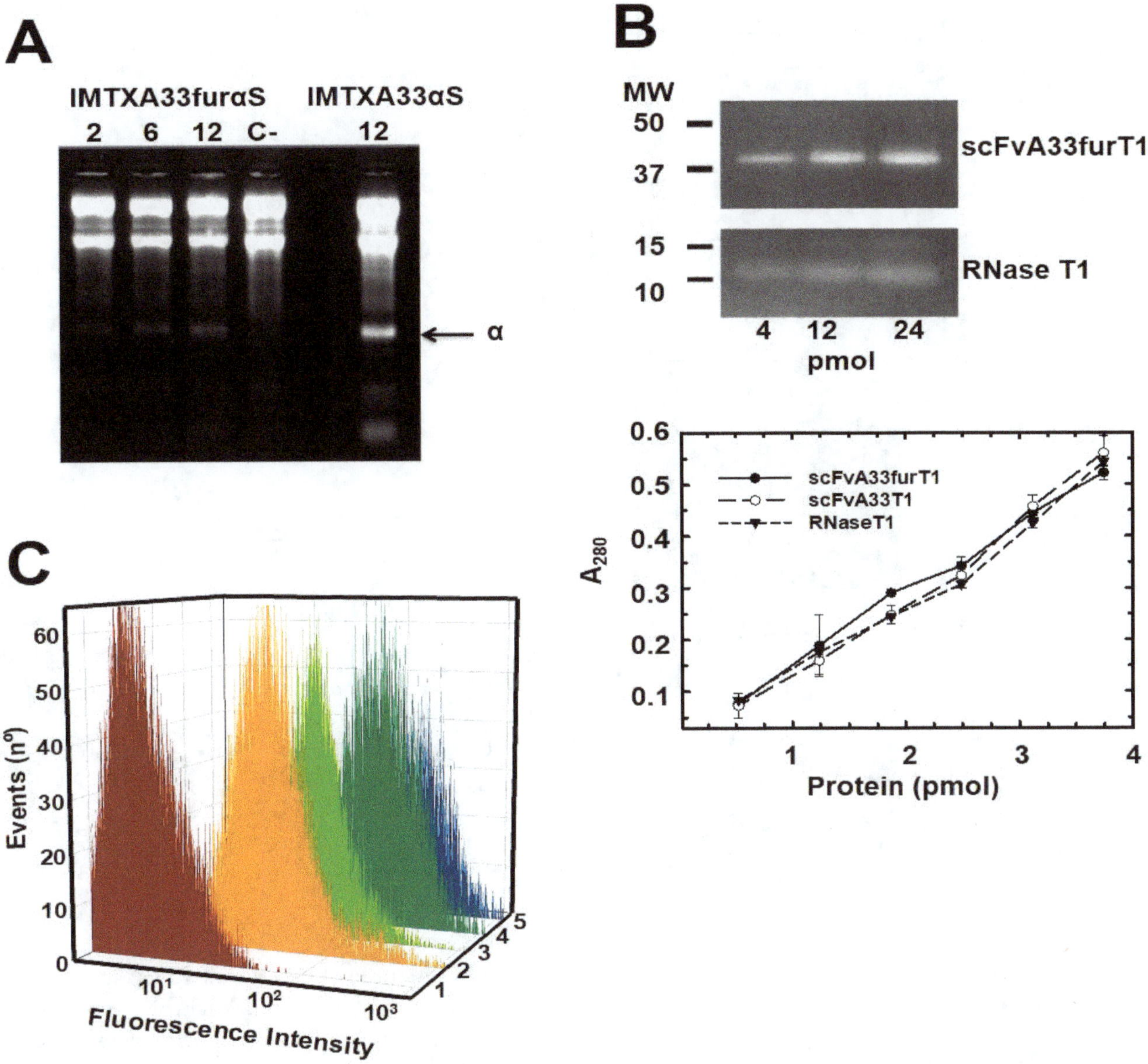

Figure 4. Functional characterization: (**A**) RNase activity assay of purified IMTXA33furαS using rabbit ribosomes as substrate. The characteristic α-fragment, as product of the specific RNase activity of α-sarcin is shown (indicated by an arrow). For IMTXA33furαS, 2, 6, and 12 pmol were assayed and 12 pmol of IMTXA33αS were used as a control. (**B**) RNase activity assays of purified scFvA33furT1. Poly(G) zymogram assay (upper panel) after SDS-PAGE of scFvA33furT1 or RNase T1. Four, 8 and 12 pmol of protein were assayed. Colorless bands were a consequence of the RNase T1 unspecific ribonucleolytic activity. MW (kDa), corresponds to electrophoretic molecular mass markers. Yeast RNA degradation assay (lower panel): The graph represents the A_{260} values versus the different amounts of scFvA33furT1 (black circles), scFvA33T1 (open circles), and RNase T1 (triangles) assayed. (**C**) Flow cytometry analysis of scFvA33furT1 (plot 2), scFvA33T1 (plot 3), IMTXA33furαS (plot 4), and (IMTXA33αS (plot 5) binding to SW1222 (GPA33-positive cells). The control curve (plot 1) corresponds to cells just treated with the anti-Histag-Alexa 488 antibody (Santa Cruz Biotechnologies, Santa Cruz, CA, USA).

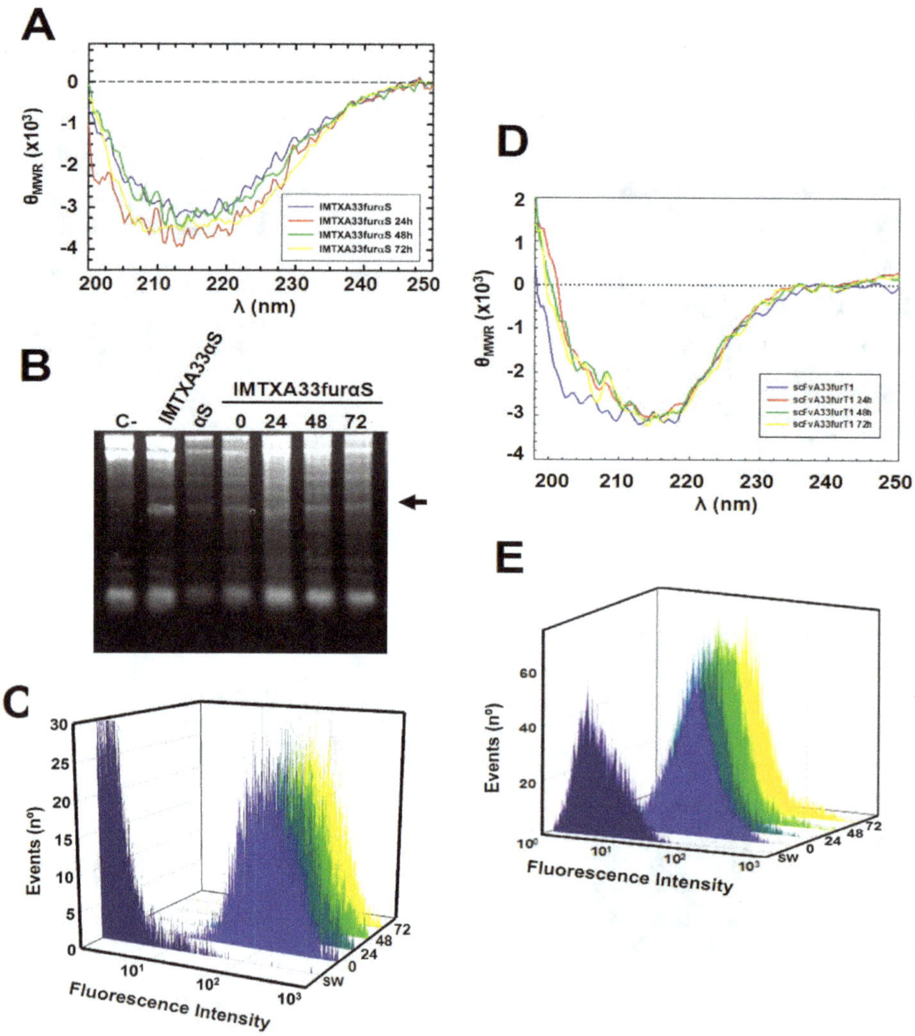

Figure 5. Stability assays of IMTXA33furαS (**A–C**) and scFvA33furT1 (**D–E**): In all cases, samples were previously incubated at 37 °C for 0, 24, 48, and 72 h. (**A**,**D**) Far-UV circular dichroism spectra (θ_{MRW}, mean residue weight ellipticities were expressed as degree × cm^2 × dmol^{-1}). Spectra were made with protein at 0.15 mg/mL in RPMI 1640 medium. (**B**) Specific ribonucleolytic activity against rabbit ribosomes. Samples were previously incubated at 37 °C in the absence of the substrate. The appearance of the α-fragment was indicated by an arrow. IMTXA33αS and α-sarcin wild type were used as controls. In all cases, 6 pmol of protein were assayed. (**C**,**E**) Binding assay o GPA33-positive SW1222 cells by flow cytometry analysis. Control curves (as in Figure 4).

2.2. IMTXA33furαS and scFVA33furT1 Follow Different Intracellular Pathway

Once it was established that the new immunoconjugate variants kept intact their antigen-specific binding capacity, as well as their ribonucleolytic activities, the next step was to analyze the effect of the furin cleavage site on the intracellular pathway followed after their internalization. In order to study this aspect, first the new constructs were labeled with Alexa 555. Both modified proteins remained fully structured, in comparison with the unlabeled versions (Figure S1), according to their far-UV CD spectra.

Internalization and intracellular localization of both labeled constructs were then studied. As shown for IMTXA33furαS (Figure 6A) and scFvA33furT1 (Figure 6B), very low colocalization was observed for both immunoconjugates with early endosomes. Although, no substantial differences were found between both constructs, interestingly, IMTXA33furαS colocalization was detected at shorter incubation times, 20 min or 2 h, than that observed for scFvA33furT1, at 5 or 24 h.

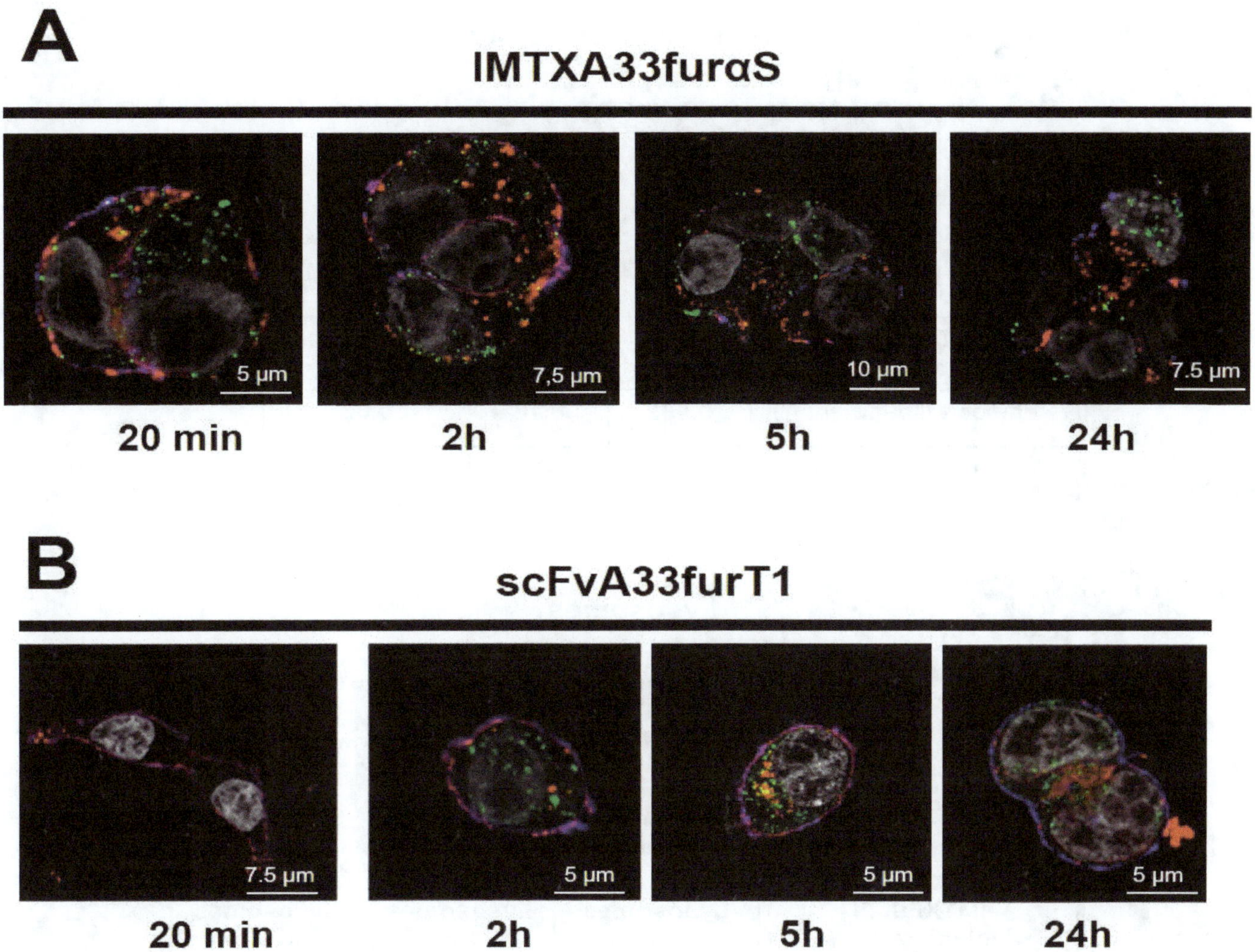

Figure 6. Endosomes colocalization analysis: Immunofluorescence confocal microscopy images obtained from cells incubated with IMTXA33furαS-555 and scFvA33furT1-555. Immunofluorescence confocal microscopy images of SW1222 cells after incubation for 20 min, 2 h, 5 h, or 24 h (from left to right) with IMTXA33furαS-555 (**A**) or scFvA33furT1-Alexa 555 (**B**). In all cases, images correspond to merging of nuclei labeled with DAPI (grey), plasmatic membrane were visualized with anti-CD44 plus GAM-Alexa 647 (blue), early endosomes were visualized with anti-EEA1 plus GAR-Alexa 488 (green), IMTXA33furαS-555 or scFvA33furT1-555 (red). The appearance of yellow dots indicates colocalization with endosomes, while violet dots correspond to colocalization with the plasmatic membrane.

As previously described for IMTXA33αS and scFvA33T1, two main intracellular pathways are followed by the toxic domain once the endosomes have been reached, via lysosomes or via Golgi-apparatus. On the one hand, for IMTXA33furαS, partial colocalization degree (22%, overlap coefficient) with Golgi apparatus at 4 h was observed, remaining at similar levels after 16 h of incubation (18%) (Figure 7A). However, colocalization with lysosomes was almost negligible. On the other hand, taken into account that for RNase T1-based immunoconjugates a significant colocalization with lysosomes was previously described [39], lysosome colocalization for scFvA33furT1 was measured. In this case, a significant colocalization was observed at 4 h, with degrees of 84%, but was dramatically decreased after 16 h (23%), and nearly disappeared when cells were treated with the antibiotic bafimolycin (<1%) (Figure 7B).

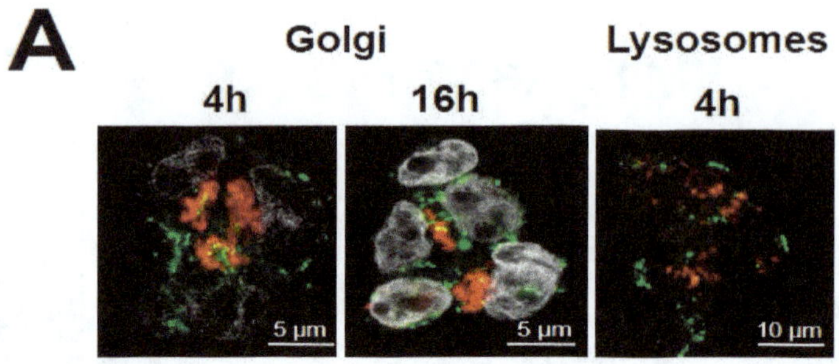

IMTXFurαS colocalization	Golgi 4h	Golgi 16h	Lysosomes 4h
Pearson's Coefficient (r)	0.192	0.18	0.03
Overlap Coefficient (%)	22.3	18.2	2.76

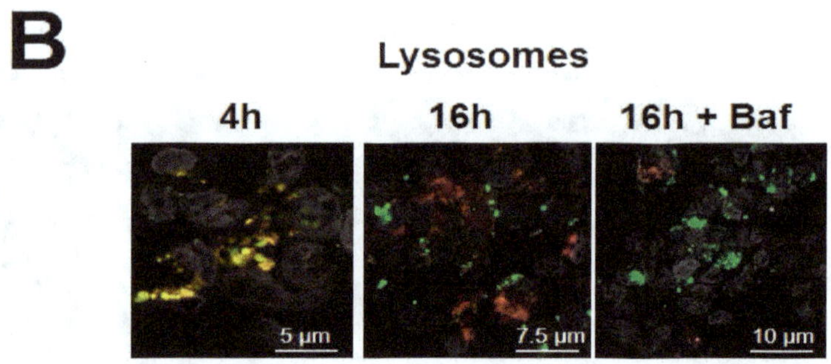

IMTXFurT1 colocalization	Lysosomes 4h	Lysosomes 16h	Lysosomes 16h + baf
Pearson's Coefficient (r)	0.824	0.177	0.055
Overlap coefficient (%)	84.5	23.4	0.71

Figure 7. Golgi apparatus and lysosomes colocalization analysis: Immunofluorescence confocal microscopy images obtained from cells incubated with IMTXA33furαS-Alexa-555 (**A**) or scFvA33furT1-Alexa-555 (**B**). (**A**) SW1222 cells were incubated for 4 or 16 h with both immunoconjugates as indicated in the figure. In all cases, images correspond to merging of nuclei labeled with DAPI (grey), Golgi with agglutinin or lysosomes with Lysotracker (red) and IMTXA33furαS-555 or scFvA33furT1-555 (green). (**B**) In the case of scFvA33T1-555, incubation was also made adding bafilomycin at 5 ng·mL^{-1}. Quantitative colocalization analysis was made as indicated in Methods. The appearance of yellow dots indicates colocalization with Golgi (**A**) or lysosomes (**B**).

The results obtained with the furin variants, compared to those described previously for the original constructions, show significant differences in the degree of colocalization with the cellular organelles involved in their intracellular pathways. On the one hand, in the case of IMTXA33furαS, although it follows the endosomas-Golgi route, just like the original construct [39], its detection in endosomes and Golgi apparatus is significantly lower, suggesting a greater or better release to the cytosol. On the other hand, for scFvA33furT1, there is a very significant increase in colocalization with the Golgi and a decrease in the case of lysosomes. As later discussed, these results would suggest that the presence of the furin cleavage site facilitates the release to the cytosol of the toxic domain of both immunoconjugates.

2.3. The Presence of the Furin Cleavage Site Significantly Increases the Cytotoxicity of Both Immunoconjugates

In vitro cytotoxicity assays were performed, to assess the effect of furin cleavage at the specific site included in these new designs. IMTXA33furαS showed an enhanced cytotoxicity with an IC_{50} two-times lower than that described for IMTXA33αS (Figure 8A). Even more interesting, cytotoxicity was increased by an additional three times when brefeldin A, that causes disassembly of Golgi-apparatus, was added (Figure 8A). However, the addition of bafilomycin that inhibits lysosomal acidification, resulted in no change in the cytotoxicity of this construction (data not shown). On the other hand, scFvA33furT1 toxicity was increased up to three times as compared to that described for scFvA33T1, being even greater when bafilomycin was added (Figure 8B). In this case no significant effect was observed with brefeldin A (data not shown).

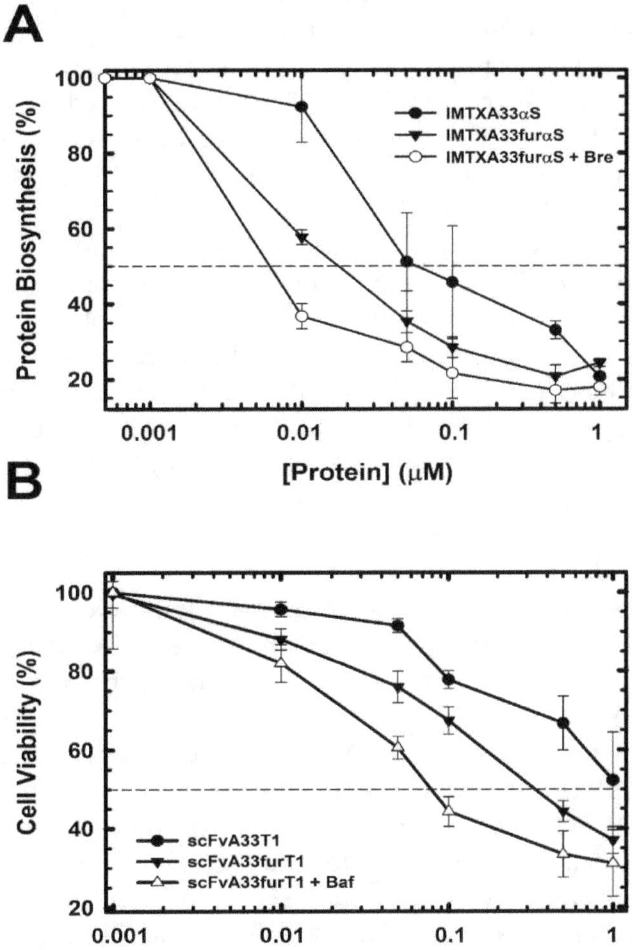

Figure 8. Cytotoxic characterization of IMTXA33furαS (**A**) and scFvA33furT1 (**B**). (**A**) Protein biosynthesis inhibition assay. SW1222 cells were incubated for 72 h with IMTXA33αS (●), IMTXA33furαS (▼), and IMTXA33aS + brefeldin A (○). (**B**) MTT viability assay of SW1222 cells incubated for 72 h with scFvA33T1 (●), scFvA33furT1 (▼), and scFvA33furT1+ bafilomycin (Δ). The 50% level of protein biosynthesis inhibition or cell viability were indicated (dashed line).

3. Discussion

We have purified and characterized two new optimized immunoconjugates, IMTXA33furαS and scFvA33furT1, which include a specific cleavage site for furin in the linker between the targeting and toxic domains of both constructs. They were purified to homogeneity from *P. pastoris* cultures, showing the expected size and folding, according to their biophysical characterization. This structural characterization yielded results which were consistent with the features previously described for their original counterparts, IMTXA33αS and scFvA33T1 [30,36], results that also were fully consistent, regarding to the nature and content of the secondary structure elements described for α-sarcin, RNase T1, and A33 scFv, their native domains [63–67]. Both constructs were also able to specifically bind to GPA33 expressed on the surface of the membrane and be internalized into SW1222 colorectal cancer cells, indicating that the targeting domain was fully functional.

Furthermore, they kept the original α-sarcin and RNase T1 ribonucleolytic activities, needed for ribosome inactivation and RNA hydrolysis, respectively. Moreover, when physiological-like conditions were analyzed, both IMTXA33αS and scFvA33T1, were stable and functional. In this sense, we could conclude that both immunoconjugates were correctly folded in terms of their structural and functional features, at least to the same extent as their original designs, IMTXA33αS and scFvA33T1.

As mentioned before, there is a close relationship between the intracellular route followed by the proteins included in the toxic domains of immunoconjugates and the antitumor efficiency of the immunotoxins [1]. Accordingly, this relationship had been previously reported for IMTXA33αS and scFvA33T1 [39]. Thus, once internalized, IMTXA33αS mainly followed the endosome-Golgi-apparatus network, whereas scFvA33T1 appeared indistinctly distributed between the lysosomes and the Golgi-apparatus. It is precisely this difference in the internalization pathway followed that led to a greater cytotoxic efficiency of IMTXA33αS [39].

Different designs of immunotoxins have been described including linkers with a furin cleavage site showing an increase in cytotoxic efficacy [51–54], confirming that intracellular processing and release of the toxic moiety is one of the key optimization spots in immunotoxin design [55–57]. Within this context, the main purpose driving this work was to evaluate the effect of including a furin linker in the previously characterized α-sarcin- and RNaseT1-based immunoconjugates [30,36,39]. The starting hypothesis was that this protease-specific site would ease the toxic moieties release and, consequently, would improve the cytotoxic efficiency of IMTXA33furαS and scFvA33furT1. Quite surprisingly, and although the results obtained for both constructs confirmed the preferred intracellular route used by each of the constructs [39], they, nevertheless, showed significant differences from what had been described for their parental designs.

The results herein presented further confirm that the cytotoxic mechanism of α-sarcin-based immunotoxins, IMTXA33furαS and IMTXA33αS, involves the endosome-Golgi intracellular pathway. The differences observed between both immunotoxins concerning the colocalization rate with the Golgi apparatus are in good agreement with their cytotoxic efficiency (Table 1). IMTXA33furαS cytotoxicity was two-fold higher than that observed for IMTXA33αS. Interestingly, the furin variant and its parent counterpart exhibited completely different behavior when traffic through the Golgi was blocked by the addition of brefeldin A. Whereas in the case of the original immunotoxin its cytotoxicity was dramatically reduced as an effect of brefeldin A, for the furin variant the cytotoxicity was significantly increased. These differences can only be explained by the presence of the furin cleavage site in the design of the immunotoxin. Furin protease activity would produce an increase in the amount of free α-sarcin that can interact with endosomal membranes and thus be released more efficiently to the cytosol, even without reaching the Golgi apparatus. It has been proven a long time ago that wild-type α-sarcin has the ability to translocate across a lipid bilayer rich in negatively charged phospholipids [68]. However, in the case of the original immunotoxin, most of the chimeric protein would reach the Golgi, and therefore the action of brefeldin A would negatively affect the release of the toxin. It must be emphasized that the inner membranes from both endosomes and Golgi apparatus have a high content of negative charges [69–72], contributing to α-sarcin translocation to the cytosol directly from endosomes or from Golgi apparatus [42,43]. Moreover, furin exert its protease activity not only in the Golgi but also in the endosomes [58]. Thus, α-sarcin release to the cytosol is facilitated by the presence of the furin cleavage site.

Table 1. Comparison of the results obtained for the furin variants vs. their originals counterparts, in relation to: level of colocalization with the Golgi apparatus and lysosomes; as well as the IC_{50} values obtained in the different cytotoxicity assays performed with just IMTXA33furαS or scFvA33furT1, or adding bafilomycin or brefeldin A, as described in Figure 8.

	IMTXA33furαS	**IMTXA33αS ***
Golgi colocalizationOverlap coefficient at 16 h (%)	18.2	46.3
IC_{50} (nM)	15	30–40
IC_{50} (nM) + Bafilomycin	15–20	30
IC_{50} (nM) + Brefefeldin A	5	>500
	IMTXA33furT1	**IMTXA33T1 ***
Lysosomes colocalizationOverlap coefficient at 16 h (%)	23.4	58.1
IC_{50} (nM)	300	>1 mM
IC_{50} (nM) + Bafilomycin	70–90	70–90
IC_{50} (nM) + Brefefeldin A	300	>1 mM

* Data from IMTXA33αS and scFVA33T1 used for comparison [39].

For scFvA33furT1, significant enhanced cytotoxicity was also observed when compared to the original design, scFvA33T1. As observed in the internalization assays, the degree of colocalization with lysosomes was significantly lower when compared to that previously described for scFVA33T1 [39] (Table 1), suggesting that most of scFvA33fur1 could follow the Golgi pathway or that the inclusion of the furin cleavage site would again favor its accumulation in endosomes. Within this, addition of bafilomycin, which impaired the recycling in the lysosomes, produced and increased in the cytotoxic effectiveness. However, the best IC_{50} value obtained for scFvA33furT1 (70–90 nM) after incubation with bafilomycin did not improve the cytotoxic effectiveness obtained by its original equivalent in the presence of the same antibiotic. Regarding this, it must be noted that the acidic pI value of RNase T1 [50,73] hamper its interaction with the endosome or Golgi membranes. Even if the lysosome pathway was partially blocked, the release into the cytosol was impaired. In fact, there is not any published account of RNase T1 being able to translocate a biological membrane on its own.

In summary, our results confirm the different routes followed by α-sarcin and RNaseT1 when included as part of the toxic domain of an immunotoxin and how we can take advantage of their features including a furin cleavage site in its design. Both furin-variant immunoconjugates exhibit enhanced antitumor effectiveness than that described for their original parents. Therefore, in vivo assays with IMTXA33furαS, exhibiting increased antitumor activity than that based in RNase T1, must be addressed.

4. Conclusions

This work not only represents a step forward in optimizing the cytotoxic efficacy of immunotoxins based on α-sarcin and RNase T1, but also highlights the development of an immunotoxin design platform based on these ribonucleases, including new designs with different specificities, with monomeric or trimeric formats [74,75], or including the use of non-immunogenic variants of α-sarcin [38]. The combination of all these optimization approaches will represent a very important boost for its application in the clinic.

5. Materials and Methods

5.1. Plasmid Design

Plasmids encoding IMTXA33αS and scFvA33T1 were previously obtained [30,36]. PCR was used to amplify the cDNA sequences of interest, using the necessary oligos to incorporate the sequence coding for the furin cleavage site between the target and the toxic domains, and also the restriction sites needed for cloning. Once purified, the resultant IMTXA33furαS and scFvA33furT1 cDNAs were cloned in pPICZαA (Invitrogen), for their expression in the methylotrophic yeast *P. pastoris KM71*. To facilitate protein detection and purification, as in their original counterparts, a 6 His-tag was included at the C-terminus of both immunotoxins (Figure 2). The expression vectors were amplified in *E. coli DH5αF′* and subsequently sequenced, using the DNA sequencing service of Universidad Complutense's Genomics Unit.

5.2. Protein Production and Purification

Electrocompetent *P. pastoris KM71* cells were used to electroporate 5–10 μg of the corresponding linearized plasmid previously cleaved with *Pme* I. A Bio-Rad Gene pulser apparatus (Bio-Rad, Berkeley, CA, USA) was used for this purpose. Multiple independent clones were selected with different amounts of zeocin (100, 400, or 750 μg/mL) and assayed to find the most productive colonies. To carry out these screenings, cells were grown in BMGY in 24-well plates at 30 °C for 24 h, were harvested afterwards, and finally suspended in BMMY. For induction of protein production, the cuture was shaked at 25 °C and 200 rpm, as previously described [30,36,39].

Once the induction was completed, the secretion to the extracellular media of the proteins of interest was analyzed by 0.1% (*w*/*v*) sodium dodecyl sulfate (SDS)-15% (*w*/*v*) polyacrylamide gel electrophoresis (PAGE) and western blot. In this sense, for the specific detection of the toxic domain by western blot, a rabbit anti-α-sarcin serum was used. In addition, an anti-histidine tag antibody was used to check integrity of the purified proteins. Large-scale production of both immunotoxins was carried out by addition of 25 mL of preinoculum to a 2 L baffled flasks containing 350 mL of BMGY. Then the culture was incubated with shaking for 16 h at 30 °C and 220 rpm. Cells were recollected by soft centrifugation at room temperature and resuspended again in 200 mL of BMMY. For induction of protein production, cells were incubated at 25 °C, 250 rpm shaking, for 48 h, supplementing the culture with methanol every 24 h. Once finalized, dialysis of the extracellular medium containing the proteins of interest was carried out, using a 50 mM sodium phosphate buffer with 0.1 M NaCl, pH 7.5.

IMTXA33furαS and scFvA33furT1 were purified from the dialyzed extracellular medium by IMAC. A Ni^{2+}-NTA agarose column was used for this purpose (HisTrap™ FF Columns, GE Healthcare, Fairfield, CT, USA). The extracellular media was applied to the column at 1 mL/min. The flow rate was controlled by a peristaltic pump. Two consecutive washes were done with the dialysis buffer and with the same but adding 20 mM imidazole, before elution of the proteins of interest, by using the same buffer but containing 250 mM imidazole. Finally, the different aliquots containing the purified proteins were collected and dialyzed again against the dialysis buffer.

5.3. Biophysical Characterization

Absorbance measurements were performed on an Uvikon 930 spectrophotometer (Kontron). As described before [76], far-UV circular dichroism (CD) spectra were carried out using a Jasco 715 spectropolarimeter. Proteins dissolved in PBS were prepared at 0.15 mg/mL. Cells of 0.1 cm optical path were used. Four spectra were averaged to obtain the final data. For stability assays, spectra were obtained after previous incubation of both constructs at 37 °C for 0, 24, 36, 48, or 72h in RPMI 1640.

5.4. Ribonucleolytic Activity Assays

The specific ribonucleolytic activity of α-sarcin, included in the toxic domain of IMTXA33furαS, was followed as described before [73,77]. For detection of the release of the characteristic 400 nt rRNA, namely α-fragment, we used as substrate ribosomes from a rabbit cell-free reticulocyte lysate. Briefly, the lysate was diluted three-fold in 40 mM Tris-HCl buffer, pH 7.5, containing 40 mM KCl and 10 mM EDTA. Then, 50 μL aliquots were taken of this dilution (5–6 pmol of ribosomes approximately) and incubated for 15 min at room temperature with different amounts of the proteins to be assayed. Then, the reaction was finished by adding 250 μL of 50 mM Tris-HCl, pH 7.4, 0.5% (*w/v*) SDS, followed by briefly vortex. Subsequently, RNA phenol/chloroform extraction was carried out. The RNA pellet obtained by the addition of isopropanol to the aqueous phase, was then washed with 70% (*v/v*) ethanol, dried exhaustively, and finally resuspended in 10 μL of DEPC H_2O. The presence of α-fragment in the samples was detected by ethidium bromide staining after electrophoresis, on denaturing 2% agarose gels. For quantification of the bands we used the Gel Doc XR Imaging System and Quantity One 1-D analysis software (Bio-Rad, Berkeley, CA, USA). Original IMTXA33αS [36] was used as the control.

The ribonucleolytic activity of RNase T1, included in scFvA33furT1, was analyzed by two parallel assays. First, RNA degradation in solution was tested by measurement of *Torula* yeast RNA (Sigma, type VI; Sigma-aldrich, St. Louis, MI, USA) hydrolysis [73]. In this assay the absorbance values obtained are proportional to the amount of soluble small oligonucleotides resulting from the RNasa activity on RNA larger size fragments contained in the substrate sample. The results obtained for the RNA samples analyzed (2 mg/mL) without protein were used to consider nonenzymatic RNA degradation, while original scFvA33T1 [30] and free RNase T1 were used as controls. In the second assay, the activity of purified scFvA33furT1 and RNase T1 was evaluated following the zymogram method [78]. Briefly, samples were applied into SDS-PAGE in 15% polyacrylamide gels, containing 0.1% (*w/v*) SDS and embedded with 0.3 mg/mL poly(G) homopolyribonucleotide [79]. Proteins exhibiting RNase activity were visualized as colorless bands, whereas the rest of the gel appeared colored.

5.5. Cell Lines Culture

Colon carcinoma SW1222 cells were used as model for the GPA33-positive cellular line [30,36,39]. The cultures were grown as described [30], in RPMI 1640 medium (Sigma-aldrich, St. Louis, MI, USA), supplemented with glutamine (300 mg/mL), containing 50 U/mL of penicillin and 50 mg/mL of streptomycin. Finally, the media was supplemented with 10% fetal bovine serum (FBS). Incubation of the cells was carried out at 37 °C in a humidified atmosphere (CO_2:air, 1:19, *v:v*). Trypsinization was routinely done for harvesting and propagation of the cultures. A hemocytometer was used to count the cells used in all assays described.

5.6. Flow Cytometry Studies

Trypsinized cells were distributed into different aliquots, containing 3×10^5 cells/mL, and washed several times with PBS 0.1% (*w/v*) BSA containing 0.02% (*w/v*) sodium azide. The samples were incubated with gentle shaking for 1 h at room temperature, with 1 μM of IMTXA33furαS or scFvA33furT1, using their original counterparts as positive controls. A second incubation, adding anti-His-Alexa488 (Sigma-aldrich, St. Louis, MI, USA) diluted 1/100, was carried out in the dark. When necessary, between the different steps, cells were collected by centrifugation (1200× *g*, 4 °C, 10 min) and then washed with PBS for several times. Flow cytometry acquisition was done on a FACScan (Becton Dickinson, Becton Dickinson, NJ, USA) and data were obtained using the WinMDI software. For stability assays, IMTXA33furαS and scFvA33furT1 were previously incubated at 37 °C for different times (0, 24 or 72 h).

5.7. Fluorescence Microscopy

To carry out these assays, both immunotoxins were first labeled. As previously described [37], using the Alexa Fluor 555 Protein Labeling Kit (Invitrogen, Carlsbad, CA, USA). Both labeled conjugates (IMTXA33furαS-555 and scFvA33furT1-555) were purified and characterized to ensure the preservation of their structural and functional features.

SW1222 cells were first trypsinized, seeded at 8×10^5 cells/well using cover-glasses, and incubated overnight at 37 °C. For treatment, IMTXA33furαS-555 or scFvA33furT1-555, at 25 μg/mL, were added to cells for the following different periods of time: from 20 min to 24 h for endosomes colocalization assays, and 4 or 16 h when lysosomes/Golgi colocalization assays were performed. Confirmation of colocalization with lysosomes was also studied by the addition of bafilomycin at 5 ng/mL, an antibiotic that inhibits lysosomal acidification [80], in combination with the immunoRNase. To observe the plasmatic membrane, incubation with anti-CD44 mAb [81] were performed. After removing the medium, the cells were fixed for 15 min with PBS containing 3% (*v*/*v*) p-formaldehyde and incubated for 15 min in PBS containing 50 mM ammonium chloride. Cells were permeabilized by the addition of digitonine at 0.01% (*w*/*v*) in PBS and incubation for 30 min, followed by another incubation in PBS containing 1.0% (*w*/*v*) BSA for 1 h. Different probes were used for organelle labeling as follows: an Ab targeting protein EAA1, present in the early endosomes [82]; lysosomes were labeled with Lysotracker (Life Technologies, Carlsbad, CA, USA), a fluorescence acidotropic specific probe [83]; and Golgi apparatus with Wheat Germ Agglutinin (Life Technologies) that binds to the highly abundant sialic acid present in the Golgi membranes [84]. Donkey anti-mouse Alexa 647 (DAM-Alexa 647) or goat anti-rabbit Alexa 488 (GAR-Alexa 488) were also added as secondary antibodies. For nuclei labeling, 10 μL of Prolong Gold-DAPI (Life Technologies) were added. Incubations were carried out at room temperature and the final samples were kept at 4 °C. To obtain the corresponding images, a Leica TCS SP2 confocal microscope was used, followed by analysis with the LCS lite software. Images presented correspond to the optical planes concerning the internal content of the cells selected for analysis. For each sample, ten different images were taken along the Z-axis, covering all the cells, from the basal zone to the apical one, Images shown correspond to the internal content of the cells, in particular to slices 4 to 6. ImageJ software was used to performed colocalization quantification, using two coefficients, the Pearson's correlation coefficient and, as described by Mander, the overlap coefficient. Both coefficients referred to the correlation between the intensity distribution of the channels and the true degree of colocalization, respectively [85].

5.8. MTT Viability Assay

Cell viability was evaluated by using the MTT-Cell Proliferation Kit I (Roche, Basel, Switzerland) as previously described [30,39]. Briefly, 5×10^3 trypsinized cells/well were seeded and then incubated for 24 h at 37 °C. The medium was then removed and scFvA33furT1 or scFvA33T1 were added at different concentrations in 200 μL final volume. Samples where incubated for 96 h, followed by another incubation with MTT at 0.5 mg/mL during 4 h at 37 °C. Finally, the solubilization buffer was added and the viability was determined in terms of A_{595} nm, whereas the higher A_{595} values were in correspondence with increasing amounts of viable cells. Cells incubated only with medium, in the absence of the protein, were taken as 100% viability. If necessary, samples including bafilomycin at 5 ng/mL, together with the protein were also done. Control only with bafilomycin, was included to evaluate potential drug related toxicity. The results shown correspond to the average of four independent assays.

5.9. Protein Biosynthesis Inhibition

To evaluate the cytotoxicity of ribotoxins the protein biosynthesis inhibition assay is routinely used [41–43]. Briefly, cells were seeded into 96-well plates (1×10^4 cells/well) in culture medium and kept under standard culture conditions for 24 h. Different concentrations of the different immunoconjugates, in 200 μL of free-FBS fresh medium were added to the cells. After 72 h of incubation at 37 °C, the medium was removed, followed by replacement with a fresh one containing 1 mCi per well of L-[4-C-3H]-Leucine (166 Ci/mmol; GE Healthcare, Fairfield, CT, USA). The samples were incubated again for 6 h, the medium was eliminated, and cells were then fixed with 5.0% (*w*/*v*) trichloroacetic acid. Several washed with cold ethanol were done, before the pellet was finally dissolved in 200 μL of 0.1 M NaOH containing 0.1% SDS. A Beckman LS3801 liquid scintillation counter was used to measure its radioactivity. Cytotoxicity was calculated in terms of IC_{50} values (namely, protein concentration needed to produce 50% protein synthesis inhibition), expressed as the percentage of the radioactivity incorporated in the assay. Three independent replicates per two assays were performed to average the IC_{50} values. When required, brefeldin A, that causes disassembly of Golgi-apparatus by altering vesicular trafficking [86], was added at 1 ng/mL together with the immunotoxins. A control, just with brefeldin A without the proteins, was performed to evaluate drug related toxicity.

Author Contributions: Conceptualization, J.L., J.R.-d.-l.-H., and J.T.-A.; methodology, J.R.-d.-l.-H., J.T.-A., and R.L.-G.; formal analysis and investigation, J.R.-d.-l.-H., J.T.-A., R.L.-G., J.G.G., and J.L.; writing—original draft preparation, J.L.; writing—review and editing, J.L., J.R.-d.-l.-H., J.T.-A., R.L.-G., J.G.G.

Acknowledgments: We very much appreciate A. Martínez del Pozo for critically reading the manuscript. JTA was granted from Instituto de Salud Carlos III (ISCIII) co-founded by FEDER Thematic Networks and Cooperative Research Centers: ARADYAL (RD16/0006/0003, RD16/0006/0013, RD16/0006/0015).

References

1. Alewine, C.; Hassan, R.; Pastan, I. Advances in anticancer immunotoxin therapy. *Oncologist* **2015**, *20*, 176–185. [CrossRef] [PubMed]
2. Kavousipour, S.; Khademi, F.; Zamani, M.; Vakili, B.; Mokarram, P. Novel biotechnology approaches in colorectal cancer diagnosis and therapy. *Biotechnol. Lett.* **2017**, *39*, 785–803. [CrossRef] [PubMed]
3. Nasiri, H.; Valedkarimi, Z.; Aghebati-Maleki, L.; Majidi, J. Antibody-drug conjugates: Promising and efficient tools for targeted cancer therapy. *J. Cell. Physiol.* **2018**, *233*, 6441–6457. [CrossRef]
4. Frankel, A.E.; Woo, J.H.; Neville, D.M. Immunotoxins. In *Principles of Cancer Biotherapy*; Oldham, R.K., Dillman, R.O., Eds.; Springer: Dordrecht, The Netherlands, 2009; pp. 407–449.
5. Madhumathi, J.; Verma, R.S. Therapeutic targets and recent advances in protein immunotoxins. *Curr. Opin. Microbiol.* **2012**, *15*, 300–309. [CrossRef]
6. Pastan, I.; Hassan, R.; FitzGerald, D.J.; Kreitman, R.J. Immunotoxin treatment of cancer. *Annu. Rev. Med.* **2007**, *58*, 221–237. [CrossRef] [PubMed]
7. Kreitman, R.J. Recombinant immunotoxins containing truncated bacterial toxins for the treatment of hematologic malignancies. *BioDrugs* **2009**, *23*, 1–13. [CrossRef] [PubMed]
8. King, E.M.; Mazor, R.; Cuburu, N.; Pastan, I. Low-dose methotrexate prevents primary and secondary humoral immune responses and induces immune tolerance to a recombinant immunotoxin. *J. Immunol.* **2018**, *200*, 2038–2045. [CrossRef] [PubMed]
9. Becker, N.; Benhar, I. Antibody-Based Immunotoxins for the Treatment of Cancer. *Antibodies* **2012**, *1*, 39–69. [CrossRef]
10. Weldon, J.E.; Xiang, L.; Zhang, J.; Beers, R.; Walker, D.A.; Onda, M.; Hassan, R.; Pastan, I. A recombinant immunotoxin against the tumor-associated antigen mesothelin reengineered for high activity, low off-target toxicity, and reduced antigenicity. *Mol. Cancer Ther.* **2013**, *12*, 48–57. [CrossRef] [PubMed]
11. Muyldermans, S. Nanobodies: Natural Single-Domain Antibodies. *Annu. Rev. Biochem.* **2013**, *82*, 775–797. [CrossRef] [PubMed]
12. Ecker, D.M.; Jones, S.D.; Levine, H.L. The therapeutic monoclonal antibody market. *mAbs* **2015**, *1*, 9–14. [CrossRef] [PubMed]
13. Álvarez-Cienfuegos, A.; Nuñez-Prado, N.; Compte, M.; Cuesta, A.M.; Blanco-Toribio, A.; Harwood, S.L.; Villate, M.; Merino, N.; Bonet, J.; Navarro, R.; et al. Intramolecular trimerization, a novel strategy for making multispecific antibodies with controlled orientation of the antigen binding domains. *Sci. Rep.* **2016**, *6*, 28643. [CrossRef] [PubMed]
14. Kimiz-Gebologlu, I.; Gulce-Iz, S.; Biray-Avci, C. Monoclonal antibodies in cancer immunotherapy. *Mol. Biol. Rep.* **2018**, *45*, 2935–2940. [CrossRef] [PubMed]
15. Appelbaum, F.R.; Bernstein, I.D. Gemtuzumab ozogamicin for acute myeloid leukemia. *Blood* **2017**, *130*, 2373–2376. [CrossRef] [PubMed]
16. Kreitman, R.J.; Dearden, C.; Zinzani, P.L.; Delgado, J.; Karlin, L.; Robak, T.; Gladstone, D.E.; le Coutre, P.; Dietrich, S.; Gotic, M.; et al. Moxetumomab pasudotox in relapsed/refractory hairy cell leukemia. *Leukemia* **2018**, *32*, 1768–1777. [CrossRef]
17. Avila, A.D.; de Acosta, C.M.; Lage, A. A new immunotoxin built by linking a hemolytic toxin to a monoclonal antibody specific for immature T lymphocytes. *Int. J. Cancer* **1988**, *42*, 568–571. [CrossRef] [PubMed]

18. Foss, F.M.; Saleh, M.N.; Krueger, J.G.; Nichols, J.C.; Murphy, J.R. Diphtheria toxin fusion proteins. *Curr. Top. Microbiol. Immunol.* **1988**, *234*, 663–681.
19. LeMaistre, C.F.; Saleh, M.N.; Kuzel, T.M.; Foss, F.; Platanias, L.C.; Schwartz, G.; Ratain, M.; Rook, A.; Freytes, C.O.; Craig, F.; et al. Phase I Trial of a Ligand Fusion-Protein (DAB389IL-2) in Lymphomas Expressing the Receptor for Interkeukin-2. *Blood* **1998**, *91*, 399–405.
20. O'Toole, J.E.; Esseltine, D.; Lynch, T.J.; Lambert, J.M.; Grossbard, M.L. Clinical trials with blocked ricin immunotoxins. *Curr. Top. Microbiol. Immunol.* **1998**, *234*, 35–56.
21. Schnell, R.; Vitetta, E.; Schindler, J.; Barth, S.; Winkler, U.; Borchmann, P.; Hansmann, M.L.; Diehl, V.; Ghetie, V.; Engert, A. Clinical trials with an anti-CD25 ricin A-chain experimental and immunotoxin (RFT5-SMPT-dgA) in Hodgkin's lymphomaLeuk. *Lymphoma* **1998**, *30*, 525–537. [CrossRef]
22. García-Ortega, L.; Alegre-Cebollada, J.; García-Linares, S.; Bruix, M.; Martínez-Del-Pozo, A.; Gavilanes, J.G. The behavior of sea anemone actinoporins at the water-membrane interface. *Biochim. Biophys. Acta* **2011**, *1808*, 2275–2288. [CrossRef] [PubMed]
23. Pirie, C.M.; Hackel, B.J.; Rosenblum, M.G.; Wittrup, K.D. Convergent potency of internalized gelonin immunotoxins across varied cell lines, antigens, and targeting moieties. *J. Biol. Chem.* **2011**, *286*, 4165–4172. [CrossRef] [PubMed]
24. Wang, Z.; Duran-Struuck, R.; Crepeau, R.; Matar, A.; Hanekamp, I.; Srinivasan, S.; Neville, D.M., Jr.; Sachs, D.H.; Huang, C.A. Development of a diphtheria toxin based antiporcine CD3 recombinant immunotoxin. *Bioconjug. Chem.* **2011**, *22*, 2014–2020. [CrossRef] [PubMed]
25. Liu, X.F.; FitzGerald, D.J.; Pastan, I. The insulin receptor negatively regulates the action of *Pseudomonas* toxin-based immunotoxins and native *Pseudomonas* toxin. *Cancer Res.* **2013**, *73*, 2281–2288. [CrossRef] [PubMed]
26. Rivera-de-Torre, E.; Palacios-Ortega, J.; Gavilanes, J.G.; Martínez-del-Pozo, Á.; García-Linares, S. Pore-Forming Proteins from Cnidarians and Arachnids as Potential Biotechnological Tools. *Toxins (Basel)* **2019**, *11*, 370. [CrossRef] [PubMed]
27. De Lorenzo, C.; D'Alessio, G. From ImmunoToxins to ImmunoRNases. *Curr. Pharm. Biotechnol.* **2008**, *9*, 210–214. [CrossRef] [PubMed]
28. Balandin, T.G.; Edelweiss, E.; Andronova, N.V.; Treshalina, E.M.; Sapozhnikov, A.M.; Deyev, S.M. Antitumor activity and toxicity of anti-HER2 immunoRNase scFv 4D5-dibarnase in mice bearing human breast cancer xenografts. *Investig. New Drugs* **2011**, *29*, 22–32. [CrossRef] [PubMed]
29. Borriello, M.; Lacceti, P.; Terrazzano, G.; D'Alessio, G.; De Lorenzo, C. A novel fully human antitumor immunoRNase targeting ErbB2-positive tumors. *Br. J. Cancer* **2011**, *104*, 1716–1723. [CrossRef]
30. Tomé-Amat, J.; Menéndez-Méndez, A.; García-Ortega, L.; Batt, C.A.; Oñaderra, M.; Martínez-del-Pozo, A.; Gavilanes, J.G.; Lacadena, J. Production and characterization of scFvA33T1, an immunoRNase targeting colon cancer cells. *FEBS J.* **2012**, *279*, 3022–3032. [CrossRef]
31. Shirmann, T.; Frenzel, A.; Linden, L.; Stelte-Ludwig, B.; Willuda, J.; Harrenga, A.; Dübel, S.; Müller-Tiemann, B.; Trautwein, M. Evaluation of human pancreatic RNase as effector molecule in a therapeutic antibody platform. *mAbs* **2014**, *6*, 367–380. [CrossRef]
32. Sun, M.; Sun, L.; Sun, D.; Zhang, C.C.; Li, M. Targeted delivery of immuno-RNase may improve cancer therapy. *Cancer Cell Int.* **2018**, *18*, 58. [CrossRef] [PubMed]
33. Wawrzynczak, E.J.; Henry, R.V.; Cumber, A.J.; Parnell, G.D.; Derbyshire, E.J.; Ulbrich, N. Biochemical, cytotoxic and pharmacokinetic properties of an immunotoxin composed of a mouse monoclonal antibody Fib75 and the ribosome-inactivating protein α-sarcin from *Aspergillus giganteus*. *Eur. J. Biochem.* **1991**, *196*, 203–209. [CrossRef] [PubMed]
34. Rathore, D.; Batra, J.K. Construction, expression and characterization of chimaeric toxins containing the ribonucleolytic toxin restrictocin: Intracellular mechanism of action. *Biochem. J.* **1997**, *324*, 815–822. [CrossRef] [PubMed]
35. Rathore, D.; Nayak, S.K.; Batra, J.K. Overproduction of fungal ribotoxin α-sarcin in Escherichia coli: Generation of an active immunotoxin. *Gene* **1997**, *190*, 31–35. [CrossRef]
36. Carreras-Sangrà, N.; Tomé-Amat, J.; García-Ortega, L.; Batt, C.A.; Oñaderra, M.; Martínez-del-Pozo, A.; Gavilanes, J.G.; Lacadena, J. Production and characterization of a colon cancer-specific immunotoxin based on the fungal ribotoxin α-sarcin. *Protein Eng. Des. Sel.* **2012**, *25*, 425–435. [CrossRef] [PubMed]

37. Tomé-Amat, J.; Herrero-Galán, E.; Oñaderra, M.; Martínez-del-Pozo, A.; Gavilanes, J.G.; Lacadena, J. Preparation of an engineered safer immunotoxin against colon carcinoma based on the ribotoxin hirsutellin A. *FEBS J.* **2015**, *282*, 2131–2141. [CrossRef] [PubMed]
38. Jones, T.D.; Heam, A.R.; Holgate, R.G.; Kozub, D.; Fogg, M.H.; Carr, F.J.; Baker, M.P.; Lacadena, J.; Gehlsen, K.R. A deimmunised form of the ribotoxin, α-sarcin, lacking CD4+ T cell epitopes and its use as an immunotoxin warhead. *Protein Eng. Des. Sel.* **2016**, *29*, 531–540. [CrossRef]
39. Tomé-Amat, J.; Ruiz-de-la-Herrán, J.; Martínez-del-Pozo, Á.; Gavilanes, J.G.; Lacadena, J. α-sarcin and RNase T1 based immunoconjugates: The role of intracellular trafficking in cytotoxic efficiency. *FEBS J.* **2015**, *282*, 673–684. [CrossRef]
40. Tome-Amat, J.; Olombrada, M.; Ruiz-de-la-Herrán, J.; Pérez-Gómez, E.; Andradas, C.; Sánchez, C.; Martínez, L.; Martínez-Del-Pozo, Á.; Gavilanes, J.G.; Lacadena, J. Efficient in vivo antitumor effect of an immunotoxin based on ribotoxin α-sarcin in nude mice bearing human colorectal cancer xenografts. *Springerplus* **2015**, *4*, 168. [CrossRef]
41. Olmo, N.; Turnay, J.; González de Buitrago, G.; de Silanes, I.L.; Gavilanes, J.G.; Lizarbe, M.A. Cytotoxic mechanism of the ribotoxin α-sarcin. Induction of cell death via apoptosis. *Eur. J. Biochem.* **2001**, *268*, 2113–2123. [CrossRef]
42. Lacadena, J.; Alvarez-García, E.; Carreras-Sangrà, N.; Herrero-Galán, E.; Alegre-Cebollada, J.; García-Ortega, L.; Oñaderra, M.; Gavilanes, J.G.; Martínez-del-Pozo, A. Fungal ribotoxins: Molecular dissection of a family of natural killers. *FEMS Microbiol. Rev.* **2007**, *1*, 212–237. [CrossRef] [PubMed]
43. Olombrada, M.; Lázaro-Gorines, R.; López-Rodríguez, J.C.; Martínez-del-Pozo, A.; Oñaderra, M.; Maestro-López, M.; Lacadena, J.; Gavilanes, J.G.; García-Ortega, L. Fungal ribotoxins: A Review of Potential Biotechnological Applications. *Toxins* **2017**, *9*, 71. [CrossRef] [PubMed]
44. Weldon, J.E.; Pastan, I. A guide to taming a toxin-recombinant immunotoxins constructed from *Pseudomonas* exotoxin A for the treatment of cancer. *FEBS J.* **2011**, *278*, 4683–4700. [CrossRef] [PubMed]
45. Weng, A.; Thakur, M.; von Mallinckradt, B.; Beceren-Braun, F.; Gilabert-Oriol, R.; Wiesner, B.; Eickhart, J.; Böttger, S.; Melzig, M.F.; Fuchs, H. Saponins modulate the intracellular trafficking of protein toxins. *J. Control. Release* **2012**, *164*, 74–86. [CrossRef] [PubMed]
46. Pasetto, M.; Antignani, A.; Ormanoglu, E.; Buehler, E.; Guha, R.; Pastan, I.; Martin, S.E.; FitzGerald, D.J. Whole-genome RNAi screen highlights components of the endoplasmic reticulum/Golgi as a source of resistance to immunotoxin-mediated cytotoxicity. *Proc. Natl. Acad. Sci. USA* **2015**, *112*, E1135–E1142. [CrossRef] [PubMed]
47. Johannes, L.; Decaudin, D. Protein toxins: Intracellular trafficking for targeted therapy. *Gene Ther.* **2005**, *12*, 1360–1368. [CrossRef] [PubMed]
48. Ritter, G.; Cohen, L.S.; Nice, E.C.; Catimel, B.; Burgess, A.W.; Moritz, R.L.; Ji, H.; Heath, J.K.; White, S.J.; Welt, S.; et al. Characterization of posttranslational modifications of human A33 antigen, a novel palmitoylated surface glycoprotein of human gastrointestinal epithelium. *Biochem. Biophys. Res. Commun.* **1997**, *236*, 682–686. [CrossRef] [PubMed]
49. Pereira-Fantini, P.M.; Judd, L.M.; Kalantzis, A.; Peterson, A.; Ernst, M.; Heath, J.K.; Giraud, A.S. A33 antigen-deficient mice have defective colonic mucosal repair. *Inflamm. Bowel Dis.* **2010**, *16*, 604–612. [CrossRef] [PubMed]
50. Yoshida, H. The ribonuclease T1 family. *Methods Enzymol.* **2001**, *341*, 28–41.
51. Goyal, A.; Batra, J.K. Inclusion of a furin-sensitive spacer enhances the cytotoxicity of ribotoxin restrictocin containing recombinant single-chain immunotoxins. *Biochem. J.* **2000**, *345*, 247–254. [CrossRef]
52. Tortorella, L.L.; Pipalia, N.H.; Mukherjee, S.; Pastan, I.; Fitzgerald, D.; Maxfiled, F.R. Efficiency of Immunotoxin Cytotoxicity Is Modulated by the Intracellular Itinerary. *PLoS ONE* **2012**, *7*, e47320. [CrossRef] [PubMed]
53. Weldon, J.E.; Scarzynski, M.; Therres, J.A.; Ostovitz, J.R.; Zhou, H.; Kreitman, R.J.; Pastan, I. Designing the furin-cleavable linker in recombinant immunotoxins based on Pseudomonas exotoxin A. *Bioconjug. Chem.* **2015**, *26*, 1120–1128. [CrossRef] [PubMed]
54. Mutter, N.L.; Soskine, M.; Huang, G.; Alburquerque, I.S.; Bernardes, G.J.L.; Maglia, G. Modular Pore-Forming Immunotoxins with Caged Cytotoxicity Tailored by Directed Evolution. *ACS Chem. Biol.* **2018**, *13*, 3153–3160. [CrossRef] [PubMed]

55. Kaplan, G.; Lee, F.; Onda, M.; Kolyvas, E.; Bhardwaj, G.; Baker, D.; Pastan, I. Protection of the Furin Cleavage Site in Low-Toxicity Immunotoxins Based on Pseudomonas Exotoxin A. *Toxins* **2016**, *8*, 217. [CrossRef] [PubMed]
56. Kaplan, G.; Mazor, R.; Lee, F.; Jang, Y.; Leshem, Y.; Pastan, I. Improving the In Vivo Efficacy of an Anti-Tac (CD25) Immunotoxin by Pseudomonas Exotoxin A Domain II Engineering. *Large Mol. Ther.* **2018**. [CrossRef] [PubMed]
57. Meng, P.; Dong, Q.C.; Tan, G.G.; Wen, W.H.; Wang, H.; Zhang, G.; Wang, Y.Z.; Jing, Y.M.; Wang, C.; Qin, W.J.; et al. Anti-tumor effects of a recombinant antiprostate specific membrane antigen immunotoxin against prostate cancer cells. *BMC Urol.* **2017**, *17*, 14. [CrossRef] [PubMed]
58. Schapiro, F.B.; Soe, T.T.; Mallet, W.G.; Maxfield, F.R. Role of Cytoplasmic Domain Serines in Intracellular Trafficking of Furin. *Mol. Biol. Cell* **2014**, *15*, 2884–2894. [CrossRef]
59. Wise, R.J.; Barr, P.J.; Wong, P.A.; Kiefer, M.C.; Brake, A.J.; Kaufman, R.J. Expression of a human proprotein processing enzyme: Correct cleavage of the von Willebrand factor precursor at a paired basic amino acid site. *Proc. Natl. Acad. Sci. USA* **1990**, *87*, 9378–9382. [CrossRef]
60. Van de Ven, W.J.; Creemers, J.W.; Roebroek, A.J. Furin: The prototype mammalian subtilisin-like proprotein-processing enzyme. Endoproteolytic cleavage at paired basic residues of proproteins of the eukaryotic secretory pathway. *Enzyme* **1991**, *45*, 257–270. [CrossRef]
61. Mattia, A.; Merker, R. Regulation of probiotic substances as ingredients in foods: Premarket approval or "generally recognized as safe" notification. *Clin. Infect. Dis. Off. Publ. Infect. Dis. Soc. Am.* **2008**, *46*, S115–S118. [CrossRef]
62. Bader, O.; Krauke, Y.; Hube, B. Processing of predicted substrates of fungal Kex2 proteinases from *Candida albicans*, *C. glabrata*, *Saccharomyces cerevisiae* and *Pichia pastoris*. *BMC Microbiol.* **2008**, *8*, 116. [CrossRef] [PubMed]
63. Martínez-del-Pozo, A.; Gasset, M.; Oñaderra, M.; Gavilanes, J.G. Conformational study of the antitumor protein α-sarcin. *Biochim. Biophys. Acta* **1988**, *953*, 280–288. [CrossRef]
64. Pace, C.N.; Heinemann, U.; Hahn, U.; Saenger, W. Ribonuclease T1: Structure, function and stability. *Angew. Chem. Int. Ed. Engl.* **1991**, *30*, 343–454. [CrossRef]
65. Pérez-Cañadillas, J.M.; Santoro, J.; Campos-Olivas, R.; Lacadena, J.; del Pozo, A.M.; Gavilanes, J.G.; Rico, M.; Bruix, M. The highly refined solution structure of the cytotoxic ribonuclease alpha-sarcin reveals the structural requirements for substrate recognition and ribonucleolytic activity. *J. Mol. Biol.* **2000**, *299*, 1061–1073. [CrossRef] [PubMed]
66. Carmichael, J.A.; Power, B.E.; Garrett, T.P.J.; Yazaki, P.J.; Shively, J.E.; Raubischek, A.A.; Wu, A.M.; Hudson, P.J. The crystal structure of an anti-CEA scFv diabody assembled from T84.66 scFvs in V(L)-to-V(H) orientation: Implications for diabody flexibility. *J. Mol. Biol.* **2003**, *326*, 341–351. [CrossRef]
67. Wilkinson, I.C.; Hall, C.J.; Veverka, V.; Shi, J.Y.; Muskett, F.W.; Stephens, P.E.; Taylor, R.J.; Henry, A.J.; Carr, M.D. High resolution NMR-based model for the structure of a scFv-IL-1beta complex: Potential for NMR as a key tool in therapeutic antibody design and development. *J. Biol. Chem.* **2009**, *284*, 31928–31935. [CrossRef] [PubMed]
68. Oñaderra, M.; Mancheño, J.M.; Gasset, M.; Lacadena, J.; Schiavo, G.; del Pozo, A.M.; Gavilanes, J.G. Translocation of α-sarcin across the lipid bilayer of asolectin vesicle. *Biochem. J.* **1993**, *295*, 221–225. [CrossRef]
69. Gruenberg, J. Lipids in endocytic membrane transport and sorting. *Curr. Opin. Cell Biol.* **2003**, *15*, 382–388. [CrossRef]
70. Bissing, C.; Gruenberg, J. Lipid sorting and multivesicular endosome biogenesis. *Cold Spring Harb. Perspect. Biol.* **2013**, *5*, a016816.
71. Van Meer, G.; Voelker, D.R.; Feigenson, G.W. Membrane lipids: Wherethey are and how they behave. *Nat. Rev. Mol. Cell Biol.* **2008**, *9*, 112–124. [CrossRef]
72. Zhao, P.; Liu, F.; Zhang, B.; Liu, X.; Wang, B.; Gong, J.; Yu, G.; Ma, M.; Lu, Y.; Sun, J.; et al. MAIGO2 is involved in abscisic acid-mediated response to abiotic stresses and Golgi-to-ER retrograde transport. *Physiol. Plant.* **2013**, *148*, 246–260. [CrossRef] [PubMed]
73. Martínez-Ruiz, A.; García-Ortega, L.; Kao, R.; Lacadena, J.; Oñaderra, M.; Mancheño, J.M.; Davies, J.; del Pozo, A.M.; Gavilanes, J.G. RNAse U2 and α-sarcin: A study of relationships. *Methods Enzimol.* **2001**, *341*, 335–351.

74. Blanco-Toribio, A.; Lacadena, J.; Nuñez-Prado, N.; Álvarez-Ciénfuegos, A.; Villate, M.; Compte, M.; Sanz, L.; Blanco, F.J.; Álvarez-Vallina, L. Efficient production of single-chain fragment variable-based N-terminal trimerbodies in *Pichia pastoris*. *Microb. Cell Factories* **2014**, *13*, 116–124. [CrossRef] [PubMed]
75. Lázaro-Gorines, R.; Ruiz-de-la-Herrán, J.; Navarro, R.; Sanz, L.; Álvarez-Vallina, L.; Martínez-del-Pozo, A.; Gavilanes, J.G.; Lacadena, J. A novel Carcinoembryonic Antigen (CEA)-Targeted Trimeric Immunotoxin shows significantly enhanced Antitumor Activity in Human Colorectal Cancer Xenografts. *Sci. Rep.* **2019**, *9*, 11680. [CrossRef] [PubMed]
76. Lacadena, J.; Martínez del Pozo, A.; Martínez-Ruiz, A.; Pérez-Cañadillas, J.M.; Bruix, M.; Mancheño, J.M.; Oñaderra, M.; Gavilanes, J.G. Role of histidine-50, glutamic acid-96, and histidine-137 in the ribonucleolytic mechanism of the ribotoxin alpha-sarcin. *Proteins* **1999**, *37*, 474–484. [CrossRef]
77. Kao, R.; Martínez-Ruiz, A.; Martínez del Pozo, A.; Crameri, R.; Davies, J. Mitogillin and related fungal ribotoxins. *Methods Enzymol.* **2001**, *341*, 324–335. [PubMed]
78. García-Ortega, L.; Masip, M.; Mancheño, J.M.; Oñaderra, M.; Lizarbe, M.A.; García-Mayoral, M.F.; Bruix, M.; Martínez-del-Pozo, A.; Gavilanes, J.G. Deletion of the NH2-terminal beta-hairpin of the ribotoxin alpha-sarcin produces a nontoxic but active ribonuclease. *J. Biol. Chem.* **2002**, *277*, 18632–18639. [CrossRef]
79. Steyaert, J. A decade of protein engineering on ribonuclease T1-atomic dissection of the enzyme-substrate interactions. *Eur. J. Biochem.* **1997**, *247*, 1–11. [CrossRef]
80. Yoshimori, T.; Yamamoto, A.; Moriyama, Y.; Futai, M.; Tashiro, Y. Bafilomycin A1, a Specific Inhibitor of Vacuolar-type H^+-ATPase, Inhibits Acidification and Protein Degradation in Lysosomes of Cultured Cell. *J. Biol. Chem.* **1991**, *266*, 17707–17712.
81. Yeung, T.M.; Shaan, C.G.; Wilding, J.L.; Muschel, R.; Bodmer, W.F. Cancer stem cells from colorectal cancer-derived cell lines. *Proc. Natl. Acad. Sci. USA* **2009**, *107*, 3722–3727. [CrossRef]
82. Nazarewicz, R.R.; Salazar, G.; Patrushev, N.; San Martin, A.; Hilenski, L.; Xiong, S.; Alexander, R.W. Early endosomal antigen 1 (EEA1) is an obligate scaffold for angiotensin II-induced, PKC-α-dependent Akt activation in endosomes. *J. Biol. Chem.* **2011**, *286*, 2886–2895. [CrossRef] [PubMed]
83. Anderson, R.G.; Orci, L. A view of acidic intracellular compartments. *J. Cell Biol.* **1988**, *106*, 539–543. [CrossRef] [PubMed]
84. Zhao, W.; Chen, T.L.; Vertel, B.M.; Colley, K.J. The CMP-syalic acid transporter is localized in the medial-trans Golgi and possesses two specific endoplasmic reticulum export motifs in its carboxyl-terminal cytoplasmic tail. *J. Biol. Chem.* **2006**, *281*, 31106–31118. [CrossRef] [PubMed]
85. Zinchuk, V.; Zinchuk, O.; Okada, T. Quantitative Colocalization Analysis of Multicolor Confocal Immunofluorescence Microscopy Images: Pushing Pixels to Explore Biological Phenomena. *Acta Histochem. Cytochem.* **2007**, *40*, 101–111. [CrossRef] [PubMed]
86. Fujiwara, T.; Oda, K.; Yokota, S.; Takatsuki, A.; Ikehara, Y. Brefeldin A Causes Disassembly of the Golgi Complex and Accumulation of Secretory Proteins in the Endoplasmic Reticulum. *J. Biol. Chem.* **1988**, *263*, 18545–18552. [PubMed]

11

Cancer Acidity and Hypertonicity Contribute to Dysfunction of Tumor-Associated Dendritic Cells: Potential Impact on Antigen Cross-Presentation Machinery

Sven Burgdorf [1,†], Stefan Porubsky [2,3,†], Alexander Marx [3] and Zoran V. Popovic [3,*]

1. Department of Cellular Immunology, LIMES Institute, University of Bonn, 53115 Bonn, Germany; burgdorf@uni-bonn.de
2. Institute of Pathology, University Hospital, Johannes-Gutenberg University Mainz, 55131 Mainz, Germany; Stefan.Porubsky@unimedizin-mainz.de
3. Institute of Pathology, University Hospital Mannheim, University of Heidelberg, 68167 Mannheim, Germany; Alexander.Marx@umm.de

* Correspondence: Zoran.Popovic@umm.de

† Authors contribute equally.

Abstract: Macrophages (MΦ) and dendritic cells (DC), major players of the mononuclear phagocyte system (MoPh), are potent antigen presenting cells that steadily sense and respond to signals from the surrounding microenvironment, leading to either immunogenic or tolerogenic outcomes. Next to classical MHC-I/MHC-II antigen-presentation pathways described in the vast majority of cell types, a subset of MoPh ($CD8^+$, $XCR1^+$, $CLEC9A^+$, $BDCA3^+$ conventional DCs in human) is endowed with a high competence to cross-present external (engulfed) antigens on MHC-I molecules to $CD8^+$ T-cells. This exceptional DC function is thought to be a crucial crossroad in cytotoxic antitumor immunity and has been extensively studied in the past decades. Biophysical and biochemical fingerprints of tumor micromilieus show significant spatiotemporal differences in comparison to non-neoplastic tissue. In tumors, low pH (mainly due to extracellular lactate accumulation via the Warburg effect and via glutaminolysis) and high oncotic and osmotic pressure (resulting from tumor debris, increased extracellular matrix components but in part also triggered by nutritive aspects) are—despite fluctuations and difficulties in measurement—likely the most constant general hallmarks of tumor microenvironment. Here, we focus on the influence of acidic and hypertonic micromilieu on the capacity of DCs to cross-present tumor-specific antigens. We discuss complex and in part controversial scientific data on the interference of these factors with to date reported mechanisms of antigen uptake, processing and cross-presentation, and we highlight their potential role in cancer immune escape and poor clinical response to DC vaccines.

Keywords: cancer acidity; hyperosmolarity; tumor microenvironment; cross-presentation

---

1. The Role of Mononuclear Phagocytes in the Tumor Microenvironment

The mononuclear phagocyte system (MoPh) with its most important and most broadly explored players—macrophages (MΦ) and dendritic cells (DC)—comprises a major population of immune cells that migrate to and infiltrate tumor tissue. Crucial influence of continuous, highly plastic interaction between MoPh, tumor cells and surrounding milieu has been well-documented in the past decades [1]. The opposing role of different MΦ/DC subsets to this regard has highlighted the need to define (from a quantitative point of view) more and more 'smaller' genotypic, phenotypic and functional

MoPh subgroups in order to decipher their possible role in antitumor immunity. The former strict differentiation between MΦ- and DC-expression profiles has meanwhile been updated and replaced by current concept based on the understanding that an expression signature and functional specialization of MoPh cells represents a rather unstable momentum that depends on interplay between cellular and molecular microenvironmental factors [2,3]. Due to an extraordinary instability and fluctuations in tumor microenvironment (TME), the categorization of tumor-associated MoPh profiles thus remains a challenging task. A number of scientific reports and excellent up-to-date reviews have addressed the question of receptor expression profiling of tumor-associated MΦ and DC in order to classify them functionally [4–6]. Thus, we do not intend to address MoPh classification algorithms; instead, we focus in this review on the cross-presentation by a subtype of tumor-associated DCs as an important functional link in triggering the cytotoxic antitumor response, and highlight the influence of low pH and high osmolarity of the TME on the cross-presenting capacities of these cells.

2. Modules of Efficient Antigen Presentation by MHC Molecules

Classical antigen-presentation pathways are not limited to professional phagocytes and imply two well-described antigen-presentation modules: (1) engulfment and processing of exogenous antigens for endosomal digestion and surface presentation in the complex with MHC-II-molecules to $CD4^+$ T cells—an unspecific mechanism present in a vast majority of cell types; and (2) processing and presentation of endogenous (intracellular) antigens on MHC-I molecules in order to activate $CD8^+$ T cell and induce their proliferation and cytotoxic response.

A third, special form of antigen-presentation can be seen (not exclusively, but most prominently) in a subset of DC: it is termed cross-presentation and is characterized as the capacity to present an external, phagocytosed antigen in the complex with MHC-I molecules to $CD8^+$ T cells [7], thereby sensing the tumor- (or virus-) specific antigens and exposing them to induce an effective cytotoxic antitumor response [8].

2.1. Cross-Presenting Capacity of DC Subsets

Generally, DCs are categorized into conventional DCs (cDCs with previously defined cDC1 and cDC2 categories) and plasmacytoid DCs (pDCs), as reviewed elsewhere [9,10]. cDC2 ($BDCA1^+$) have—especially in humans—at least a minor capacity to cross-present, even though there is evidence that cDC2 prefer classical MHC-II antigen presentation module [5,11]. By contrast, the role of cross-presentation by pDC is controversial: there are experiments showing intact clearance of viral antigens in a pDC-depleted system [12], indicating that pDCs likely do not have a major role in cross-presentation.

The cDC1 subtype seems to be the most potent cross-presenting DC population. The development of cDC1 has been reported to depend on IRF8- and Batf3- transcription factors and is characterized in humans by expression of the chemokine receptor XCR1, efficient uptake of apoptotic particles via CLEC9A (DNGR1) or necrotic debris via BDCA3 (CD141), prominent TLR3-reactivity with high IL-12 output, high intraendosomal reactive oxygen species and low acidification of endosomes [8,13,14]. In several animal models, the failure of cDC1-deficient mice to reject transplanted immunogenic tumors (for example, using Batf3-/- mice) underscores the importance of these cells in cross-presentation and consecutive $CD8^+$ T cell priming [5,15]. Next, high expression of MHC-I pathway related genes has been reported as a hallmark of the cDC1 subset [16]. These cells also show enhanced expression of NADPH-oxidase 2 (NOX2), which has been linked to ROS production and active alkalization of endosomes, together with synchronous, low-level expression of the c-type lectin, Siglec-G (a potent NOX2-inhibitor). Both features are required for efficient cross-presentation and are critically responsible for the enhanced cross-presentation capacities of cDC1 cells [14,17].

Of relevance, compared to other intratumoral/peritumoral leukocytes, the cDC1 population is generally small in tumor tissue. Additionally, in contrast to the immunosuppressive role of tumor-associated macrophages (TAM), a high cDC1-load in malignant tumors has been shown to have a positive prognostic and predictive value [5,18]. Accordingly, if augmentation of the cytotoxic antitumor response through attraction of cDC1 to the cancer site and prolongation of their retention there is a therapeutic goal, induction of specific chemokine secretion by tumor cells and other immune cells (CCL4, CCL5, XCL1) might be the appropriate strategy [19,20]. Especially tumor-associated NK cells might be a key factor in this regard. Next to the aforementioned chemokines, NK cells secrete fms-like tyrosine kinase 3 ligand (FLT3-L) as well, which is regarded as a factor that prolongs cDC1 viability [5,21].

2.2. Subcellular Pathways of Cross-Presentation

On a subcellular level, two general cross-presentation pathways are described to date: the vacuolar pathway and the endosome-to-cytosol pathway [22,23]. In the vacuolar pathway, internalized antigens are degraded within endosomal compartments by lysosomal proteases and loaded onto MHC-I molecules there [24,25]. In the endosome-to-cytosol pathway, internalized antigens need to be translocated from endosomes into the cytosol, where they are degraded by the proteasome [26,27]. Afterwards, antigen-derived peptides are retranslocated by the transporter associated with antigen processing (TAP) into the ER or into endosomes for loading onto MHC-I [28–30]. Although both cross-presentation pathways have been well-documented in the past [31,32], most of the published data point to the endosome-to-cytosol pathway as a dominant mechanism of cross-presentation. The proteosomal antigen degradation seems to be a step of crucial importance for an efficient activation of CD8$^+$ T cells to recognize and kill the target tumor cells or virus-carrying cells (reviewed in [8]). A recent study pointed out that proteasomes might also be present in antigen-containing endosomes and hence, proteasomal degradation might also play a role in the vacuolar cross-presentation pathway [33]. However, the physiological relevance of endosomal proteasomes still needs to be determined. In addition to the vacuolar and the endosome-to-cytosol pathway, 'alternative', endocytosis-independent mechanisms of cross-presentation have been suggested, such as the transfer of preprocessed antigens via a gap junction-meditated contact between a 'donor cell' and a DC [34] or 'cross-dressing', which assumes the acquisition of a peptide-loaded MHC-I molecule via membrane transfer [35]. Yet, the in vivo relevance of such models in the tumor setting remains unclear and needs further investigation.

3. Acidity and Hypertonicity as Biophysical Hallmarks of the TME

In addition to varying biochemical and cellular parameters, physical stress plays an important role in tumor spreading and therapy response [36]. The typical microenvironment of solid tumors is characterized by hypoxia (mainly due to insufficient blood perfusion), low extracellular pH and high intratumoral pressure (Figure 1).

3.1. Mechanisms of TME Acidification

Acidity of the TME has been traditionally linked to hypoxia, as both phenomena are synchronous hallmarks of the TME. Briefly, normal human cells under aerobic conditions produce required amounts of ATP molecules from energy-rich glucose via cellular respiration process down to CO_2 molecules resulting in the production of 32 molecules of ATP from one molecule of glucose. In normal cells under anaerobic conditions—but constitutively also in many tumors due to the Warburg effect (i.e., aerobic glycolysis; first described by Otto Warburg and his team in the 1923)—NADH is re-oxidized, leading to a reduction of pyruvate into lactate, the production of only two ATP molecules per molecule of glucose and resulting in local accumulation of lactate (reviewed in [37]). Thereby, even though the synthesis of lactate is not necessarily associated with hypoxic conditions, excessive lactate production and accumulation inside many tumors is responsible for their well described acidic TME. Specifically, melanomas, squamous cell carcinomas, breast cancer and many other adenocarcinomas as well as brain tumors show low pH values in their milieu, ranging from pH 5.8 to pH 7.4, as reviewed by Diaz et al. [38]. Other substrates next to glucose may also result in tumor-associated lactate production:

for example, glutaminolysis pathway via citric acid cycle may be even a major source of lactate in cancer microenvironment [39]. Functionally, acidosis of the tumor interstitium has been shown to be a crucial factor of tumor survival, local progression and metastasis [40].

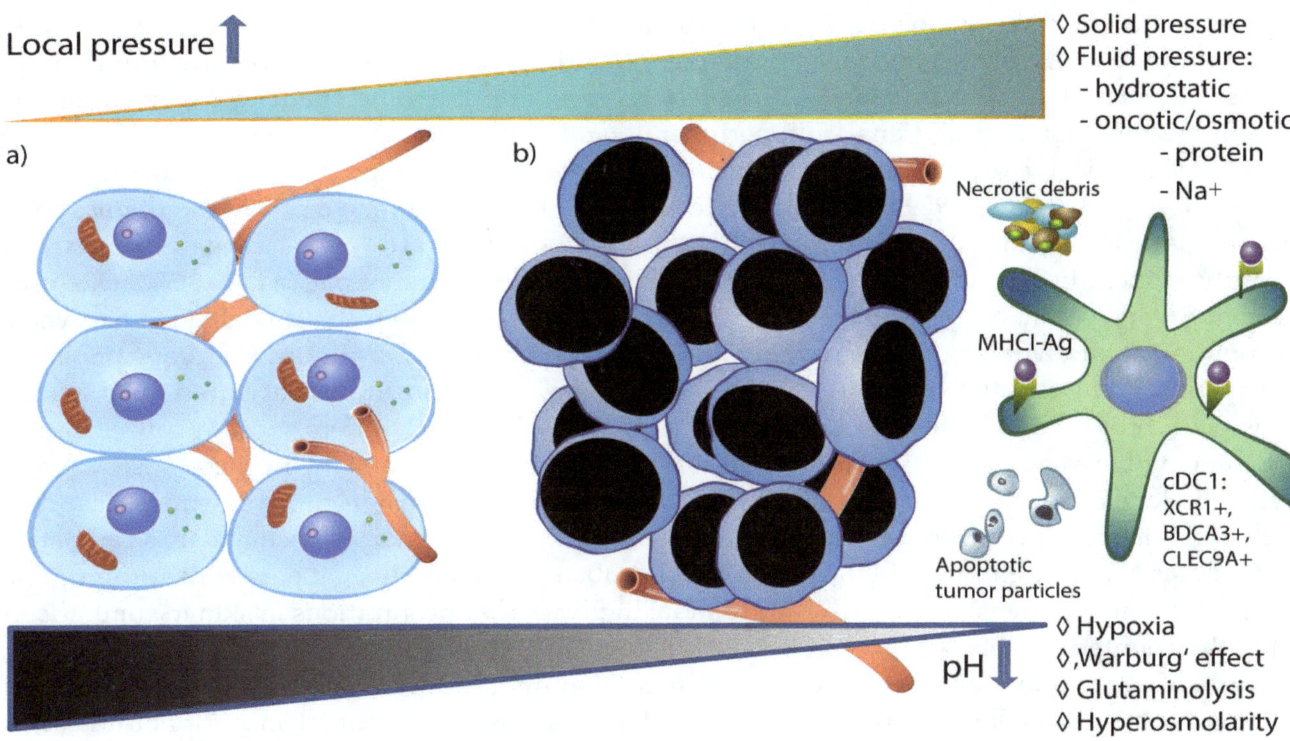

Figure 1. Typical microenvironment of tumor-associated cDC1 is acidic and hypertonic. In comparison to physiologic conditions (**a**), malignant neoplastic tissue (**b**) is characterized by lactate-induced decrease of pH value via hypoxia, aerobic glycolysis and glutaminolysis. On the other hand, increased (fluid and solid) pressure of tumor interstitium depends on biophysical characteristics of tumor mass, tumor cell death rate, abnormal blood supply but also nutritive aspects, like high-salt diet. Increased extracellular Na^+ may further enhance lactate accumulation via supporting aerobic glycolysis.

3.2. Elevated TME Pressure—Biophysical Prediction Models

On the other hand, very few reports are available on the role of high pressure in tumor micromilieus. It has been reported and reviewed that many solid tumors demonstrate an elevated interstitial pressure [1], forming a physical barrier to transcapillary transport and thereby affecting the antitumor therapy. Still, as a result of technical difficulties to directly measure intratumoral pressure in different tissue compartments, its relevance for tumor progression (involving immune escape mechanisms) has remained largely unexplored to date. In general, pressure-induced stress in tumors can be divided into two categories: fluid-phase and solid-phase stress. Further, fluid-phase stress can be roughly categorized into hydrostatic fluid pressure of the tumor interstitium and osmotic/oncotic pressure [41]. Increased osmotic pressure results from increased ionic and protein load of distinct etiologies. Limited available data in this regard demonstrate a general hypertonicity of some TMEs (for instance, in a pancreatic adenocarcinoma murine subcutaneous tumor graft model) [42–44]. In the absence of direct in vivo measurement techniques, a compelling biomechanical approach to predict an intratumoral osmotic pressure has been proposed [42]. In this approach, based on previously published data on increased hyaluron (and other glycosaminoglycan) content in melanomas, sarcomas and adenocarcinomas, the authors developed a triphasic mathematical and biomechanical model that takes into account solid and fluid tumor pressure together with transport of anions and cations. Interestingly, the authors suggest that increased hydraulic conductivity of the tumor-associated blood vessels (defined as interstitial fluid flow through the interstitial compartment [45]) elevates the intratumoral concentration of free ions and thereby osmotic pressure [42].

3.3. *Potential Contribution of Increased Na^+ Uptake to Hypertonicity of TME*

Regulation of tissue osmolarity in regard to interstitial Na^+ concentration has been extensively explored in the past decade. In order to understand and discuss a plausible Na^+ accumulation in the tumor insterstitium, it is necessary to understand recent updates and challenges concerning the (patho)physiology of 'central' (renal) and peripheral regulation of Na^+ metabolism:

First, historically, despite the documentation of interstitial storage of chloride in preclinical studies (observed already 1909 by Padtberg; reviewed in [46]) more than a century ago, for a long time it was assumed that the regulatory function of kidney in regard to Na^+ keeps osmolarity of interstitium including peripheral tissue in a tight range, similar to that of plasma (290–300 mOsm/L). The concept of constant Na^+ concentration of extracellular tissue has been challenged in the past years and pointed at alternative pathways of Na^+ regulation, especially nonosmotic Na storage pools via electrolytic binding to sulfated glucosaminoglycans, i.e., important constituents of extracellular matrix. It has been proposed that this mechanism prevents water loss and buffers sodium concentration by balancing between free and stored (bound) Na^+ [47]. In concordance with these observations, a recently developed MRI-based approach (Na-MRI) enabled precise detection of extracellular Na^+ -fluctuations in time and space and revealed that peripheral tissue indeed does not maintain steady-state extracellular Na^+ concentration [48]. As detected in subcutaneous tissue, patients with autoimmune disease, arterial hypertension, or renal failure show higher Na^+ concentrations in skin in comparison to healthy counterparts [49,50].

Second, as mainly demonstrated in experimental animal models, a shift of nutritional habits towards high salt uptake may provoke a markedly increased Na^+ content in peripheral tissues, independent on a putative preexisting pathologic condition [51,52].

4. Cross-Presentation Cascade in Acidic and Hypertonic Milieu: Current Data and Possible Implications

A successful cross-presentation of tumor antigen requires efficient binding and processing of engulfed material. The cascade of antigen processing (starting with antigen uptake, delayed degradation, translocation into the cytosol, transport and loading on MHC-I molecules and transport of endoplasmatic reticulum components to endosome) has been recently reviewed [8]. Therefore, we focus here on the scarce currently available data on pH- and Na^+- dependent modifications of the cross-presentation pathway.

4.1. *Cross-Presentation in Low Extracellular pH*

4.1.1. The Influence of Low pH on Antigen Uptake

DCs in the tumor micromilieu screen and bind soluble and particular antigens via a wide range of surface receptors. The abundancy and type of endocytic receptor in combination with the presented antigen likely have a significant influence on efficacy of cross-presentation per se. It is reasonable to assume, that binding and processing of apoptotic and necrotic tumor material via binding to different receptors like e.g., DEC205 will be a dominant mechanism of uptake in apoptotic particles-rich or necrotic tumors. DEC205, a member of mannose receptor family typically expressed on cross-presenting dendritic cells and on thymic epithelial cells [53,54], is a well-characterized endocytic receptor that may induce either tolerance or immunity, depending on external signals [55]. An in vitro study has shown a pH-dependent recognition of apoptotic particles and necrotic tumor cells by DEC205 via formation of a double-ringed receptor conformation in the acidic microenvironment, implying enhanced engulfment of tumor-associated material in acidic TME [53].

In dendritic cells, mannose receptor (MR) is another effective endocytic carbohydrate-binding damage-associated-molecular-pattern (DAMP) receptor with a variety of ligands (endogenous and microbial) [56]. MR has been reported to target the endocytosed material via pH-dependent steps for cross-presentation [57]. At physiological pH, the MR acquires an extended conformation. A decrease in pH (6–7, corresponding to early endosomes or pH 5–6 in late endosomes), results in a continuous conformational change of the receptor, which mediates ligand release [58]. Based on these data, it can be hypothesized that tumor-associated extracellular low pH decreases the capacity of MR to form stable receptor-antigen complexes and thus can be responsible for reduced cross-presentation in acidic micromilieu. Indeed, it has been shown that antigenic targeting of the human MR is capable of inducing antitumor immunity [59].

Of note, although both DEC205 and MR belong to the mannose receptor family, their pathways after antigen internalization seem to diverge. Whereas MR-mediated antigen engulfment in human DCs leads to its routing into early endosomes, delayed degradation and potent cross-presentation, internalization via the DEC205-pathway favors antigen-processing in lysosomes and rather poor cross-presentation [60]. Thus, summarizing these data, it can be discussed that an acidic cancer milieu may abrogate successful antigen internalization and processing within tumor-associated dendritic cell by favorizing less efficient DEC205-dependent cross-presentation model (Figure 2).

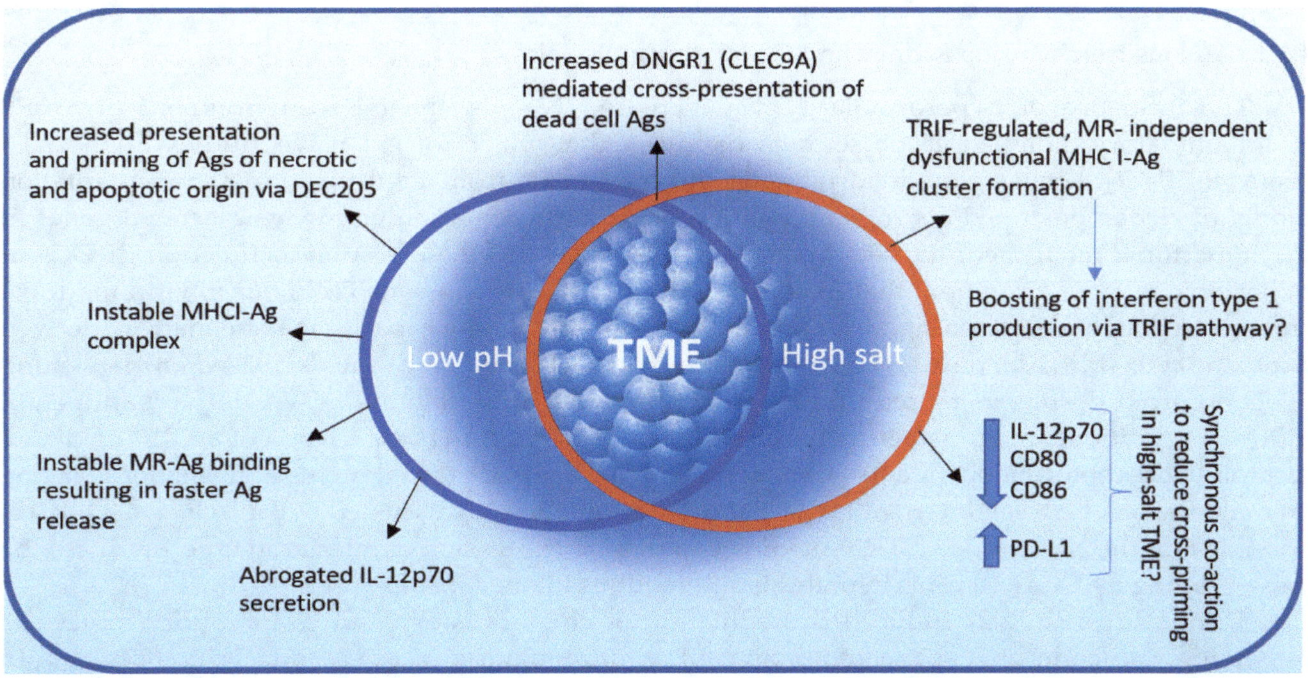

Figure 2. Impact of acidic and hyperosmolar tumor microenvironment (TME) on cross-presentation and cross-priming cascade is dynamic and complex. Interplay of low pH- and high Na^+- triggered phenomena likely decides the fate and efficacy of cross-presentation. Also here can be postulated that tumor nature and viability (in regard to apoptotic and necrotic rate) partially shape the receptor–antigen binding signature and thus contribute to the response of cDC1 to biophysical TME stresses.

It is evident that low pH influences other DC receptors as well, not necessarily leading to a similar outcome, adding to the complexity of the phenomenon. An example is the pH- and ionic load- dependent alteration of another marker of type 1 classical DCs, DNGR1 [61]. DNGR1 (synonym: CLEC9A) is a DAMP-receptor typically expressed on cross-presenting DCs, facilitating cross-presentation of dead-cell-associated antigens. Hanc et al. have convincingly shown that low pH and increased ionic content of the microenvironment lead to a conformational change of the neck region and induction of so-called reduction-sensitive receptor dimers to trigger more efficient cross-presentation and cross-priming [61]. The detailed role of DNGR1 in regulation of the necrotic-cargo intracellular compartment [62] via directing the necrotic antigen material to nonlysosomal, rather alkaline, nondegradative niche, thereby facilitating CD8$^+$ T cell activation [63] has been reviewed by Cueto et al. [64].

4.1.2. The Influence of Low pH on Antigen-MHC-I Stability and Costimulatory Signals

Supporting the theory of damaged cross-presentation at low pH, older studies have documented that peptide-MHC-I complexes are more stable at neutral than at acidic pH [65]; still, no recent data are available to this regard. In addition, lactate has been reported to modulate cytokine secretion by monocyte-derived DCs. Lactic acid has triggered a significant reduction of IL-12p70 in tumor associated dendritic cells, hence blocking an important stimulatory signal in the cross-priming cascade [66,67]. In the same experimental setting no significant impact on secretion of 'anti-inflammatory' IL-10 could be seen.

Interestingly, both high salt and acidic milieu have been shown to trigger IL-1β secretion via activation of inflammasome pathway ([68]; also recent publication from Pitzer et al., FASEB, April 2020). Although recently published ovalbumine-based in vitro models suggest that NLRP3 inflammasome activation may trigger (MHC-I- and MHC-II- dependent) antigen presentation in general [69], its role in an efficient cross-presentation remains to be further investigated.

4.2. Cross-Presentation in Hyperosmolar Micromilieu

4.2.1. Lessons from Murine Kidney and Cell Culture Models

The influence of hyperosmolarity via increased Na$^+$ in the microenvironment of MoPh in inflammatory, non-neoplastic settings has been the subject of extensive studies in the past years [46,70–77]. Focusing on dendritic cells, our initial data from a murine kidney transplantation model have demonstrated a strong abrogation of cross-presentation pathway associated genes in the hypertonic renal medullary compartment [71]. Linking these results to function of DCs in hypertonic microenvironment that may reflect the osmolarity range of TME, our in vitro model of cross-presentation showed a significant reduction of cross-priming capacity in bone marrow derived dendritic cells (BMDCs) developed in hyperosmolarity [78]. Notably, the decreased cross-priming effect occurred despite increased uptake, processing and presentation of OVA-derived antigen in high salt conditions. In our experiments, blockade of cross-priming was a result of a TRIF-mediated (yet toll-like receptor-independent) dysfunctional MHC-I-peptide complex cluster formation. Having on mind the link between Interferon type 1 and TRIF signaling, as discussed by Jantsch et al. [46], it is possible that the Na$^+$ induced, TRIF-mediated excessive expression of interferon type 1 reduces the cross-priming by DCs [79]. This hypothesis still requires further examination.

To our surprise, Na$^+$-induced dysregulation of co-stimulatory and co-inhibitory molecules (including reduction of IL-12 secretion as well as upregulation of PD-L1 and inhibition of both CD80 and CD86 expression upon exposure to high salt) was not responsible for the reduction of cross-priming—at least not in a 'single-parameter'-dependent manner. Nevertheless, we cannot exclude a coaction of the abovementioned regulatory molecules in high-salt induced blockade of cross-priming [78]. Intriguingly, the salt-induced cross-presentation phenotype was in this experimental setting independent of MR, suggesting that also the hypertonic TME may redirect MR-mediated antigen uptake towards other, in the light of cross-presentation less efficient DAMP receptors [78].

4.2.2. Linking TME Hyperosmolarity to Lactate-Induced Acidosis

High salt content of TME may also modify cancer metabolism towards supporting aerobic glycolysis and consequent accumulation of lactate, highlighting the complexity of metabolic tumor surveillance [80]. It has been suggested that hypertonic extracellular stress induces the Warburg effect by enhancing glucose transport and lactic acidosis in tumor cells [81]; these results were concordant with older observations from breast cancer and liver tumor mouse models [82].

Taken together, limited and in part discordant published data indicate that interplay between acidic and hypertonic stress results in modification of cancer cell metabolism and dendritic cell function towards blockade of efficient cross-presentation and cross-priming (Figure 2).

5. Conclusions

Dendritic cells (specifically cDC1) are the most efficient antigen-presenting cells. Their unique cross-presentation capacity has been extensively explored in attempts to boost cytotoxic tumor immunity via DC vaccine strategies, albeit with rather poor clinical results to date. We reviewed here focused, limited and to some extent discordant data on the role of hypertonicity and acidity on DC function that largely go in line with other published observations regarding a general suppression of antitumor immunity via tumor metabolites [67,83,84].

In general, available evidence on the effects of low pH and hypertonicity on dendritic cells is (a) mainly focused on single steps of antigen uptake and presentation per se (to our knowledge without available data on subcellular antigen processing cascade) and thus poorly explored to date; (b) mostly related to in vitro or animal models, hence not automatically applicable to clinical situation and (c) in part based on older scientific studies that do not necessarily follow the current state of immunological knowledge. Specifically, methodological issues in measurement of pH and osmolarity of extracellular microenvironment in situ—in time and space—represent to our opinion the major obstacle to be addressed to this regard.

It must be pointed out that—independent of subcellular pathways—the effect of TME on immune cell activation should be finally observed in the context of tumor survival as the most relevant clinical endpoint. Clearly, antitumor immunity is a result of coaction of all parts of immune system at the tumor site and in regional draining lymph nodes and cannot be determined via observation of single components alone. Indeed, opposing data from two in vivo mouse tumor models based on subcutaneous injection of murine melanoma and lung carcinoma cells reported significant reduction of tumor growth upon high-salt intake via depletion of myeloid-derived suppressor cells [85]. On the other hand, in humans, highly malignant nature of tumors rising in hypertonic organ compartments (like collecting duct carcinoma of kidney and medullary renal cell cancer) with an extraordinary metastatic potential speak in favor of high salt-induced immune escape mechanisms. In the same line, a large set of epidemiologic data clearly indicates that high salt diet (independent on Helicobacter pylori infection) represents an independent high-risk factor for the development and progression of gastric cancer [86]. Nonetheless, mechanisms underlying the development and progression of potentially salt-induced malignancies remain unclear.

Finally, further interdisciplinary investigations of molecular and physical mechanisms of pH- and Na^+-mediated modulation of DC function together with appreciation of dynamic, complex, species-, tissue- and tumor-type-specific relationships between immune system compartments and tumor microenvironments are necessary for a better understanding of and fighting against the immune escape of cancer.

Author Contributions: Z.V.P. designed and took the lead in writing the manuscript with critical input from S.B. and S.P. A.M. contributed to the design and aided in interpreting literature data. All authors provided feedback and contributed to the final manuscript. All authors have read and agreed to the published version of the manuscript.

References

1. Heldin, C.H.; Rubin, K.; Pietras, K.; Ostman, A. High interstitial fluid pressure-an obstacle in cancer therapy. *Nat. Rev. Cancer* **2004**, *4*, 806–813. [CrossRef] [PubMed]
2. Laviron, M.; Boissonnas, A. Ontogeny of Tumor-Associated Macrophages. *Front. Immunol.* **2019**, *10*, 1799. [CrossRef] [PubMed]

3. Murray, P.J.; Allen, J.E.; Biswas, S.K.; Fisher, E.A.; Gilroy, D.W.; Goerdt, S.; Gordon, S.; Hamilton, J.A.; Ivashkiv, L.B.; Lawrence, T.; et al. Macrophage activation and polarization: Nomenclature and experimental guidelines. *Immunity* **2014**, *41*, 14–20. [CrossRef] [PubMed]
4. Blander, J.M. Regulation of the Cell Biology of Antigen Cross-Presentation. *Annu. Rev. Immunol.* **2018**, *36*, 717–753. [CrossRef] [PubMed]
5. Bottcher, J.P.; Reis e Sousa, C. The Role of Type 1 Conventional Dendritic Cells in Cancer Immunity. *Trends. Cancer* **2018**, *4*, 784–792. [CrossRef] [PubMed]
6. Olingy, C.E.; Dinh, H.Q.; Hedrick, C.C. Monocyte heterogeneity and functions in cancer. *J. Leukoc. Biol.* **2019**, *106*, 309–322. [CrossRef]
7. Huang, A.Y.; Golumbek, P.; Ahmadzadeh, M.; Jaffee, E.; Pardoll, D.; Levitsky, H. Role of bone marrow-derived cells in presenting MHC class I-restricted tumor antigens. *Science* **1994**, *264*, 961–965. [CrossRef]
8. Embgenbroich, M.; Burgdorf, S. Current Concepts of Antigen Cross-Presentation. *Front. Immunol.* **2018**, *9*, 1643. [CrossRef]
9. Guilliams, M.; Ginhoux, F.; Jakubzick, C.; Naik, S.H.; Onai, N.; Schraml, B.U.; Segura, E.; Tussiwand, R.; Yona, S. Dendritic cells, monocytes and macrophages: A unified nomenclature based on ontogeny. *Nat. Rev. Immunol.* **2014**, *14*, 571–578. [CrossRef]
10. Guilliams, M.; Malissen, B. A Death Notice for In-Vitro-Generated GM-CSF Dendritic Cells? *Immunity* **2015**, *42*, 988–990. [CrossRef]
11. Savina, A.; Jancic, C.; Hugues, S.; Guermonprez, P.; Vargas, P.; Moura, I.C.; Lennon-Dumenil, A.M.; Seabra, M.C.; Raposo, G.; Amigorena, S. NOX2 controls phagosomal pH to regulate antigen processing during crosspresentation by dendritic cells. *Cell* **2006**, *126*, 205–218. [CrossRef] [PubMed]
12. Savina, A.; Peres, A.; Cebrian, I.; Carmo, N.; Moita, C.; Hacohen, N.; Moita, L.F.; Amigorena, S. The small GTPase Rac2 controls phagosomal alkalinization and antigen crosspresentation selectively in CD8(+) dendritic cells. *Immunity* **2009**, *30*, 544–555. [CrossRef] [PubMed]
13. Spranger, S.; Dai, D.; Horton, B.; Gajewski, T.F. Tumor-Residing Batf3 Dendritic Cells Are Required for Effector T Cell Trafficking and Adoptive T Cell Therapy. *Cancer Cell* **2017**, *31*, 711–723. [CrossRef] [PubMed]
14. Dudziak, D.; Kamphorst, A.O.; Heidkamp, G.F.; Buchholz, V.R.; Trumpfheller, C.; Yamazaki, S.; Cheong, C.; Liu, K.; Lee, H.W.; Park, C.G.; et al. Differential antigen processing by dendritic cell subsets in vivo. *Science* **2007**, *315*, 107–111. [CrossRef] [PubMed]
15. Ding, Y.; Guo, Z.; Liu, Y.; Li, X.; Zhang, Q.; Xu, X.; Gu, Y.; Zhang, Y.; Zhao, D.; Cao, X. The lectin Siglec-G inhibits dendritic cell cross-presentation by impairing MHC class I-peptide complex formation. *Nat. Immunol.* **2016**, *17*, 1167–1175. [CrossRef] [PubMed]
16. Merad, M.; Sathe, P.; Helft, J.; Miller, J.; Mortha, A. The dendritic cell lineage: Ontogeny and function of dendritic cells and their subsets in the steady state and the inflamed setting. *Annu. Rev. Immunol.* **2013**, *31*, 563–604. [CrossRef]
17. GeurtsvanKessel, C.H.; Willart, M.A.; van Rijt, L.S.; Muskens, F.; Kool, M.; Baas, C.; Thielemans, K.; Bennett, C.; Clausen, B.E.; Hoogsteden, H.C.; et al. Clearance of influenza virus from the lung depends on migratory langerin+CD11b- but not plasmacytoid dendritic cells. *J. Exp. Med.* **2008**, *205*, 1621–1634. [CrossRef]
18. Ma, Y.; Shurin, G.V.; Peiyuan, Z.; Shurin, M.R. Dendritic cells in the cancer microenvironment. *J. Cancer* **2013**, *4*, 36–44. [CrossRef]
19. Halama, N.; Zoernig, I.; Berthel, A.; Kahlert, C.; Klupp, F.; Suarez-Carmona, M.; Suetterlin, T.; Brand, K.; Krauss, J.; Lasitschka, F.; et al. Tumoral Immune Cell Exploitation in Colorectal Cancer Metastases Can Be Targeted Effectively by Anti-CCR5 Therapy in Cancer Patients. *Cancer Cell* **2016**, *29*, 587–601. [CrossRef]
20. Tan, M.C.; Goedegebuure, P.S.; Belt, B.A.; Flaherty, B.; Sankpal, N.; Gillanders, W.E.; Eberlein, T.J.; Hsieh, C.S.; Linehan, D.C. Disruption of CCR5-dependent homing of regulatory T cells inhibits tumor growth in a murine model of pancreatic cancer. *J. Immunol.* **2009**, *182*, 1746–1755. [CrossRef]
21. Barry, K.C.; Hsu, J.; Broz, M.L.; Cueto, F.J.; Binnewies, M.; Combes, A.J.; Nelson, A.E.; Loo, K.; Kumar, R.; Rosenblum, M.D.; et al. A natural killer-dendritic cell axis defines checkpoint therapy-responsive tumor microenvironments. *Nat. Med.* **2018**, *24*, 1178–1191. [CrossRef] [PubMed]
22. Burgdorf, S.; Kurts, C. Endocytosis mechanisms and the cell biology of antigen presentation. *Curr. Opin. Immunol.* **2008**, *20*, 89–95. [CrossRef] [PubMed]

23. Burgdorf, S.; Scholz, C.; Kautz, A.; Tampe, R.; Kurts, C. Spatial and mechanistic separation of cross-presentation and endogenous antigen presentation. *Nat. Immunol.* **2008**, *9*, 558–566. [CrossRef] [PubMed]
24. Bertholet, S.; Goldszmid, R.; Morrot, A.; Debrabant, A.; Afrin, F.; Collazo-Custodio, C.; Houde, M.; Desjardins, M.; Sher, A.; Sacks, D. Leishmania antigens are presented to CD8+ T cells by a transporter associated with antigen processing-independent pathway in vitro and in vivo. *J. Immunol.* **2006**, *177*, 3525–3533. [CrossRef] [PubMed]
25. Shen, L.; Sigal, L.J.; Boes, M.; Rock, K.L. Important role of cathepsin S in generating peptides for TAP-independent MHC class I crosspresentation in vivo. *Immunity* **2004**, *21*, 155–165. [CrossRef]
26. Ackerman, A.L.; Kyritsis, C.; Tampe, R.; Cresswell, P. Early phagosomes in dendritic cells form a cellular compartment sufficient for cross presentation of exogenous antigens. *Proc. Natl. Acad. Sci. USA* **2003**, *100*, 12889–12894. [CrossRef]
27. Kovacsovics-Bankowski, M.; Rock, K.L. Presentation of exogenous antigens by macrophages: Analysis of major histocompatibility complex class I and II presentation and regulation by cytokines. *Eur. J. Immunol.* **1994**, *24*, 2421–2428. [CrossRef]
28. Ackerman, A.L.; Giodini, A.; Cresswell, P. A role for the endoplasmic reticulum protein retrotranslocation machinery during crosspresentation by dendritic cells. *Immunity* **2006**, *25*, 607–617. [CrossRef]
29. Guermonprez, P.; Saveanu, L.; Kleijmeer, M.; Davoust, J.; Van Endert, P.; Amigorena, S. ER-phagosome fusion defines an MHC class I cross-presentation compartment in dendritic cells. *Nature* **2003**, *425*, 397–402. [CrossRef]
30. Houde, M.; Bertholet, S.; Gagnon, E.; Brunet, S.; Goyette, G.; Laplante, A.; Princiotta, M.F.; Thibault, P.; Sacks, D.; Desjardins, M. Phagosomes are competent organelles for antigen cross-presentation. *Nature* **2003**, *425*, 402–406. [CrossRef]
31. Liu, T.; Zhou, X.; Abdel-Motal, U.M.; Ljunggren, H.G.; Jondal, M. MHC class I presentation of live and heat-inactivated Sendai virus antigen in T2Kb cells depends on an intracellular compartment with endosomal characteristics. *Scand. J. Immunol.* **1997**, *45*, 527–533. [CrossRef]
32. Pfeifer, J.D.; Wick, M.J.; Roberts, R.L.; Findlay, K.; Normark, S.J.; Harding, C.V. Phagocytic processing of bacterial antigens for class I MHC presentation to T cells. *Nature* **1993**, *361*, 359–362. [CrossRef] [PubMed]
33. Sengupta, D.; Graham, M.; Liu, X.; Cresswell, P. Proteasomal degradation within endocytic organelles mediates antigen cross-presentation. *EMBO J.* **2019**, *38*, e99266. [CrossRef] [PubMed]
34. Neijssen, J.; Herberts, C.; Drijfhout, J.W.; Reits, E.; Janssen, L.; Neefjes, J. Cross-presentation by intercellular peptide transfer through gap junctions. *Nature* **2005**, *434*, 83–88. [CrossRef] [PubMed]
35. Dolan, B.P.; Gibbs, K.D., Jr.; Ostrand-Rosenberg, S. Dendritic cells cross-dressed with peptide MHC class I complexes prime CD8+ T cells. *J. Immunol.* **2006**, *177*, 6018–6024. [CrossRef]
36. Jain, R.K.; Martin, J.D.; Stylianopoulos, T. The role of mechanical forces in tumor growth and therapy. *Annu. Rev. Biomed. Eng.* **2014**, *16*, 321–346. [CrossRef]
37. Liberti, M.V.; Locasale, J.W. The Warburg Effect: How Does it Benefit Cancer Cells? *Trends. Biochem. Sci.* **2016**, *41*, 211–218. [CrossRef]
38. Erra Diaz, F.; Dantas, E.; Geffner, J. Unravelling the Interplay between Extracellular Acidosis and Immune Cells. *Mediat. Inflamm.* **2018**, *2018*, 1218297. [CrossRef]
39. DeBerardinis, R.J.; Mancuso, A.; Daikhin, E.; Nissim, I.; Yudkoff, M.; Wehrli, S.; Thompson, C.B. Beyond aerobic glycolysis: Transformed cells can engage in glutamine metabolism that exceeds the requirement for protein and nucleotide synthesis. *Proc. Natl. Acad. Sci. USA* **2007**, *104*, 19345–19350. [CrossRef]
40. Corbet, C.; Feron, O. Tumour acidosis: From the passenger to the driver's seat. *Nat. Rev. Cancer* **2017**, *17*, 577–593. [CrossRef]
41. Stylianopoulos, T.; Martin, J.D.; Snuderl, M.; Mpekris, F.; Jain, S.R.; Jain, R.K. Coevolution of solid stress and interstitial fluid pressure in tumors during progression: Implications for vascular collapse. *Cancer Res.* **2013**, *73*, 3833–3841. [CrossRef] [PubMed]
42. Voutouri, C.; Stylianopoulos, T. Evolution of osmotic pressure in solid tumors. *J. Biomech.* **2014**, *47*, 3441–3447. [CrossRef] [PubMed]

43. DuFort, C.C.; DelGiorno, K.E.; Carlson, M.A.; Osgood, R.J.; Zhao, C.; Huang, Z.; Thompson, C.B.; Connor, R.J.; Thanos, C.D.; Scott Brockenbrough, J.; et al. Interstitial Pressure in Pancreatic Ductal Adenocarcinoma Is Dominated by a Gel-Fluid Phase. *Biophys. J.* **2016**, *110*, 2106–2119. [CrossRef] [PubMed]
44. DuFort, C.C.; DelGiorno, K.E.; Hingorani, S.R. Mounting Pressure in the Microenvironment: Fluids, Solids, and Cells in Pancreatic Ductal Adenocarcinoma. *Gastroenterology* **2016**, *150*, 1545–1557. [CrossRef] [PubMed]
45. Stylianopoulos, T.; Munn, L.L.; Jain, R.K. Reengineering the Physical Microenvironment of Tumors to Improve Drug Delivery and Efficacy: From Mathematical Modeling to Bench to Bedside. *Trends. Cancer* **2018**, *4*, 292–319. [CrossRef] [PubMed]
46. Neubert, P.; Schroder, A.; Muller, D.N.; Jantsch, J. Interplay of Na(+) Balance and Immunobiology of Dendritic Cells. *Front. Immunol.* **2019**, *10*, 599. [CrossRef]
47. Titze, J.; Shakibaei, M.; Schafflhuber, M.; Schulze-Tanzil, G.; Porst, M.; Schwind, K.H.; Dietsch, P.; Hilgers, K.F. Glycosaminoglycan polymerization may enable osmotically inactive Na+ storage in the skin. *Am. J. Physiol. Heart Circ. Physiol.* **2004**, *287*, H203–H208. [CrossRef]
48. Linz, P.; Santoro, D.; Renz, W.; Rieger, J.; Ruehle, A.; Ruff, J.; Deimling, M.; Rakova, N.; Muller, D.N.; Luft, F.C.; et al. Skin sodium measured with (2)(3)Na MRI at 7.0 T. *NMR Biomed.* **2015**, *28*, 54–62. [CrossRef]
49. Jantsch, J.; Schatz, V.; Friedrich, D.; Schroder, A.; Kopp, C.; Siegert, I.; Maronna, A.; Wendelborn, D.; Linz, P.; Binger, K.J.; et al. Cutaneous Na+ storage strengthens the antimicrobial barrier function of the skin and boosts macrophage-driven host defense. *Cell Metab.* **2015**, *21*, 493–501. [CrossRef]
50. Kopp, C.; Beyer, C.; Linz, P.; Dahlmann, A.; Hammon, M.; Jantsch, J.; Neubert, P.; Rosenhauer, D.; Muller, D.N.; Cavallaro, A.; et al. Na+ deposition in the fibrotic skin of systemic sclerosis patients detected by 23Na-magnetic resonance imaging. *Rheumatology* **2017**, *56*, 556–560. [CrossRef]
51. Titze, J.; Lang, R.; Ilies, C.; Schwind, K.H.; Kirsch, K.A.; Dietsch, P.; Luft, F.C.; Hilgers, K.F. Osmotically inactive skin Na+ storage in rats. *Am. J. Physiol. Renal. Physiol.* **2003**, *285*, F1108–F1117. [CrossRef] [PubMed]
52. Wiig, H.; Schroder, A.; Neuhofer, W.; Jantsch, J.; Kopp, C.; Karlsen, T.V.; Boschmann, M.; Goss, J.; Bry, M.; Rakova, N.; et al. Immune cells control skin lymphatic electrolyte homeostasis and blood pressure. *J. Clin. Investig.* **2013**, *123*, 2803–2815. [CrossRef] [PubMed]
53. Cao, L.; Shi, X.; Chang, H.; Zhang, Q.; He, Y. pH-Dependent recognition of apoptotic and necrotic cells by the human dendritic cell receptor DEC205. *Proc. Natl. Acad. Sci. USA* **2015**, *112*, 7237–7242. [CrossRef] [PubMed]
54. Jiang, W.; Swiggard, W.J.; Heufler, C.; Peng, M.; Mirza, A.; Steinman, R.M.; Nussenzweig, M.C. The receptor DEC-205 expressed by dendritic cells and thymic epithelial cells is involved in antigen processing. *Nature* **1995**, *375*, 151–155. [CrossRef] [PubMed]
55. Hawiger, D.; Inaba, K.; Dorsett, Y.; Guo, M.; Mahnke, K.; Rivera, M.; Ravetch, J.V.; Steinman, R.M.; Nussenzweig, M.C. Dendritic cells induce peripheral T cell unresponsiveness under steady state conditions in vivo. *J. Exp. Med.* **2001**, *194*, 769–779. [CrossRef]
56. Martinez-Pomares, L. The mannose receptor. *J. Leukoc. Biol.* **2012**, *92*, 1177–1186. [CrossRef]
57. Burgdorf, S.; Lukacs-Kornek, V.; Kurts, C. The mannose receptor mediates uptake of soluble but not of cell-associated antigen for cross-presentation. *J. Immunol.* **2006**, *176*, 6770–6776. [CrossRef]
58. Hu, Z.; Shi, X.; Yu, B.; Li, N.; Huang, Y.; He, Y. Structural Insights into the pH-Dependent Conformational Change and Collagen Recognition of the Human Mannose Receptor. *Structure* **2018**, *26*, 60–71. [CrossRef]
59. He, L.Z.; Crocker, A.; Lee, J.; Mendoza-Ramirez, J.; Wang, X.T.; Vitale, L.A.; O'Neill, T.; Petromilli, C.; Zhang, H.F.; Lopez, J.; et al. Antigenic targeting of the human mannose receptor induces tumor immunity. *J. Immunol.* **2007**, *178*, 6259–6267. [CrossRef]
60. Chatterjee, B.; Smed-Sorensen, A.; Cohn, L.; Chalouni, C.; Vandlen, R.; Lee, B.C.; Widger, J.; Keler, T.; Delamarre, L.; Mellman, I. Internalization and endosomal degradation of receptor-bound antigens regulate the efficiency of cross presentation by human dendritic cells. *Blood* **2012**, *120*, 2011–2020. [CrossRef]
61. Hanc, P.; Schulz, O.; Fischbach, H.; Martin, S.R.; Kjaer, S.; Reis e Sousa, C. A pH- and ionic strength-dependent conformational change in the neck region regulates DNGR-1 function in dendritic cells. *EMBO J.* **2016**, *35*, 2484–2497. [CrossRef] [PubMed]
62. Zelenay, S.; Keller, A.M.; Whitney, P.G.; Schraml, B.U.; Deddouche, S.; Rogers, N.C.; Schulz, O.; Sancho, D.; Reis e Sousa, C. The dendritic cell receptor DNGR-1 controls endocytic handling of necrotic cell antigens to favor cross-priming of CTLs in virus-infected mice. *J. Clin. Investig.* **2012**, *122*, 1615–1627. [CrossRef] [PubMed]

63. Burgdorf, S.; Kautz, A.; Bohnert, V.; Knolle, P.A.; Kurts, C. Distinct pathways of antigen uptake and intracellular routing in CD4 and CD8 T cell activation. *Science* **2007**, *316*, 612–616. [CrossRef] [PubMed]
64. Cueto, F.J.; Del Fresno, C.; Sancho, D. DNGR-1, a Dendritic Cell-Specific Sensor of Tissue Damage That Dually Modulates Immunity and Inflammation. *Front. Immunol.* **2019**, *10*, 3146. [CrossRef]
65. Stryhn, A.; Pedersen, L.O.; Romme, T.; Olsen, A.C.; Nissen, M.H.; Thorpe, C.J.; Buus, S. pH dependence of MHC class I-restricted peptide presentation. *J. Immunol.* **1996**, *156*, 4191–4197.
66. Gottfried, E.; Kunz-Schughart, L.A.; Ebner, S.; Mueller-Klieser, W.; Hoves, S.; Andreesen, R.; Mackensen, A.; Kreutz, M. Tumor-derived lactic acid modulates dendritic cell activation and antigen expression. *Blood* **2006**, *107*, 2013–2021. [CrossRef] [PubMed]
67. Romero-Garcia, S.; Moreno-Altamirano, M.M.; Prado-Garcia, H.; Sanchez-Garcia, F.J. Lactate Contribution to the Tumor Microenvironment: Mechanisms, Effects on Immune Cells and Therapeutic Relevance. *Front. Immunol.* **2016**, *7*, 52. [CrossRef] [PubMed]
68. Rajamaki, K.; Nordstrom, T.; Nurmi, K.; Akerman, K.E.; Kovanen, P.T.; Oorni, K.; Eklund, K.K. Extracellular acidosis is a novel danger signal alerting innate immunity via the NLRP3 inflammasome. *J. Biol. Chem.* **2013**, *288*, 13410–13419. [CrossRef] [PubMed]
69. Li, T.; Zehner, M.; He, J.; Prochnicki, T.; Horvath, G.; Latz, E.; Burgdorf, S.; Takeoka, S. NLRP3 inflammasome-activating arginine-based liposomes promote antigen presentations in dendritic cells. *Int. J. Nanomed.* **2019**, *14*, 3503–3516. [CrossRef]
70. Chessa, F.; Hielscher, T.; Mathow, D.; Grone, H.J.; Popovic, Z.V. Transcriptional profiling of dendritic cells matured in different osmolarities. *Genom. Data* **2016**, *7*, 64–66. [CrossRef] [PubMed]
71. Chessa, F.; Mathow, D.; Wang, S.; Hielscher, T.; Atzberger, A.; Porubsky, S.; Gretz, N.; Burgdorf, S.; Grone, H.J.; Popovic, Z.V. The renal microenvironment modifies dendritic cell phenotype. *Kidney Int.* **2016**, *89*, 82–94. [CrossRef] [PubMed]
72. Machnik, A.; Neuhofer, W.; Jantsch, J.; Dahlmann, A.; Tammela, T.; Machura, K.; Park, J.K.; Beck, F.X.; Muller, D.N.; Derer, W.; et al. Macrophages regulate salt-dependent volume and blood pressure by a vascular endothelial growth factor-C-dependent buffering mechanism. *Nat. Med.* **2009**, *15*, 545–552. [CrossRef]
73. Muller, D.N.; Wilck, N.; Haase, S.; Kleinewietfeld, M.; Linker, R.A. Sodium in the microenvironment regulates immune responses and tissue homeostasis. *Nat. Rev. Immunol.* **2019**, *19*, 243–254. [CrossRef]
74. Schatz, V.; Neubert, P.; Schroder, A.; Binger, K.; Gebhard, M.; Muller, D.N.; Luft, F.C.; Titze, J.; Jantsch, J. Elementary immunology: Na(+) as a regulator of immunity. *Pediatr. Nephrol.* **2017**, *32*, 201–210. [CrossRef] [PubMed]
75. Titze, J. Interstitial fluid homeostasis and pressure: News from the black box. *Kidney Int.* **2013**, *84*, 869–871. [CrossRef]
76. Titze, J.; Dahlmann, A.; Lerchl, K.; Kopp, C.; Rakova, N.; Schroder, A.; Luft, F.C. Spooky sodium balance. *Kidney Int.* **2014**, *85*, 759–767. [CrossRef] [PubMed]
77. Wiig, H.; Luft, F.C.; Titze, J.M. The interstitium conducts extrarenal storage of sodium and represents a third compartment essential for extracellular volume and blood pressure homeostasis. *Acta Physiol.* **2018**, *222*, e13006. [CrossRef]
78. Popovic, Z.V.; Embgenbroich, M.; Chessa, F.; Nordstrom, V.; Bonrouhi, M.; Hielscher, T.; Gretz, N.; Wang, S.; Mathow, D.; Quast, T.; et al. Hyperosmolarity impedes the cross-priming competence of dendritic cells in a TRIF-dependent manner. *Sci. Rep.* **2017**, *7*, 311. [CrossRef]
79. Pfaender, S.; Grabski, E.; Detje, C.N.; Riebesehl, N.; Lienenklaus, S.; Steinmann, E.; Kalinke, U.; Pietschmann, T. Hepatitis C Virus Stimulates Murine CD8alpha-Like Dendritic Cells to Produce Type I Interferon in a TRIF-Dependent Manner. *PLoS Pathog.* **2016**, *12*, e1005736. [CrossRef]
80. Amara, S.; Tiriveedhi, V. Inflammatory role of high salt level in tumor microenvironment (Review). *Int. J. Oncol.* **2017**, *50*, 1477–1481. [CrossRef]
81. Epstein, T.; Xu, L.; Gillies, R.J.; Gatenby, R.A. Separation of metabolic supply and demand: Aerobic glycolysis as a normal physiological response to fluctuating energetic demands in the membrane. *Cancer Metab.* **2014**, *2*, 7. [CrossRef] [PubMed]
82. Sparks, R.L.; Pool, T.B.; Smith, N.K.; Cameron, I.L. Effects of amiloride on tumor growth and intracellular element content of tumor cells in vivo. *Cancer Res.* **1983**, *43*, 73–77. [PubMed]

83. Huber, V.; Camisaschi, C.; Berzi, A.; Ferro, S.; Lugini, L.; Triulzi, T.; Tuccitto, A.; Tagliabue, E.; Castelli, C.; Rivoltini, L. Cancer acidity: An ultimate frontier of tumor immune escape and a novel target of immunomodulation. *Semin. Cancer Biol.* **2017**, *43*, 74–89. [CrossRef]
84. Lee, J.H.; Choi, S.Y.; Jung, N.C.; Song, J.Y.; Seo, H.G.; Lee, H.S.; Lim, D.S. The Effect of the Tumor Microenvironment and Tumor-Derived Metabolites on Dendritic Cell Function. *J. Cancer* **2020**, *11*, 769–775. [CrossRef] [PubMed]
85. Willebrand, R.; Hamad, I.; Van Zeebroeck, L.; Kiss, M.; Bruderek, K.; Geuzens, A.; Swinnen, D.; Corte-Real, B.F.; Marko, L.; Lebegge, E.; et al. High Salt Inhibits Tumor Growth by Enhancing Anti-tumor Immunity. *Front. Immunol.* **2019**, *10*, 1141. [CrossRef]
86. Peleteiro, B.; Lopes, C.; Figueiredo, C.; Lunet, N. Salt intake and gastric cancer risk according to Helicobacter pylori infection, smoking, tumour site and histological type. *Br. J. Cancer* **2011**, *104*, 198–207. [CrossRef]

12

Tumor Microenvironment as a Regulator of Radiation Therapy: New Insights into Stromal-Mediated Radioresistance

Varintra E. Krisnawan [1,2], Jennifer A. Stanley [3,4], Julie K. Schwarz [3,4,5] and David G. DeNardo [1,2,4,*]

1 Department of Medicine, Washington University School of Medicine, St. Louis, MO 63110, USA; varintra@wustl.edu
2 Department of Pathology and Immunology, Washington University School of Medicine, St. Louis, MO 63110, USA
3 Department of Radiation Oncology, Washington University School of Medicine, St. Louis, MO 63110, USA; jastanley@wustl.edu (J.A.S.); jschwarz@wustl.edu (J.K.S.)
4 Siteman Cancer Center, Washington University School of Medicine, St. Louis, MO 63110, USA
5 Department of Cell Biology and Physiology, Washington University School of Medicine, St. Louis, MO 63110, USA
* Correspondence: ddenardo@wustl.edu

Simple Summary: Cancer is multifaceted and consists of more than just a collection of mutated cells. These cancerous cells reside along with other non-mutated cells in an extracellular matrix which together make up the tumor microenvironment or tumor stroma. The composition of the tumor microenvironment plays an integral role in cancer initiation, progression, and response to treatments. In this review, we discuss how the tumor microenvironment regulates the response and resistance to radiation therapy and what targeted agents have been used to combat stromal-mediated radiation resistance.

Abstract: A tumor is a complex "organ" composed of malignant cancer cells harboring genetic aberrations surrounded by a stroma comprised of non-malignant cells and an extracellular matrix. Considerable evidence has demonstrated that components of the genetically "normal" tumor stroma contribute to tumor progression and resistance to a wide array of treatment modalities, including radiotherapy. Cancer-associated fibroblasts can promote radioresistance through their secreted factors, contact-mediated signaling, downstream pro-survival signaling pathways, immunomodulatory effects, and cancer stem cell-generating role. The extracellular matrix can govern radiation responsiveness by influencing oxygen availability and controlling the stability and bioavailability of growth factors and cytokines. Immune status regarding the presence of pro- and anti-tumor immune cells can regulate how tumors respond to radiation therapy. Furthermore, stromal cells including endothelial cells and adipocytes can modulate radiosensitivity through their roles in angiogenesis and vasculogenesis, and their secreted adipokines, respectively. Thus, to successfully eradicate cancers, it is important to consider how tumor stroma components interact with and regulate the response to radiation. Detailed knowledge of these interactions will help build a preclinical rationale to support the use of stromal-targeting agents in combination with radiotherapy to increase radiosensitivity.

Keywords: stroma; cancer-associated fibroblast (CAF); extracellular matrix (ECM); cytokine/chemokine; growth factors; pro- and anti-tumor immune cells; immunomodulatory roles; radiotherapy dose fractionation; radioresistance; radiosensitivity

1. Introduction

The field of oncology has evolved from a malignant mutated cancer cell-centered view to the understanding of cancer as a complex "organ" composed of both malignant cells and diverse nonmalignant cellular and non-cellular components termed the tumor stroma or tumor microenvironment (TME) [1–5]. The concept of cancer as a disease focusing only on malignant tumor cells has been deemed inaccurate; in some cancers, stromal cells represent the majority of cell types, as is frequently seen in pancreatic and breast cancers [6]. These cellular stromal components often include activated cancer-associated fibroblasts (CAFs), leukocytes, and vascular cells, but they also sometimes include other adjacent normal tissue/cells such as non-transformed epithelia, adipose tissue, or neurons [1–5]. The non-cellular compartment of the tumor stroma comprises extracellular matrix (ECM) components like collagens, laminins, fibrinogen, elastin, and proteoglycan, and secreted factors such as cytokines, chemokines, and sequestered growth factors [1–11]. Accumulating evidence highly suggests that malignant cancer cells and the tumor stroma reciprocally communicate with and influence one another, but this relationship is complex and remains poorly understood. To treat cancer as a disease, we cannot single-mindedly focus on cancer cells with their autonomous genetic mutations; we need to simultaneously consider the TME because its interactions with tumor cells often contribute to disease initiation, progression, and treatment response [2–4,6,12].

Radiation therapy (RT) is a powerful anti-cancer therapeutic used to treat up to 50–60% of cancer patients [12,13]. The goal of RT is to target highly proliferative cancer cells while sparing normal tissue. The concept of dose fractionation—delivering small daily RT doses over several days—is designed to exploit cancer cells' vulnerabilities in repairing DNA damage, leading to their demise, while giving normal healthy cells a chance to activate their DNA repair and cell cycle mechanisms [13–16]. Historically, radiobiology has utilized linear quadratic modeling to estimate the therapeutic treatment ratio, with increasing radiation toxicity to cancer cells while avoiding surrounding normal tissue. This "therapeutic ratio" is based on differences between the DNA damage and repair kinetics of cancer and normal cells. The linear-quadratic model utilizes the α and β parameters to describe the linear and quadratic portions of the cell survival curve, respectively, and experimental evidence suggests that these parameters and the α:β ratio differ widely across and even within some tumor types [17,18]. Classical modeling predicts that delivering small doses of radiation over the course of multiple treatments (i.e., conventional dose fractionation) can increase the therapeutic ratio compared to single-dose delivery, and early studies using small and large animal models confirmed these effects [17–19]. However, recent evidence has called into question whether small doses of radiation delivered over a protracted treatment course (conventional fractionation) are required to achieve these effects.

Standard of care for the majority of solid tumors requires 50 to 70 Gy total radiation dose delivered with conventionally fractionated schedules, most commonly utilizing 1.8 to 2 Gy per fraction. Over the past decade significant technologic advances in image-guided radiation, tumor tracking, beam intensity modulation, and beam shaping have facilitated the capacity to precisely deliver higher dose per fraction to the tumor while sparing larger volumes of surrounding normal structures. This concept of hypofractionation, or higher fractional doses of radiation over fewer total fractions and commonly delivered with stereotactic guidance via stereotactic body radiotherapy (SBRT) or stereotactic radiosurgery (SRS), has demonstrated safety and efficacy in many tumor types [20–23]. However, data also suggest that the clinical effects of hypofractionation are not solely due to differences in tumor and normal tissue DNA repair kinetics but also to the effects of radiotherapy on the TME. Although largely anecdotal, TME alterations can be demonstrated through the observation of "out-of-field" or abscopal responses to focused radiation as first described in the early 1950s [24]. Since then, additional work has demonstrated that the abscopal response is dependent on alterations in the immune system and the surrounding stromal tissue. Radiation can result in immune cell priming, neoantigen and cytokine release, modification of tumor vasculature, and alteration of the ECM, all of which have the potential to be optimized to enhance RT efficacy [25–29].

Despite RT designed to target malignant tumor cells, and the knowledge that RT can be used to prime the immune system, the complex interaction between malignant tumor cells and other cells within the TME is important because the stroma can impact malignant cells' response and contribute to treatment resistance [12]. Additionally, there are reports that RT can cause numerous changes in stromal cells within the TME that further promote undesirable tumor growth, invasion, and treatment resistance [12]. To successfully eradicate cancers, these reciprocal interactions between the tumor cells and tumor stroma must be characterized in detail. Moreover, the use of stromal-targeting agents in combination with RT is a largely unaddressed therapeutic option. These topics deserve more attention to broaden our knowledge to design better treatment strategies to combat cancers, particularly those characterized by a high density of stromal cells and other stromal components within the TME. In this review, we summarize the roles of stromal components and the TME that contribute to cancer cell radioresistance (Figure 1) and discuss how they may be targeted for possible therapeutic benefit (Figure 2).

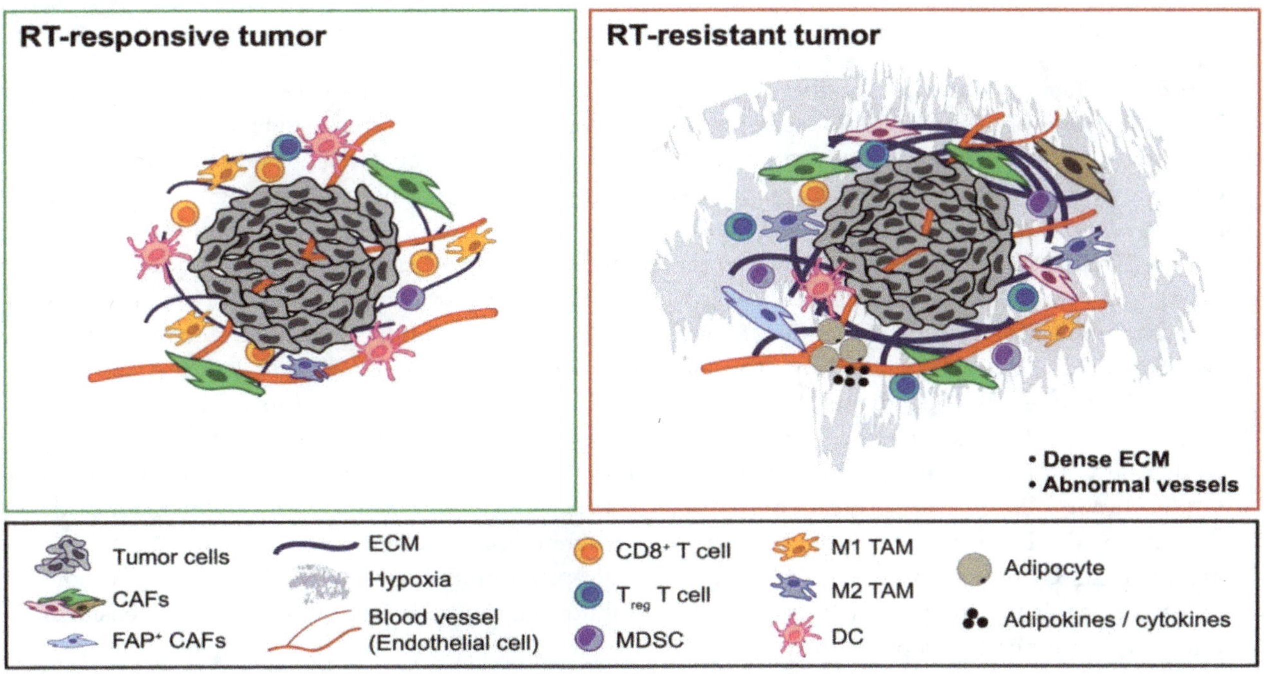

Figure 1. Components of the tumor microenvironment governing radiotherapy responsiveness. Components of the tumor stroma differentially dictate whether tumor cells are radiotherapy (RT)-responsive (Left) vs. RT-resistant (Right). Some tumor-promoting cancer-associated fibroblast (CAF) populations can cause tumors to be resistant to RT, such as fibroblast activated protein (FAP)$^+$ CAFs. While immune cells such as CD8$^+$ T cells, dendritic cells, and M1-like tumor-associated macrophages (TAMs) have been linked with RT-responsive tumors, pro-tumorigenic immune cells such as CD4$^+$ T regulatory (T_{reg}) cells, myeloid-derived suppressor cells, and M2-like TAMs have been associated with RT-resistant tumors. Dense extracellular matrix and abnormal endothelial cells and vessel formation, which contribute to tumor hypoxia, have been associated with RT-resistant tumors. Likewise, adipokines secreted by cancer-associated adipocytes can similarly cause tumors to be resistant to RT.

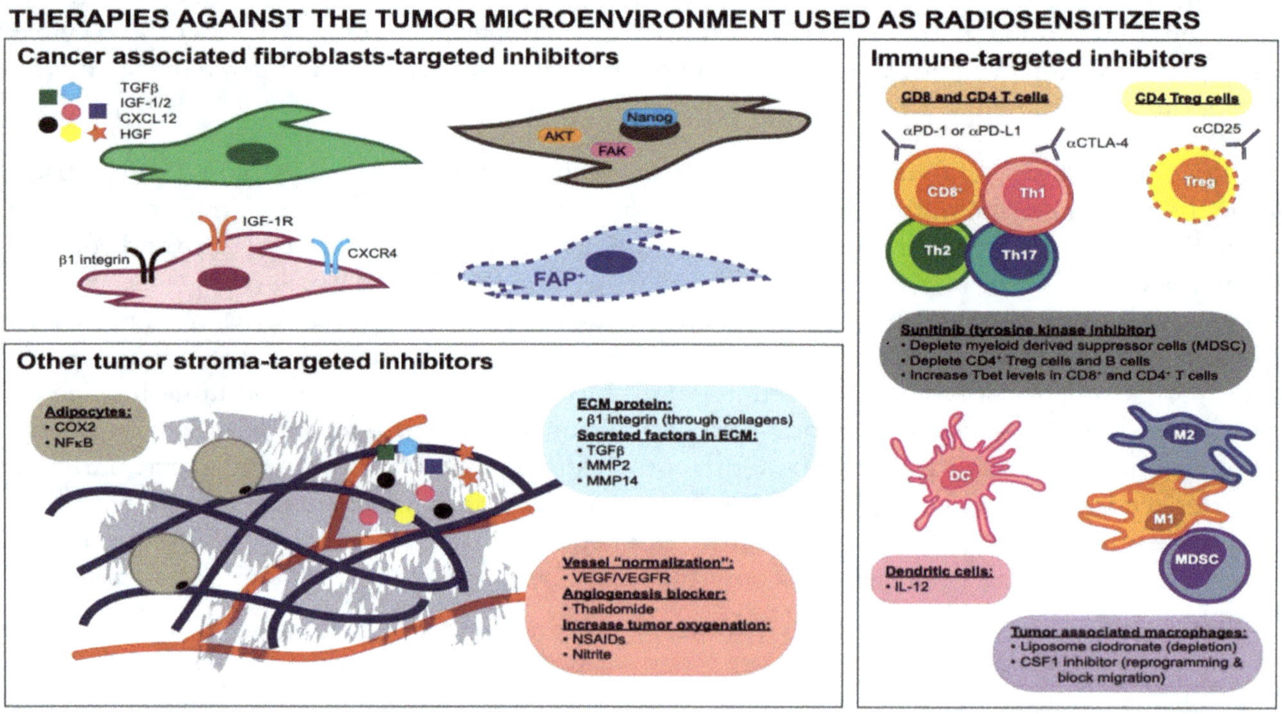

Figure 2. Therapies directed against distinct tumor stromal components used as radiosensitizers. Targeted inhibitors against CAFs' secretory molecules, CAFs' downstream cytosolic and nuclear signaling pathways, and CAFs' receptors can increase RT efficacy. Targeting a unique population of CAFs, FAP$^+$ CAFs, specifically for depletion can also radiosensitize tumors. Components of the ECM can activate β1 integrin receptor on CAFs and targeting β1 integrin can reverse tumor radioresistance. Targeted inhibitors against secreted factors reserved in the ECM have been shown to be radiosensitizing agents. "Normalizing" tumor vessels using VEGF/VEGFR inhibitors and Thalidomide can reverse tumor radioresistance. NSAIDs and nitrite have also been used as radiosensitizers due to their ability to increase tumor oxygenation. Inhibitors of COX-2 and NFκB targeted against cancer-associated adipocytes can reverse the radioresistance in tumors. Immune checkpoint inhibitors (αPD-1 or αPD-L1 and αCTLA-4 antibodies) can rescue "dysfunctional" CD8$^+$ and/or CD4$^+$ T cells and are beneficial when combined with RT. Depletion antibody αCD25 targeted against CD4$^+$ T regulatory cells (T$_{regs}$) can render tumor cells more radiosensitive. Interleukin-12 capable of enhancing the function of dendritic cells can increase the efficacy of RT. TAMs depletion agent, liposome clodronate, and CSF1 inhibitor can increase RT sensitivity. CSF1 inhibitor can also reprogram/polarize TAMs into having a more anti-tumorigenic phenotype. The tyrosine kinase inhibitor, sunitinib, has been used as a radiosensitizer due to its immunomodulatory ability.

2. The Impact of RT on the Tumor Stroma

RT seeks to exploit DNA repair deficiencies in malignant tumor cells, but even in perfect scenarios, it invariably affects stromal cells within the tumor mass or at its boundaries [30]. Although many RT-mediated stromal changes are beneficial, such as the revival of or polarization toward tumor-suppressing immunity, RT can act as a double-edged sword in tumors [13]. Specifically, deleterious side effects could facilitate cancer progression and treatment resistance. These are the byproducts of RT we hope to avoid by carefully designing and planning RT dose regimens and combinatorial treatments.

One impact of RT on the tumor stroma is chronic inflammation that drives RT-induced fibrosis marked by an increased number of stromal cells and ECM components, through several mechanisms that have been reviewed elsewhere [31]. RT-induced fibrosis is a well-known side effect that can arise in some patients [1,31,32]. RT can completely transform the TME by inducing rapid and chronic loss of hyaluronic acid [33] and collagen remodeling [34] by altering how CAFs regulate their collagen production [10,35]. Furthermore, RT-treated CAF populations can undergo modifications and alterations in terms of their diversity, secretome, and phenotype [36]. Additionally, RT enhances activation of proliferating machinery involving the RAS and mitogen-activated protein kinase (MAPK) cascades; the invasion pathways, which involve matrix metalloproteins (MMPs), laminin 5, and filamin A; transforming growth factor beta (TGFβ) signaling, which is involved in tumor progression, resistance, and metastasis [2,7,37]. Likewise, RT to the stroma can increase tumor invasiveness due to increased hepatocyte growth factor (HGF)/c-Met (HGF receptor) signaling and MAPK activity, which enhances tumor mobility and can be deleterious [38]. Taken together, these reports suggest that RT can activate stromal features indicative of potential stromal-mediated treatment resistance.

It is still unclear how different fractionated RT regimens alter the stromal components of the TME and how these changes affect subsequent responses of cancer cells to RT. Similarly, the attempts to combine stromal-disrupting agents with RT to overcome stromal-mediated radioresistance remain unclear and merit further study.

3. The Impact of CAFs on RT Efficacy

CAFs are heterogeneous and the major contributors to the tumor stroma [3,4]. CAFs have been shown to control tumor phenotype at all stages of tumor progression. Their roles have been reviewed elsewhere and include the ability to shape the ECM; modulate innate and adaptive immune microenvironments; recruit and regulate leukocyte migration and inflammation via cytokines, chemokines, and growth factors; provide metabolic support (amino acids, lipids, and tricarboxylic acid cycle intermediates); and contribute to paracrine activation of mitogenic and pro-survival cellular signaling via cell surface receptor-ligand interaction and secreted proteins or exosomes [3,4,39]. The mechanisms by which CAFs contribute to radioresistance are likely mediated through their secreted factors, contact-mediated signaling, immunomodulatory effects, and ECM alterations [40].

CAFs secrete a number of different active factors that have diverse effects on tumor phenotype [3,4]. For example, through their active secretory function, tumor stromal fibroblasts can transfer RNA within exosomes to cancer cells. This exosome transfer mechanism has been implicated in paracrine anti-viral RIG-I and juxtacrine NOTCH (NOTCH3-JAG1) signaling pathways, which both contributed to the expansion of therapy-resistant tumor-initiating cells. Stromal cells, which include CAFs and some bone marrow cells, protected breast cancer cells by inducing an interferon (IFN)-related DNA damage resistance signature in a STAT1-dependent manner and caused the tumors to be chemo- and radio-resistant [41]. In another model, conditioned media (CM) from pancreatic stellate cells (PSCs), which are the central mediator of desmoplasia and major contributors of pancreatic CAFs, dose-dependently enhanced pancreatic tumor cell proliferation, migration, invasion, and colony formation and caused resistance to gemcitabine and RT. The CM was found to activate the MAPK AKT pathways in tumor cells, and the authors postulated that factors such as interleukin-1β (IL-1β) and TGFβ were responsible [42]. The TME of glioblastoma is known to produce abundant TGFβ, a pleiotropic cytokine that promotes an effective DNA damage response. Glioma-initiating cells were protected from RT-induced cell death by this increase in TGFβ production, which promoted an effective DNA damage response and self-renewal via C-X-C chemokine receptor type 4 (CXCR4) and NOTCH1. TGFβ inhibition prevented tumor cell DNA repair and enhanced RT efficacy in this glioblastoma model [43]. Furthermore, CAFs can promote irradiated cancer cell recovery and tumor relapse after RT by producing insulin-like growth factor-1/2 (IGF-1/2), C-X-C motif chemokine ligand 12 (CXCL12), and β-hydroxybutyrate. These secreted factors increase reactive oxygen species (ROS) levels post-RT, which enhanced protein phosphatase 2A activity and repressed the mammalian target of rapamycin activation, therefore inducing autophagy in cancer cells to promote cancer cell recovery. It was argued that blocking IGF-2 and autophagy can reduce CAF-promoted tumor relapse in mice after RT and could be a promising RT sensitization therapeutic strategy (Figure 2) [44].

CAF-secreted factors trigger many downstream autocrine and/or paracrine signaling pathways that regulate treatment response. A network of paracrine signaling among cancer cells, myeloid cells, and stromal cells such as endothelial cells can drive the processes of treatment resistance and metastasis [45]. CXCL1 signaling is an example of paracrine signaling that contributes to radioresistance. Along with cancer cells, CAFs highly express and secrete CXCL1, which inhibits expression of the ROS-scavenging enzyme superoxide dismutase 1, leading to ROS accumulation following RT [46]. In this scenario, tumor cells take advantage of ROS accumulation to enhance DNA damage repair mechanisms and ultimately cause radioresistance. This radioresistance is also mediated by activation of the mitogen-activated protein kinase ERK kinase/extracellular-signal-regulated kinase (MEK/ERK) signaling pathway important for malignant transformation [47,48]. Crosstalk between CAFs and tumor cells through CXCL1 expression in an autocrine/paracrine signaling loop is responsible for the radioresistance phenotype [46]. Together, these studies showed that through their secreted active factors, CAFs can confer radioresistance to tumor cells.

CAFs are embedded in the tumor stroma, allowing them to actively communicate with other cells present in their surrounding environment through various mechanisms [3,4]. Besides acting through their secreted factors, CAFs also induce radioresistance through direct contact-mediated signaling between cancer cells and CAFs [3]. In pancreatic cancer, PSCs promote radioprotection and stimulate the proliferation of pancreatic cancer cells through β1 integrin signaling. β1 integrin is known to modulate the cellular response to genotoxic stress including RT [49]. It was found that this effect is independent of phosphoinositide 3-kinase (PI3K) but depends on focal adhesion kinase (FAK). β1 integrin inhibition or FAK knockout can abolish PSC-mediated radioprotection in pancreatic cancer cells to single-dose and fractionated RT [50]. These findings indicate that downstream cellular signaling pathways activated due to direct interactions between CAFs and tumor cells can mediate radioresistance.

Additionally, CAFs can work through paracrine networking to enrich cancer stem cells (CSCs), which have been implicated in chemo- and radioresistance. In pancreatic cancer, the presence of PSCs can induce CSC characteristics by increasing the epithelial-mesenchymal transition (EMT) phenotype. A proteomic screen revealed that TGFβ is involved in the radioresistance phenotype, and TGFβ neutralizing antibody can inhibit the EMT and CSC phenotype, thus sensitizing tumor cells to RT and reducing tumorigenicity in vivo [51]. In another setting, IGF-1 receptor (IGF-1R) signaling activation in cancer cells in the presence of CAFs expressing IGF-2 induced Oct3/4, Nanog, and Sox2 expression and promoted stemness pathways related to IGF-1R, EMT, PI3K, TGFβ, WNT, and Hedgehog signaling. This group showed that CAF-derived HGF, IGF-2, basic fibroblast growth factor (bFGF), WNT, and oncostatin M regulated CSC-like characteristics in a paracrine manner through counterpart receptor signaling components and stemness factors. They found that blocking IGF-2/IGF-1R/AKT/Nanog signaling reduced CSC stemness and concluded that there were potential clinical applications of targeted therapy to improve chemo- and radioresistance (Figure 2) [52]. Furthermore, CSCs play an important role in disease recurrence after RT as a result of their high DNA repair and antioxidative capabilities. Fractionated RT can enhance IGF-1 secretion and subsequent upregulation of IGF-1R in CSCs. IGF-1R upregulation exerts a dual radioprotective effect by inducing upregulation of AKT/ERK survival signaling and FoxO3 activation, which results in radiation protection. Additionally, they showed that inhibition of IGF-1R signaling reverses CSC radioresistance [53]. Collectively, these findings showed that CAFs can trigger radioresistance through their CSC-promoting roles.

In addition to CAFs' de novo roles in mediating radioresistance, changes in CAFs due to RT can mediate further treatment resistance. This is important because most anti-cancer treatment regimens, including RT, are given in multiple treatment cycles with gaps to allow for normal cell recovery [32]. These gaps between treatment cycles can be exploited by both the tumor and stromal cells to take advantage of survival mechanisms. Thus, changes in the TME in between treatment cycles are important to consider with regard to the subsequent treatment response and resistance [32]. CAFs are not usually killed by RT; they are highly radioresistant due to the defective p53/p21 response pathway and high expression of the cancer marker Survivin [54]. Irradiated fibroblasts can promote the invasive growth of squamous cell carcinoma through the induction of c-Met, RAS, MAPK cascade (Raf-1, MEK1, ERK-1/2), MMP-1, MMP-9, laminin 5, and filamin A. Irradiated fibroblasts also express high levels of TGFβ1 [37]. The effects these irradiated fibroblasts can have on non-irradiated neighboring cells are referred to as radiation-induced bystander effects [55], and there is evidence that many of these factors can promote radioresistance.

There are several examples by which RT-induced changes in CAFs contribute to radioresistance. After genotoxic stress, CAFs can secrete WNT16B to the TME and promote prostate cancer therapy resistance. WNT16B, a secreted protein that is activated in fibroblasts through the nuclear factor (NF)κB pathway after DNA damage, subsequently activates the canonical WNT program and promotes EMT in neoplastic cells through paracrine signaling. This process attenuates the effects of both chemo- and radiotherapies and promotes tumor cell survival and disease progression [56]. Moreover, exposure to low-dose RT (<20 cGy) can induce premature senescence in stromal fibroblasts. In one setting, these senescent CAFs are responsible for stimulating enhanced proliferation of breast carcinoma cells and are correlated with radioresistance, which is partly mediated by the AKT pathway [57]. In addition, senescent CAFs can induce a senescence-associated secretory phenotype that includes the production of IL-6, IL-8, and osteopontin that are considered to be pro-tumorigenic factors and have been associated with immunosuppression and stromal-mediated therapeutic resistance [3,6,58]. RT can also promote EMT transition and invasion of pancreatic cancer cells by activating CAFs. CAF-derived CXCL12 directly promoted tumor cell EMT and invasion by acting through CXCR4 on tumor cells and downstream activation of the P38 pathway. Blocking CXCL12/CXCR4 signaling between pancreatic cancer cells and CAFs could attenuate RT-induced tumor cell invasion [59]. Indeed, HGF secretion by irradiated CAFs can increase phosphorylation of c-Met and MAPK activity in pancreatic tumor cells, which translates into enhanced invasion. This unwanted byproduct of RT can be overcome by blocking HGF signaling with an HGF antagonist [38]. Finally, exposure of CAFs to 18 Gy RT resulted in potent induction of multiple DNA damage response (DDR) foci; induced premature cellular senescence; and inhibited proliferative, migrative, and invasive capacity of CAFs. This RT dose increased the expression of integrins α2, β1, and α5 and dramatically augmented and redistributed focal contacts [60]. The increase in β1 integrin has been correlated with radioresistance [50]. All of these examples point to RT-induced changes in CAFs that can promote further radioresistance. This should encourage us to find therapeutic regimens that target both the tumor and stroma to successfully deliver anti-cancer treatment.

CAF-secreted factors, contact-mediated signaling, downstream pro-survival signaling pathways, CSC-generating role, and changes due to RT all comprise intricate crosstalk between CAFs and cancer cells to render tumor cells radioresistant. While we understand that CAFs play a critical role in shaping responses to RT, there are several areas where we do not fully understand their impact. First, CAFs in tumors are a diverse heterogeneous population that can have opposing roles [3,4,39]. While an abundance of literature supports the tumor-supporting roles of CAFs, some studies also suggest that certain CAF subsets may have tumor-restraining abilities [61,62]. These diverse CAF subsets may have differential effects on radioresistance and, in turn, be shaped differently by RT. Second, the plasticity, diverse origins, and spatial location of CAFs [40,63–65] may complicate things further in terms of their contributions to radioresistance. RT may alter CAF phenotypes temporally and spatially, and this will also affect cancer cells' responses to RT. Lastly, RT dose fractionation may differentially impact CAF diversification. Our understanding of CAF diversity and plasticity is still limited, but it is logical to assume that CAF-mediated radioresistance is a problem in RT success and needs further study.

4. The Impact of ECM on RT Efficacy

The ECM plays an essential role in regulating cancer progression and radiosensitivity. Tumor ECMs are dynamic structures that are remodeled during tumor progression and/or treatment [8]. Among the approximately 300 proteins present in the ECM that are known to regulate tissue homeostasis, inflammation, and disease, collagen is the most abundant, constituting up to 90% of the tumor ECM. In addition to collagens, other prominent fibrous proteins are elastins, fibronectins, and laminins, which are also involved in controlling tumor phenotype [8]. Tumor ECM is typically denser and mechanically stiffer than normal ECM, due to the quantity of ECM as well as structural changes in molecular architecture such as the extent of crosslinking [66]. These changes in ECM density, composition, and stiffness significantly impact malignant cell invasion, survival, and proliferation [67,68]. Variations in ECM stiffness and density have been correlated with disease aggressiveness, progression-free survival, and in some cases, resistance to different treatment modalities [8].

The ability of tumor-promoting ECM to drive treatment resistance is particularly applicable to RT. Tumor cells can interact with the ECM through direct interaction (cell-protein contact), and one major way is through the engagement with integrins [49]. ECM stiffness can facilitate integrin clustering, which can lead to activation of downstream FAK activation and MAP/ERK kinase signaling pathways leading to cell survival, proliferation, migration, and invasion. Integrin-mediated adhesions can also activate transcription factors NFκB, inositol lipid metabolism, and MMP activity [49], in addition to the activation of PI3K/AKT and RAS/MAPK pathways. Integrin activation is important in regulating tumor phenotypes and has been associated with processes such as angiogenesis, survival, invasion, metastasis, and treatment resistance [2,4]. Further complicating this is the fact that RT can increase the expression of integrins α2, α5, β1, and β6; therefore, we need to consider how RT fractionation controls subsequent treatment resistance [60,69,70]. For example, it was found that β1 integrin controls radioresistance by resisting cellular apoptosis from RT through the activation of AKT signaling. Inhibition of β1 integrin can resensitize tumor cells to RT by decreasing proliferation and increasing apoptosis (Figure 2) [71,72]. Another group also found that β1 integrin-mediated adhesion confers RT resistance through downstream FAK-interacting proteins (p130Cas and paxillin) and PI3K/AKT-mediated pro-survival signaling pathways [73]. Together, these examples showed that contact-mediated signaling between tumor cells and ECM proteins in cancers can contribute to radioresistance.

The ECM also contains secreted soluble signaling molecules from tumor and stromal cells. The ECM acts as a reservoir for these cytokines, chemokines, and growth factors. Two prominent examples of these secreted factors that control tumor phenotype are TGFβ and various members of the MMP family. Besides interacting directly with the stromal cells and surface proteins in the ECM, tumor cells are constantly and sophisticatedly communicating with these secreted regulatory molecules [10]. Many of these proteins are already known to be capable of inducing radioresistance, such as TGFβ [42,43,51]. Moreover, RT can further increase TGFβ levels, which can accelerate tumor progression. Inhibition with TGFβ neutralizing antibodies has been shown to prevent radiation-induced metastatic progression [74]. Another class of secreted proteins that are highly abundant in the ECM and mediate tumor progression are the different MMPs [2,8,75]. MMP2 is known to degrade collagen IV and plays a role in RT-induced lung injury. MMP2 inhibition prior to RT abrogated the induction of FoxM1 expression, reduced p53 and p21 expression, decreased expression of DNA repair genes XRCC1 and Chk2/1, and abrogated G2 cell cycle arrest, leading to apoptosis and enhanced radiosensitivity [76]. These examples showed that the ECM serves as a tumor growth factor and cytokine sink, which contributes to tumor radioresistance and worthy of consideration in future therapeutic planning.

Besides controlling the stability and bioavailability of numerous growth factors and cytokines, ECM structure and integrity also influence oxygen availability, acidity, and interstitial fluid pressure in tumors, through its regulation of the tumor vascular system, so it has important effects in terms of controlling treatment response (Figure 1) [8,66]. Oxygen availability is critical for RT response as hypoxic cells are generally 2.5–3 times less radiosensitive than normoxic cells [77–80]. The indirect effects of RT produce ROS through the hydrolysis of water, which then propagate and modify lipids, membranes, and proteins [10]. Using nitric oxide-dependent arteriole vasorelaxation as a way to increase the partial pressure of oxygen in tumors, multiple groups found that low-dose nitrite can sensitize tumors to RT, leading to a significant tumor growth delay and longer survival [81,82].

Antiangiogenic therapy such as vascular endothelial growth factor (VEGF) receptor 2 blockade, which can create a "normalization window" that increases tumor oxygenation, has also been shown to enhance the RT response (Figure 2). This effect is dependent on the increased pericyte coverage of tumor vessels via the upregulation of angiopoietin 1 and degradation of the pathologically thick basement membrane via MMP activation [83]. Thalidomide, an angiogenesis inhibitor, can also increase tumor reoxygenation correlated with reduced interstitial fluid pressure and increased perfusion, sufficient to radiosensitize tumors [84]. Non-steroidal anti-inflammatory drugs (NSAIDs) are another radiosensitizing drug class that works through increasing tumor oxygenation via either a decrease in macrophage recruitment or inhibiting mitochondrial respiration. Using four different NSAIDs (diclofenac, indomethacin, piroxicam, and NS-398), radiation sensitivity in tumor cells can be increased by enhancing radioinduced apoptosis and inhibiting repair of sublethal RT damage [85]. These studies showed that tumor ECM governs oxygen bioavailability in cancers, controls radiosensitivity, and that RT requires sufficient tumor oxygenation to avoid radioresistance (Figure 1).

In most cancers, tumor cells are embedded in stromal cells with abundant ECM components, that, as described above, govern radioresistance through direct interaction with tumor cells and the ECM's roles as protein reservoirs and a major controller of tumor oxygen bioavailability. Even though many of these factors negatively impact RT efficacy, there are known inhibitors that can successfully reverse ECM-mediated radioresistance. As with CAFs, our current knowledge is still lacking on how RT dose fractionation may differentially impact ECM alterations and how they contribute to radioresistance.

5. The Impact of Immune Cells on RT Efficacy

RT is a powerful therapeutic approach used in many patients due to its numerous beneficial effects leading to tumor cell eradication. Besides the direct killing of highly proliferating tumor cells by mitotic catastrophe or apoptosis or necrosis, RT is increasingly appreciated to have immunomodulatory effects, which can take advantage of the fact that our immune cells can target and kill abnormal cancerous cells [11,13,30,32,86]. RT modulates the immunogenicity and adjuvanticity of tumors by increasing the expression and release of tumor-associated antigens, increasing the expression of major histocompatibility complex I (MHC-I), inducing immunogenic cell death (ICD) and its downstream anti-tumor pathways, and releasing danger signals and chemokines that recruit inflammatory anti-tumor immune cells to the TME, including antigen-presenting cells that can activate cytolytic T cells [75,87,88]. RT can also enhance tumor killing by increasing the number of tumor-infiltrating immunostimulatory cells and neoantigen expression [89–91]. However, there are reports that RT can induce immunosuppression on top of anti-tumor immune promoting effects [12,32]. The balance between the two variables predicts the treatment response. Due to its double-edged sword effects on immune modulation, precise dosing regimens and combinatorial treatments of RT must be carefully considered to avoid unwanted immunosuppressive effects [7,9–11,13,30,32,86,87].

As we have discussed with CAFs and ECM, radiosensitivity depends on the complex interaction of malignant cancer cells with their immune TME [86]. Notably, the host immune status also determines the efficacy of treatments, including RT (Figure 1). The presence and activation status of dendritic cells (DCs) and $CD8^+$ T cells and anti-tumor cytokines such as IFNγ determine the responsiveness to RT [92–95]. IFN-related DNA damage resistance signature (IRDS) genes including STAT1, IFN-stimulated genes 15 (ISG15), and IFN-induced protein with tetratricopeptide repeats 1 (IFIT1) are associated with resistance to chemotherapy and/or RT across different tumor cell lines [69]. Additionally, the intratumoral immune response after RT also determines the therapeutic response. RT success is dependent on the antigen-specific nature of immune activation, which can be enhanced by combining RT with immune checkpoint blockade therapies like αPD-1 and αCTLA-4 [26,87,96,97]. Increases in intratumoral anti-tumor immune cells and IFNγ were found to imbue $CD8^+$ T cells with lytic activity against tumor cells, and the addition of IL-12 as immunotherapy can augment this RT-induced anti-tumor immunity [94,98]. Radiation can upregulate the expression of programmed death ligand 1 (PD-L1) on tumor cells in numerous in vivo models, which binds with immune checkpoint receptor PD-1 expressed by CTLs and thereby promotes their dysfunction. The combination of radiation and inhibition of this immune checkpoint has been shown to improve the radiation-induced anti-tumor response through activation of cytotoxic T cells and diminished the influx of myeloid-derived suppressive cells (MDSCs) into the TME [99–101]. Interestingly, several studies in mice and humans have demonstrated abscopal effects, with response of both the primary tumor and distant disease to combination therapy of RT and immune checkpoint blockade [102]. Although most of these studies were conducted utilizing hypofractionated or single-dose ablative radiation schemes, the optimal dose, fractionation, and timing to achieve this effect are unknown [103]. In vivo studies have demonstrated that PD-L1 expression peaks at 3 days post-irradiation, and that concurrent but not sequential treatment with checkpoint inhibitors is necessary for a T cell-mediated tumor response [93,101]. Interestingly, in the KEYNOTE-001 trial, patients who received radiation at any time prior to immune checkpoint therapy had significantly increased progression-free survival, with median time ranging from 9.5 to 11.5 months [104,105]. Despite these appealing data, larger studies demonstrating sufficient survival benefits to lead to approval of regimens containing RT in combination with immune checkpoints have not been published. However, these findings showed the importance of the host's immune status as one major contributor that can predict radiosensitivity.

Like CAFs, immune cells in the TME are very diverse and have different roles. Tumor-associated macrophages (TAMs), MDSCs, and $CD4^+$ regulatory T cells (T_{regs}) are known to be immune suppressive and pro-tumorigenic; on the other hand, immune cells such as DCs, $CD8^+$ T cells, and NK cells are anti-tumorigenic [12]. Likewise, these immune cells also differentially regulate radiosensitivity in cancers (Figure 1). The presence of TAMs correlates with increased radioresistance in many different tumors [106]. Radiation plays a role in the recruitment and phenotype modulation of TAMs in the TME. Recruitment of TAMs occurs irrespective of dose and fractionation [107]. Conventional fractionation leads to transcription of colony-stimulating factor 1 (CSF1), which when blocked in prostate cancer models reduces TAM recruitment. Conversely, hypofractionated regimens promote TAM recruitment in hypoxic conditions, where in glioma models radiation-induced hypoxia-inducible factor 1 (HIF-1) expression leads to the increased density of TAMs [108,109]. Co-implantation of tumor cells with bone marrow-derived macrophages increased tumor radioresistance, so depletion of TAMs using a systemic or local injection of macrophage-depleting liposomal clodronate before RT can increase anti-tumor effects in different RT dosing regimens. Radioresistance coming from TAMs is mediated by the tumor necrosis factor (TNF) signaling-dependent upregulation of VEGF, and anti-VEGF or anti-TNF therapy can reverse this radioresistance (Figure 2) [110]. The effect of the radiation-induced influx of TAMs in the TME depends on the exact phenotype they acquire once infiltrated. The decision tree for macrophage polarization, unlike recruitment, does appear to be dependent on the radiation dose and fraction. Anti-tumor phenotypes may be favored in conventionally fractionated dosing, which can in turn enhance T cell-mediated tumor control [111,112]. Importantly, this effect may be lost in hypofractionated and single-dose ablative regimens. One reason may be that hypoxia which results from vascular impairment by RT promotes macrophage immunosuppressive and pro-tumorigenic tissue remodeling functions [113–115]. However, this is likely an oversimplification, and the true impact of TAMs may depend on the organ- and cancer-specific context in which radiation is employed. RT itself can cause an influx of MDSCs into tumors that eventually polarize the TME into an immune-suppressive environment. This polarization is dependent on transcriptional regulation by the NFκB p50 subunit, as mice lacking NFκB p50 are much more sensitive to RT [116]. Additionally, MDSCs can be recruited further into the TME from RT in a fractionated RT regimen due to the recruitment of DNA damage-induced kinase ABL1 into cell nuclei where it binds the CSF1 gene promoter and enhances its transcription. Hence, blocking macrophage migration with a CSF1 inhibitor radiosensitizes tumors [46]. Another group also found that a neutralizing antibody to CSF1 or a small molecular inhibitor to the CSF1 receptor kinase efficiently depletes macrophages and delays tumor regrowth following RT (Figure 2). This delay is a reflection of the increased presence of $CD8^+$

T cells and reduced presence of $CD4^+$ T cells, the main source of T helper 2 (Th2) cytokines IL-4 and IL-13. The authors proposed that the response to RT could be enhanced by reducing TAMs in tumors or blocking their induction of Th2 polarization [117]. Moreover, treatment with the small tyrosine kinase inhibitor sunitinib resulted in a significant reduction of MDSCs and phospho-STAT3 and increased T cell proliferative activity in cancer patients. Sunitinib's ability to increase RT efficacy in tumors is mediated through the reduction in the number and function of immunosuppressive MDSCs and is significantly correlated with lower $CD4^+$ T_{reg} and B cell numbers and augmentation of Tbet expression in primary $CD4^+$ and $CD8^+$ T cells [118,119]. Finally, due to the intrinsic radioresistant nature of $CD4^+$ T_{regs} and its immunosuppressive roles, $CD4^+$ T_{reg} presence in tumors has also been correlated with radioresistance [120,121]. T_{regs} are essential to generating immune tolerance, are radioresistant compared to other T cell subtypes, and demonstrate a relative increase in the TME after irradiation. T_{regs} are known to increase in mice receiving whole-body radiation [122], and studies of human cervical cancers treated with 10-30 Gy demonstrate decreased $CD8^+$ and $CD4^+$ T cells, without any effect on T_{reg} numbers [123]. In vivo tumor models with systemically depleted T_{regs} demonstrate significant determent of primary and metastatic tumor progression. When these tumors are irradiated, these models demonstrate significantly reduced tumor burden post-RT and improved overall survival [124–129]. Dose and fractionation have also been demonstrated to play a role in the balance of immune priming and immunosuppression post-RT. A B16 murine model receiving a single 5 Gy dose of irradiation showed a relative increase in the T_{reg} population compared to cytotoxic T cells. However, a single 10 Gy dose resulted in a relative decrease of T_{regs}, while a single 15 Gy dose increased both T_{reg} and effector T cells [130]. Systemic elimination of $CD4^+$ T_{regs} using anti-CD25 monoclonal antibody enhances radiotherapeutic benefits via immune modulation (Figure 2) [122]. Collectively, these studies showed that pro-tumorigenic immune cells can modulate radioresistance in many cancers.

While initially thought to create an immunosuppressive TME, radiation has recently gained momentum clinically as a means to prime the immune system to recognize and remove tumor cells. To achieve this end, cross-presentation of tumor antigen by DCs to cytotoxic T cells must be upregulated. Radiation has been shown to increase IFN-I signaling, leading to expansion and activation of DCs, through induction of the stimulator of IFN genes (STING) pathway [26,93,131,132]. Additionally, tumor cell removal requires the induction of cell death pathways, which can be variable, and include apoptosis, necrosis, autophagy, and mitotic catastrophe. Immunogenic cell death upregulation is frequently observed following irradiation. This involves three key molecular signals: calreticulin, which undergoes translocation from the endoplasmic reticulum to the plasma membrane to signal uptake of dying tumor cells by DCs; high-mobility group protein B1 (HMGB1), which is released from the dying cells to bind Toll-like receptor 4 on DCs promoting antigen cross-presentation; and adenosine triphosphate (ATP), which activates cytotoxic T cells through inflammasome activation via the P2XR7 pathway [86,132–135]. In vitro experiments have demonstrated that the generation of these three key signaling molecules is dependent on irradiation dose [88]. However, the optimal dose and fractionation of irradiation required to induce ICD in vivo is influenced by the TME [75,86,133]. Utilizing a B16 melanoma mouse model expressing ovalbumin antigen, several groups have demonstrated that single-dose, 15-20 Gy irradiation was more effective in generating activated cytotoxic T cells than more conventional fractionated schedules of 15 Gy in 5 daily fractions and 20 Gy in 4 bi-weekly fractions. This indicated that the prescribed dose per fraction and also the specific timing of individual dose delivery are important to elicit RT-induced immune responses [26,131]. Clinical investigations of this mechanism in patients with colorectal and prostate cancer demonstrated a detectable increase in circulating cytotoxic T cells (Survivin- and/or prostate-specific antigen-specific) in post-irradiation blood samples [136,137]. Additionally, early-stage non-small cell lung cancer patients treated with SBRT, 48 Gy in 6-8 fractions, showed increased circulating cytotoxic T cells [138]. Many studies have indicated that ablative radiation doses are required for activation of T cell immunity, and this is corroborated by clinical evidence suggesting that conventional fractionation can have a detrimental effect on the

TME as a result of the death of infiltrating anti-tumor lymphocytes [32,139–141]. In preclinical studies, mice bearing bilateral flank implants of CT26 colon carcinoma treated with conventional fractionation (10 Gy in 5 fractions) initially demonstrated T cell reductions after each dose of radiation; however, this regimen at 7 days post-therapy led to an expansion of local polyclonal T cells responses and infiltrating T cells, revealing a treatment duration effect in this model system [142]. Several groups have moved away from flank models, due to the prevailing theory that to initiate tumor growth you create a wound stimulating a subsequent acute immune response. Instead, several groups have adopted genetically-engineered mouse models (GEMMs) that spontaneously form tumors. Recent publications utilizing GEMMs of pancreatic cancer and sarcoma have demonstrated that reprogramming the TME can induce T cell immunity and sensitize tumors to radiation [143–145] from both single high-dose and hypofractionated RT schemes.

Radiation also plays an important role in overcoming T cell exclusion from the TME. One barrier is the dampened homing of effector T cells, which is modulated by cytokines released from tumor cells and the surrounding stroma. Irradiation can significantly enhance the secretion of CXCL16 by mouse and human breast cancer cells; this chemokine binds to CXCR6 on activated cytotoxic T cells and plays an important role in their recruitment to inflammation sites. CXCL16 can be induced in vitro by a single fraction dose of 5 Gy; while in vivo induction was found to be dose-dependent, reaching a plateau at 12 Gy [146,147]. In another study, mice deficient in IFNγ, a cytokine that is critical for innate and adaptive immunity, received tumor-localized irradiation and demonstrated decreased expression of MHC-I and CXCL9/CXCL10, which are important chemoattractants for cytotoxic T cells [147,148]. TNFα can also be induced by single-fraction irradiation in tumor cell lines [149]. Radiation also leads to upregulation of anti-inflammatory cytokines, like TGFβ, which will suppress the function of DCs and cytotoxic T cells and promote maturation of T_{regs}. Single fraction radiation from 5–10 Gy in mouse mammary tumors upregulated TGFβ in both tumor cells and the surrounding adipose stroma [34,150]. In irradiated tissues, there is a relative increase in ROS, leading to activation of TGFβ. Mouse models of mammary carcinoma demonstrate that activation of DCs and priming of cytotoxic T cells during RT can be improved by administering TGFβ-neutralizing antibodies [99,150].

Tumors counteract this influx of activated cytotoxic T cells through the downregulation of antigen-presenting MHC-I proteins. Historical studies revealed that radiation increases MHC-I protein expression on tumor cells, leading to restored antigen recognition by cytotoxic T cells. In primary glioblastoma lines, increasing doses of radiation up to 12 Gy led to increased MHC-I expression, and a similar effect was demonstrated in ovarian and cervical cancer cell lines with doses of 25 to 100 Gy [151–154]. Conventionally fractionated radiation also can induce MHC-I expression, where conditioned media from breast cancer lines treated with 6-10 Gy delivered in 3-5 fractions was able to stimulate expression of total cellular and surface MHC-I in recipient cells [155].

The interactions between tumor cells and their immune microenvironment is very complex due to their abundance, diversity, and varying roles. Evidence showing the presence of anti-tumor immune cells and IRDS genes being important to determine RT efficacy and the roles of pro-tumor immune cells to promote radioresistance should inspire us to design therapeutic regimens with different immune-modulating drugs to synergize with RT. However, it is still unclear how different RT fractions affect immune TME. Additionally, it was recently discovered that distinct immune cell origins (bone marrow or embryonic) have different roles in controlling tumor phenotype [156]. How the immune cell origin contributes to immune-mediated radioresistance is still a largely unaddressed question in the field and needs to be studied [157,158].

6. Immunomodulatory Roles of CAFs and the ECM and How Their Interactions Regulate RT Efficacy

With recent discoveries, it is increasingly appreciated that malignant tumor cells interact with their TME in a complex and reciprocal manner to regulate tumor progression and treatment response [1–5]. In addition to the ability of the individual stromal components to directly control tumor cell phenotype, interactions among the components of the TME themselves can also exert the same effects [6,66]. Immune cells in the TME are regulated by their microenvironment, including the CAFs and ECM in addition to the tumor cells. These communal interactions in the TME are important to consider because they can inadvertently affect treatment response [11,32,86].

CAFs have various pro-tumorigenic roles by regulating tumor immunity, ECM, and hypoxia, among many other factors [66]. One group reported that fibroblast activation protein (FAP)$^+$ CAFs, one subtype of CAFs, are responsible for suppressing anti-tumor immunity and thus contribute to uncontrollable tumor growth. Depleting FAP-expressing cells provides some tumor growth control through a process involving IFNγ and TNFα [159]. In a cervical cancer model, mesenchymal stromal cells were responsible for immunosuppression through their ability to dampen CD8$^+$ T cell proliferation, activation, and effector functions. This was found to be mediated by the expression of CD39 and CD73 ectonucleotidases and the generation of adenosine by the stromal cells [160]. Lastly, CAFs can support tumorigenesis and mediate tumor-enhancing inflammation by enhancing tumor angiogenesis, proliferation, and invasion. These tumor-promoting characteristics are mediated by NFκB pathways [161]. These tumor-promoting roles of CAFs, through their modulation of tumor immunity, may apply to the mechanisms of stromal-mediated radioresistance.

CAFs can control tumor immunity through multiple mechanisms [66,162]. CAFs regulate both adaptive and innate immune cell functions, including T cell and immunosuppressive myeloid cells. CAFs can negatively impair the function of CD8$^+$ T cells including cytolytic activity and cytokine production through the production of soluble factors, such as TGFβ and VEGF, metabolic reprogramming via indoleamine 2,3-dioxygenase and arginase, and expression of checkpoint inhibitors like PD-L1 [66,163]. Many of these factors were discussed previously in the other sections as they are implicated in radioresistance [42,43,51,110]. CAFs can also affect myeloid cell and DC maturation status and function [164–167]. These immune cells are essential mediators of radiosensitivity [92–95,106]. More importantly, many recent discoveries have shown how targeting the stroma can reawaken anti-tumor immunity and synergize with immunotherapy [168–170], as reviewed elsewhere [66]. The concept of how stromal interactions with the immune microenvironment affect immunotherapy response may also hold true for RT responses.

One way by which CAFs regulate the immune TME is through their secreted factors. CAFs secrete many active factors to the TME which are eventually stored in the ECM reservoir, including the various MMPs [2,8,10,75]. MMP14 mediates tumor progression through vascular and immune-modulatory effects. The anti-MMP14 inhibitory antibody can inhibit tumor growth, reduce tissue hypoxia, increase macrophage number, and shift cell phenotype towards the more anti-tumor M1-like phenotype due to reduced active TGFβ and SMAD2/3 signaling, hence synergistically enhancing RT effects (Figure 2) [171]. This example demonstrates that CAF interactions with the ECM and the immune microenvironment can regulate tumor cell radiosensitivity.

CAFs and the ECM have many immunomodulatory functions, which can control tumor cells' treatment response, including RT efficacy. Even on their own, CAFs, ECM, and immune cells can directly confer a radioresistance phenotype to tumor cells, and their interactions among themselves also affect how tumor cells respond to RT. It is presently unclear how these relationships among the tumor stroma components are affected by host immune status and vice versa. Similarly, it is not known how different RT doses and fractionations change these complex interactions and their ensuing tumor-regulating phenotype. It will be fascinating to see how new technologies such as single-cell RNA sequencing will help us discover novel stromal and immune cells and shape our understanding of the immunomodulatory functions of stromal cells in cancers.

7. The Impact of Other Stromal Cells on RT Efficacy

The TME contains other stromal cells present besides CAFs: blood endothelial cells, lymphatic endothelial cells, adipocytes, mesenchymal stem cells, fibrocytes, pericytes, neurons, etc. Although their contribution is small in terms of their numbers in the TME, they still play important roles in tumor progression, treatment response, treatment resistance, and cancer metastasis [1,7].

Endothelial cells are important players in many different types of cancer. They supply nutrients for tumor growth, provide routes for metastatic dissemination, and contribute to chemo- and radioresistance [80,172,173]. Hence, it is important to understand the tumor vasculature to comprehend endothelial cell-mediated radioresistance. Tumors have two main ways to develop vasculature: angiogenesis and vasculogenesis. Angiogenesis is the process in which vessels are developed from nearby endothelial cells, while vasculogenesis is the formation of blood vessels from circulating cells postulated to come from the bone marrow [80]. It is clear that angiogenesis is an important process fundamental to treatment refractoriness, but vasculogenesis is especially imperative in RT resistance due to the fact that local RT abrogates local angiogenesis, forcing tumors to rely heavily on the vasculogenesis pathway for blood vessel regrowth post-RT. This mechanism poses another barrier to T cell infiltration. Dysfunctional tumor-associated vasculature has endothelial cells lining the vessels that suppress T cell activity, target them for destruction, and block entry into the TME [174]. Studies of ablative doses of radiation as high as 25 Gy led to the infiltration of TAMs expressing immunosuppressive enzymes [175]. Notably, single-fraction ablative doses also induce significant endothelial cell death, causing reduced vascular flow, hampering T cell recruitment, and inducing a hypoxic and immunosuppressive TME [176,177]. These ablative doses have been evaluated by bioinformatic studies, demonstrating that alteration of tumor vasculature post-irradiation accounts for 20–30% of the radiographic response of brain metastases in stereotactic radiosurgery cases [178]. In contrast, radiation doses <10 Gy have been shown to promote vascular relaxation and increase tumor oxygenation, with fractionated schedules providing the maximal benefit on tumor growth delay due to tumor reoxygenation [179,180]. Low-dose radiation also plays a role in the reprogramming of macrophages, which are important during the angiogenesis process, allowing increased T cell extravasation in vivo through inducible nitric oxide synthetase [112]. There is an influx of $CD11b^+$ myeloid cells following tumor irradiation, and increased tumor hypoxia increases HIF-1 levels and subsequently upregulates stromal cell-derived factor 1 (SDF1, also known as CXCL12) to initiate vasculogenesis [80]. Many angiogenic inhibitors have been used in the clinic and have proven efficacy as radiosensitizing agents because of multiple different mechanisms related to the "normalization" of tumor vessels and their subsequent oxygen content and acidity (Figure 2) [2,6,32]. One group claims that the use of the VEGF receptor inhibitor axitinib radiosensitized tumor endothelium and enabled tumor control [181]. Another group found that angiogenesis-promoting factors that protect against endothelial damage can diminish the RT response. Reversing this effect with a VEGF inhibitor promotes RT-induced endothelial injury through the generation of the second messenger ceramide through acid sphingomyelinase trafficking to the plasma membrane. This tumor endothelial cell RT resensitization was shown to mediate tumor control [181]. These studies demonstrated that endothelial cells are important mediators of tumor radioresistance due to their ability to form vessels and control tumor oxygen content.

Adipocytes are also active players in the TME that control cancer development, progression, metastasis, and treatment response, especially in cancers that interact closely with adipose tissue-like breast cancers [182]. Cancer-associated adipocytes (CAAs) are energetic cells capable of secreting a heterogeneous group of molecules known as adipokines that include hormones, growth factors, and cytokines. Some examples of adipokines are leptin, adiponectin, autotaxin, IL-6, TNFα, IGF-1, and HGF. In addition, CAAs actively participate in metabolic remodeling that supports cancer cell growth by regulating the fatty acid reservoir to increase mitochondrial β-oxidation. They also interact closely with CAFs and ECM molecules through ECM remodeling. More importantly, they act as obstacles to various anti-cancer therapies as they are involved in diverse resistance mechanisms [1,7].

One mechanism of adipocyte-mediated radioresistance is through their secreted adipokines. Some of these adipokines such as TNFα, IGF-1, and HGF were discussed earlier with regard to their contributions to stromal-mediated radioresistance (Figure 1) [38,52,110,159]. Another group reported that these adipokines can increase the gene expression of NFκB and cyclin D to induce anti-apoptotic transcription and stabilize pro-oncogenic factors such as β-catenin and cyclin-dependent kinases [182]. It was also found that breast cancer cells co-cultured with adipocytes are radioresistant, and the mechanism is through adipocyte secretion of IL-6 resulting in the phosphorylation of Chk1 associated with decreased cancer cell death [182,183]. Another mechanism of adipocyte-mediated radioresistance is the initiation of autotaxin (ATX)–lysophosphatidic acid (LPA) signaling. This group found that CAAs, which closely interact with adjacent tumor cells, can become inflamed from tumor-derived cytokines, which results in the stimulation of adipocytes' ATX secretion and subsequent LPA production. This further promotes inflammatory cytokine production in a vicious feed-forward cycle. RT-induced adipocyte injury triggers increased levels of ATX, cyclooxygenase-2 (COX-2), IL-1β, IL-6, IL-10, TNFα, and LPA1 and LPA2 receptors. This inflammatory response depends on the DNA damage response pathways ATM, ATR, and PARP-1 and inflammatory mediators COX-2 and NFκB, which can potentially be inhibited to reverse radioresistance. Induction of LPA signaling enhances lymphocyte invasion and cytokine and VEGF production to stimulate angiogenesis required for tumor growth [184]. As detailed earlier, angiogenesis is one factor that contributes to tumor cell radioresistance [8]. These studies showed that adipocytes are not dormant "fat" cells; they are active contributors to tumor phenotype through their active metabolism and secreted factors.

Even though endothelial cells and adipocytes do not make up a significant portion of the tumor stroma, they contribute to tumor radioresistance. Multiple groups have shown that we should not negate their roles in controlling RT response to prevent the formation of radioresistant cancer cells. However, the complexity of different RT doses and fractionation regimens has left the field with an unanswered question regarding their effect on stromal cells present in cancers.

8. Forward Looking Conclusions

Malignant tumor cells that harbor genetic aberrations are in close proximity with the tumor stroma composed of diverse cellular and non-cellular entities including CAFs, ECM components, immune cells, endothelial cells, adipocytes, and secreted bioactive molecules. At every step of the tumor lifecycle, there is reciprocal communication between these malignant cancer cells and their neighbors. Their highly dynamic interactions control tumor initiation, progression, invasion, metastasis, and treatment resistance, which complicates cancer therapeutic planning [1–6,8,10–13,185]. Here, we reviewed how the tumor stroma can contribute to cancer radioresistance; many of which are mediated through secreted factors, cell surface receptors, and downstream pro-survival and/or anti-apoptotic signaling pathways. The tumor stroma is very diverse, and our current knowledge of distinct cell types is still lacking. It will be interesting to see how new technologies to discover novel CAFs and immune cell types will broaden our knowledge of tumor-stromal interactions.

Further complicating the concept of stromal-mediated radioresistance is the fact that with successive treatments tumor and stromal cells can become more resistant, which could be a problem for many anti-cancer treatment regimens given in cycles, such as chemo- and radiotherapies. Based on the potential of these tumor stroma to induce radioresistance, it seems plausible to include stromal-targeted agents in combination with RT for therapeutic benefit. Multi-directed treatments toward both the tumor cells and the tumor stroma could help eradicate cancers and prevent therapeutic resistance and tumor relapse.

Lastly, RT is a rapidly evolving field. Ultra-high dose rate of RT (FLASH-RT) is a new technology that enables the ultra-fast delivery of doses while sparing normal tissues [186,187]. It will be important to see how FLASH-RT influences tumor-stroma communications and stromal-mediated radioresistance. Despite many recent discoveries, there are still many remaining questions in the field to be addressed, such as how CAF diversity affects radioresistance and how the tumor stroma changes with different RT dosing and fractionation regimens. Future discoveries about these mechanisms can be used for the design of novel RT and drug combinations to target stromal-mediated RT resistance.

Author Contributions: V.E.K., J.A.S., J.K.S., and D.G.D. wrote the manuscript; V.E.K. and D.G.D. prepared the figures. All authors contributed to the writing of the manuscript. All authors have read and agreed to the published version of the manuscript.

References

1. Valkenburg, K.C.; De Groot, A.E.; Pienta, K.J. Targeting the tumour stroma to improve cancer therapy. *Nat. Rev. Clin. Oncol.* **2018**, *15*, 366–381. [CrossRef] [PubMed]
2. Mueller, M.M.; Fusenig, N.E. Friends or foes—Bipolar effects of the tumour stroma in cancer. *Nat. Rev. Cancer* **2004**, *4*, 839–849. [CrossRef] [PubMed]
3. Kalluri, R. The biology and function of fibroblasts in cancer. *Nat. Rev. Cancer* **2016**, *16*, 582–598. [CrossRef] [PubMed]
4. Kalluri, R.; Zeisberg, M. Fibroblasts in cancer. *Nat. Rev. Cancer* **2006**, *6*, 392–401. [CrossRef]
5. D'Arcangelo, E.; Wu, N.C.; Cadavid, J.L.; McGuigan, A.P. The life cycle of cancer-associated fibroblasts within the tumour stroma and its importance in disease outcome. *Br. J. Cancer* **2020**. [CrossRef]
6. Junttila, M.R.; De Sauvage, F.J. Influence of tumour micro-environment heterogeneity on therapeutic response. *Nature* **2013**, *501*, 346–354. [CrossRef]
7. Turley, S.J.; Cremasco, V.; Astarita, J.L. Immunological hallmarks of stromal cells in the tumour microenvironment. *Nat. Rev. Immunol.* **2015**, *15*, 669–682. [CrossRef]
8. Gilkes, D.M.; Semenza, G.L.; Wirtz, D. Hypoxia and the extracellular matrix: Drivers of tumour metastasis. *Nat. Rev. Cancer* **2014**, *14*, 430–439. [CrossRef]
9. Iyer, S.P.; Hunt, C.R.; Pandita, T.K. Cross Talk between Radiation and Immunotherapy: The Twain Shall Meet. *Radiat. Res.* **2018**, *189*, 219–224. [CrossRef]
10. Barcellos-Hoff, M.H.; Park, C.; Wright, E.G. Radiation and the microenvironment—Tumorigenesis and therapy. *Nat. Rev. Cancer* **2005**, *5*, 867–875. [CrossRef]
11. McLaughlin, M.; Patin, E.C.; Pedersen, M.; Wilkins, A.; Dillon, M.T.; Melcher, A.A.; Harrington, K.J. Inflammatory microenvironment remodelling by tumour cells after radiotherapy. *Nat. Rev. Cancer* **2020**. [CrossRef] [PubMed]
12. Barker, H.E.; Paget, J.T.E.; Khan, A.A.; Harrington, K.J. The tumour microenvironment after radiotherapy: Mechanisms of resistance and recurrence. *Nat. Rev. Cancer* **2015**, *15*, 409–425. [CrossRef] [PubMed]
13. Weichselbaum, R.R.; Liang, H.; Deng, L.; Fu, Y.X. Radiotherapy and immunotherapy: A beneficial liaison? *Nat. Rev. Clin. Oncol.* **2017**, *14*, 365–379. [CrossRef] [PubMed]
14. Hwang, W.L.; Pike, L.R.G.; Royce, T.J.; Mahal, B.A.; Loeffler, J.S. Safety of combining radiotherapy with immune-checkpoint inhibition. *Nat. Rev. Clin. Oncol.* **2018**, *15*, 477–494. [CrossRef]
15. Schaue, D.; McBride, W.H. Opportunities and challenges of radiotherapy for treating cancer. *Nat. Rev. Clin. Oncol.* **2015**, *12*, 527–540. [CrossRef]
16. Grassberger, C.; Ellsworth, S.G.; Wilks, M.Q.; Keane, F.K.; Loeffler, J.S. Assessing the interactions between radiotherapy and antitumour immunity. *Nat. Rev. Clin. Oncol.* **2019**, *16*, 729–745. [CrossRef]
17. Van Leeuwen, C.M.; Oei, A.L.; Crezee, J.; Bel, A.; Franken, N.A.P.; Stalpers, L.J.A.; Kok, H.P. The alfa and beta of tumours: A review of parameters of the linear-quadratic model, derived from clinical radiotherapy studies. *Radiat. Oncol.* **2018**, *13*, 96. [CrossRef]
18. Hall, E.; Giaccia, A. Cell survival curves. In *Radiobiology for the Radiologist*, 7th ed.; Lippincott Williams & Wilkins: Philadelphia, PA, USA, 2012; pp. 35–53.
19. Papiez, L.; Timmerman, R. Hypofractionation in radiation therapy and its impact. *Med. Phys.* **2008**, *35*, 112–118. [CrossRef]
20. Mahajan, A.; Ahmed, S.; McAleer, M.F.; Weinberg, J.S.; Li, J.; Brown, P.; Settle, S.; Prabhu, S.S.; Lang, F.F.; Levine, N.; et al. Post-operative stereotactic radiosurgery versus observation for completely resected brain metastases: A single-centre, randomised, controlled, phase 3 trial. *Lancet Oncol.* **2017**, *18*, 1040–1048. [CrossRef]
21. Qiu, H.; Moravan, M.J.; Milano, M.T.; Usuki, K.Y.; Katz, A.W. SBRT for Hepatocellular Carcinoma: 8-Year Experience from a Regional Transplant Center. *J. Gastrointest. Cancer* **2018**, *49*, 463–469. [CrossRef]
22. Kishan, A.U.; King, C.R. Stereotactic Body Radiotherapy for Low- and Intermediate-Risk Prostate Cancer. *Semin. Radiat. Oncol.* **2017**, *27*, 268–278. [CrossRef] [PubMed]

23. Aridgides, P.; Bogart, J. Stereotactic Body Radiation Therapy for Stage I Non-Small Cell Lung Cancer. *Thorac. Surg. Clin.* **2016**, *26*, 261–269. [CrossRef] [PubMed]
24. Mole, R.H. Whole body irradiation; radiobiology or medicine? *Br. J. Radiol.* **1953**, *26*, 234–241. [CrossRef] [PubMed]
25. Dewan, M.Z.; Galloway, A.E.; Kawashima, N.; Dewyngaert, J.K.; Babb, J.S.; Formenti, S.C.; Demaria, S. Fractionated but not single-dose radiotherapy induces an immune-mediated abscopal effect when combined with anti-CTLA-4 antibody. *Clin. Cancer Res.* **2009**, *15*, 5379–5388. [CrossRef] [PubMed]
26. Lee, Y.; Auh, S.L.; Wang, Y.; Burnette, B.; Wang, Y.; Meng, Y.; Beckett, M.; Sharma, R.; Chin, R.; Tu, T.; et al. Therapeutic effects of ablative radiation on local tumor require CD8+ T cells: Changing strategies for cancer treatment. *Blood* **2009**, *114*, 589–595. [CrossRef]
27. Reits, E.A.; Hodge, J.W.; Herberts, C.A.; Groothuis, T.A.; Chakraborty, M.; Wansley, E.K.; Camphausen, K.; Luiten, R.M.; de Ru, A.H.; Neijssen, J.; et al. Radiation modulates the peptide repertoire, enhances MHC class I expression, and induces successful antitumor immunotherapy. *J. Exp. Med.* **2006**, *203*, 1259–1271. [CrossRef]
28. Reynders, K.; Illidge, T.; Siva, S.; Chang, J.Y.; De Ruysscher, D. The abscopal effect of local radiotherapy: Using immunotherapy to make a rare event clinically relevant. *Cancer Treat. Rev.* **2015**, *41*, 503–510. [CrossRef]
29. Riaz, N.; Morris, L.; Havel, J.J.; Makarov, V.; Desrichard, A.; Chan, T.A. The role of neoantigens in response to immune checkpoint blockade. *Int. Immunol.* **2016**, *28*, 411–419. [CrossRef]
30. Leroi, N.; Lallemand, F.; Coucke, P.; Noel, A.; Martinive, P. Impacts of ionizing radiation on the different compartments of the tumor microenvironment. *Front. Pharmacol.* **2016**, *7*, 1–9. [CrossRef]
31. Straub, J.M.; New, J.; Hamilton, C.D.; Lominska, C.; Shnayder, Y.; Thomas, S.M. Radiation-induced fibrosis: Mechanisms and implications for therapy. *J. Cancer Res. Clin. Oncol.* **2015**, *141*, 1985–1994. [CrossRef]
32. Arnold, K.M.; Flynn, N.J.; Raben, A.; Romak, L.; Yu, Y.; Dicker, A.P.; Mourtada, F.; Sims-Mourtada, J. The Impact of Radiation on the Tumor Microenvironment: Effect of Dose and Fractionation Schedules. *Cancer Growth Metastasis* **2018**, *11*. [CrossRef] [PubMed]
33. Penney, D.P.; Wayne, A.; Rosenkrans, J. Cell-Cell Matrix Interactions in Induced Lung Injury: I. The Effects of X-Irradiation on Basal Laminar Proteoglycans. *Radiat. Res.* **1984**, *99*, 410–419. [CrossRef] [PubMed]
34. Barcellos-Hoff, M.H. Radiation-induced Transforming Growth Factor β and Subsequent Extracellular Matrix Reorganization in Murine Mammary Gland. *Cancer Res.* **1993**, *53*, 3880–3886. [PubMed]
35. Remy, J.; Wegrowski, J.; Crechet, F.; Martin, M.; Daburon, F. Long-Term Overproduction of Collagen in Radiation-Induced Fibrosis. *Radiat. Res.* **1991**, *125*, 14–19. [CrossRef]
36. Chargari, C.; Clemenson, C.; Martins, I.; Perfettini, J.-L.; Deutsch, E. Understanding the functions of tumor stroma in resistance to ionizing radiation: Emerging targets for pharmacological modulation. *Drug Resist. Updat.* **2013**, *16*, 10–21. [CrossRef]
37. Kamochi, N.; Nakashima, M.; Aoki, S.; Uchihashi, K.; Sugihara, H.; Toda, S.; Kudo, S. Irradiated fibroblast-induced bystander effects on invasive growth of squamous cell carcinoma under cancer-stromal cell interaction. *Cancer Sci.* **2008**, *99*, 2417–2427. [CrossRef]
38. Ohuchida, K.; Mizumoto, K.; Murakami, M.; Qian, L.W.; Sato, N.; Nagai, E.; Matsumoto, K.; Nakamura, T.; Tanaka, M. Radiation to Stromal Fibroblasts Increases Invasiveness of Pancreatic Cancer Cells through Tumor-Stromal Interactions. *Cancer Res.* **2004**, *64*, 3215–3222. [CrossRef]
39. Tommelein, J.; Verset, L.; Boterberg, T.; Demetter, P.; Bracke, M.; De Wever, O. Cancer-Associated Fibroblasts Connect Metastasis-Promoting Communication in Colorectal Cancer. *Front. Oncol.* **2015**, *5*, 1–11. [CrossRef]
40. Wang, Z.; Tang, Y.; Tan, Y.; Wei, Q.; Yu, W. Cancer-associated fibroblasts in radiotherapy: Challenges and new opportunities. *Cell Commun. Signal.* **2019**, *17*, 1–12. [CrossRef]
41. Boelens, M.C.; Wu, T.J.; Nabet, B.Y.; Xu, B.; Qiu, Y.; Yoon, T.; Azzam, D.J.; Twyman-Saint Victor, C.; Wiemann, B.Z.; Ishwaran, H.; et al. Exosome transfer from stromal to breast cancer cells regulates therapy resistance pathways. *Cell* **2014**, *159*, 499–513. [CrossRef]
42. Hwang, R.F.; Moore, T.; Arumugam, T.; Ramachandran, V.; Amos, K.D.; Rivera, A.; Ji, B.; Evans, D.B.; Logsdon, C.D. Cancer-associated stromal fibroblasts promote pancreatic tumor progression. *Cancer Res.* **2008**, *68*, 918–926. [CrossRef] [PubMed]
43. Hardee, M.E.; Marciscano, A.E.; Medina-Ramirez, C.M.; Zagzag, D.; Narayana, A.; Lonning, S.M.; Barcellos-Hoff, M.H. Resistance of glioblastoma-initiating cells to radiation mediated by the tumor microenvironment can be abolished by inhibiting transforming growth factor-β. *Cancer Res.* **2012**, *72*, 4119–4129. [CrossRef] [PubMed]

44. Wang, Y.; Gan, G.; Wang, B.; Wu, J.; Cao, Y.; Zhu, D.; Xu, Y.; Wang, X.; Han, H.; Li, X.; et al. Cancer-associated Fibroblasts Promote Irradiated Cancer Cell Recovery Through Autophagy. *EBioMedicine* **2017**, *17*, 45–56. [CrossRef] [PubMed]
45. Acharyya, S.; Oskarsson, T.; Vanharanta, S.; Malladi, S.; Kim, J.; Morris, P.G.; Manova-Todorova, K.; Leversha, M.; Hogg, N.; Seshan, V.E.; et al. A CXCL1 paracrine network links cancer chemoresistance and metastasis. *Cell* **2012**, *150*, 165–178. [CrossRef]
46. Zhang, H.; Yue, J.; Jiang, Z.; Zhou, R.; Xie, R.; Xu, Y.; Wu, S. CAF-secreted CXCL1 conferred radioresistance by regulating DNA damage response in a ROS-dependent manner in esophageal squamous cell carcinoma. *Cell Death Dis.* **2017**, *8*, e2790. [CrossRef]
47. Downward, J. Targeting RAS signalling pathways in cancer therapy. *Nat. Rev. Cancer* **2003**, *3*, 11–22. [CrossRef]
48. Dhillon, A.S.; Hagan, S.; Rath, O.; Kolch, W. MAP kinase signalling pathways in cancer. *Oncogene* **2007**, *26*, 3279–3290. [CrossRef]
49. Cordes, N. Integrin-mediated cell-matrix interactions for prosurvival and antiapoptotic signaling after genotoxic injury. *Cancer Lett.* **2006**, *242*, 11–19. [CrossRef]
50. Mantoni, T.S.; Lunardi, S.; Al-Assar, O.; Masamune, A.; Brunner, T.B. Pancreatic stellate cells radioprotect pancreatic cancer cells through β1-integrin signaling. *Cancer Res.* **2011**, *71*, 3453–3458. [CrossRef]
51. Al-Assar, O.; Demiciorglu, F.; Lunardi, S.; Gaspar-Carvalho, M.M.; McKenna, W.G.; Muschel, R.M.; Brunner, T.B. Contextual regulation of pancreatic cancer stem cell phenotype and radioresistance by pancreatic stellate cells. *Radiother. Oncol.* **2014**, *111*, 243–251. [CrossRef]
52. Chen, W.J.; Ho, C.C.; Chang, Y.L.; Chen, H.Y.; Lin, C.A.; Ling, T.Y.; Yu, S.L.; Yuan, S.S.; Louisa Chen, Y.J.; Lin, C.Y.; et al. Cancer-associated fibroblasts regulate the plasticity of lung cancer stemness via paracrine signalling. *Nat. Commun* **2014**, *5*. [CrossRef] [PubMed]
53. Osuka, S.; Sampetrean, O.; Shimizu, T.; Saga, I.; Onishi, N.; Sugihara, E.; Okubo, J.; Fujita, S.; Takano, S.; Matsumura, A.; et al. IGF1 receptor signaling regulates adaptive radioprotection in glioma stem cells. *Stem Cells* **2013**, *31*, 627–640. [CrossRef] [PubMed]
54. Hawsawi, N.M.; Ghebeh, H.; Hendrayani, S.F.; Tulbah, A.; Al-Eid, M.; Al-Tweigeri, T.; Ajarim, D.; Alaiya, A.; Dermime, S.; Aboussekhra, A. Breast carcinoma-associated fibroblasts and their counterparts display neoplastic-specific changes. *Cancer Res.* **2008**, *68*, 2717–2725. [CrossRef] [PubMed]
55. Tang, F.R.; Loke, W.K. Molecular mechanisms of low dose ionizing radiation-induced hormesis, adaptive responses, radioresistance, bystander effects, and genomic instability. *Int. J. Radiat. Biol.* **2015**, *91*, 13–27. [CrossRef]
56. Sun, Y.; Campisi, J.; Higano, C.; Beer, T.M.; Porter, P.; Coleman, I.; True, L.; Nelson, P.S. Treatment-induced damage to the tumor microenvironment promotes prostate cancer therapy resistance through WNT16B. *Nat. Med.* **2012**, *18*, 1359–1368. [CrossRef]
57. Tsai, K.K.C.; Stuart, J.; Chuang, Y.-Y.E.; Little, J.B.; Yuan, Z.-M. Low-Dose Radiation-Induced Senescent Stromal Fibroblasts Render Nearby Breast Cancer Cells Radioresistant. *Radiat. Res.* **2009**, *172*, 306–313. [CrossRef]
58. Pazolli, E.; Alspach, E.; Milczarek, A.; Prior, J.; Piwnica-Worms, D.; Stewart, S.A. Chromatin remodeling underlies the senescence- associated secretory phenotype of tumor stromal fibroblasts that supports cancer progression. *Cancer Res.* **2012**, *72*, 2251–2261. [CrossRef]
59. Li, D.; Qu, C.; Ning, Z.; Wang, H.; Zang, K.; Zhuang, L.; Chen, L.; Wang, P.; Meng, Z. Radiation promotes epithelial-to-mesenchymal transition and invasion of pancreatic cancer cell by activating carcinoma-associated fibroblasts. *Am. J. Cancer Res.* **2016**, *6*, 2192–2206.
60. Hellevik, T.; Pettersen, I.; Berg, V.; Winberg, J.O.; Moe, B.T.; Bartnes, K.; Paulssen, R.H.; Busund, L.T.; Bremnes, R.; Chalmers, A.; et al. Cancer-associated fibroblasts from human NSCLC survive ablative doses of radiation but their invasive capacity is reduced. *Radiat. Oncol.* **2012**, *7*. [CrossRef]
61. Özdemir, B.C.; Pentcheva-Hoang, T.; Carstens, J.L.; Zheng, X.; Wu, C.C.; Simpson, T.R.; Laklai, H.; Sugimoto, H.; Kahlert, C.; Novitskiy, S.V.; et al. Depletion of carcinoma-associated fibroblasts and fibrosis induces immunosuppression and accelerates pancreas cancer with reduced survival. *Cancer Cell* **2014**, *25*, 719–734. [CrossRef]
62. Rhim, A.D.; Oberstein, P.E.; Thomas, D.H.; Mirek, E.T.; Palermo, C.F.; Sastra, S.A.; Dekleva, E.N.; Saunders, T.; Becerra, C.P.; Tattersall, I.W.; et al. Stromal elements act to restrain, rather than support, pancreatic ductal adenocarcinoma. *Cancer Cell* **2014**, *25*, 735–747. [CrossRef] [PubMed]

63. Biffi, G.; Oni, T.E.; Spielman, B.; Hao, Y.; Elyada, E.; Park, Y.; Preall, J.; Tuveson, D.A. IL1-Induced JAK/STAT Signaling Is Antagonized by TGFβ to Shape CAF Heterogeneity in Pancreatic Ductal Adenocarcinoma. *Cancer Discov.* **2019**, *9*, 282. [CrossRef] [PubMed]
64. Elyada, E.; Bolisetty, M.; Laise, P.; Flynn, W.F.; Courtois, E.T.; Burkhart, R.A.; Teinor, J.A.; Belleau, P.; Biffi, G.; Lucito, M.S.; et al. Cross-species single-cell analysis of pancreatic ductal adenocarcinoma reveals antigen-presenting cancer-associated fibroblasts. *Cancer Discov.* **2019**. [CrossRef] [PubMed]
65. Öhlund, D.; Handly-Santana, A.; Biffi, G.; Elyada, E.; Almeida, A.S.; Ponz-Sarvise, M.; Corbo, V.; Oni, T.E.; Hearn, S.A.; Lee, E.J.; et al. Distinct populations of inflammatory fibroblasts and myofibroblasts in pancreatic cancer. *J. Exp. Med.* **2017**, *214*, 579–596. [CrossRef]
66. Jiang, H.; Hegde, S.; DeNardo, D.G. Tumor-associated fibrosis as a regulator of tumor immunity and response to immunotherapy. *Cancer Immunol. Immunother.* **2017**, *66*, 1037–1048. [CrossRef]
67. Lu, P.; Weaver, V.M.; Werb, Z. The extracellular matrix: A dynamic niche in cancer progression. *J. Cell Biol.* **2012**, *196*, 395–406. [CrossRef]
68. Poltavets, V.; Kochetkova, M.; Pitson, S.M.; Samuel, M.S. The Role of the Extracellular Matrix and Its Molecular and Cellular Regulators in Cancer Cell Plasticity. *Front. Oncol.* **2018**, *8*, 431. [CrossRef]
69. Weichselbaum, R.R.; Ishwaran, H.; Yoon, T.; Nuyten, D.S.A.; Baker, S.W.; Khodarev, N.; Su, A.W.; Shaikh, A.Y.; Roach, P.; Kreike, B.; et al. An interferon-related gene signature for DNA damage resistance is a predictive marker for chemotherapy and radiation for breast cancer. *Proc. Natl. Acad. Sci. USA* **2008**, *105*, 18490–18495. [CrossRef]
70. Puthawala, K.; Hadjiangelis, N.; Jacoby, S.C.; Bayongan, E.; Zhao, Z.; Yang, Z.; Devitt, M.L.; Horan, G.S.; Weinreb, P.H.; Lukashev, M.E.; et al. Inhibition of integrin αvβ6, an activator of latent transforming growth factor-β, prevents radiation-induced lung fibrosis. *Am. J. Respir. Crit. Care Med.* **2008**, *177*, 82–90. [CrossRef]
71. Park, C.C.; Zhang, H.; Pallavicini, M.; Gray, J.W.; Baehner, F.; Park, C.J.; Bissell, M.J. B1 Integrin Inhibitory Antibody Induces Apoptosis of Breast Cancer Cells, Inhibits Growth, and Distinguishes Malignant from Normal Phenotype in Three Dimensional Cultures and in Vivo. *Cancer Res.* **2006**, *66*, 1526–1535. [CrossRef]
72. Park, C.C.; Zhang, H.J.; Yao, E.S.; Park, C.J.; Bissell, M.J. B1 Integrin Inhibition Dramatically Enhances Radiotherapy Efficacy in Human Breast Cancer Xenografts. *Cancer Res.* **2008**, *68*, 4398–4405. [CrossRef] [PubMed]
73. Cordes, N.; Seidler, J.; Durzok, R.; Geinitz, H.; Brakebusch, C. B1-Integrin-Mediated Signaling Essentially Contributes to Cell Survival After Radiation-Induced Genotoxic Injury. *Oncogene* **2006**, *25*, 1378–1390. [CrossRef] [PubMed]
74. Biswas, S.; Freeman, M.L.; Arteaga, C.L.; Biswas, S.; Guix, M.; Rinehart, C.; Dugger, T.C.; Chytil, A.; Moses, H.L.; Freeman, M.L.; et al. Inhibition of TGF Beta with neutralizing antibodies prevents radiation-induced acceleration of metastatic cancer progression Find the latest version: Inhibition of TGF- β with neutralizing antibodies prevents radiation-induced acceleration of metastatic. *J. Clin. Investig.* **2007**, *117*, 1305–1313. [CrossRef] [PubMed]
75. Hellevik, T.; Martinez-Zubiaurre, I. Radiotherapy and the tumor stroma: The importance of dose and fractionation. *Front. Oncol.* **2014**, *4*, 1–12. [CrossRef]
76. Chetty, C.; Bhoopathi, P.; Rao, J.S.; Lakka, S.S. Inhibition of matrix metalloproteinase-2 enhances radiosensitivity by abrogating radiation-induced FoxM1-mediated G2/M arrest in A549 lung cancer cells. *Int. J. Cancer* **2009**, *124*, 2468–2477. [CrossRef]
77. Bertout, J.A.; Patel, S.A.; Simon, M.C. The impact of O2 availability on human cancer. *Nat. Rev. Cancer* **2008**, *8*, 967–975. [CrossRef]
78. Gray, L.H.; Conger, A.D.; Ebert, M.; Hornsey, S.; Scott, O.C.A. The Concentration of Oxygen Dissolved in Tissues at the Time of Irradiation as a Factor in Radiotherapy. *Br. J. Radiol.* **1953**, *26*, 638–648. [CrossRef]
79. Brown, J.M. The hypoxic cell: A target for selective cancer therapy—Eighteenth Bruce F. Cain Memorial Award Lecture. *Cancer Res.* **1999**, *59*, 5863–5870.
80. Brown, J.M. Vasculogenesis: A crucial player in the resistance of solid tumours to radiotherapy. *Br. J. Radiol.* **2014**, *87*. [CrossRef]
81. Frérart, F.; Sonveaux, P.; Rath, G.; Smoos, A.; Meqor, A.; Charlier, N.; Jordan, B.F.; Saliez, J.; Noel, A.; Dessy, C.; et al. The acidic tumor microenvironment promotes the reconversion of nitrite into nitric oxide: Towards a new and safe radiosensitizing strategy. *Clin. Cancer Res.* **2008**, *14*, 2768–2774. [CrossRef]
82. Mitchell, J.B.; Wink, D.A.; DeGraff, W.; Gamson, J.; Keefer, L.K.; Krishna, M.C. Hypoxic mammalian cell radiosensitization by nitric oxide. *Cancer Res.* **1993**, *53*, 5845–5848. [PubMed]

83. Winkler, F.; Kozin, S.V.; Tong, R.T.; Chae, S.-S.; Booth, M.F.; Garkavtsev, I.; Xu, L.; Hicklin, D.J.; Fukumura, D.; di Tomaso, E.; et al. Kinetics of vascular normalization by VEGFR2 blockade governs brain tumor response to radiation. *Cancer Cell* **2004**, *6*, 553–563. [CrossRef] [PubMed]
84. Ansiaux, R.; Baudelet, C.; Jordan, B.F.; Beghein, N.; Sonveaux, P.; De Wever, J.; Martinive, P.; Grégoire, V.; Feron, O.; Gallez, B. Thalidomide radiosensitizes tumors through early changes in the tumor microenvironment. *Clin. Cancer Res.* **2005**, *11*, 743–750.
85. Crokart, N.; Radermacher, K.; Jordan, B.F.; Baudelet, C.; Cron, G.O.; Grégoire, V.; Beghein, N.; Bouzin, C.; Feron, O.; Gallez, B. Tumor radiosensitization by antiinflammatory drugs: Evidence for a new mechanism involving the oxygen effect. *Cancer Res.* **2005**, *65*, 7911–7916. [CrossRef] [PubMed]
86. Demaria, S.; Formenti, S.C. Radiation as an immunological adjuvant: Current evidence on dose and fractionation. *Front. Oncol.* **2012**, *2*, 1–7. [CrossRef]
87. Formenti, S.C.; Rudqvist, N.P.; Golden, E.; Cooper, B.; Wennerberg, E.; Lhuillier, C.; Vanpouille-Box, C.; Friedman, K.; Ferrari de Andrade, L.; Wucherpfennig, K.W.; et al. Radiotherapy induces responses of lung cancer to CTLA-4 blockade. *Nat. Med.* **2018**, *24*, 1845–1851. [CrossRef]
88. Golden, E.B.; Frances, D.; Pellicciotta, I.; Demaria, S.; Helen Barcellos-Hoff, M.; Formenti, S.C. Radiation fosters dose-dependent and chemotherapy-induced immunogenic cell death. *Oncoimmunology* **2014**, *3*, e28518. [CrossRef]
89. Harding, S.M.; Benci, J.L.; Irianto, J.; Discher, D.E.; Minn, A.J.; Greenberg, R.A. Mitotic progression following DNA damage enables pattern recognition within micronuclei. *Nature* **2017**, *548*, 466–470. [CrossRef]
90. Dillon, M.T.; Bergerhoff, K.F.; Pedersen, M.; Whittock, H.; Crespo-Rodriguez, E.; Patin, E.C.; Pearson, A.; Smith, H.G.; Paget, J.T.E.; Patel, R.R.; et al. ATR Inhibition Potentiates the Radiation-induced Inflammatory Tumor Microenvironment. *Clin. Cancer Res.* **2019**, *25*, 3392–3403. [CrossRef]
91. Mackenzie, K.J.; Carroll, P.; Martin, C.A.; Murina, O.; Fluteau, A.; Simpson, D.J.; Olova, N.; Sutcliffe, H.; Rainger, J.K.; Leitch, A.; et al. cGAS surveillance of micronuclei links genome instability to innate immunity. *Nature* **2017**, *548*, 461–465. [CrossRef]
92. Blair, T.C.; Bambina, S.; Alice, A.F.; Kramer, F.; Medler, T.R.; Baird, J.R.; Broz, M.L.; Tormoen, G.W.; Troesch, V.; Crittenden, M.R.; et al. Dendritic Cell Maturation Defines Immunological Responsiveness of Tumors to Radiation Therapy. *J. Immunol.* **2020**, *204*. [CrossRef] [PubMed]
93. Gupta, A.; Probst, H.C.; Vuong, V.; Landshammer, A.; Muth, S.; Yagita, H.; Schwendener, R.; Pruschy, M.; Knuth, A.; van den Broek, M. Radiotherapy Promotes Tumor-Specific Effector CD8 + T Cells via Dendritic Cell Activation. *J. Immunol.* **2012**, *189*, 558–566. [CrossRef] [PubMed]
94. Gerber, S.A.; Sedlacek, A.L.; Cron, K.R.; Murphy, S.P.; Frelinger, J.G.; Lord, E.M. IFN-γ mediates the antitumor effects of radiation therapy in a murine colon tumor. *Am. J. Pathol.* **2013**, *182*, 2345–2354. [CrossRef] [PubMed]
95. Filatenkov, A.; Baker, J.; Mueller, A.M.S.; Kenkel, J.; Ahn, G.O.; Dutt, S.; Zhang, N.; Kohrt, H.; Jensen, K.; Dejbakhsh-Jones, S.; et al. Ablative tumor radiation can change the tumor immune cell microenvironment to induce durable complete remissions. *Clin. Cancer Res.* **2015**, *21*, 3727–3739. [CrossRef]
96. Sharabi, A.B.; Nirschl, C.J.; Kochel, C.M.; Nirschl, T.R.; Francica, B.J.; Velarde, E.; Deweese, T.L.; Drake, C.G. Stereotactic radiation therapy augments antigen-specific PD-1-mediated antitumor immune responses via cross-presentation of tumor antigen. *Cancer Immunol. Res.* **2015**, *3*, 345–355. [CrossRef]
97. Yoshimoto, Y.; Suzuki, Y.; Mimura, K.; Ando, K.; Oike, T.; Sato, H.; Okonogi, N.; Maruyama, T.; Izawa, S.; Noda, S.E.; et al. Radiotherapy-induced anti-tumor immunity contributes to the therapeutic efficacy of irradiation and can be augmented by CTLA-4 blockade in a mouse model. *PLoS ONE* **2014**, *9*, e92572. [CrossRef]
98. Gerber, S.A.; Lim, J.Y.H.; Connolly, K.A.; Sedlacek, A.L.; Barlow, M.L.; Murphy, S.P.; Egilmez, N.K.; Lord, E.M. Radio-responsive tumors exhibit greater intratumoral immune activity than nonresponsive tumors. *Int. J. Cancer* **2014**, *134*, 2383–2392. [CrossRef]
99. Vanpouille-Box, C.; Diamond, J.M.; Pilones, K.A.; Zavadil, J.; Babb, J.S.; Formenti, S.C.; Barcellos-Hoff, M.H.; Demaria, S. TGFβ Is a Master Regulator of Radiation Therapy-Induced Antitumor Immunity. *Cancer Res.* **2015**, *75*, 2232–2242. [CrossRef]
100. Deng, L.; Liang, H.; Burnette, B.; Beckett, M.; Darga, T.; Weichselbaum, R.R.; Fu, Y.X. Irradiation and anti-PD-L1 treatment synergistically promote antitumor immunity in mice. *J. Clin. Investig.* **2014**, *124*, 687–695. [CrossRef]

101. Dovedi, S.J.; Adlard, A.L.; Lipowska-Bhalla, G.; McKenna, C.; Jones, S.; Cheadle, E.J.; Stratford, I.J.; Poon, E.; Morrow, M.; Stewart, R.; et al. Acquired resistance to fractionated radiotherapy can be overcome by concurrent PD-L1 blockade. *Cancer Res.* **2014**, *74*, 5458–5468. [CrossRef]
102. Park, S.S.; Dong, H.; Liu, X.; Harrington, S.M.; Krco, C.J.; Grams, M.P.; Mansfield, A.S.; Furutani, K.M.; Olivier, K.R.; Kwon, E.D. PD-1 Restrains Radiotherapy-Induced Abscopal Effect. *Cancer Immunol. Res.* **2015**, *3*, 610–619. [CrossRef] [PubMed]
103. Formenti, S.C.; Demaria, S. Systemic effects of local radiotherapy. *Lancet Oncol.* **2009**, *10*, 718–726. [CrossRef]
104. Shaverdian, N.; Lisberg, A.E.; Bornazyan, K.; Veruttipong, D.; Goldman, J.W.; Formenti, S.C.; Garon, E.B.; Lee, P. Previous radiotherapy and the clinical activity and toxicity of pembrolizumab in the treatment of non-small-cell lung cancer: A secondary analysis of the KEYNOTE-001 phase 1 trial. *Lancet Oncol.* **2017**, *18*, 895–903. [CrossRef]
105. Kang, J.; Demaria, S.; Formenti, S. Current clinical trials testing the combination of immunotherapy with radiotherapy. *J. Immunother. Cancer* **2016**, *4*, 51. [CrossRef] [PubMed]
106. Milas, L. Tumor Bed Effect in Murine Tumors: Relationship to Tumor Take and Tumor Macrophage Content. *Radiat. Res.* **1990**, *123*, 232. [CrossRef] [PubMed]
107. Vatner, R.E.; Formenti, S.C. Myeloid-derived cells in tumors: Effects of radiation. *Semin. Radiat. Oncol.* **2015**, *25*, 18–27. [CrossRef] [PubMed]
108. Xu, J.; Escamilla, J.; Mok, S.; David, J.; Priceman, S.; West, B.; Bollag, G.; McBride, W.; Wu, L. CSF1R signaling blockade stanches tumor-infiltrating myeloid cells and improves the efficacy of radiotherapy in prostate cancer. *Cancer Res.* **2013**, *73*, 2782–2794. [CrossRef]
109. Ceradini, D.J.; Kulkarni, A.R.; Callaghan, M.J.; Tepper, O.M.; Bastidas, N.; Kleinman, M.E.; Capla, J.M.; Galiano, R.D.; Levine, J.P.; Gurtner, G.C. Progenitor cell trafficking is regulated by hypoxic gradients through HIF-1 induction of SDF-1. *Nat. Med.* **2004**, *10*, 858–864. [CrossRef]
110. Meng, Y.; Beckett, M.A.; Liang, H.; Mauceri, H.J.; Van Rooijen, N.; Cohen, K.S.; Weichselbaum, R.R. Blockade of tumor necrosis factor α signaling in tumor-associated macrophages as a radiosensitizing strategy. *Cancer Res.* **2010**, *70*, 1534–1543. [CrossRef]
111. Prakash, H.; Klug, F.; Nadella, V.; Mazumdar, V.; Schmitz-Winnenthal, H.; Umansky, L. Low doses of gamma irradiation potentially modifies immunosuppressive tumor microenvironment by retuning tumor-associated macrophages: Lesson from insulinoma. *Carcinogenesis* **2016**, *37*, 301–313. [CrossRef]
112. Klug, F.; Prakash, H.; Huber, P.E.; Seibel, T.; Bender, N.; Halama, N.; Pfirschke, C.; Voss, R.H.; Timke, C.; Umansky, L.; et al. Low-dose irradiation programs macrophage differentiation to an iNOS^{+}/M1 phenotype that orchestrates effective T cell immunotherapy. *Cancer Cell* **2013**, *24*, 589–602. [CrossRef] [PubMed]
113. Chiang, C.S.; Fu, S.Y.; Wang, S.C.; Yu, C.F.; Chen, F.H.; Lin, C.M.; Hong, J.H. Irradiation promotes an m2 macrophage phenotype in tumor hypoxia. *Front. Oncol.* **2012**, *2*, 89. [CrossRef] [PubMed]
114. Okubo, M.; Kioi, M.; Nakashima, H.; Sugiura, K.; Mitsudo, K.; Aoki, I.; Taniguchi, H.; Tohnai, I. M2-polarized macrophages contribute to neovasculogenesis, leading to relapse of oral cancer following radiation. *Sci. Rep.* **2016**, *6*, 27548. [CrossRef] [PubMed]
115. Seifert, L.; Werba, G.; Tiwari, S.; Giao Ly, N.N.; Nguy, S.; Alothman, S.; Alqunaibit, D.; Avanzi, A.; Daley, D.; Barilla, R.; et al. Radiation Therapy Induces Macrophages to Suppress T-Cell Responses Against Pancreatic Tumors in Mice. *Gastroenterology* **2016**, *150*, 1659–1672. [CrossRef] [PubMed]
116. Crittenden, M.R.; Cottam, B.; Savage, T.; Nguyen, C.; Newell, P.; Gough, M.J. Expression of NF-κb p50 in tumor stroma limits the control of tumors by radiation therapy. *PLoS ONE* **2012**, *7*, e39295. [CrossRef] [PubMed]
117. Shiao, S.L.; Ruffell, B.; DeNardo, D.G.; Faddegon, B.A.; Park, C.C.; Coussens, L.M. TH2-polarized CD4+ T Cells and macrophages limit efficacy of radiotherapy. *Cancer Immunol. Res.* **2015**, *3*, 518–525. [CrossRef]
118. Chen, H.M.; Ma, G.; Gildener-Leapman, N.; Eisenstein, S.; Coakley, B.A.; Ozao, J.; Mandeli, J.; Divino, C.; Schwartz, M.; Sung, M.; et al. Myeloid-derived suppressor cells as an immune parameter in patients with concurrent sunitinib and stereotactic body radiotherapy. *Clin. Cancer Res.* **2015**, *21*, 4073–4085. [CrossRef] [PubMed]
119. Ko, J.S.; Zea, A.H.; Rini, B.I.; Ireland, J.L.; Elson, P.; Cohen, P.; Golshayan, A.; Rayman, P.A.; Wood, L.; Garcia, J.; et al. Sunitinib mediates reversal of myeloid-derived suppressor cell accumulation in renal cell carcinoma patients. *Clin. Cancer Res.* **2009**, *15*, 2148–2157. [CrossRef]

120. Persa, E.; Balogh, A.; Sáfrány, G.; Lumniczky, K. The effect of ionizing radiation on regulatory T cells in health and disease. *Cancer Lett.* **2015**, *368*, 252–261. [CrossRef]
121. Facciabene, A.; Motz, G.T.; Coukos, G. T-Regulatory cells: Key players in tumor immune escape and angiogenesis. *Cancer Res.* **2012**, *72*, 2162–2171. [CrossRef]
122. Kachikwu, E.L.; Iwamoto, K.S.; Liao, Y.P.; Demarco, J.J.; Agazaryan, N.; Economou, J.S.; McBride, W.H.; Schaue, D. Radiation enhances regulatory T cell representation. *Int. J. Radiat. Oncol. Biol. Phys.* **2011**, *81*, 1128–1135. [CrossRef] [PubMed]
123. Qinfeng, S.; Depu, W.; Xiaofeng, Y.; Shah, W.; Hongwei, C.; Yili, W. In situ observation of the effects of local irradiation on cytotoxic and regulatory T lymphocytes in cervical cancer tissue. *Radiat. Res.* **2013**, *179*, 584–589. [CrossRef] [PubMed]
124. Komatsu, N.; Hori, S. Full restoration of peripheral Foxp3+ regulatory T cell pool by radioresistant host cells in scurfy bone marrow chimeras. *Proc. Natl. Acad. Sci. USA* **2007**, *104*, 8959–8964. [CrossRef] [PubMed]
125. Schaue, D.; Xie, M.W.; Ratikan, J.A.; McBride, W.H. Regulatory T cells in radiotherapeutic responses. *Front. Oncol.* **2012**, *2*, 90. [CrossRef] [PubMed]
126. Bos, P.D.; Plitas, G.; Rudra, D.; Lee, S.Y.; Rudensky, A.Y. Transient regulatory T cell ablation deters oncogene-driven breast cancer and enhances radiotherapy. *J. Exp. Med.* **2013**, *210*, 2435–2466. [CrossRef] [PubMed]
127. Oweida, A.J.; Darragh, L.; Phan, A.; Binder, D.; Bhatia, S.; Mueller, A.; Court, B.V.; Milner, D.; Raben, D.; Woessner, R.; et al. STAT3 Modulation of Regulatory T Cells in Response to Radiation Therapy in Head and Neck Cancer. *J. Natl. Cancer Inst.* **2019**, *111*, 1339–1349. [CrossRef] [PubMed]
128. Oweida, A.; Hararah, M.K.; Phan, A.; Binder, D.; Bhatia, S.; Lennon, S.; Bukkapatnam, S.; Van Court, B.; Uyanga, N.; Darragh, L.; et al. Resistance to Radiotherapy and PD-L1 Blockade Is Mediated by TIM-3 Upregulation and Regulatory T-Cell Infiltration. *Clin. Cancer Res.* **2018**, *24*, 5368–5380. [CrossRef] [PubMed]
129. Bhatia, S.; Oweida, A.; Lennon, S.; Darragh, L.B.; Milner, D.; Phan, A.V.; Mueller, A.C.; Van Court, B.; Raben, D.; Serkova, N.J.; et al. Inhibition of EphB4-Ephrin-B2 Signaling Reprograms the Tumor Immune Microenvironment in Head and Neck Cancers. *Cancer Res.* **2019**, *79*, 2722–2735. [CrossRef]
130. Schaue, D.; Ratikan, J.A.; Iwamoto, K.S.; McBride, W.H. Maximizing tumor immunity with fractionated radiation. *Int. J. Radiat. Oncol. Biol. Phys.* **2012**, *83*, 1306–1310. [CrossRef]
131. Lugade, A.A.; Moran, J.P.; Gerber, S.A.; Rose, R.C.; Frelinger, J.G.; Lord, E.M. Local radiation therapy of B16 melanoma tumors increases the generation of tumor antigen-specific effector cells that traffic to the tumor. *J. Immunol.* **2005**, *174*, 7516–7523. [CrossRef]
132. Apetoh, L.; Ghiringhelli, F.; Tesniere, A.; Obeid, M.; Ortiz, C.; Criollo, A.; Mignot, G.; Maiuri, M.C.; Ullrich, E.; Saulnier, P.; et al. Toll-like receptor 4-dependent contribution of the immune system to anticancer chemotherapy and radiotherapy. *Nat. Med.* **2007**, *13*, 1050–1059. [CrossRef] [PubMed]
133. Demaria, S.; Golden, E.B.; Formenti, S.C. Role of Local Radiation Therapy in Cancer Immunotherapy. *JAMA Oncol.* **2015**, *1*, 1325–1332. [CrossRef] [PubMed]
134. Obeid, M.; Tesniere, A.; Ghiringhelli, F.; Fimia, G.M.; Apetoh, L.; Perfettini, J.L.; Castedo, M.; Mignot, G.; Panaretakis, T.; Casares, N.; et al. Calreticulin exposure dictates the immunogenicity of cancer cell death. *Nat. Med.* **2007**, *13*, 54–61. [CrossRef]
135. Ghiringhelli, F.; Apetoh, L.; Tesniere, A.; Aymeric, L.; Ma, Y.; Ortiz, C.; Vermaelen, K.; Panaretakis, T.; Mignot, G.; Ullrich, E.; et al. Activation of the NLRP3 inflammasome in dendritic cells induces IL-1beta-dependent adaptive immunity against tumors. *Nat. Med.* **2009**, *15*, 1170–1178. [CrossRef] [PubMed]
136. Gulley, J.L.; Arlen, P.M.; Bastian, A.; Morin, S.; Marte, J.; Beetham, P.; Tsang, K.Y.; Yokokawa, J.; Hodge, J.W.; Ménard, C.; et al. Combining a recombinant cancer vaccine with standard definitive radiotherapy in patients with localized prostate cancer. *Clin. Cancer Res.* **2005**, *11*, 3353–3362. [CrossRef]
137. Schaue, D.; Comin-Anduix, B.; Ribas, A.; Zhang, L.; Goodglick, L.; Sayre, J.W.; Debucquoy, A.; Haustermans, K.; McBride, W.H. T-cell responses to survivin in cancer patients undergoing radiation therapy. *Clin. Cancer Res.* **2008**, *14*, 4883–4890. [CrossRef]
138. Rutkowski, J.; Ślebioda, T.; Kmieć, Z.; Zaucha, R. Changes in systemic immune response after stereotactic ablative radiotherapy. Preliminary results of a prospective study in patients with early lung cancer. *Pol. Arch. Intern. Med.* **2017**, *127*, 245–253. [CrossRef]

139. Wasserman, J.; Blomgren, H.; Rotstein, S.; Petrini, B.; Hammarström, S. Immunosuppression in irradiated breast cancer patients: In vitro effect of cyclooxygenase inhibitors. *Bull. N. Y. Acad. Med.* **1989**, *65*, 36–44.
140. Rödel, F.; Frey, B.; Manda, K.; Hildebrandt, G.; Hehlgans, S.; Keilholz, L.; Seegenschmiedt, M.H.; Gaipl, U.S.; Rödel, C. Immunomodulatory properties and molecular effects in inflammatory diseases of low-dose x-irradiation. *Front. Oncol.* **2012**, *2*, 120. [CrossRef]
141. Trowell, O.A. The sensitivity of lymphocytes to ionising radiation. *J. Pathol. Bacteriol.* **1952**, *64*, 687–704. [CrossRef]
142. Frey, B.; Rückert, M.; Weber, J.; Mayr, X.; Derer, A.; Lotter, M.; Bert, C.; Rödel, F.; Fietkau, R.; Gaipl, U.S. Hypofractionated Irradiation Has Immune Stimulatory Potential and Induces a Timely Restricted Infiltration of Immune Cells in Colon Cancer Tumors. *Front. Immunol.* **2017**, *8*, 231. [CrossRef] [PubMed]
143. Panni, R.Z.; Herndon, J.M.; Zuo, C.; Hegde, S.; Hogg, G.D.; Knolhoff, B.L.; Breden, M.A.; Li, X.; Krisnawan, V.E.; Khan, S.Q.; et al. Agonism of CD11b reprograms innate immunity to sensitize pancreatic cancer to immunotherapies. *Sci. Transl. Med.* **2019**, *11*. [CrossRef] [PubMed]
144. Hegde, S.; Krisnawan, V.E.; Herzog, B.H.; Zuo, C.; Breden, M.A.; Knolhoff, B.L.; Hogg, G.D.; Tang, J.P.; Baer, J.M.; Mpoy, C.; et al. Dendritic Cell Paucity Leads to Dysfunctional Immune Surveillance in Pancreatic Cancer. *Cancer Cell* **2020**, *37*, 289–307. [CrossRef] [PubMed]
145. Wisdom, A.J.; Hong, C.S.; Lin, A.J.; Xiang, Y.; Cooper, D.E.; Zhang, J.; Xu, E.S.; Kuo, H.C.; Mowery, Y.M.; Carpenter, D.J.; et al. Neutrophils promote tumor resistance to radiation therapy. *Proc. Natl. Acad. Sci. USA* **2019**, *116*, 18584–18589. [CrossRef] [PubMed]
146. Matsumura, S.; Demaria, S. Up-regulation of the pro-inflammatory chemokine CXCL16 is a common response of tumor cells to ionizing radiation. *Radiat. Res.* **2010**, *173*, 418–425. [CrossRef]
147. Matsumura, S.; Wang, B.; Kawashima, N.; Braunstein, S.; Badura, M.; Cameron, T.O.; Babb, J.S.; Schneider, R.J.; Formenti, S.C.; Dustin, M.L.; et al. Radiation-induced CXCL16 release by breast cancer cells attracts effector T cells. *J. Immunol.* **2008**, *181*, 3099–3107. [CrossRef]
148. Lugade, A.A.; Sorensen, E.W.; Gerber, S.A.; Moran, J.P.; Frelinger, J.G.; Lord, E.M. Radiation-induced IFN-gamma production within the tumor microenvironment influences antitumor immunity. *J. Immunol.* **2008**, *180*, 3132–3139. [CrossRef]
149. Hallahan, D.E.; Spriggs, D.R.; Beckett, M.A.; Kufe, D.W.; Weichselbaum, R.R. Increased tumor necrosis factor alpha mRNA after cellular exposure to ionizing radiation. *Proc. Natl. Acad. Sci. USA* **1989**, *86*, 10104–10107. [CrossRef]
150. Barcellos-Hoff, M.H.; Derynck, R.; Tsang, M.L.; Weatherbee, J.A. Transforming growth factor-beta activation in irradiated murine mammary gland. *J. Clin. Investig.* **1994**, *93*, 892–899. [CrossRef]
151. Marincola, F.M.; Jaffee, E.M.; Hicklin, D.J.; Ferrone, S. Escape of human solid tumors from T-cell recognition: Molecular mechanisms and functional significance. *Adv. Immunol.* **2000**, *74*, 181–273. [CrossRef]
152. Klein, B.; Loven, D.; Lurie, H.; Rakowsky, E.; Nyska, A.; Levin, I.; Klein, T. The effect of irradiation on expression of HLA class I antigens in human brain tumors in culture. *J. Neurosurg.* **1994**, *80*, 1074–1077. [CrossRef] [PubMed]
153. Santin, A.D.; Hermonat, P.L.; Hiserodt, J.C.; Chiriva-Internati, M.; Woodliff, J.; Theus, J.W.; Barclay, D.; Pecorelli, S.; Parham, G.P. Effects of irradiation on the expression of major histocompatibility complex class I antigen and adhesion costimulation molecules ICAM-1 in human cervical cancer. *Int. J. Radiat. Oncol. Biol. Phys.* **1997**, *39*, 737–742. [CrossRef]
154. Santin, A.D.; Hiserodt, J.C.; Fruehauf, J.; DiSaia, P.J.; Pecorelli, S.; Granger, G.A. Effects of irradiation on the expression of surface antigens in human ovarian cancer. *Gynecol. Oncol.* **1996**, *60*, 468–474. [CrossRef] [PubMed]
155. Wan, S.; Pestka, S.; Jubin, R.G.; Lyu, Y.L.; Tsai, Y.C.; Liu, L.F. Chemotherapeutics and radiation stimulate MHC class I expression through elevated interferon-beta signaling in breast cancer cells. *PLoS ONE* **2012**, *7*, e32542. [CrossRef]
156. Zhu, Y.; Herndon, J.M.; Sojka, D.K.; Kim, K.W.; Knolhoff, B.L.; Zuo, C.; Cullinan, D.R.; Luo, J.; Bearden, A.R.; Lavine, K.J.; et al. Tissue-Resident Macrophages in Pancreatic Ductal Adenocarcinoma Originate from Embryonic Hematopoiesis and Promote Tumor Progression. *Immunity* **2017**, *47*, 323–338. [CrossRef]
157. Wynn, T.A.; Chawla, A.; Pollard, J.W. Macrophage biology in development, homeostasis and disease. *Nature* **2013**, *496*, 445–455. [CrossRef]

158. DeNardo, D.G.; Ruffell, B. Macrophages as regulators of tumour immunity and immunotherapy. *Nat. Rev. Immunol.* **2019**, *19*, 369–382. [CrossRef]
159. Kraman, M.; Bambrough, P.J.; Arnold, J.N.; Roberts, E.W.; Magiera, L.; Jones, J.O.; Gopinathan, A.; Tuveson, D.A.; Fearon, D.T. Suppression of Antitumor. *Science* **2010**, *330*, 827–830. [CrossRef]
160. Lourdes Mora-García, M.; García-Rocha, R.; Morales-Ramírez, O.; Montesinos, J.J.; Weiss-Steider, B.; Hernández-Montes, J.; Ávila-Ibarra, L.R.; Don-López, C.A.; Velasco-Velázquez, M.A.; Gutiérrez-Serrano, V.; et al. Mesenchymal stromal cells derived from cervical cancer produce high amounts of adenosine to suppress cytotoxic T lymphocyte functions. *J. Transl. Med.* **2016**, *14*, 1–14. [CrossRef]
161. Erez, N.; Truitt, M.; Olson, P.; Hanahan, D. Cancer-Associated Fibroblasts Are Activated in Incipient Neoplasia to Orchestrate Tumor-Promoting Inflammation in an NF-κB-Dependent Manner. *Cancer Cell* **2010**, *17*, 135–147. [CrossRef]
162. Liu, T.; Han, C.; Wang, S.; Fang, P.; Ma, Z.; Xu, L.; Yin, R. Cancer-associated fibroblasts: An emerging target of anti-cancer immunotherapy. *J. Hematol. Oncol.* **2019**, *12*, 86. [CrossRef] [PubMed]
163. Wynn, T.A.; Ramalingam, T.R. Mechanisms of fibrosis: Therapeutic translation for fibrotic disease. *Nat. Med.* **2012**, *18*, 1028–1040. [CrossRef] [PubMed]
164. Cheng, J.t.; Deng, Y.n.; Yi, H.m.; Wang, G.y.; Fu, B.s.; Chen, W.j.; Liu, W.; Tai, Y.; Peng, Y.w.; Zhang, Q. Hepatic carcinoma-associated fibroblasts induce IDO-producing regulatory dendritic cells through IL-6-mediated STAT3 activation. *Oncogenesis* **2016**, *5*, e198. [CrossRef]
165. Khosravi-Maharlooei, M.; Pakyari, M.; Jalili, R.B.; Salimi-Elizei, S.; Lai, J.C.Y.; Poormasjedi-Meibod, M.; Kilani, R.T.; Dutz, J.; Ghahary, A. Tolerogenic effect of mouse fibroblasts on dendritic cells. *Immunology* **2016**, *148*, 22–33. [CrossRef] [PubMed]
166. Mace, T.A.; Ameen, Z.; Collins, A.; Wojcik, S.; Mair, M.; Young, G.S.; Fuchs, J.R.; Eubank, T.D.; Frankel, W.L.; Bekaii-Saab, T.; et al. Pancreatic Cancer-Associated Stellate Cells Promote Differentiation of Myeloid-Derived Suppressor Cells in a STAT3-Dependent Manner. *Cancer Res.* **2013**, *73*, 3007. [CrossRef]
167. Kim, J.H.; Oh, S.-H.; Kim, E.-J.; Park, S.J.; Hong, S.P.; Cheon, J.H.; Kim, T.I.; Kim, W.H. The role of myofibroblasts in upregulation of S100A8 and S100A9 and the differentiation of myeloid cells in the colorectal cancer microenvironment. *Biochem. Biophys. Res. Commun.* **2012**, *423*, 60–66. [CrossRef]
168. Feig, C.; Jones, J.O.; Kraman, M.; Wells, R.J.B.; Deonarine, A.; Chan, D.S.; Connell, C.M.; Roberts, E.W.; Zhao, Q.; Caballero, O.L.; et al. Targeting CXCL12 from FAP-expressing carcinoma-associated fibroblasts synergizes with anti–PD-L1 immunotherapy in pancreatic cancer. *PNAS* **2013**, *110*, 20212. [CrossRef]
169. Jiang, H.; Hegde, S.; Knolhoff, B.L.; Zhu, Y.; Herndon, J.M.; Meyer, M.A.; Nywening, T.M.; Hawkins, W.G.; Shapiro, I.M.; Weaver, D.T.; et al. Targeting focal adhesion kinase renders pancreatic cancers responsive to checkpoint immunotherapy. *Nat. Med.* **2016**, *22*, 851–860. [CrossRef]
170. Serrels, A.; Lund, T.; Serrels, B.; Byron, A.; McPherson, R.C.; von Kriegsheim, A.; Gómez-Cuadrado, L.; Canel, M.; Muir, M.; Ring, J.; et al. Nuclear FAK Controls Chemokine Transcription, Tregs, and Evasion of Anti-tumor Immunity. *Cell* **2015**, *163*, 160–173. [CrossRef]
171. Ager, E.I.; Kozin, S.V.; Kirkpatrick, N.D.; Seano, G.; Kodack, D.P.; Askoxylakis, V.; Huang, Y.; Goel, S.; Snuderl, M.; Muzikansky, A.; et al. Blockade of MMP14 activity in murine breast carcinomas: Implications for macrophages, vessels, and radiotherapy. *J. Natl. Cancer Inst.* **2015**, *107*, 1–12. [CrossRef]
172. Shibuya, M. Vascular endothelial growth factor and its receptor system: Physiological functions in angiogenesis and pathological roles in various diseases. *J. Biochem.* **2013**, *153*, 13–19. [CrossRef] [PubMed]
173. Kibria, G.; Hatakeyama, H.; Harashima, H. Cancer multidrug resistance: Mechanisms involved and strategies for circumvention using a drug delivery system. *Arch. Pharm. Res.* **2014**, *37*, 4–15. [CrossRef] [PubMed]
174. Lanitis, E.; Irving, M.; Coukos, G. Targeting the tumor vasculature to enhance T cell activity. *Curr. Opin. Immunol.* **2015**, *33*, 55–63. [CrossRef] [PubMed]
175. Tsai, C.S.; Chen, F.H.; Wang, C.C.; Huang, H.L.; Jung, S.M.; Wu, C.J.; Lee, C.C.; McBride, W.H.; Chiang, C.S.; Hong, J.H. Macrophages from irradiated tumors express higher levels of iNOS, arginase-I and COX-2, and promote tumor growth. *Int. J. Radiat. Oncol. Biol. Phys.* **2007**, *68*, 499–507. [CrossRef] [PubMed]
176. Park, H.J.; Griffin, R.J.; Hui, S.; Levitt, S.H.; Song, C.W. Radiation-induced vascular damage in tumors: Implications of vascular damage in ablative hypofractionated radiotherapy (SBRT and SRS). *Radiat. Res.* **2012**, *177*, 311–327. [CrossRef]

177. Hasmim, M.; Noman, M.Z.; Messai, Y.; Bordereaux, D.; Gros, G.; Baud, V.; Chouaib, S. Cutting edge: Hypoxia-induced Nanog favors the intratumoral infiltration of regulatory T cells and macrophages via direct regulation of TGF-β1. *J. Immunol.* **2013**, *191*, 5802–5806. [CrossRef]
178. Kocher, M.; Treuer, H.; Voges, J.; Hoevels, M.; Sturm, V.; Müller, R.P. Computer simulation of cytotoxic and vascular effects of radiosurgery in solid and necrotic brain metastases. *Radiother. Oncol.* **2000**, *54*, 149–156. [CrossRef]
179. Sonveaux, P.; Dessy, C.; Brouet, A.; Jordan, B.F.; Grégoire, V.; Gallez, B.; Balligand, J.L.; Feron, O. Modulation of the tumor vasculature functionality by ionizing radiation accounts for tumor radiosensitization and promotes gene delivery. *FASEB J.* **2002**, *16*, 1979–1981. [CrossRef]
180. Crokart, N.; Jordan, B.F.; Baudelet, C.; Ansiaux, R.; Sonveaux, P.; Grégoire, V.; Beghein, N.; DeWever, J.; Bouzin, C.; Feron, O.; et al. Early reoxygenation in tumors after irradiation: Determining factors and consequences for radiotherapy regimens using daily multiple fractions. *Int. J. Radiat. Oncol. Biol. Phys.* **2005**, *63*, 901–910. [CrossRef]
181. Rao, S.S.; Thompson, C.; Cheng, J.; Haimovitz-Friedman, A.; Powell, S.N.; Fuks, Z.; Kolesnick, R.N. Axitinib sensitization of high Single Dose Radiotherapy. *Radiother. Oncol.* **2014**, *111*, 88–93. [CrossRef]
182. Choi, J.; Cha, Y.J.; Koo, J.S. Adipocyte biology in breast cancer: From silent bystander to active facilitator. *Prog. Lipid Res.* **2018**, *69*, 11–20. [CrossRef] [PubMed]
183. Bochet, L.; Meulle, A.; Imbert, S.; Salles, B.; Valet, P.; Muller, C. Cancer-associated adipocytes promotes breast tumor radioresistance. *Biochem. Biophys. Res. Commun* **2011**, *411*, 102–106. [CrossRef] [PubMed]
184. Meng, G.; Tang, X.; Yang, Z.; Benesch, M.G.K.; Marshall, A.; Murray, D.; Hemmings, D.G.; Wuest, F.; McMullen, T.P.W.; Brindley, D.N. Implications for breast cancer treatment from increased autotaxin production in adipose tissue after radiotherapy. *FASEB J.* **2017**, *31*, 4064–4077. [CrossRef] [PubMed]
185. Begg, A.C.; Stewart, F.A.; Vens, C. Strategies to improve radiotherapy with targeted drugs. *Nat. Rev. Cancer* **2011**, *11*, 239–253. [CrossRef] [PubMed]
186. Vozenin, M.C.; Hendry, J.H.; Limoli, C.L. Biological Benefits of Ultra-high Dose Rate FLASH Radiotherapy: Sleeping Beauty Awoken. *Clin. Oncol.* **2019**, *31*, 407–415. [CrossRef]
187. Harrington, K.J. Ultrahigh dose-rate radiotherapy: Next steps for FLASH-RT. *Clin. Cancer Res.* **2019**, *25*, 3–5. [CrossRef]

13

Histone Demethylase KDM5B as a Therapeutic Target for Cancer Therapy

Anmi Jose [1], Gautham G. Shenoy [2], Gabriel Sunil Rodrigues [3], Naveena A. N. Kumar [4], Murali Munisamy [1], Levin Thomas [1], Jill Kolesar [5], Ganesha Rai [6], Praveen P. N. Rao [7] and Mahadev Rao [1,*]

1. Department of Pharmacy Practice, Manipal College of Pharmaceutical Sciences, Manipal Academy of Higher Education, Manipal, Karnataka 576104, India; anmi.jose@learner.manipal.edu (A.J.); murali.m@manipal.edu (M.M.); levin.thomas@learner.manipal.edu (L.T.)
2. Department of Pharmaceutical Chemistry, Manipal College of Pharmaceutical Sciences, Manipal Academy of Higher Education, Manipal, Karnataka 576104, India; gautham.gs@manipal.edu
3. Department of Surgery, Kasturba Medical College, Manipal Academy of Higher Education, Manipal, Karnataka 576104, India; gaby.rodrigues@manipal.edu
4. Department of Surgical Oncology, Kasturba Medical College, Manipal Academy of Higher Education, Manipal, Karnataka 576104, India; naveenkumar.an@manipal.edu
5. Department of Pharmacy Practice & Science, 567 TODD Building, 789 South Limestone Street, Lexington, KY 40539-0596, USA; jill.kolesar@uky.edu
6. National Center for Advancing Translational Sciences, National Institutes of Health, 9800 Medical Center Drive, MSC 3370, Bethesda, MD 20892, USA; bantukallug@mail.nih.gov
7. School of Pharmacy, Health Sciences Campus, 200 University Avenue West, University of Waterloo, Waterloo, ON N2L 3G1, Canada; praopera@uwaterloo.ca

* Correspondence: mahadev.rao@manipal.edu

Abstract: Lysine-specific demethylase 5B (KDM5B/PLU1/JARID1B) is found to be overexpressed in numerous malignancies, including breast, lung, skin, liver, and prostate cancer. Identification of molecules targeting the KDM5B enzyme could be a potential lead in cancer research. Although many KDM5B inhibitors with promising outcomes have been developed so far, its further application in clinical practice is limited due to toxicity and lack of target specificity. Here, we summarize the significance of targeting KDM5B in anticancer therapy and report the molecular docking studies of some known anti-viral agents, decitabine, entecavir, abacavir, penciclovir, and 3-deazaneplanocin A in the catalytic domain JmjC of KDM5B. These studies show the repurposing potential of identified anti-viral agents in cancer therapy.

Keywords: cancer; histone modification; inhibitor; KDM5B; molecular docking; repurposing

1. Introduction

Studies over the past few decades and ongoing research reveal that, along with genetic alterations, epigenetic aberrations play a vital part in the evolution and progress of numerous diseases, including several types of cancers [1]. Epigenetic changes, including DNA methylation and histone modifications, cause altered gene expression without changing the DNA sequence [2,3].

Histone, being the functional protein, not only actively takes part in gene expression, but also acts as a spool for DNA to wind around. Any modification on histone molecules via methylation, acetylation, phosphorylation, ubiquitylation, or sumoylation alters the compact chromatin architecture, leading to abnormal gene expression [4]. Histone methylation on arginine or lysine, which are abundantly present on N- and C- terminal tails of histones, can either turn on or off transcription based on the degree and location of methylation [5].

Lysine-specific demethylation is finely tuned by two enzyme categories, called lysine-specific demethylase (KDM1/LSD1) and the JumonjiC (JmjC) domain, encompassing histone demethylases (KDMs). JmjC, being the largest among two families, displays high substrate specificity, with demethylase activity targeting histones H3 and H4 [6]. In mammals, around thirty KDMs have been identified and grouped as phylogenetically distinct subfamilies from KDM2-8 with numerous subcategories [7].

The KDM5/JARID1 subfamily consists of four interrelated histone demethylase enzymes—KDM5A, KDM5B, KDM5C and KDM5D—involved in several human biological processes, including hormonal response, stem cell regeneration, genomic stability, cellular proliferation, and differentiation [8,9]. KDM5B (also known as PLU1 or JARID1B), demethylates lysine 4 of histone 3 (H3K4), and acts as a transcriptional repressor on certain tumor suppressor genes, thus converting it into the transcriptionally inactive state [10]. The deregulated expression of KDM5B has been implicated in numerous cancer types, including breast, lung, skin, prostate, testis, and liver [11]. Figure 1 depicts the top ten cancers, with high KDM5B mRNA expression data extracted from cBioPortal for cancer genomics—TCGA, PanCancer Atlas study [12–14]. Thus, KDM5B could be considered as a potential therapeutic target in precision oncology. Hence, drugs that can selectively inhibit KDM5B could be of substantial importance as a therapeutic intervention for such cancer types. This review attempts to comprehend, as thoroughly as possible, the oncogenic role of KDM5B in major cancer types and the drug repurposing potential of some known small molecules by targeting KDM5B's catalytic domain through molecular docking studies.

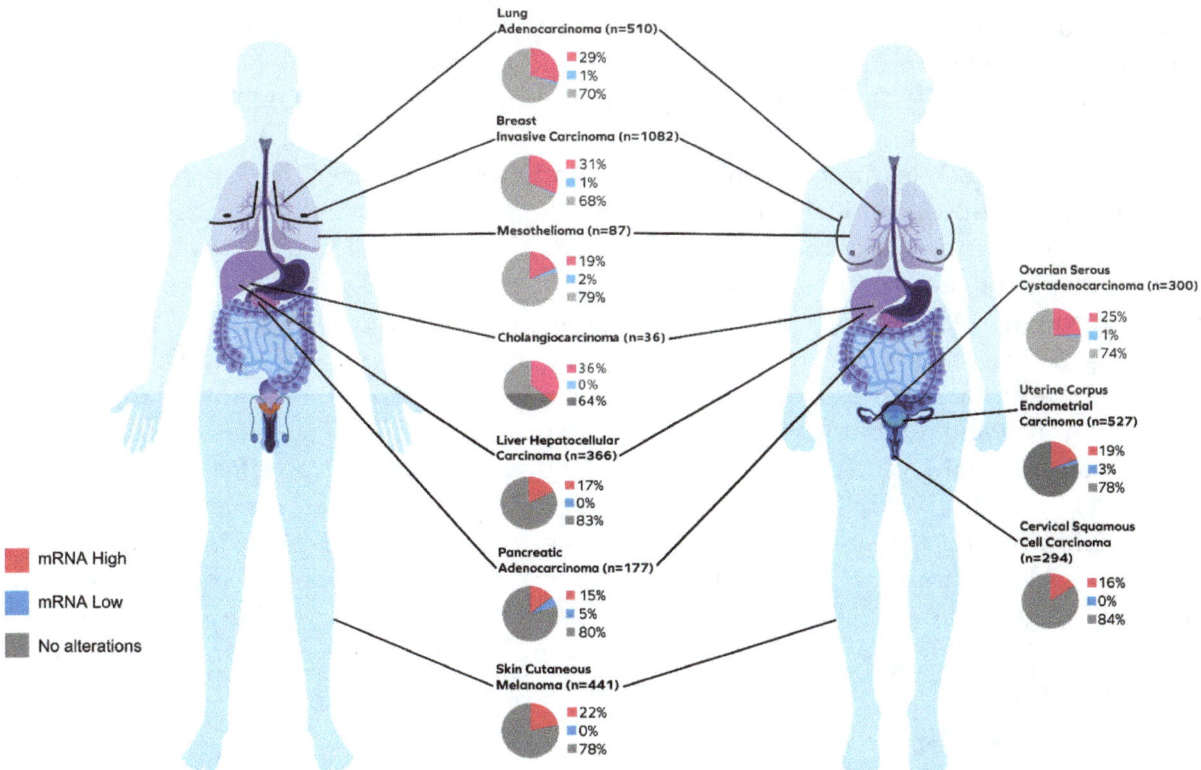

Figure 1. Pictorial representation of the top ten cancers with high KDM5B mRNA expression. Data extracted from the cBioPortal for cancer genomics—TCGA, PanCancer Atlas (n = number of patients).

2. Structure and Enzymatic Function of KDM5B

The JmjC family is reliant on Fe (II) and α- ketoglutarate co-factors for its demethylating activity. KDM5B gene consists of 4632 bases, positioned on chromosome 1, in the cytogenetic band of 1q32.1 with a molecular mass of 175 kilodaltons. It encodes a protein of 1544 amino acids [15] comprising an *N*-terminal Jumonji (JmjN) domain, a catalytic JmjC domain, an AT-rich domain (ARID), a C5HC2 zinc finger domain, a PLU1 motif and three plant homeobox domain (PHD1, PHD2, and PHD3). The domain architecture of KDM5B is highly conserved and homologous from yeast to humans. JmjN and JmjC are vital domains required for enzymatic activity, whereas AT-rich domain binds to GC rich DNA sequences. PHD domains contribute to substrate recognition in which it prevents reverse reaction [16–21]. ARID and PHD domains have very less influence, whereas JmjN and JmjC along with C5HC2 zinc finger domain have more impact on the KDM5B's catalytic activity. The overall catalytic core is composed of three conserved domains consisting of: (i) the JmjN, JmjC, and ARID domains (residues 31–72, 375–602 and 94–100, respectively); (ii) a C-terminal helical domain (residues 604–671 and 737–753); (iii) a β-sheet composed of three β-strands (residues 673–734) that harbored a C5HC2 zinc finger motif [20].

3. Significance of KDM5B in Various Cancers

3.1. Breast Cancer

Although the consistent expression of KDM5B in breast cancer was established by Lu P.J. et al. [22] in 1999, Yamane K. et al. in 2007 revealed the salient role of KDM5B in breast cancer cell proliferation via the transcriptional repression of tumor suppressor genes, including BRCA1 [19]. Subsequent studies both in vitro and in vivo, involving gene expression and KDM5B knockdown, confirmed its putative role in breast tumorigenesis [19,23–25]. One of the proposed mechanisms of KDM5B-mediated tumor cell proliferation was by repressing tumor suppressor miRNA let-7e [26]. Besides, the TFAP2C-Myc-KDM5B complex can repress p21, leading to tumorigenesis and therapy failure [27]. A recent study showed that estrogen receptor-positive (ER^+) tumors, with KDM5B overexpression, had poor clinical outcomes and resistance to hormonal therapy [25]. Moreover, KDM5B expression was found to be negatively correlated with p16 protein expression [28]. Significantly, microRNA hsa-miR-448 can suppress KDM5B expression through MALAT1 and can prevent triple-negative breast cancer (TNBC) progression [29]. The downregulation of KDM5B led to 3'UTR lengthening of the cyclin D1 (CCND1) oncogene and lengthening of a tumor suppressor gene, DICER1, suggesting KDM5B as a novel target for 3'UTR processing [30]. KDM5B inhibition promoted the re-expression of tumor suppressor protein HEXIM1, and upregulated HEXIM1 aided in the inhibition of breast cancer cell proliferation using KDM5B inhibitors [31]. Recently, Paroni G. et al. showed that HER2–positive breast cancer cells were sensitive to KDM5 inhibition and KDM5 inhibitors exhibited a synergistic effect with HER2 targeting drugs, trastuzumab and lapatinib [32]. Similarly, numerous studies have reported the oncogenic role of KDM5B, where gene expression levels were related with poor prognosis, cancer cell proliferation, and metastasis [33–35]. Figure 2 shows the KDM5B mRNA overexpression in breast cancer from various studies retrieved from the cBioPortal for cancer genomics [12–14,36–38].

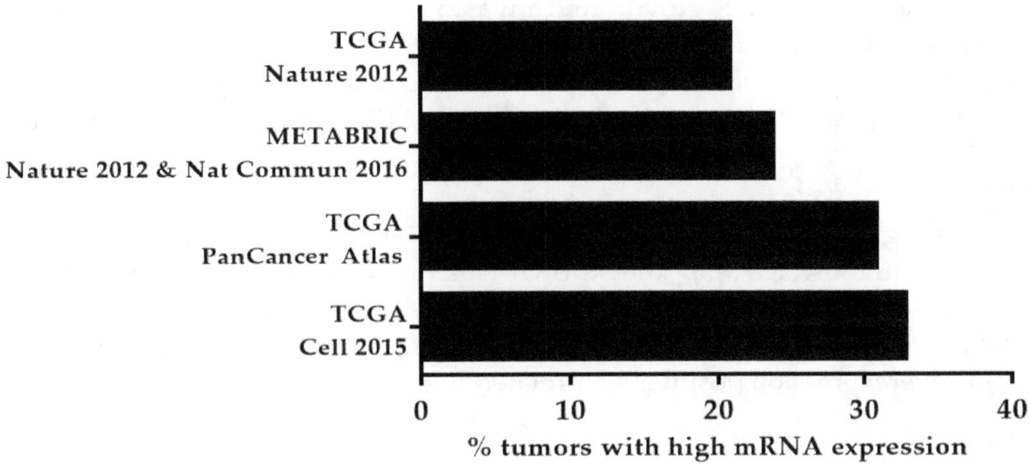

Figure 2. A graphical representation of the high KDM5B mRNA expression among breast cancer patients. Data extracted from the cBioPortal for cancer genomics.

3.2. Lung Cancer

KDM5B expression rate was found to be highly elevated in neoplastic tissues, in contrast to normal tissues, irrespective of lung carcinoma histology [39–41]. The suppression of KDM5B expression showed a significant reduction in cancer cell growth via the E2F/RB1 pathway [40]. Han L. et al. reported in 2013 that KDM5B positively regulates brain metastasis in NSCLC [42]. Moreover, KDM5B aids in the proliferation, invasion, and metastasis activities of lung cancer cells through downregulated p53 [39]. Besides, Shen X. et al. reported that KDM5B overexpression positively correlated with size and stage of the tumor, lymph node metastasis, and reduced survival rate [39]. A recent study by Lu Y. et al. established that KDM5B plays crucial roles in hypoxia-induced gefitinib (EGFR TKI) resistance and epithelial–mesenchymal transition (EMT) [43].

3.3. Melanoma

The role of KDM5B in melanoma is still controversial. Roesch A. et al., in their studies, showed that KDM5B promoted tumor cell maintenance and metastasis, and its knockdown led to the exhaustion of melanoma cells [44]. However, KDM5B has also been suggested as a tumor-suppressive agent in melanocytic cells through the regulation of activities of the retinoblastoma protein [45,46]. Interestingly, it is evident that, in melanoma cells, KDM5B expression is dynamically regulated. However, KDM5B was overexpressed in certain benign tumors, whereas downregulated in aggressive and metastatic melanomas [47]. The relevance of KDM5B in chemo-resistance was confirmed when KDM5B depletion led to the increased sensitivity of melanocytes to anti-melanoma treatment [48].

3.4. Hepatocellular Carcinoma

KDM5B was often upregulated in hepatocellular carcinoma (HCC) samples, compared to corresponding non-neoplastic tissues. Besides, the gene expression level was associated with tumor properties and stages of cancer. HCC patients with KDM5B overexpression had more tumor metastasis, poor prognosis, and significantly shorter overall survival [49–52]. KDM5B exerts its oncogenic function by inactivating PTEN transcription [49] and by silencing KDM5B, which, remarkably, hinders cancer cell proliferation through p15 and p27 up-regulation [50].

3.5. Gastric Cancer

The aberrant expression of KDM5B mRNA was detected in gastric tumor specimens and cell lines in comparison with normal tissues. The expression rate also correlated with TNM stage and depth of invasion [53]. Various studies confirm the contribution of KDM5B in various signaling pathways for tumor cell development and migration [53,54]. Bao J. et al. reported that miR-194, which obstructs gastric cancer cell growth and invasion, directly targets and negatively regulates KDM5B [55]. These findings revealed the potential role of KDM5B, as a tumor promoter in gastric cancer. A recent study by Xu W. et al. described that increased KDM5B expression, associated with cisplatin resistance in gastric cancer cell lines and targeting KDM5B, reversed the phenotype [56].

3.6. Colorectal Cancer

The functional significance of KDM5B in colorectal cancer (CRC) stem cells was confirmed through in vitro and in vivo studies. KDM5B knockdown was found to surge H3K4 trimethylation at the p16/INK4A tumor suppressor's promoter region, which subsequently induced cellular senescence [57]. Besides, KDM5B was found to be overexpressed in CRC tumor tissue compared with normal colon samples and this overexpression positively correlated with cancer progression [58].

3.7. Bladder Cancer

Knockdown and apoptosis studies demonstrated the close link of KDM5B, in cell cycle regulation and cancer cell maintenance, in bladder cancer cell lines. Overexpression of KDM5B was noted in the early and advanced stages of bladder cancer, irrespective of cancer grade [40]. A potential inverse connection between KDM5B and connexin 26 (CX26) in the progression of bladder cancer was reported, where KDM5B was found to be upregulated in contrast to CX26 [59].

3.8. Prostate Cancer

KDM5B was found to be overexpressed in prostate cancer tissues, compared to benign tissues, and has been suggested as a potential therapeutic target [15,60]. Various studies evaluated the role of microRNAs in regulating KDM5B. The forced miR-29a expression inhibited proliferation, and induced apoptosis in prostate cancer cells, by repressing KDM5B expression, whereas, by KDM5B targeting, miR-137 aided as a tumor suppressor in prostate carcinogenesis [61,62].

3.9. KDM5B in Other Cancers

KDM5B showed significantly high expression levels in patients with B-cell precursor acute lymphoblastic leukemia (B-ALL), compared to normal bone marrow [63]. The suppression of KDM5B hindered metastasis and the invasion of human oral squamous cell carcinoma and sensitized radiation therapy [64]. KDM5B overexpression was significantly associated with tumor cell proliferation in head and neck cancer, and KDM5B silencing caused cell growth suppression both in vitro and in vivo [65]. Similar studies supporting the oncogenic role of KDM5B were observed in other malignancies, such as esophageal squamous cell carcinoma [66], cervical cancer [67], renal cell carcinoma [68], epithelial ovarian cancer [69] and neuroblastoma [70].

3.10. KDM5B as a Therapeutic Target

Apart from the oncogenic and tumorigenic role, KDM5B is also considered as a cancer-testis antigen (CTA), where gene expression is restricted in normal tissues except adult testes [22,71]. Therefore, abnormal overexpression of KDM5B in any neoplastic tissue, in comparison with corresponding non-neoplastic tissues, makes it an ideal therapeutic target. Furthermore, CTA properties suggest that targeting KDM5B may be associated with reduced toxicity. Therefore, the development of specific KDM5B inhibitors will offer a deeper insight into the therapeutic potential for many types of cancers.

As Fe (II) and α- ketoglutarate are the two vital co-factors of KDM5B in demethylation, studies are focusing on the development of compounds that mimic α-ketoglutarate or compounds that chelate with Fe (II). Over the years, many KDM5B inhibitors have been developed (Figure 3) and have provided promising outcomes [72]. The 2,4-pyridinedicarboxylic acid (2,4-PDCA) inhibits KDM5B in vitro with an IC_{50} value of 3 ± 1 μM [5], whereas GSK-J1 with an IC_{50} of 0.55 μM [20,73]. GSK467 displayed an inhibitory concentration of 0.026 μM. The crystalline structure of KDM5B with GSK467 provides a possible template for the development of selective KDM5B inhibitors [20,74]. Compounds 54j and 54k are potent, cell permeable dual inhibitors of the KDM4 and KDM5 subfamilies. Compounds 54j and 54k inhibit KDM5B with IC_{50} values 0.014 μM and 0.023 μM, respectively, and have shown adequate cellular permeability [75]. CPI-455 with IC_{50} of 0.003 μM, was identified as a pan-KDM5 inhibitor that competitively binds to the two cofactor binding sites [76]. KDM5-C49, a 2,4-PDCA analogue, and further modified KDOAM-25 have shown acceptable inhibitory potency on KDM5B, in which KDOAM-25 exhibited good stability, high selectivity and low cytotoxicity [20,77]. An orally available, potent inhibitor of KDM5B, named compound 33, was identified through structure activity relationship exploration and presented promising selectivity compared to early inhibitors [78]. Recently, a pyrazole derivative, compound 27ab, was discovered, which inhibited MKN45 cell proliferation, wound healing and migration [79]. All these inhibitors are in their initial stage of development and have not made it to the clinics yet.

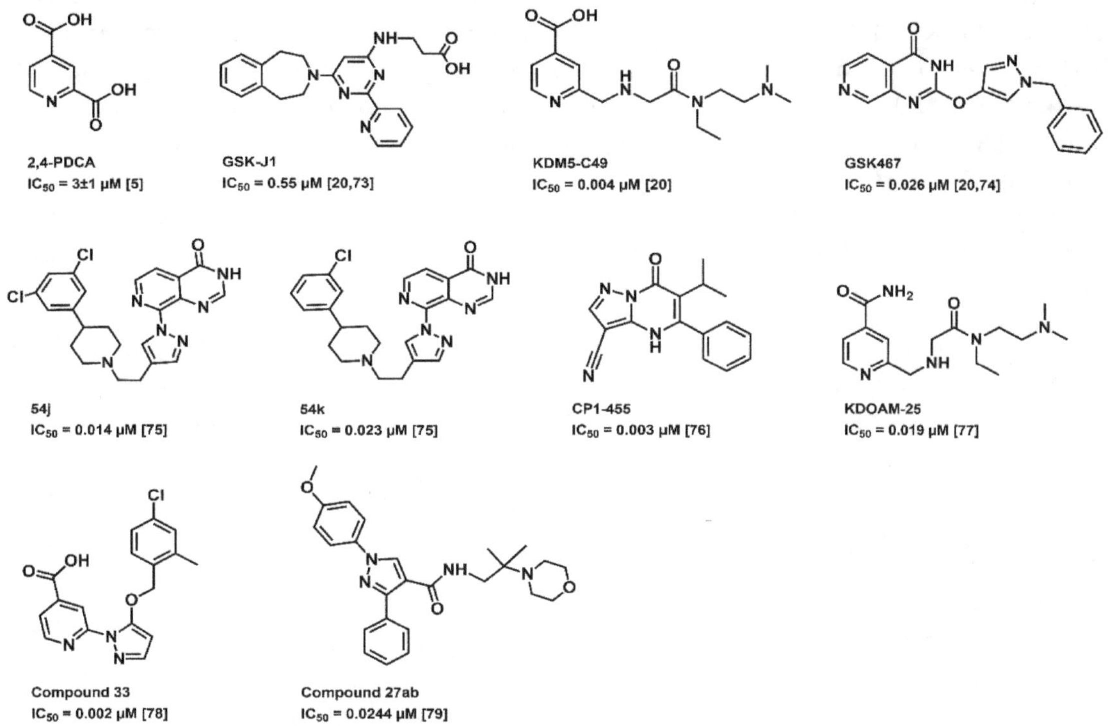

Figure 3. Previously reported KDM5B inhibitors (IC_{50}: half maximal inhibitory concentration).

4. Molecular Docking Studies

The JmjC domain of native KDM5B, which is involved in histone demethylation, contains Fe (II) ion and α-ketoglutarate as cofactors. This site is an attractive target to develop KDM5B inhibitors. One of the solved crystal structures of KDM5B, with an inhibitor GSK467 in the JmjC domain, contains Mn (II) instead of Fe (II) [20]. This structure provides an excellent starting point to develop novel KDM5B inhibitors using computational tools. Accordingly, we used computational modeling to explore the potential of known drugs to inhibit KDM5B. Drug repurposing is an approach where new therapeutic indications for already marketed drugs are discovered. This approach aims to lessen the price and time involved in drug discovery process [80,81]. On this note, we considered the drug repurposing potential of nucleoside derivatives, which are well known as antiviral agents [82]. Several studies in the past have shown that nucleoside derivatives, with monocyclic or bicyclic ring systems, exhibit anticancer properties [83–85]. We investigated the drug repurposing potential of known compounds, such as decitabine, entecavir, abacavir, penciclovir, and 3-deazaneplanocin A (DZNep) (Figure 4), which are all nucleoside derivatives, as inhibitors of KDM5B, by conducting molecular docking experiments. In addition, we compared the binding modes of previously reported KDM5B inhibitors containing planar bicyclic rings, such as GSK467, 54j, and CPI-455, with penciclovir and DZNep, to determine their interactions in the JmjC domain of KDM5B. It should be noted that decitabine (Dacogen®) is currently used to treat myelodysplastic syndrome (MDS), entecavir (Baraclude®) is used as an anti-hepatitis B agent, abacavir (Ziagen®) is used to treat HIV infections and penciclovir (Denavir®) is a known drug used in the treatment of herpes infections. The carbocyclic adenosine derivative DZNep, is a known inhibitor of histone methyltransferase EZH2 and is a promising compound in cancer immunotherapy [86]. Molecular docking studies were carried out using the computational software, Discovery Studio (DS) Structure-Based-Design (BIOVIA Inc, Dassault Systemes, USA). Moreover, previous studies have shown that nucleoside derivatives with either a monocyclic or bicyclic ring exhibit anticancer property. The ligands decitabine, entecavir, abacavir, penciclovir, and DZNep were built in 3D, using the Small Molecules module in DS using CHARMm force field. The X-ray crystal structure of human KDM5B was obtained from PDB (pdb id: 5FUN) [20]. This KDM5B structure contains a pyridopyrimidine ligand GSK467 and the catalytic site contains Mn^{2+} ion. All the water molecules were removed and a 10 Å binding site sphere was defined by selecting the bound ligand GSK467, after which it was deleted. The KDM5B protein was prepared using the Macromolecules module in DS using CHARMm force field. Docking was carried out using the LibDock algorithm by employing 100 hotspots, a docking tolerance of 0.25 Å, and an implicit solvent model, with a distance-dependent dielectric constant and CHARMm force field. The binding poses obtained, were further energy minimized using Smart minimizer (1000 steps and an RMS gradient of 0.001 kcal/mol) and ranked using the LibDock scoring function. The ligand-binding interactions were further studied by considering the polar and nonpolar contacts in the KDM5B binding site. The general computational methods applied were as per our previously reported method [87].

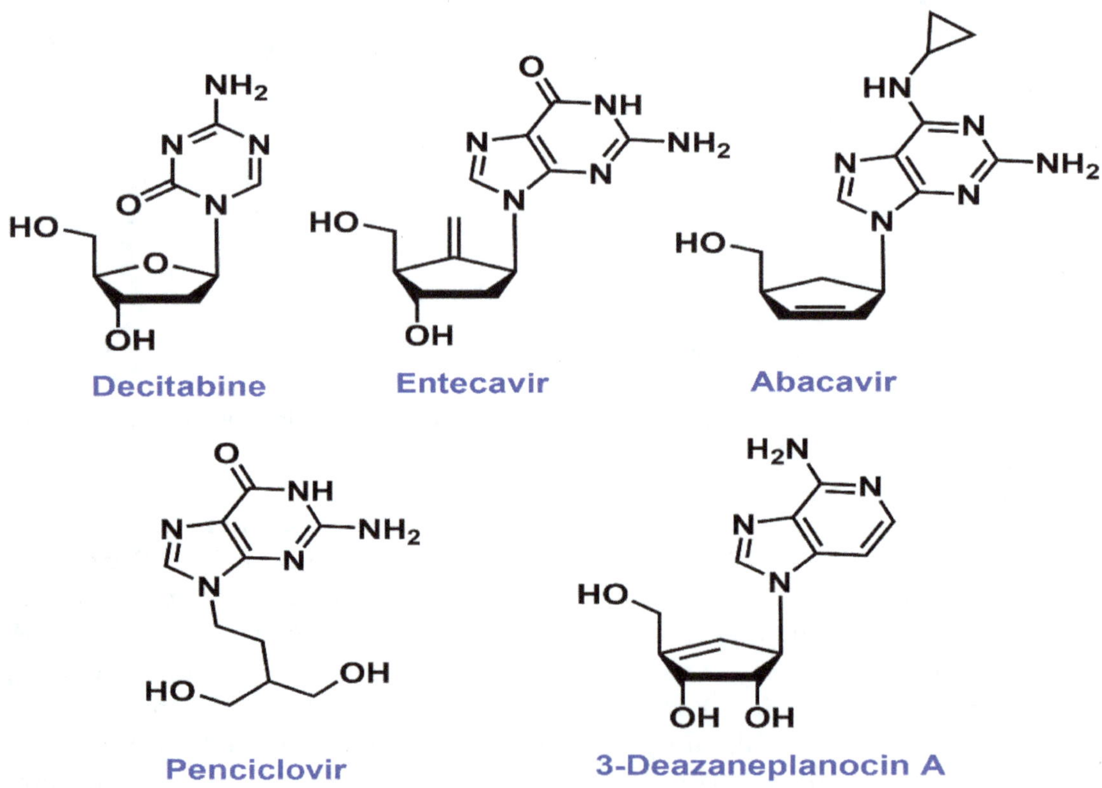

Figure 4. Selected antiviral drugs targeting KDM5B.

Docking the nucleoside decitabine in the KDM5B catalytic site shows that the 6-member azacytidine ring was in the α-ketoglutarate binding pocket and underwent π–π stacked hydrophobic interactions with aromatic rings of Tyr488 and Phe496, respectively (distance < 4.1 Å). The azacytidine N3 was not forming any metal-ligand bonding with Mn^{2+} center (distance ≈ 5.0 Å, Figure 5, Panel A). The deoxy sugar moiety was in a region comprised of Tyr425, Gly426, and Ser495. The hydroxy and the hydroxymethyl groups were in contact with Ser495 and Gly426 backbones, via hydrogen bonding interaction (distance < 1.9 Å, Figure 5, Panel A). These studies suggest that decitabine can undergo favorable interactions with KDM5B.

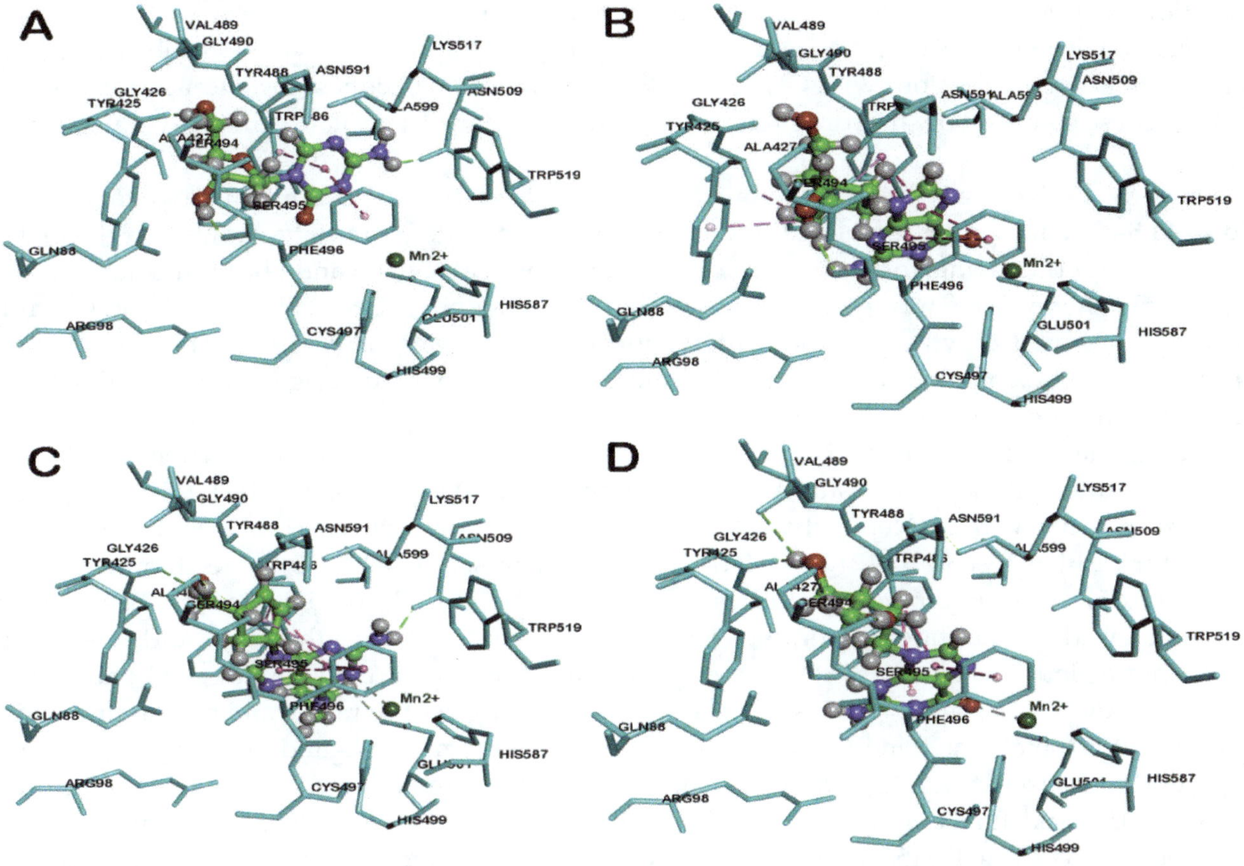

Figure 5. The binding modes of decitabine (**A**), entecavir (**B**), abacavir (**C**) and penciclovir (**D**) in ball and stick cartoon within the JmjC domain of human KDM5B (pdb id: 5FUN). Mn^{2+} ion is shown as a green circle. Hydrogen atoms are removed to enhance clarity. Polar and nonpolar interactions are color-coded.

Docking entecavir in KDM5B shows that the bicyclic guanosine ring was oriented in the α-ketoglutarate binding pocket, where it underwent some favorable interactions. The pyrimidine and imidazole rings were in contact with Tyr488 and Phe496 via four π–π stacked hydrophobic interactions (distance < 4.5 Å, Figure 5, Panel B). Interestingly, the guanosine C6 ketone (C = O) underwent metal–ligand bonding with the Mn^{2+} center (distance = 2.6 Å). The exocyclic alkene was in contact with Tyr425, Ala427, and Tyr488 (distance < 5.0 Å), whereas the hydroxy group of the cyclopentenyl ring formed a hydrogen bond with the backbone of Ser495 (distance < 2.0 Å, Figure 5, Panel B). In general, entecavir exhibited better binding interactions with KDM5B compared to decitabine. This can be attributed to the presence of a planar bicyclic guanosine ring in entecavir, and the metal–ligand bond with the guanosine ketone.

Docking the anti-HIV agent abacavir with KDM5B shows that it was buried in the α-ketoglutarate binding pocket closer to the metal center similar to entecavir, and the purine ring underwent π–π stacking interactions with aromatic rings of Tyr488 and Phe496 (distance < 4.8 Å) and the N1 of purine ring was in contact with Mn^{2+} (distance = 2.6 Å). Furthermore, the C2 amino substituent underwent hydrogen bonding interaction with the backbone of Asn509 (distance < 1.9 Å, Figure 5, Panel C). The cyclopentenyl ring was in contact with Tyr488 and Phe496 via hydrophobic interactions (distance < 4.8 Å).

Docking another purine-based drug penciclovir, which contains a guanosine ring similar to entecavir in the KDM5B, shows that it was exhibiting a similar binding mode as entecavir, and the guanosine ring was in hydrophobic contact with Tyr488 and Phe496 by forming several π–π stacking interactions (distance < 4.4 Å, Figure 5, Panel D). The guanosine ketone forms a metal–ligand interaction with Mn^{2+} (distance = 2.4 Å). The acyclic sugar moiety was closer to a polar region comprised of Gly426, Ser494, Val489, and Asn591. The hydroxy and hydroxymethyl substituents form hydrogen-bonding interactions with Gly429, Ser494, and Val489 backbones (distance < 2.8 Å, Figure 5, Panel D). These studies show that drugs containing a bicyclic purine template exhibit favorable binding in KDM5B.

Docking DZNep, an investigational drug molecule, which also contains a planar bicyclic imidazo[4,5-c]pyridine ring template (Figure 4), and a cyclopentenyl moiety, shows that the bicyclic imidazo[4,5-c]pyridine ring, forms a π–π stacking interaction with Tyr488 and Phe496 (distance < 4.3 Å). Interestingly, the pyridine nitrogen, chelated with Mn^{2+} (distance = 2.8 Å, Figure 6A) and C2 amino substituents formed a hydrogen bond interaction with backbone of Asn509. The cyclopentenyl hydroxyl and hydroxymethyl substituents also underwent hydrogen bonding interactions with Gly426 and Ser495 (distance < 2.0 Å).

Among these compounds, DZNep exhibited the most favorable binding interaction with KDM5B. The binding interaction was measured by calculating the LibDock scores for the best binding poses. The ranking order was DZNep (LibDock score = 131.60) > penciclovir (LibDock score = 129.84) > entecavir (LibDock score = 121.26) > abacavir (LibDock score = 118.10) > decitabine (LibDock score = 109.55). Molecular docking studies of known KDM5B inhibitor, 54j (Figure 6B), shows that its bicyclic pyridopyrimidine ring underwent van der Waal's contact with Tyr488 and Phe496 (π–π stacked interactions, distance < 5 Å) and the pyrimidinone ketone formed a hydrogen bond with the side chain of Lys517 (distance = 1.55 Å). Interestingly, the nitrogen of pyrazole and pyrimidinone rings was close to the metal center, indicating the ability of 54j to form metal–ligand interactions (Figure 6B). The piperidine benzene with 3,5-dichloro substituents, was oriented in a hydrophobic pocket made up of Ile500, Val553 and Tyr586. Furthermore, 54j is a much larger molecule (molecular volume = 345.7 Å^3) compared to GSK467, CPI-455, decitabine, entecavir, abacavir, penciclovir, and DZNep (molecular volume range ~ 168.7–231.5 Å^3). Therefore, 54j is able to bind in the entire span of the JmjC domain (Figure 6B), which is not possible for the antivirals investigated in this study, as they are smaller. This is also supported by a superior LibDock score obtained for 54j (LibDock score = 145.08). However, similar to 54j, all the bicyclic ring-containing agents, entecavir, abacavir, penciclovir, and DZNep, are able to undergo metal–ligand interaction (Figures 5 and 6), which is a common feature observed.

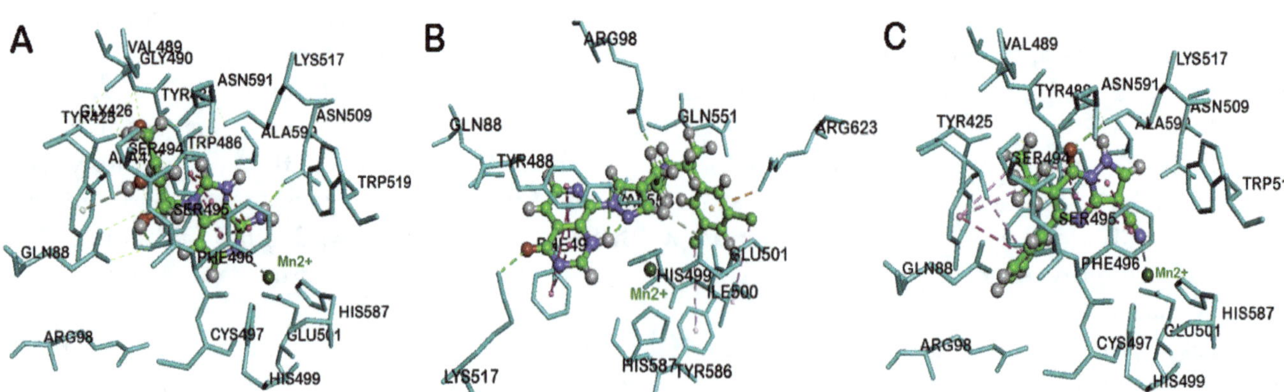

Figure 6. The binding mode of DZNep (**A**), 54j (**B**) and CPI-455 (**C**) (ball and stick cartoon) within JmjC domain of human KDM5B (pdb id: 5FUN). Mn^{2+} ion is shown as a green circle. Hydrogen atoms are removed to enhance clarity. Polar and nonpolar interactions are color-coded.

Molecular docking studies of the known KDM5B inhibitor, CPI-455 (Figure 6C), shows that it was oriented in a similar region compared to molecules containing the planar bicyclic ring investigated in this study. The bicyclic pyrazolopyrimidinone ring of CPI-455 was in van der Waal's contact with Tyr488 and Phe496 (distance < 5 Å), and the pyrimidinone ketone underwent a hydrogen-bonding interaction with the Lys517 side chain (distance = 2.48 Å). The C6 isopropyl substituent was in a hydrophobic pocket and underwent multiple interactions with Tyr425 and Ala427 (distance < 5 Å), whereas the C5 phenyl ring underwent π–π stacking interactions with Tyr425 (distance < 5 Å). Interestingly, the C3 nitrile substituent was able to chelate with the metal center (distance = 2.6 Å, Figure 6C) which shows the significance of a nitrile substituent in KDM5B binding (LibDock score = 120.19). These molecular docking studies also show that bicyclic ring-containing agents (e.g., 54j, CPI-455, entecavir, abacavir, penciclovir, and DZNep), exhibit better binding in the JmjC domain of KDM5B, compared to monocyclic ring-containing decitabine, which is also reflected in a lower LibDock score (109.55) obtained for decitabine compared to other molecules.

The binding modes of DZNep and penciclovir, which exhibited superior LibDock scores, were compared with the known X-ray structure of GSK467 (Figure 3), bound to KDM5B. This investigation shows that, similar to GSK467, the planar bicyclic rings of DZNep and penciclovir were oriented in the α-ketoglutarate binding pocket, and more significantly, the pyridine nitrogen of DZNep and guanosine ketone of penciclovir were in contact with the metal center Mn^{2+} (Figure 7). These observations were similar to the binding mode of GSK467 in the JmjC domain of human KDM5B, where the pyridopyrimidine nitrogen interacts with the metal center (Figure 7) [20].

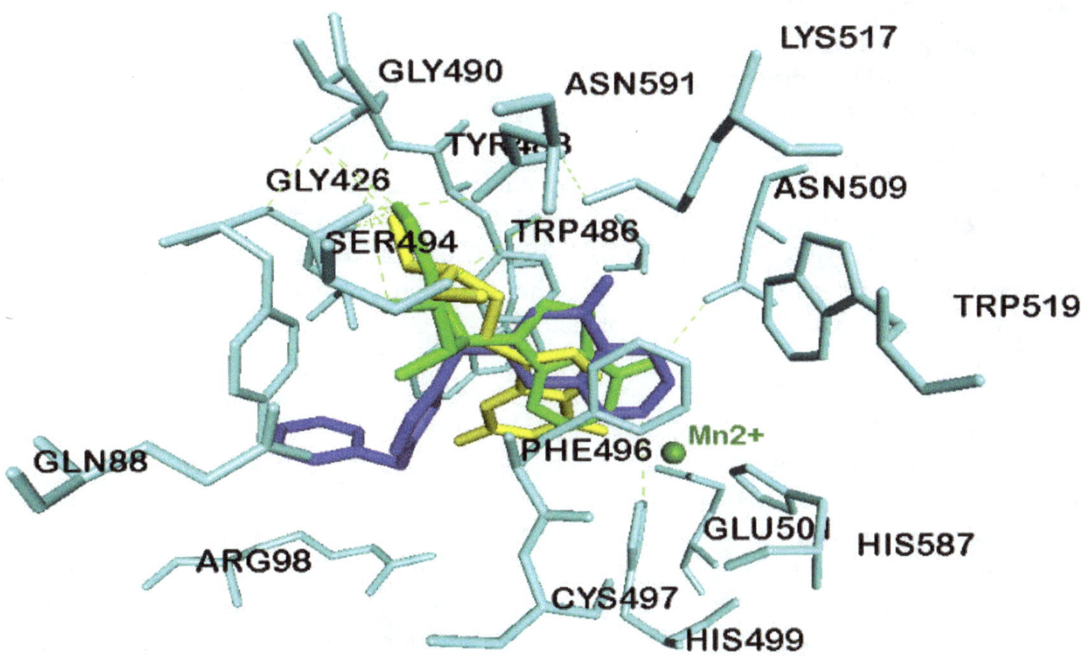

Figure 7. Comparison of binding modes of GSK467 (blue stick cartoon), penciclovir (yellow stick cartoon) and DZNep (green stick cartoon) in the JmjC domain of human KDM5B (pdb id: 5FUN). Mn^{2+} ion is shown as a green circle. Hydrogen atoms are removed to enhance clarity.

These results also show that small molecules, which possess planar bicyclic heterocyclic rings, exhibit favorable binding toward the JmjC domain of human KDM5B. This is due to their ability to undergo interactions with the catalytic site metal ion, which is an important criterion in KDM5 inhibition and is consistent with previous studies [20,77,88]. Our molecular docking investigations show that decitabine, entecavir, abacavir, penciclovir, and DZNep have the potential to be repurposed as KDM5B inhibitors to treat various types of cancers.

5. Conclusions

The leading role of KDM5B oncogene in tumorigenesis and cancer progression is well established in various malignancies and is therefore, considered as a potential therapeutic target. Although many small molecule inhibitors of KDM5B have been identified so far, their possible clinical application in cancer treatment is a work in progress. This study provides a rationale on how repurposing antiviral drugs could contribute to the discovery and development of KDM5B inhibitors. We anticipate that these studies will stimulate further research in considering drug repurposing approaches to target KDM5B, and to discover novel therapies for various cancers.

Author Contributions: Conceptualization, M.R., P.P.N.R., and A.J.; writing—original draft preparation, A.J., P.P.N.R., and M.R.; writing—review and editing, A.J., M.R., P.P.N.R., G.R., G.G.S., J.K., N.A.N.K., G.S.R., M.M., and L.T. All authors have read and agreed to the published version of the manuscript.

Acknowledgments: A.J. and L.T. are thankful for the TMA Pai PhD Scholarship from Manipal Academy of Higher Education, Manipal, India.

References

1. Sharma, S.; Kelly, T.K.; Jones, P.A. Epigenetics in cancer. *Carcinogenesis* **2010**, *31*, 27–36. [CrossRef] [PubMed]
2. Feinberg, A.P.; Tycko, B. The history of cancer epigenetics. *Nat. Rev. Cancer* **2004**, *4*, 143–153. [CrossRef] [PubMed]
3. Dupont, C.; Armant, D.R.; Brenner, C.A. Epigenetics: Definition, mechanisms and clinical perspective. *Semin. Reprod. Med.* **2009**, *27*, 351–357. [CrossRef] [PubMed]
4. Wang, G.G.; Allis, C.D.; Chi, P. Chromatin remodeling and cancer, Part I: Covalent histone modifications. *Trends Mol. Med.* **2007**, *13*, 363–372. [CrossRef] [PubMed]
5. Kristensen, L.H.; Nielsen, A.L.; Helgstrand, C.; Lees, M.; Cloos, P.; Kastrup, J.S.; Helin, K.; Olsen, L.; Gajhede, M. Studies of H3K4me3 demethylation by KDM5B/Jarid1B/PLU1 reveals strong substrate recognition in vitro and identifies 2, 4-pyridine-dicarboxylic acid as an in vitro and in cell inhibitor. *FEBS J.* **2012**, *279*, 1905–1914. [CrossRef]
6. Agger, K.; Christensen, J.; Cloos, P.A.; Helin, K. The emerging functions of histone demethylases. *Curr. Opin. Genet. Dev.* **2008**, *18*, 159–168. [CrossRef]
7. Allis, C.D.; Berger, S.L.; Cote, J.; Dent, S.; Jenuwien, T.; Kouzarides, T.; Pillus, L.; Reinberg, D.; Shi, Y.; Shiekhattar, R. New nomenclature for chromatin-modifying enzymes. *Cell* **2007**, *131*, 633–636. [CrossRef]
8. Shi, Y.; Whetstine, J.R. Dynamic regulation of histone lysine methylation by demethylases. *Mol. Cell.* **2007**, *25*, 1–14. [CrossRef]
9. Harmeyer, K.M.; Facompre, N.D.; Herlyn, M.; Basu, D. JARID1 histone demethylases: Emerging targets in cancer. *Trends Cancer* **2017**, *3*, 713–725. [CrossRef]
10. Benevolenskaya, E.V. Histone H3K4 demethylases are essential in development and differentiation. *Biochem. Cell Biol.* **2007**, *85*, 435–443. [CrossRef]
11. Rotili, D.; Mai, A. Targeting histone demethylases: A new avenue for the fight against cancer. *Genes Cancer* **2011**, *2*, 663–679. [CrossRef] [PubMed]
12. Cerami, E.; Gao, J.; Dogrusoz, U.; Gross, B.E.; Sumer, S.O.; Aksoy, B.A.; Jacobsen, A.; Byrne, C.J.; Heuer, M.L.; Larsson, E. The cBio cancer genomics portal: An open platform for exploring multidimensional cancer genomics data. *AACR* **2012**, 401–404. [CrossRef] [PubMed]
13. Gao, J.; Aksoy, B.A.; Dogrusoz, U.; Dresdner, G.; Gross, B.; Sumer, S.O.; Sun, Y.; Jacobsen, A.; Sinha, R.; Larsson, E. Integrative analysis of complex cancer genomics and clinical profiles using the cBioPortal. *Sci. Signal.* **2013**, *6*, pl1. [CrossRef]
14. Hoadley, K.A.; Yau, C.; Hinoue, T.; Wolf, D.M.; Lazar, A.J.; Drill, E.; Shen, R.; Taylor, A.M.; Cherniack, A.D.; Thorsson, V. Cell-of-origin patterns dominate the molecular classification of 10,000 tumors from 33 types of cancer. *Cell* **2018**, *173*, 291–304.e6. [CrossRef] [PubMed]
15. Xiang, Y.; Zhu, Z.; Han, G.; Ye, X.; Xu, B.; Peng, Z.; Ma, Y.; Yu, Y.; Lin, H.; Chen, A.P. JARID1B is a histone H3 lysine 4 demethylase up-regulated in prostate cancer. *Proc. Natl. Acad. Sci. USA.* **2007**, *104*, 19226–19231. [CrossRef] [PubMed]
16. Wilsker, D.; Probst, L.; Wain, H.M.; Maltais, L.; Tucker, P.W.; Moran, E. Nomenclature of the ARID family of DNA-binding proteins. *Genomics* **2005**, *86*, 242–251. [CrossRef] [PubMed]

17. Wysocka, J.; Swigut, T.; Xiao, H.; Milne, T.A.; Kwon, S.Y.; Landry, J.; Kauer, M.; Tackett, A.J.; Chait, B.T.; Badenhorst, P. A PHD finger of NURF couples histone H3 lysine 4 trimethylation with chromatin remodelling. *Nature* **2006**, *442*, 86–90. [CrossRef] [PubMed]
18. Pilka, E.S.; James, T.; Lisztwan, J.H. Structural definitions of Jumonji family demethylase selectivity. *Drug Discov. Today.* **2015**, *20*, 743–749. [CrossRef]
19. Yamane, K.; Tateishi, K.; Klose, R.J.; Fang, J.; Fabrizio, L.A.; Erdjument-Bromage, H.; Taylor-Papadimitriou, J.; Tempst, P.; Zhang, Y. PLU-1 is an H3K4 demethylase involved in transcriptional repression and breast cancer cell proliferation. *Mol. Cell* **2007**, *25*, 801–812. [CrossRef]
20. Johansson, C.; Velupillai, S.; Tumber, A.; Szykowska, A.; Hookway, E.S.; Nowak, R.P.; Strain-Damerell, C.; Gileadi, C.; Philpott, M.; Burgess-Brown, N. Structural analysis of human KDM5B guides histone demethylase inhibitor development. *Nat. Chem. Biol.* **2016**, *12*, 539–545. [CrossRef]
21. Dorosz, J.; Kristensen, L.H.; Aduri, N.G.; Mirza, O.; Lousen, R.; Bucciarelli, S.; Mehta, V.; Sellés-Baiget, S.; Solbak, S.M.Ø.; Bach, A. Molecular architecture of the Jumonji C family histone demethylase KDM5B. *Sci. Rep.* **2019**, *9*, 4019. [CrossRef]
22. Lu, P.J.; Sundquist, K.; Baeckstrom, D.; Poulsom, R.; Hanby, A.; Meier-Ewert, S.; Jones, T.; Mitchell, M.; Pitha-Rowe, P.; Freemont, P. A novel gene (PLU-1) containing highly conserved putative DNA/chromatin binding motifs is specifically up-regulated in breast cancer. *J. Biol. Chem.* **1999**, *274*, 15633–15645. [CrossRef] [PubMed]
23. Scibetta, A.G.; Santangelo, S.; Coleman, J.; Hall, D.; Chaplin, T.; Copier, J.; Catchpole, S.; Burchell, J.; Taylor-Papadimitriou, J. Functional analysis of the transcription repressor PLU-1/JARID1B. *Mol. Cell Biol.* **2007**, *27*, 7220–7235. [CrossRef] [PubMed]
24. Catchpole, S.; Spencer-Dene, B.; Hall, D.; Santangelo, S.; Rosewell, I.; Guenatri, M.; Beatson, R.; Scibetta, A.G.; Burchell, J.M.; Taylor-Papadimitriou, J. PLU-1/JARID1B/KDM5B is required for embryonic survival and contributes to cell proliferation in the mammary gland and in ER+ breast cancer cells. *Int. J. Oncol.* **2011**, *38*, 1267–1277. [CrossRef] [PubMed]
25. Yamamoto, S.; Wu, Z.; Russnes, H.G.; Takagi, S.; Peluffo, G.; Vaske, C.; Zhao, X.; Vollan, H.K.M.; Maruyama, R.; Ekram, M.B. JARID1B is a luminal lineage-driving oncogene in breast cancer. *Cancer Cell* **2014**, *25*, 762–777. [CrossRef]
26. Mitra, D.; Das, P.M.; Huynh, F.C.; Jones, F.E. Jumonji/ARID1 B (JARID1B) protein promotes breast tumor cell cycle progression through epigenetic repression of microRNA let-7e. *J. Biol. Chem.* **2011**, *286*, 40531–40535. [CrossRef] [PubMed]
27. Wong, P.-P.; Miranda, F.; Chan, K.V.; Berlato, C.; Hurst, H.C.; Scibetta, A.G. Histone demethylase KDM5B collaborates with TFAP2C and Myc to repress the cell cycle inhibitor p21cip (CDKN1A). *Mol. Cell. Biol.* **2012**, *32*, 1633–1644. [CrossRef]
28. Zhao, L.; Liu, H. Immunohistochemical detection and clinicopathological significance of JARID1B/KDM5B and P16 expression in invasive ductal carcinoma of the breast. *Genet. Mol. Res.* **2015**, *14*, 5417–5426. [CrossRef]
29. Bamodu, O.A.; Huang, W.-C.; Lee, W.-H.; Wu, A.; Wang, L.S.; Hsiao, M.; Yeh, C.-T.; Chao, T.-Y. Aberrant KDM5B expression promotes aggressive breast cancer through MALAT1 overexpression and downregulation of hsa-miR-448. *BMC Cancer* **2016**, *16*, 160. [CrossRef]
30. Blair, L.P.; Liu, Z.; Labitigan, R.L.D.; Wu, L.; Zheng, D.; Xia, Z.; Pearson, E.L.; Nazeer, F.I.; Cao, J.; Lang, S.M. KDM5 lysine demethylases are involved in maintenance of 3′ UTR length. *Sci. Adv.* **2016**, *2*, e1501662. [CrossRef]
31. Montano, M.M.; Yeh, I.J.; Chen, Y.; Hernandez, C.; Kiselar, J.G.; de la Fuente, M.; Lawes, A.M.; Nieman, M.T.; Kiser, P.D.; Jacobberger, J.; et al. Inhibition of the histone demethylase, KDM5B, directly induces re-expression of tumor suppressor protein HEXIM1 in cancer cells. *Breast Cancer Res.* **2019**, *21*, 138. [CrossRef]
32. Paroni, G.; Bolis, M.; Zanetti, A.; Ubezio, P.; Helin, K.; Staller, P.; Gerlach, L.O.; Fratelli, M.; Neve, R.M.; Terao, M. HER2-positive breast-cancer cell lines are sensitive to KDM5 inhibition: Definition of a gene-expression model for the selection of sensitive cases. *Oncogene* **2019**, *38*, 2675–2689. [CrossRef]
33. Hinohara, K.; Wu, H.-J.; Vigneau, S.; McDonald, T.O.; Igarashi, K.J.; Yamamoto, K.N.; Madsen, T.; Fassl, A.; Egri, S.B.; Papanastasiou, M. KDM5 histone demethylase activity links cellular transcriptomic heterogeneity to therapeutic resistance. *Cancer Cell* **2018**, *34*, 939–953.e9. [CrossRef]

34. Tang, D.; Zhao, X.; Zhang, L.; Wang, Z.; Wang, C. Identification of hub genes to regulate breast cancer metastasis to brain by bioinformatics analyses. *J. Cell. Biochem.* **2019**, *120*, 9522–9531. [CrossRef] [PubMed]
35. Zhang, Z.-G.; Zhang, H.-S.; Sun, H.-L.; Liu, H.-Y.; Liu, M.-Y.; Zhou, Z. KDM5B promotes breast cancer cell proliferation and migration via AMPK-mediated lipid metabolism reprogramming. *Exp. Cell Res.* **2019**, *379*, 182–190. [CrossRef] [PubMed]
36. Ciriello, G.; Gatza, M.L.; Beck, A.H.; Wilkerson, M.D.; Rhie, S.K.; Pastore, A.; Zhang, H.; McLellan, M.; Yau, C.; Kandoth, C. Comprehensive molecular portraits of invasive lobular breast cancer. *Cell* **2015**, *163*, 506–519. [CrossRef] [PubMed]
37. Cancer Genome Atlas Network. Comprehensive molecular portraits of human breast tumours. *Nature* **2012**, *490*, 61–70. [CrossRef]
38. Pereira, B.; Chin, S.-F.; Rueda, O.M.; Vollan, H.-K.M.; Provenzano, E.; Bardwell, H.A.; Pugh, M.; Jones, L.; Russell, R.; Sammut, S.-J. The somatic mutation profiles of 2433 breast cancers refine their genomic and transcriptomic landscapes. *Nat. Commun.* **2016**, *7*, 11479. [CrossRef]
39. Shen, X.; Zhuang, Z.; Zhang, Y.; Chen, Z.; Shen, L.; Pu, W.; Chen, L.; Xu, Z. JARID1B modulates lung cancer cell proliferation and invasion by regulating p53 expression. *Tumor Biol.* **2015**, *36*, 7133–7142. [CrossRef]
40. Hayami, S.; Yoshimatsu, M.; Veerakumarasivam, A.; Unoki, M.; Iwai, Y.; Tsunoda, T.; Field, H.I.; Kelly, J.D.; Neal, D.E.; Yamaue, H. Overexpression of the JmjC histone demethylase KDM5B in human carcinogenesis: Involvement in the proliferation of cancer cells through the E2F/RB pathway. *Mol. Cancer* **2010**, *9*, 59. [CrossRef]
41. Kuo, K.-T.; Huang, W.-C.; Bamodu, O.A.; Lee, W.-H.; Wang, C.-H.; Hsiao, M.; Wang, L.-S.; Yeh, C.-T. Histone demethylase JARID1B/KDM5B promotes aggressiveness of non-small cell lung cancer and serves as a good prognostic predictor. *Clin. Epigenetics.* **2018**, *10*, 107. [CrossRef] [PubMed]
42. Han, L.; Liang, X.-H.; Chen, L.-X.; Bao, S.-M.; Yan, Z.-Q. SIRT1 is highly expressed in brain metastasis tissues of non-small cell lung cancer (NSCLC) and in positive regulation of NSCLC cell migration. *Int. J. Clin. Exp. Pathol.* **2013**, *6*, 2357–2365. [PubMed]
43. Lu, Y.; Liu, Y.; Oeck, S.; Glazer, P.M. Hypoxia promotes resistance to EGFR inhibition in NSCLC cells via the histone demethylases, LSD1 and PLU-1. *Mol. Cancer Res.* **2018**, *16*, 1458–1469. [CrossRef] [PubMed]
44. Roesch, A.; Fukunaga-Kalabis, M.; Schmidt, E.C.; Zabierowski, S.E.; Brafford, P.A.; Vultur, A.; Basu, D.; Gimotty, P.; Vogt, T.; Herlyn, M. A temporarily distinct subpopulation of slow-cycling melanoma cells is required for continuous tumor growth. *Cell* **2010**, *141*, 583–594. [CrossRef] [PubMed]
45. Roesch, A.; Mueller, A.M.; Stempfl, T.; Moehle, C.; Landthaler, M.; Vogt, T. RBP2-H1/JARID1B is a transcriptional regulator with a tumor suppressive potential in melanoma cells. *Int. J. Cancer* **2008**, *122*, 1047–1057. [CrossRef] [PubMed]
46. Roesch, A.; Becker, B.; Schneider-Brachert, W.; Hagen, I.; Landthaler, M.; Vogt, T. Re-expression of the retinoblastoma-binding protein 2-homolog 1 reveals tumor-suppressive functions in highly metastatic melanoma cells. *J. Invest. Dermatol.* **2006**, *126*, 1850–1859. [CrossRef]
47. Roesch, A.; Becker, B.; Meyer, S.; Wild, P.; Hafner, C.; Landthaler, M.; Vogt, T. Retinoblastoma-binding protein 2-homolog 1: A retinoblastoma-binding protein downregulated in malignant melanomas. *Mod. Pathol.* **2005**, *18*, 1249–1257. [CrossRef]
48. Roesch, A.; Vultur, A.; Bogeski, I.; Wang, H.; Zimmermann, K.M.; Speicher, D.; Körbel, C.; Laschke, M.W.; Gimotty, P.A.; Philipp, S.E. Overcoming intrinsic multidrug resistance in melanoma by blocking the mitochondrial respiratory chain of slow-cycling JARID1B(high) cells. *Cancer Cell* **2013**, *23*, 811–825. [CrossRef]
49. Tang, B.; Qi, G.; Tang, F.; Yuan, S.; Wang, Z.; Liang, X.; Li, B.; Yu, S.; Liu, J.; Huang, Q. JARID1B promotes metastasis and epithelial-mesenchymal transition via PTEN/AKT signaling in hepatocellular carcinoma cells. *Oncotarget* **2015**, *6*, 12723–12739. [CrossRef]
50. Wang, D.; Han, S.; Peng, R.; Jiao, C.; Wang, X.; Yang, X.; Yang, R.; Li, X. Depletion of histone demethylase KDM5B inhibits cell proliferation of hepatocellular carcinoma by regulation of cell cycle checkpoint proteins p15 and p27. *J. Exp. Clin. Cancer Res.* **2016**, *35*, 37. [CrossRef]
51. Shigekawa, Y.; Hayami, S.; Ueno, M.; Miyamoto, A.; Suzaki, N.; Kawai, M.; Hirono, S.; Okada, K.-I.; Hamamoto, R.; Yamaue, H. Overexpression of KDM5B/JARID1B is associated with poor prognosis in hepatocellular carcinoma. *Oncotarget* **2018**, *9*, 34320–34335. [CrossRef] [PubMed]

52. Gong, J.; Yan, S.; Yu, H.; Zhang, W.; Zhang, D. Increased Expression of Lysine-Specific Demethylase 5B (KDM5B) Promotes Tumor Cell Growth in Hep3B Cells and is an Independent Prognostic Factor in Patients with Hepatocellular Carcinoma. *Med. Sci. Monit.* **2018**, *24*, 7586–7594. [CrossRef] [PubMed]
53. Wang, Z.; Tang, F.; Qi, G.; Yuan, S.; Zhang, G.; Tang, B.; He, S. KDM5B is overexpressed in gastric cancer and is required for gastric cancer cell proliferation and metastasis. *Am. J. Cancer Res.* **2015**, *5*, 87–100. [PubMed]
54. Li, Y.; Chen, L.; Feng, L.; Zhu, M.; Shen, Q.; Fang, Y.; Liu, X.; Zhang, X. NEK2 promotes proliferation, migration and tumor growth of gastric cancer cells via regulating KDM5B/H3K4me3. *Am. J. Cancer Res.* **2019**, *9*, 2364–2378.
55. Bao, J.; Zou, J.; Li, C.; Zheng, G. miR-194 inhibits gastric cancer cell proliferation and tumorigenesis by targeting KDM5B. *Eur. Rev. Med. Pharmacol. Sci.* **2016**, *20*, 4487–4493.
56. Xu, W.; Zhou, B.; Zhao, X.; Zhu, L.; Xu, J.; Jiang, Z.; Chen, D.; Wei, Q.; Han, M.; Feng, L. KDM5B demethylates H3K4 to recruit XRCC1 and promote chemoresistance. *Int. J. Biol. Sci.* **2018**, *14*, 1122–1132. [CrossRef]
57. Ohta, K.; Haraguchi, N.; Kano, Y.; Kagawa, Y.; Konno, M.; Nishikawa, S.; Hamabe, A.; Hasegawa, S.; Ogawa, H.; Fukusumi, T. Depletion of JARID1B induces cellular senescence in human colorectal cancer. *Int. J. Oncol.* **2013**, *42*, 1212–1218. [CrossRef]
58. Tarnowski, M.; Czerewaty, M.; Deskur, A.; Safranow, K.; Marlicz, W.; Urasińska, E.; Ratajczak, M.Z.; Starzyńska, T. Expression of cancer testis antigens in colorectal cancer: New prognostic and therapeutic implications. *Dis. Markers* **2016**, *2016*, 1987505. [CrossRef]
59. Li, X.; Su, Y.; Pan, J.; Zhou, Z.; Song, B.; Xiong, E.; Chen, Z. Connexin 26 is down-regulated by KDM5B in the progression of bladder cancer. *Int. J. Mol. Sci.* **2013**, *14*, 7866–7879. [CrossRef]
60. Lu, W.; Liu, S.; Li, B.; Xie, Y.; Adhiambo, C.; Yang, Q.; Ballard, B.R.; Nakayama, K.I.; Matusik, R.J.; Chen, Z. SKP2 inactivation suppresses prostate tumorigenesis by mediating JARID1B ubiquitination. *Oncotarget* **2015**, *6*, 771–788. [CrossRef]
61. Li, J.; Wan, X.; Qiang, W.; Li, T.; Huang, W.; Huang, S.; Wu, D.; Li, Y. MiR-29a suppresses prostate cell proliferation and induces apoptosis via KDM5B protein regulation. *Int. J. Clin. Exp. Med.* **2015**, *8*, 5329–5339. [PubMed]
62. Nilsson, E.M.; Laursen, K.B.; Whitchurch, J.; McWilliam, A.; Ødum, N.; Persson, J.L.; Heery, D.M.; Gudas, L.J.; Mongan, N.P. MiR137 is an androgen regulated repressor of an extended network of transcriptional coregulators. *Oncotarget* **2015**, *6*, 35710–35725. [CrossRef] [PubMed]
63. Wang, H.; Song, C.; Ding, Y.; Pan, X.; Ge, Z.; Tan, B.-H.; Gowda, C.; Sachdev, M.; Muthusami, S.; Ouyang, H. Transcriptional regulation of JARID1B/KDM5B histone demethylase by ikaros, histone deacetylase 1 (HDAC1), and casein kinase 2 (CK2) in B-cell acute lymphoblastic leukemia. *J. Biol.* **2016**, *291*, 4004–4018. [CrossRef]
64. Lin, C.-S.; Lin, Y.-C.; Adebayo, B.O.; Wu, A.; Chen, J.-H.; Peng, Y.-J.; Cheng, M.-F.; Lee, W.-H.; Hsiao, M.; Chao, T.-Y. Silencing JARID1B suppresses oncogenicity, stemness and increases radiation sensitivity in human oral carcinoma. *Cancer Lett.* **2015**, *368*, 36–45. [CrossRef] [PubMed]
65. Cui, Z.; Song, L.; Hou, Z.; Han, Y.; Hu, Y.; Wu, Y.; Chen, W.; Mao, L. PLU-1/JARID1B overexpression predicts proliferation properties in head and neck squamous cell carcinoma. *Oncol. Rep.* **2015**, *33*, 2454–2460. [CrossRef] [PubMed]
66. Kano, Y.; Konno, M.; Ohta, K.; Haraguchi, N.; Nishikawa, S.; Kagawa, Y.; Hamabe, A.; Hasegawa, S.; Ogawa, H.; Fukusumi, T. Jumonji/Arid1b (Jarid1b) protein modulates human esophageal cancer cell growth. *Mol. Clin. Oncol.* **2013**, *1*, 753–757. [CrossRef]
67. Zhou, Y.; An, Q.; Guo, R.-X.; Qiao, Y.-H.; Li, L.-X.; Zhang, X.-Y.; Zhao, X.-L. miR424-5p functions as an anti-oncogene in cervical cancer cell growth by targeting KDM5B via the Notch signaling pathway. *Life Sci.* **2017**, *171*, 9–15. [CrossRef]
68. Kumar, A.; Kumari, N.; Nallabelli, N.; Sharma, U.; Rai, A.; Singh, S.K.; Kakkar, N.; Prasad, R. Expression profile of H3K4 demethylases with their clinical and pathological correlation in patients with clear cell renal cell carcinoma. *Gene* **2020**, *739*, 144498. [CrossRef]
69. Wang, L.; Mao, Y.; Du, G.; He, C.; Han, S. Overexpression of JARID1B is associated with poor prognosis and chemotherapy resistance in epithelial ovarian cancer. *Tumor Biol.* **2015**, *36*, 2465–2472. [CrossRef]

70. Kuo, Y.-T.; Liu, Y.-L.; Adebayo, B.O.; Shih, P.-H.; Lee, W.-H.; Wang, L.-S.; Liao, Y.-F.; Hsu, W.-M.; Yeh, C.-T.; Lin, C.-M. JARID1B expression plays a critical role in chemoresistance and stem cell-like phenotype of neuroblastoma cells. *PLoS ONE* **2015**, *10*, e0125343. [CrossRef]
71. Barrett, A.; Madsen, B.; Copier, J.; Lu, P.J.; Cooper, L.; Scibetta, A.G.; Burchell, J.; Taylor-Papadimitriou, J. PLU-1 nuclear protein, which is upregulated in breast cancer, shows restricted expression in normal human adult tissues: A new cancer/testis antigen? *Int. J. Cancer* **2002**, *101*, 581–588. [CrossRef] [PubMed]
72. Zheng, Y.-C.; Chang, J.; Wang, L.-C.; Ren, H.-M.; Pang, J.-R.; Liu, H.-M. Lysine demethylase 5B (KDM5B): A potential anti-cancer drug target. *Eur. J. Med. Chem.* **2019**, *161*, 131–140. [CrossRef] [PubMed]
73. Heinemann, B.; Nielsen, J.M.; Hudlebusch, H.R.; Lees, M.J.; Larsen, D.V.; Boesen, T.; Labelle, M.; Gerlach, L.-O.; Birk, P.; Helin, K. Inhibition of demethylases by GSK-J1/J4. *Nature* **2014**, *514*, E1–E2. [CrossRef] [PubMed]
74. Westaway, S.M.; Preston, A.G.; Barker, M.D.; Brown, F.; Brown, J.A.; Campbell, M.; Chung, C.-W.; Drewes, G.; Eagle, R.; Garton, N. Cell penetrant inhibitors of the KDM4 and KDM5 families of histone lysine demethylases. 2. Pyrido [3–d] pyrimidin-4 (3 H)-one derivatives. *J. Med. Chem.* **2016**, *59*, 1370–1387. [CrossRef]
75. Bavetsias, V.; Lanigan, R.M.; Ruda, G.F.; Atrash, B.; McLaughlin, M.G.; Tumber, A.; Mok, N.Y.; Le Bihan, Y.-V.; Dempster, S.; Boxall, K.J. 8-Substituted Pyrido [3, 4-d] pyrimidin-4 (3 H)-one Derivatives as Potent, Cell Permeable, KDM4 (JMJD2) and KDM5 (JARID1) Histone Lysine Demethylase Inhibitors. *J. Med. Chem.* **2016**, *59*, 1388–1409. [CrossRef]
76. Vinogradova, M.; Gehling, V.S.; Gustafson, A.; Arora, S.; Tindell, C.A.; Wilson, C.; Williamson, K.E.; Guler, G.D.; Gangurde, P.; Manieri, W. An inhibitor of KDM5 demethylases reduces survival of drug-tolerant cancer cells. *Nat. Chem. Biol.* **2016**, *12*, 531–538. [CrossRef]
77. Tumber, A.; Nuzzi, A.; Hookway, E.S.; Hatch, S.B.; Velupillai, S.; Johansson, C.; Kawamura, A.; Savitsky, P.; Yapp, C.; Szykowska, A. Potent and selective KDM5 inhibitor stops cellular demethylation of H3K4me3 at transcription start sites and proliferation of MM1S myeloma cells. *Cell Chem. Biology* **2017**, *24*, 371–380. [CrossRef]
78. Nie, Z.; Shi, L.; Lai, C.; O'Connell, S.M.; Xu, J.; Stansfield, R.K.; Hosfield, D.J.; Veal, J.M.; Stafford, J.A. Structure-based design and discovery of potent and selective KDM5 inhibitors. *Bioorg. Med. Chem. Lett.* **2018**, *28*, 1490–1494. [CrossRef]
79. Zhao, B.; Liang, Q.; Ren, H.; Zhang, X.; Wu, Y.; Zhang, K.; Ma, L.-Y.; Zheng, Y.-C.; Liu, H.-M. Discovery of pyrazole derivatives as cellular active inhibitors of histone lysine specific demethylase 5B (KDM5B/JARID1B). *Eur. J. Med. Chem.* **2020**, *192*, 112161. [CrossRef]
80. Pushpakom, S.; Iorio, F.; Eyers, P.A.; Escott, K.J.; Hopper, S.; Wells, A.; Doig, A.; Guilliams, T.; Latimer, J.; McNamee, C. Drug repurposing: Progress, challenges and recommendations. *Nat. Rev. Drug Discov.* **2019**, *18*, 41–58. [CrossRef]
81. Sleire, L.; Førde, H.E.; Netland, I.A.; Leiss, L.; Skeie, B.S.; Enger, P.Ø. Drug repurposing in cancer. *Pharmacol. Res.* **2017**, *124*, 74–91. [CrossRef] [PubMed]
82. Eyer, L.; Nencka, R.; De Clercq, E.; Seley-Radtke, K.; Růžek, D. Nucleoside analogs as a rich source of antiviral agents active against arthropod-borne flaviviruses. *Antivir. Chem. Chemother.* **2018**, *26*, 2040206618761299. [CrossRef] [PubMed]
83. Damaraju, V.L.; Damaraju, S.; Young, J.D.; Baldwin, S.A.; Mackey, J.; Sawyer, M.B.; Cass, C.E. Nucleoside anticancer drugs: The role of nucleoside transporters in resistance to cancer chemotherapy. *Oncogene* **2003**, *22*, 7524–7536. [CrossRef] [PubMed]
84. Tănase, C.I.; Drăghici, C.; Cojocaru, A.; Galochkina, A.V.; Orshanskaya, J.R.; Zarubaev, V.V.; Shova, S.; Enache, C.; Maganu, M. New carbocyclic N6-substituted adenine and pyrimidine nucleoside analogues with a bicyclo [2.2. 1] heptane fragment as sugar moiety; synthesis, antiviral, anticancer activity and X-ray crystallography. *Bioorg. Med. Chem.* **2015**, *23*, 6346–6354. [CrossRef] [PubMed]
85. Guinan, M.; Benckendorff, C.; Smith, M.; Miller, G.J. Recent Advances in the Chemical Synthesis and Evaluation of Anticancer Nucleoside Analogues. *Molecules* **2020**, *25*, E2050. [CrossRef]
86. Rao, M.; Chinnasamy, N.; Hong, J.A.; Zhang, Y.; Zhang, M.; Xi, S.; Liu, F.; Marquez, V.E.; Morgan, R.A.; Schrump, D.S. Inhibition of histone lysine methylation enhances cancer–testis antigen expression in lung cancer cells: Implications for adoptive immunotherapy of cancer. *Cancer Res.* **2011**, *71*, 4192–4204. [CrossRef]

87. Mohamed, T.; Rao, P.P. 2, 4-Disubstituted quinazolines as amyloid-β aggregation inhibitors with dual cholinesterase inhibition and antioxidant properties: Development and structure-activity relationship (SAR) studies. *Eur. J. Med. Chem.* **2017**, *126*, 823–843. [CrossRef]
88. Horton, J.R.; Liu, X.; Gale, M.; Wu, L.; Shanks, J.R.; Zhang, X.; Webber, P.J.; Bell, J.S.; Kales, S.C.; Mott, B.T. Structural basis for KDM5A histone lysine demethylase inhibition by diverse compounds. *Cell Chem. Biol.* **2016**, *23*, 769–781. [CrossRef]

Permissions

All chapters in this book were first published by MDPI; hereby published with permission under the Creative Commons Attribution License or equivalent. Every chapter published in this book has been scrutinized by our experts. Their significance has been extensively debated. The topics covered herein carry significant findings which will fuel the growth of the discipline. They may even be implemented as practical applications or may be referred to as a beginning point for another development.

The contributors of this book come from diverse backgrounds, making this book a truly international effort. This book will bring forth new frontiers with its revolutionizing research information and detailed analysis of the nascent developments around the world.

We would like to thank all the contributing authors for lending their expertise to make the book truly unique. They have played a crucial role in the development of this book. Without their invaluable contributions this book wouldn't have been possible. They have made vital efforts to compile up to date information on the varied aspects of this subject to make this book a valuable addition to the collection of many professionals and students.

This book was conceptualized with the vision of imparting up-to-date information and advanced data in this field. To ensure the same, a matchless editorial board was set up. Every individual on the board went through rigorous rounds of assessment to prove their worth. After which they invested a large part of their time researching and compiling the most relevant data for our readers.

The editorial board has been involved in producing this book since its inception. They have spent rigorous hours researching and exploring the diverse topics which have resulted in the successful publishing of this book. They have passed on their knowledge of decades through this book. To expedite this challenging task, the publisher supported the team at every step. A small team of assistant editors was also appointed to further simplify the editing procedure and attain best results for the readers.

Apart from the editorial board, the designing team has also invested a significant amount of their time in understanding the subject and creating the most relevant covers. They scrutinized every image to scout for the most suitable representation of the subject and create an appropriate cover for the book.

The publishing team has been an ardent support to the editorial, designing and production team. Their endless efforts to recruit the best for this project, has resulted in the accomplishment of this book. They are a veteran in the field of academics and their pool of knowledge is as vast as their experience in printing. Their expertise and guidance has proved useful at every step. Their uncompromising quality standards have made this book an exceptional effort. Their encouragement from time to time has been an inspiration for everyone.

The publisher and the editorial board hope that this book will prove to be a valuable piece of knowledge for researchers, students, practitioners and scholars across the globe.

List of Contributors

Catarina Nascimento, Ana Catarina Urbano, Andreia Gameiro, Jorge Correia and Fernando Ferreira
CIISA – Centro de Investigação Interdisciplinar em Sanidade Animal, Faculdade de Medicina Veterinária, Universidade de Lisboa, Avenida da Universidade Técnica, Lisboa 1300-477, Portugal

João Ferreira
Instituto de Medicina Molecular, Faculdade de Medicina, Universidade de Lisboa, Lisboa 1649-028, Portugal

Gyeongyun Go
Department of Biochemistry, Soonchunhyang University College of Medicine, Cheonan 31151, Korea

Sang Hun Lee
Department of Biochemistry, Soonchunhyang University College of Medicine, Cheonan 31151, Korea
Medical Science Research Institute, Soonchunhyang University Seoul Hospital, Seoul 04401, Korea

Flávia Martins
i3S-Institute for Research and Innovation in Health, University of Porto, 4200-135 Porto, Portugal
INEB-Institute of Biomedical Engineering, University of Porto, 4200-135 Porto, Portugal
IPATIMUP-Institute of Molecular Pathology and Immunology, University of Porto, 4200-135 Porto, Portugal
Department of Pathology and Oncology, Faculty of Medicine, University of Porto, 4200-319 Porto, Portugal

Luísa Pereira
i3S-Institute for Research and Innovation in Health, University of Porto, 4200-135 Porto, Portugal
IPATIMUP-Institute of Molecular Pathology and Immunology, University of Porto, 4200-135 Porto, Portugal
Department of Pathology and Oncology, Faculty of Medicine, University of Porto, 4200-319 Porto, Portugal

Ana João Silva, Diogo Adão, Ana Patrícia Cardoso, Rosa Oliveira and Angela Margarida Costa
i3S-Institute for Research and Innovation in Health, University of Porto, 4200-135 Porto, Portugal
INEB-Institute of Biomedical Engineering, University of Porto, 4200-135 Porto, Portugal

Bruno Cavadas, Filipe Pinto, Bárbara Sousa and Nicole Pedro
i3S-Institute for Research and Innovation in Health, University of Porto, 4200-135 Porto, Portugal
IPATIMUP-Institute of Molecular Pathology and Immunology, University of Porto, 4200-135 Porto, Portugal

Maria José Oliveira
i3S-Institute for Research and Innovation in Health, University of Porto, 4200-135 Porto, Portugal
INEB-Institute of Biomedical Engineering, University of Porto, 4200-135 Porto, Portugal
Department of Pathology and Oncology, Faculty of Medicine, University of Porto, 4200-319 Porto, Portugal
ICBAS-Institute of Biomedical Sciences Abel Salazar, University of Porto, 4050-313 Porto, Portugal

Flávia Castro
i3S-Institute for Research and Innovation in Health, University of Porto, 4200-135 Porto, Portugal
INEB-Institute of Biomedical Engineering, University of Porto, 4200-135 Porto, Portugal
ICBAS-Institute of Biomedical Sciences Abel Salazar, University of Porto, 4050-313 Porto, Portugal

Marta Laranjeiro Pinto
i3S-Institute for Research and Innovation in Health, University of Porto, 4200-135 Porto, Portugal
INEB-Institute of Biomedical Engineering, University of Porto, 4200-135 Porto, Portugal
CNC-Center for Neuroscience and Cell Biology, University of Coimbra, 3004-517 Coimbra, Portugal

José Pedro Loureiro
i3S-Institute for Research and Innovation in Health, University of Porto, 4200-135 Porto, Portugal
IBMC-Institute of Molecular and Cellular Biology, University of Porto, 4200-135 Porto, Portugal

Rui Manuel Reis
Molecular Oncology Research Center, Barretos Cancer Hospital, 14.784-400 Barretos-SP, Brazil
Life and Health Sciences Research Institute (ICVS), School of Medicine, University of Minho, 4710-057 Braga, Portugal
ICVS/3B's-PT Government Associate Laboratory, 4710-057 Braga, Portugal

Robert D. Carlson, John C. Flickinger, Jr. and Adam E. Snook
Department of Pharmacology and Experimental Therapeutics, Thomas Jefferson University, 1020 Locust Street, Philadelphia, PA 19107, USA

Shuhui Cheng and Eleanor J. Cheadle
Manchester Academic Health Science Centre, Manchester NIHR Biomedical Research Centre, Division of Cancer Sciences, Faculty of Biology, Medicine and Health, University of Manchester, Manchester M13 9PL, UK

Timothy M. Illidge
Manchester Academic Health Science Centre, Manchester NIHR Biomedical Research Centre, Division of Cancer Sciences, Faculty of Biology, Medicine and Health, University of Manchester, Manchester M13 9PL, UK
The Christie NHS Foundation Trust, Manchester M20 4BX, UK

Shivam O. Mittal
Section for Parkinson's Disease and Movement Disorders, Cleveland Clinic Abu Dhabi, Abu Dhabi 112412, UAE

Bahman Jabbari
Department of Neurology, Yale University School of Medicine, New Haven, CT 06519, USA

Ru Li, Annie Wen and Jun Lin
Department of Anesthesiology, Stony Brook University Health Sciences Center, Stony Brook, NY 11794-8480, USA

Andrea Colarusso, Zaira Maroccia, Ermenegilda Parrilli and Maria Luisa Tutino
Department of Chemical Sciences, University of Naples Federico II, Complesso Universitario M. S. Angelo, Via Cintia, 80126 Napoli, Italy

Alessia Fabbri, Elena Angela Pia Germinario, Andrea Fortuna, Stefano Loizzo and Laura Ricceri
Istituto Superiore di Sanità, Viale Regina Elena 299, 00161 Rome, Italy

Carla Fiorentini
Istituto Superiore di Sanità, Viale Regina Elena 299, 00161 Rome, Italy
Association for Research on Integrative Oncological Therapies (ARTOI), 00165 Rome, Italy

Lara Dura-Perez, Suneil Jain, Paul B. Mullan, Rich Williams, Simon S. McDade and Sharon L. Eddie
Patrick G Johnston Centre for Cancer Research, Queen's University, Belfast BT9 7AE, UK

Charles M. Haughey and Ian G. Mills
Patrick G Johnston Centre for Cancer Research, Queen's University, Belfast BT9 7AE, UK
Nuffield Department of Surgical Sciences, John Radcliffe Hospital, University of Oxford, Oxford OX3 9DU, UK

Debayan Mukherjee, Amy Popple, Mehjabin Patel and Jamie Honeychurch
Targeted Therapy Group, Division of Cancer Sciences, Faculty of Biology Medicine and Health, The University of Manchester, Manchester M13 9PL, UK

Timothy Illidge
Targeted Therapy Group, Division of Cancer Sciences, Faculty of Biology Medicine and Health, The University of Manchester, Manchester M13 9PL, UK
The Christie Hospital Foundation Trust, Manchester M20 4BX, UK

Adam Pickard
Patrick G Johnston Centre for Cancer Research, Queen's University, Belfast BT9 7AE, UK
Wellcome Centre for Cell Matrix Research, University of Manchester, Manchester M13 9PL, UK

Rebecca E. Steele
Patrick G Johnston Centre for Cancer Research, Queen's University, Belfast BT9 7AE, UK
The Breast Cancer Now Toby Robins Breast Cancer Research Centre, The Institute of Cancer Research, London SM2 5NG, UK

Pedro Oliveira
The Christie Hospital Foundation Trust, Manchester M20 4BX, UK

Niamh E. Buckley
Patrick G Johnston Centre for Cancer Research, Queen's University, Belfast BT9 7AE, UK
School of Pharmacy, Queen's University Belfast, Belfast BT9 7BL, UK

Javier Ruiz-de-la-Herrán, Rodrigo Lázaro-Gorines, José G. Gavilanes and Javier Lacadena
Departamento de Bioquímica y Biología Molecular, Facultad de Ciencias Químicas, Universidad Complutense de Madrid, Madrid 28040, Spain

Jaime Tomé-Amat
Departamento de Bioquímica y Biología Molecular, Facultad de Ciencias Químicas, Universidad Complutense de Madrid, Madrid 28040, Spain
Centre for Plant Biotechnology and Genomics (UPM-INIA), Universidad Politécnica de Madrid, Pozuelo de Alarcón, Madrid 28223, Spain

Sven Burgdorf
Department of Cellular Immunology, LIMES Institute, University of Bonn, 53115 Bonn, Germany

Alexander Marx and Zoran V. Popovic
Institute of Pathology, University Hospital Mannheim, University of Heidelberg, 68167 Mannheim, Germany

Stefan Porubsky
Institute of Pathology, University Hospital, Johannes-Gutenberg University Mainz, 55131 Mainz, Germany
Institute of Pathology, University Hospital Mannheim, University of Heidelberg, 68167 Mannheim, Germany

Varintra E. Krisnawan
Department of Medicine, Washington University School of Medicine, St. Louis, MO 63110, USA
Department of Pathology and Immunology, Washington University School of Medicine, St. Louis, MO 63110, USA

David G. DeNardo
Department of Medicine, Washington University School of Medicine, St. Louis, MO 63110, USA
Department of Pathology and Immunology, Washington University School of Medicine, St. Louis, MO 63110, USA
Siteman Cancer Center, Washington University School of Medicine, St. Louis, MO 63110, USA

Julie K. Schwarz
Department of Radiation Oncology, Washington University School of Medicine, St. Louis, MO 63110, USA Siteman Cancer Center, Washington University School of Medicine, St. Louis, MO 63110, USA
Department of Cell Biology and Physiology, Washington University School of Medicine, St. Louis, MO 63110, USA

Jennifer A. Stanley
Department of Radiation Oncology, Washington University School of Medicine, St. Louis, MO 63110, USA
Siteman Cancer Center, Washington University School of Medicine, St. Louis, MO 63110, USA

Anmi Jose, Murali Munisamy, Levin Thomas and Mahadev Rao
Department of Pharmacy Practice, Manipal College of Pharmaceutical Sciences, Manipal Academy of Higher Education, Manipal, Karnataka 576104, India

Gautham G. Shenoy
Department of Pharmaceutical Chemistry, Manipal College of Pharmaceutical Sciences, Manipal Academy of Higher Education, Manipal, Karnataka 576104, India

Gabriel Sunil Rodrigues
Department of Surgery, Kasturba Medical College, Manipal Academy of Higher Education, Manipal, Karnataka 576104, India

Naveena A. N. Kumar
Department of Surgical Oncology, Kasturba Medical College, Manipal Academy of Higher Education, Manipal, Karnataka 576104, India

Jill Kolesar
Department of Pharmacy Practice & Science, 567 TODD Building, 789 South Limestone Street, Lexington, KY 40539-0596, USA

Ganesha Rai
National Center for Advancing Translational Sciences, National Institutes of Health, 9800 Medical Center Drive, MSC 3370, Bethesda, MD 20892, USA

Praveen P. N. Rao
School of Pharmacy, Health Sciences Campus, 200 University Avenue West, University of Waterloo, Waterloo, ON N2L 3G1, Canada

Index

A

Adenocarcinoma, 19, 25, 47, 72, 101, 121, 143, 151, 153, 157, 183, 190, 210-211, 215

Adipocytes, 32, 193, 195-196, 205-207, 217

Adjuvant Chemotherapy, 2, 14, 20, 28

Adoptive Cell Therapy, 54, 62, 66, 73, 75

Animal Models, 2, 63, 105, 159, 181, 184, 187, 194

Anti-neoplastic Agent, 127-128

Antibodies, 1-2, 11, 15-16, 22-23, 29, 48-49, 58, 60, 85, 115, 118, 126, 138, 155, 161, 174-175, 196, 200, 204, 211

Atezolizumab, 2, 14, 60, 71, 94

Autophagy, 82, 91-92, 139, 197, 203, 210

B

Biomarkers, 1-2, 14, 22, 60, 70, 77-78, 83, 86-89, 92-93, 95

Bone Marrow, 62-63, 74, 111-112, 117, 122-123, 125, 186, 188, 197, 202, 204, 206, 214, 222

Botulinum Neurotoxins, 97, 99, 105-106

Breast Cancer, 1-2, 8-9, 12-16, 18, 20-24, 26-29, 32, 45, 50-51, 72, 78, 85, 105, 107, 109-110, 114-116, 118, 121, 123-126, 141, 145, 176, 182, 186, 197, 204, 207, 209-211, 214-215, 217, 220-221, 229-230, 232

Brefeldin A, 18, 169-171, 175, 179

C

Calcitonin, 97, 105

Calreticulin, 80, 91, 203, 214

Cancer Cells, 1-2, 6-9, 12-13, 15-29, 31-32, 36-37, 44-48, 50-51, 56, 59-60, 63, 75, 78, 82, 85, 97-98, 109, 111-117, 122-125, 153, 160, 170, 176, 178, 189, 193-194, 197-199, 201, 204, 207, 209-211, 215, 220-222, 229-232

Cancer Stem Cell, 17-18, 21, 23, 28-29, 193, 210

Cell Adhesion, 18, 116

Cell Death, 1-6, 14-15, 18, 20, 24-25, 27, 49, 59, 62, 70-71, 79-82, 91-94, 177, 183, 197, 201, 203, 206-207, 210, 212, 214

Cellular Differentiation, 17-18

Circadian Rhythm, 17-18

Clinical Trials, 24, 58-62, 64-66, 72, 88-89, 92, 95, 97, 99, 111, 117-118, 122, 176, 213

Colon Cancer, 15, 19-20, 22-23, 25, 27-29, 31-33, 40, 42-48, 51-52, 140, 176, 215

Colorectal Cancer, 14, 19-22, 27-29, 50-52, 62-63, 68-69, 74-75, 78, 82, 86, 90, 94, 114-115, 117-118, 121, 123, 125, 145, 160, 170, 175, 177, 179, 188, 209, 216, 222, 231

Cytokines, 2, 15, 40-41, 45-46, 51, 58-59, 64, 66, 68, 78, 80, 88-89, 111-112, 114-117, 122-124, 189, 193-194, 197, 200-201, 203-204, 206-207

Cytoskeleton, 19, 135

D

Dendritic Cells, 2, 9, 45, 61, 72, 78, 80, 112, 180, 184-191, 195-196, 201, 214, 216

Doxorubicin, 2, 16, 23, 27, 87

Drug Discovery, 127

Drug Resistance, 17-18, 20-23, 27-29, 52, 92

E

Endoplasmic Reticulum, 9, 17, 24-25, 177, 179, 189, 203

Epithelial-mesenchymal Transition, 19, 28, 123, 128, 198, 221, 230

Escherichia Coli, 127-128, 139-140, 176

Extracellular Matrix, 19, 21, 32, 81, 111-112, 114, 122, 124, 180, 184, 193-195, 208-209, 211

Extracellular Vesicles, 112, 114, 122, 124

F

Fibroblasts, 32, 78, 81, 91, 114-115, 124, 135, 153, 193-194, 197, 199, 208-211, 216

G

Gastric Cancer, 8-9, 14, 19, 25-27, 187, 192, 221-222, 231

Glioblastoma, 18, 27-28, 52, 61, 65, 73, 91-92, 109, 127, 139, 197, 204, 209

Glioma, 65, 73, 118, 127-128, 139, 197, 202, 210

Glutamate, 97, 105, 110

Glycoprotein, 2, 17, 20, 27, 75, 177

H

Heat-killed Bacteria, 54, 56, 66

Homeostasis, 17-18, 59, 68, 190-191, 199, 215

Hyperhidrosis, 97-98, 105-106

Hypoxia, 20, 28, 31-33, 36-37, 39-40, 44-46, 50-52, 67, 81, 114, 122, 157, 182-183, 195, 202, 205-206, 208, 213, 217, 221, 230

I

Immune Checkpoint Blockade, 59, 66, 70, 77, 92, 95-96, 201-202, 209

Immune Checkpoint Inhibitors, 54, 59-60, 70-71, 78, 95, 151, 196

Immunocytochemistry, 143, 154

Immunohistochemistry, 44, 94, 142, 144-145, 149-150, 154

Immunosuppression, 2, 9, 13, 16, 67, 79-81, 199, 201, 203, 205, 210, 215

Immunotherapy, 1-2, 13, 15, 51, 54-57, 60, 66-78, 87-95, 126, 157-158, 175, 201, 205, 208-209, 211, 213-214, 216, 223-224, 232

Integrins, 18, 199-200

Interleukin, 52, 58, 68, 70, 74, 80, 111, 115, 121-126, 196-197

L
Laminin, 18, 24, 26, 139, 197, 199
Leukocytes, 112, 181, 194
Lung Cancer, 2, 9, 15, 28, 60, 71, 88, 93-96, 114-115, 118, 126, 151, 203, 209-214, 221, 230, 232
Lymph Nodes, 2, 12, 59, 62, 69, 114, 187
Lymphocytes, 1-2, 7, 12-16, 57-59, 62-63, 67, 69, 71-75, 85-86, 93-94, 115, 145, 152, 175, 204, 214-215

M
Macrophages, 2, 31-32, 36-39, 44-52, 78-80, 112, 116, 145, 149-152, 155-156, 180-181, 187-189, 191, 195, 202, 206, 213, 215-217
Mammary Carcinoma, 1-4, 8-10, 13-14, 16, 204
Mastectomy, 10, 106
Metastasis, 11, 13, 17-24, 27-29, 32, 51, 67, 86-87, 111-112, 114-118, 122-126, 159, 183, 197-198, 200, 206-210, 220-222, 230-231
Metastatic Melanoma, 2, 9, 15, 58, 60, 62, 68-70, 74, 118, 230
Mitochondria, 17-18, 20, 133-136, 138
Murine Cell Lines, 143, 151, 158
Myelin, 17-18, 24
Myeloid Cells, 51, 78-80, 89, 112, 114-116, 125, 142, 145, 149, 158, 198, 205-206, 213, 216

N
Necrosis, 1-2, 6, 10, 12, 20, 45, 79-82, 112, 201-203, 213, 215

O
Osteosarcoma, 45, 54, 56, 65-66

P
Pancreatic Cancer, 9, 15, 18, 25, 27, 109, 114-115, 117-118, 121, 125, 188, 198-199, 204, 209-211, 215-216
Pre-clinical Models, 141, 151
Pre-metastatic Niche, 111-112, 114, 122-123, 125
Primary Tumor, 19, 111, 113-117, 122, 202
Prion Disease, 17, 23, 30
Prognosis, 1, 25, 31-33, 37, 40-43, 45-46, 50-51, 78, 81, 86, 115, 118, 123, 141, 220-221, 230-231
Prostate Cancer, 61, 69, 72-73, 90, 92, 109, 117-118, 121, 125-126, 141-142, 146, 151-154, 156-159, 178, 199, 202-203, 208, 210, 213-214, 218, 222, 228

R
Radiotherapy, 77, 79-80, 82-83, 85-87, 90-93, 95, 101, 106, 110, 115, 141-142, 146-150, 155, 157-159, 193-195, 208-209, 211-214, 216-217
Reactive Oxygen Species, 32, 81, 181, 197
Regulatory T Cells, 8-9, 59, 67-68, 78, 90, 188, 202, 214, 217
Rett Syndrome, 128, 136, 139

S
Secretome, 31-32, 46, 197
Sialorrhea, 97-98, 105, 110
Somatic Mutations, 1, 8-9, 23, 30
Stromal Cells, 78, 80, 111-117, 193-198, 200-201, 205, 207-208, 216

T
Therapeutic Targets, 2, 22, 32, 175
Therapy Resistance, 32, 199, 209-210
Tumor Microenvironment, 1-2, 14, 31, 44, 50, 59, 64, 66-67, 69, 90-92, 111-112, 114-115, 157, 180-181, 185, 191-195, 209-213, 215
Tumorigenesis, 2, 31, 124, 139, 205, 208, 220-221, 228, 231

W
Western Blot Analysis, 130-131, 133, 136

www.ingramcontent.com/pod-product-compliance
Lightning Source LLC
LaVergne TN
LVHW081031210926
848485LV00004B/1002